POCKET C[...]
Rob[...]
Pathologic Basis
of Disease

Eighth Edition

Richard N. Mitchell, MD, PhD
Associate Professor, Department of Pathology
Harvard Medical School and Health Sciences
   and Technology
Director, Human Pathology
Harvard-MIT Division of Health Sciences and Technology
Staff Pathologist, Brigham and Women's Hospital
Boston, Massachusetts

Vinay Kumar, MBBS, MD, FRCPath
Alice Hogge and Arthur Baer Professor
Chairman, Department of Pathology
Executive Vice Dean, Division of Biologic Sciences and
The Pritzker School of Medicine
The University of Chicago
Chicago, Illinois

Abul K. Abbas, MBBS
Professor and Chairman, Department of Pathology
University of California, San Francisco
San Francisco, California

Nelson Fausto, MD
Professor and Chairman, Department of Pathology
University of Washington School of Medicine
Seattle, Washington

Jon C. Aster, MD, PhD
Professor of Pathology
Harvard Medical School
Brigham and Women's Hospital
Boston, Massachusetts

With Illustrations by James A. Perkins, MS, MFA

ELSEVIER
SAUNDERS

ELSEVIER
SAUNDERS

1600 John F. Kennedy Blvd.
Ste 1800
Philadelphia, PA 19103-2899

POCKET COMPANION TO ROBBINS AND
COTRAN PATHOLOGIC BASIS OF DISEASE   ISBN: 978-1-4160-5454-2

Notices

Knowledge and best practice in this field are constantly changing. As new research and experience broaden our understanding, changes in research methods, professional practices, or medical treatment may become necessary.

Practitioners and researchers must always rely on their own experience and knowledge in evaluating and using any information, methods, compounds, or experiments described herein. In using such information or methods they should be mindful of their own safety and the safety of others, including parties for whom they have a professional responsibility.

With respect to any drug or pharmaceutical products identified, readers are advised to check the most current information provided (i) on procedures featured or (ii) by the manufacturer of each product to be administered, to verify the recommended dose or formula, the method and duration of administration, and contraindications. It is the responsibility of practitioners, relying on their own experience and knowledge of their patients, to make diagnoses, to determine dosages and the best treatment for each individual patient, and to take all appropriate safety precautions.

To the fullest extent of the law, neither the Publisher nor the authors, contributors, or editors, assume any liability for any injury and/or damage to persons or property as a matter of products liability, negligence or otherwise, or from any use or operation of any methods, products, instructions, or ideas contained in the material herein.

ISBN: 978-1-4160-5454-2

Executive Editor: William Schmitt
Managing Editor: Rebecca Gruliow
Publishing Services Manager: Julie Eddy
Senior Project Manager: Laura Loveall
Design Direction: Ellen Zanolle

Working together to grow
libraries in developing countries

www.elsevier.com | www.bookaid.org | www.sabre.org

ELSEVIER   BOOK AID International   Sabre Foundation

Printed in the United States
Last digit is the print number: 9 8 7 6 5 4 3 2 1

Contributors

Charles E. Alpers, MD
Professor of Pathology, Adjunct Professor of Medicine, University of Washington School of Medicine; Pathologist, University of Washington Medical Center, Seattle, WA
The Kidney

Douglas C. Anthony, MD, PhD
Professor and Chair, Department of Pathology and Anatomical Sciences, University of Missouri, Columbia, MO
Peripheral Nerve and Skeletal Muscle; The Central Nervous System

James M. Crawford, MD, PhD
Senior Vice President for Laboratory Services; Chair, Department of Pathology and Laboratory Medicine, North Shore–Long Island Jewish Health System, Manhasset, NY
Liver and Biliary Tract

Umberto De Girolami, MD
Professor of Pathology, Harvard Medical School; Director of Neuropathology, Brigham and Women's Hospital, Boston, MA
Peripheral Nerve and Skeletal Muscle; The Central Nervous System

Lora Hedrick Ellenson, MD
Weill Medical College of Cornell University, Professor of Pathology and Laboratory Medicine; Attending Pathologist, New York Presbyterian Hospital, New York, NY
The Female Genital Tract

Jonathan I. Epstein, MD
Professor of Pathology, Urology, and Oncology; The Reinhard Professor of Urologic Pathology, The Johns Hopkins University School of Medicine; Director of Surgical Pathology, The Johns Hopkins Hospital, Baltimore, MD
The Lower Urinary Tract and Male Genital System

Robert Folberg, MD
Dean, Oakland University William Beaumont School of Medicine, Rochester, MI; Chief Academic Officer, Beaumont Hospitals, Royal Oak, MI
The Eye

Matthew P. Frosch, MD, PhD
Associate Professor of Pathology, Harvard Medical School; Director, C.S. Kubik Laboratory for Neuropathology, Massachusetts General Hospital, Boston, MA
Peripheral Nerve and Skeletal Muscle; The Central Nervous System

Ralph H. Hruban, MD
Professor of Pathology and Oncology, The Sol Goldman Pancreatic Cancer Research Center, The Johns Hopkins University School of Medicine, Baltimore, MD
The Pancreas

Aliya N. Husain, MBBS
Professor, Department of Pathology, Pritzker School of Medicine,
The University of Chicago, Chicago, IL
The Lung

Christine A. Iacobuzio-Donahue, MD, PhD
Associate Professor of Pathology and Oncology, The Sol Goldman
Pancreatic Cancer Research Center, The Johns Hopkins
University School of Medicine, Baltimore, MD
The Pancreas

Alexander J.F. Lazar, MD, PhD
Assistant Professor, Department of Pathology and Dermatology,
Sections of Dermatopathology and Soft Tissue Sarcoma
Pathology, Faculty of Sarcoma Research Center, University of
Texas M.D. Anderson Cancer Center, Houston, TX
The Skin

Susan C. Lester, MD, PhD
Assistant Professor of Pathology, Harvard Medical School; Chief,
Breast Pathology, Brigham and Women's Hospital, Boston, MA
The Breast

Mark W. Lingen, DDS, PhD
Associate Professor, Department of Pathology, Pritzker School of
Medicine, The University of Chicago, Chicago, IL
Head and Neck

Chen Liu, MD, PhD
Associate Professor of Pathology, Immunology and Laboratory
Medicine; Director, Gastrointestinal and Liver Pathology, The
University of Florida College of Medicine, Gainesville, FL
Liver and Biliary Tract

Anirban Maitra, MBBS
Associate Professor of Pathology and Oncology, The Johns
Hopkins University School of Medicine; Pathologist, The Johns
Hopkins Hospital, Baltimore, MD
Diseases of Infancy and Childhood; The Endocrine System

Alexander J. McAdam, MD, PhD
Assistant Professor of Pathology, Harvard Medical School; Medical
Director, Infectious Diseases Diagnostic Laboratory, Children's
Hospital Boston, Boston, MA
Infectious Diseases

Richard N. Mitchell, MD, PhD
Associate Professor, Department of Pathology, Harvard Medical
School; Director, Human Pathology, Harvard-MIT Division of
Health Sciences and Technology, Harvard Medical School; Staff
Pathologist, Brigham and Women's Hospital, Boston, MA
*Hemodynamic Disorders, Thromboembolic Disease, and Shock;
Blood Vessels; The Heart*

George F. Murphy, MD
Professor of Pathology, Harvard Medical School; Director
of Dermatopathology, Brigham and Women's Hospital,
Boston, MA
The Skin

Edyta C. Pirog, MD
Associate Professor of Clinical Pathology and Laboratory
  Medicine, New York Presbyterian Hospital-Weil Medical College
  of Cornell University; Associate Attending Pathologist,
  New York Presbyterian Hospital, New York, NY
  The Female Genital Tract

Andrew E. Rosenberg, MD
Professor, Department of Pathology, Harvard Medical School;
  Pathologist, Massachusetts General Hospital, Boston, MA
  Bones, Joints, and Soft-Tissue Tumors

Frederick J. Schoen, MD, PhD
Professor of Pathology and Health Sciences and Technology,
  Harvard Medical School; Director, Cardiac Pathology and
  Executive Vice Chairman, Department of Pathology, Brigham
  and Women's Hospital, Boston, MA
  Blood Vessels; The Heart

Arlene H. Sharpe, MD, PhD
Professor of Pathology, Harvard Medical School; Chief,
  Immunology Research Division, Department of Pathology,
  Brigham and Women's Hospital, Boston, MA
  Infectious Diseases

Thomas Stricker, MD, PhD
Orthopedic Pathology Fellow, Department of Pathology, Pritzker
  School of Medicine, The University of Chicago, Chicago, IL
  Neoplasia

Jerrold R. Turner, MD, PhD
Professor and Associate Chair, Department of Pathology, Pritzker
  School of Medicine, The University of Chicago, Chicago, IL
  The Gastrointestinal Tract

Preface

Robbins and Cotran Pathologic Basis of Disease (AKA, the Big Book) has long been a fundamental text for students of medicine around the world; with publication of the eighth edition, it entered its Golden Jubilee 50th year—vibrant and vigorous in its illumination of the "molecular basis of human disease with clinical correlations." While the *Pocket Companion* may not (yet) have the same storied history, it nevertheless provides an important and useful adjunct to the parent volume. Initially an offspring of the fourth edition in 1991 (identified then as just *Robbins Pathologic Basis of Disease*), the *Pocket Companion* was born of the recognition that the immense wealth of information about human disease somehow needed to be succinctly organized and made accessible for the overwhelmed medical student and harried house officer. This edition of the *Pocket Companion* carries on that tradition and, as before, is intended to be much more than a simple topical outline. In assembling this update, four major objectives have guided the writing:

- Make the detailed expositions in *Robbins and Cotran Pathologic Basis of Disease* easier to digest by providing a condensed overview.
- Facilitate the use of the Big Book by providing the relevant cross-referenced page numbers.
- Help readers identify the core material that requires their primary attention.
- Serve as a handy tool for quick review of a large body of information.

In the age of Wikipedia and other online data compendiums, it is obviously not difficult to just *find* information; to be sure, the *Pocket Companion* is also available in a readily searchable digital format. However, what the 21st century student of pathology needs is an organized, pithy, and easy-to-digest synopsis of the pertinent concepts and facts with specific links to the definitive material in a more expansive volume.

This eighth edition of the *Pocket Companion* hopefully accomplishes that end. It has been completely rewritten, reflecting all the innovations and new knowledge encompassed in the parent tome. Illustrative tables and figures have also been included wherever possible to reduce the verbiage. Although as before, the beautiful gross and histologic images of the Big Book are not reproduced. Pains have also been taken to present all the material with the same stylistic voice; the organization of the material and level of detail is considerably more uniform between chapters than in previous editions. In doing so, we hope that the *Pocket Companion* retains the flavor and excitement of the Big Book—just in a more bite-size format—and truly is a suitable "companion."

In closing, the authors specifically wish to acknowledge the invaluable assistance and editing skills (and infinite patience) of Rebecca Mitchell and Becca Gruliow; without their help and collaboration, this edition of the *Pocket Companion* might still be in gestation.

Rick Mitchell

Vinay Kumar

Abul Abbas

Nelson Fausto

Jon Aster

Contents

General Pathology

Systemic Pathology: Diseases of Organ Systems

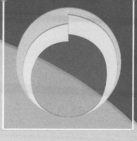

General Pathology

Cellular Responses to Stress and Toxic Insults: Adaptation, Injury, and Death

Introduction (p. 4)

Pathology is the study of the structural and functional causes of human disease. The four aspects of a disease process that form the core of pathology are:

- The cause of a disease *(etiology)*
- The mechanism(s) of disease development *(pathogenesis)*
- The structural alterations induced in cells and tissues by the disease *(morphologic change)*
- The functional consequences of the morphologic changes *(clinical significance)*

Overview (p. 5)

Normal cell function requires a balance between physiologic demands and the constraints of cell structure and metabolic capacity; the result is a steady state, or *homeostasis*. Cells can alter their functional state in response to modest stress to maintain the steady state. More excessive physiologic stresses, or adverse pathologic stimuli *(injury)*, result in (1) adaption, (2) reversible injury, or (3) irreversible injury and cell death (Table 1-1). These responses may be considered a continuum of progressive impairment of cell structure and function.

- *Adaptation* occurs when physiologic or pathologic stressors induce a new state that changes the cell but otherwise preserves its viability in the face of the exogenous stimuli. These changes include:

  Hypertrophy (increased cell mass, p. 7)
  Hyperplasia (increased cell number, p. 8)
  Atrophy (decreased cell mass, p. 9)
  Metaplasia (change from one mature cell type to another, p. 10)

- *Reversible injury* denotes pathologic cell changes that can be restored to normalcy if the stimulus is removed or if the cause of injury is mild.
- *Irreversible injury* occurs when stressors exceed the capacity of the cell to adapt (beyond a *point of no return*) and denotes permanent pathologic changes that cause cell death.
- *Cell death* occurs primarily through two morphologic and mechanistic patterns denoted *necrosis* and *apoptosis* (Table 1-2).

TABLE 1-1 Cellular Responses to Injury	
Nature of Injurious Stimulus	**Cellular Response**
Altered physiological stimuli; some nonlethal, injurious stimuli	**Cellular adaptations**
Increased demand, increased stimulation (e.g., by growth factors, hormones)	Hyperplasia, hypertrophy
Decreased nutrients, decreased stimulation	Atrophy
Chronic irritation (physical or chemical)	Metaplasia
Reduced oxygen supply; chemical injury; microbial infection	**Cell injury**
Acute and transient	Acute reversible injury Cellular swelling fatty change
	Irreversible injury → cell death Necrosis Apoptosis
Metabolic alterations, genetic or acquired; chronic injury	**Intracellular accumulations; calcification**
Cumulative, sublethal injury over long life span	**Cellular aging**

TABLE 1-2 Features of Necrosis and Apoptosis		
Feature	**Necrosis**	**Apoptosis**
Cell size	Enlarged (swelling)	Reduced (shrinkage)
Nucleus	Pyknosis → karyorrhexis → karyolysis	Fragmentation into nucleosome-size fragments
Plasma membrane	Disrupted	Intact; altered structure, especially orientation of lipids
Cellular contents	Enzymatic digestion; may leak out of cell	Intact; may be released in apoptotic bodies
Adjacent inflammation	Frequent	No
Physiologic or pathologic role	Invariable pathologic (culmination of irreversible cell injury)	Often physiologic, means of eliminating unwanted cells; may be pathologic after some forms of cell injury, especially DNA damage

Although necrosis always represents a pathologic process, apoptosis may also serve a number of normal functions (e.g., in embryogenesis) and is not necessarily associated with cell injury.

Necrosis is the more common type of cell death, involving severe cell swelling, denaturation and coagulation of proteins, breakdown of cellular organelles, and cell rupture. Usually, a large number of cells in the adjoining tissue are affected, and an inflammatory infiltrate is recruited.

Apoptosis occurs when a cell dies by activation of an internal "suicide" program, involving an orchestrated disassembly of cellular components; there is minimal disruption of the surrounding tissue and there is minimal, if any, inflammation. Morphologically, there is chromatin condensation and fragmentation.

Autophagy is an adaptive response of cells to nutrient deprivation; it is essentially a self-cannibalization to maintain viability. However, it can also culminate in cell death and is invoked as a cause for cell loss in degenerative disorders of muscle and nervous system (p. 32).

Causes of Cell Injury (p. 11)

- *Oxygen deprivation (hypoxia)* affects aerobic respiration and therefore ability to generate adenosine triphosphate (ATP). This extremely important and common cause of cell injury and death occurs as a result of:

  Ischemia (loss of blood supply)
  Inadequate oxygenation (e.g., cardiorespiratory failure)
  Loss of oxygen-carrying capacity of the blood (e.g., anemia, carbon monoxide poisoning)

- *Physical agents,* including trauma, heat, cold, radiation, and electric shock (Chapter 9)
- *Chemical agents and drugs,* including therapeutic drugs, poisons, environmental pollutants, and "social stimuli" (alcohol and narcotics)
- *Infectious agents,* including viruses, bacteria, fungi, and parasites (Chapter 8)
- *Immunologic reactions,* including autoimmune diseases (Chapter 6) and cell injury following responses to infection (Chapter 2)
- *Genetic derangements,* such as chromosomal alterations and specific gene mutations (Chapter 5)
- *Nutritional imbalances,* including protein–calorie deficiency or lack of specific vitamins, as well as nutritional excesses (Chapter 9)

Morphologic Alternations in Cell Injury (p. 12)

Injury leads to loss of cell function long before damage is morphologically recognizable. Morphologic changes become apparent only some time after a critical biochemical system within the cell has been deranged; the interval between injury and morphologic change depends on the method of detection (Fig. 1-1). However, once developed, reversible injury and irreversible injury *(necrosis)* have characteristic features.

Reversible Injury (p. 12)

- *Cell swelling* appears whenever cells cannot maintain ionic and fluid homeostasis (largely due to loss of activity in plasma membrane energy-dependent ion pumps).
- *Fatty change* is manifested by cytoplasmic lipid vacuoles, principally encountered in cells involved in or dependent on fat metabolism (e.g., hepatocytes and myocardial cells).

Necrosis (p. 14)

Necrosis is the sum of the morphologic changes that follow cell death in living tissue or organs. Two processes underlie the basic morphologic changes:

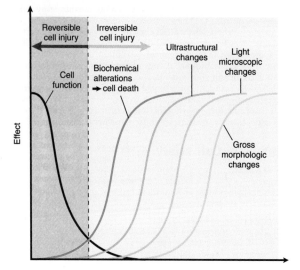

FIGURE 1-1 Timing of biochemical and morphologic changes in cell injury.

- Denaturation of proteins
- Enzymatic digestion of organelles and other cytosolic components

There are several distinctive features: necrotic cells are more *eosinophilic* (pink) than viable cells by standard hematoxylin and eosin (H&E) staining. They appear "glassy" owing to glycogen loss and may be vacuolated; cell membranes are fragmented. Necrotic cells may attract calcium salts; this is particularly true of necrotic fat cells (forming fatty soaps). Nuclear changes include *pyknosis* (small, dense nucleus), *karyolysis* (faint, dissolved nucleus), and *karyorrhexis* (fragmented nucleus). General tissue patterns of necrosis include the following:

- *Coagulative necrosis* (p. 15) is the most common pattern, predominated by protein denaturation with preservation of the cell and tissue framework. This pattern is characteristic of hypoxic death in all tissues except the brain. Necrotic tissue undergoes either *heterolysis* (digestion by lysosomal enzymes of invading leukocytes) or *autolysis* (digestion by its own lysosomal enzymes).
- *Liquefactive necrosis* (p. 15) occurs when autolysis or heterolysis predominates over protein denaturation. The necrotic area is soft and filled with fluid. This type of necrosis is most frequently seen in localized bacterial infections *(abscesses)* and in the brain.
- *Gangrenous necrosis* (p.15) is not a specific pattern but is rather just coagulative necrosis as applied to an ischemic limb; superimposed bacterial infection makes for a more liquefactive pattern called *wet gangrene.*
- *Caseous necrosis* (p. 16) is characteristic of tuberculous lesions; it appears grossly as soft, friable, "cheesy" material and microscopically as amorphous eosinophilic material with cell debris.
- *Fat necrosis* (p. 16) is seen in adipose tissue; lipase activation (e.g., from injured pancreatic cells or macrophages) releases fatty

acids from triglycerides, which then complex with calcium to create soaps. Grossly, these are white, chalky areas (*fat saponification*); histologically, there are vague cell outlines and calcium deposition.

* *Fibrinoid necrosis* (p. 16 and Chapter 6) is a pathologic pattern resulting from antigen-antibody (*immune complex*) deposition in blood vessels. Microscopically there is bright-pink amorphous material (protein deposition) in arterial walls, often with associated inflammation and thrombosis.

Mechanisms of Cell Injury (p. 17)

The biochemical pathways in cell injury can be organized around a few general principles:

* Responses to injurious stimuli depend on the type of injury, duration, and severity.
* The consequences of injury depend on the type, state, and adaptability of the injured cell.
* Cell injury results from perturbations in any of five essential cellular elements:

   ATP production (mostly through effects on mitochondrial *aerobic respiration*)
   Mitochondrial integrity independent of ATP production
   Plasma membrane integrity, responsible for ionic and osmotic homeostasis
   Protein synthesis, folding, degradation, and refolding
   Integrity of the genetic apparatus

The intracellular mechanisms of cell injury fall into one of six general pathways (Fig. 1-2). Structural and biochemical elements of the cell are so closely interrelated that regardless of the locus of initial injury, secondary effects rapidly propagate through other elements.

Depletion of ATP (p. 17)

Decreased ATP synthesis and ATP depletion are common consequences of both ischemic and toxic injury. ATP is generated through glycolysis (anaerobic, inefficient) and oxidative phosphorylation in the mitochondria (aerobic, efficient). Hypoxia leads to increased anaerobic glycolysis with glycogen depletion, increased lactic acid production, and intracellular acidosis. ATP is critical for membrane transport, maintenance of ionic gradients (particularly Na^+, K^+, and Ca^{2+}), and protein synthesis; reduced ATP synthesis dramatically affects those pathways.

Mitochondrial Damage (p. 18)

Mitochondrial damage can occur directly due to hypoxia or toxins or as a consequence of increased cytosolic Ca^{2+}, oxidative stress, or phospholipid breakdown. Damage results in formation of a high-conductance channel (*mitochondrial permeability transition pore*) that leaks protons and dissipates the electromotive potential that drives oxidative phosphorylation. Damaged mitochondria also leak cytochrome *c*, which can trigger apoptosis (see later discussion).

Influx of Calcium and Loss of Calcium Homeostasis (p. 19)

Cytosolic calcium is maintained at extremely low levels by energy-dependent transport; ischemia and toxins can cause Ca^{2+} influx across the plasma membrane and release of Ca^{2+} from mitochondria

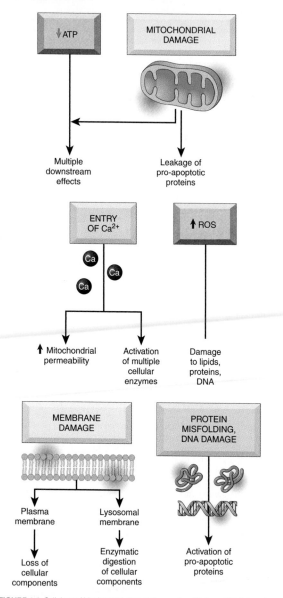

FIGURE 1-2 Cellular and biochemical sites of damage in cell injury. *ATP*, Adenosine triphosphate; *ROS*, reactive oxygen species.

and endoplasmic reticulum (ER). Increased cytosolic calcium activates phospholipases that degrade membrane phospholipids; proteases that break down membrane and cytoskeletal proteins; ATPases that hasten ATP depletion; and endonucleases that cause chromatin fragmentation.

Accumulation of Oxygen-Derived Free Radicals (Oxidative Stress) (p. 20)

Free radicals are unstable, partially reduced molecules with unpaired electrons in outer orbitals that make them particularly reactive with other molecules. Although other elements can have free radical forms, O_2-derived free radicals (also called *reactive oxygen species* or *ROS*) are the most common in biological systems. The major forms are *superoxide anion* ($O_2^{\bar{\cdot}}$, one extra electron), *hydrogen peroxide* (H_2O_2, two extra electrons), *hydroxyl ions* ($OH^{\bullet}$, three extra electrons) and *peroxynitrate ion* ($ONOO^{\cdot}$; formed by interactions of nitric oxide [NO] and $O_2^{\bar{\cdot}}$).

Free radicals readily propagate additional free radical formation with other molecules in an autocatalytic chain reaction that often breaks chemical bonds. Thus, free radicals damage lipids (peroxidizing double bonds and causing chain breakage), proteins (oxidizing and fragmenting peptide bonds), and nucleic acids (causing single strand breaks).

Free radical generation occurs by:

- Normal metabolic processes such as the reduction of oxygen to water during respiration; the sequential addition of four electrons leads to small numbers ROS intermediates.
- Absorption of radiant energy; ionizing radiation (e.g., ultraviolet light and x-rays) can hydrolyze water into hydroxyl ($OH^{\bullet}$) and hydrogen ($H^{\bullet}$) free radicals.
- Production by leukocytes during inflammation to sterilize sites of infection (Chapter 2).
- Enzymatic metabolism of exogenous chemicals or drugs (e.g., acetaminophen).
- *Transition metals* (e.g., iron and copper) can catalyze free radical formation.
- *Nitric oxide (NO)*, an important chemical mediator (Chapter 2), can act directly as a free radical or be converted to other highly reactive forms.

Fortunately, free radicals are *inherently unstable and generally decay spontaneously*. In addition, several systems contribute to free radical inactivation:

- *Antioxidants* either block the initiation of free radical formation or scavenge free radicals; these include vitamins E and A, ascorbic acid, and glutathione.
- The levels of transition metals that can participate in free radical formation are minimized by binding to storage and transport proteins (e.g., *transferrin, ferritin, lactoferrin,* and *ceruloplasmin*).
- Free radical scavenging *enzyme* systems catabolize hydrogen peroxide *(catalase, glutathione peroxidase)* and superoxide anion *(superoxide dismutase)*.

Defects in Membrane Permeability (p. 22)

Membranes can be damaged directly by toxins, physical and chemical agents, lytic complement components, and perforins, or indirectly as described by the preceding events (e.g., ROS, Ca^{2+} activation of phospholipases). Increased plasma membrane permeability affects intracellular osmolarity as well as enzymatic activity; increased mitochondrial membrane permeability reduces ATP synthesis and can drive apoptosis; altered lysosomal integrity unleashes extremely potent acid hydrolases that can digest proteins, nucleic acids, lipids, and glycogen.

Damage to DNA and Proteins (p. 23)

Damage to DNA that exceeds normal repair capacity (e.g., due to ROS, radiation, or drugs) leads to activation of apoptosis. Similarly, accumulation of large amounts of improperly folded proteins (e.g., due to ROS or heritable mutations) leads to a stress response that also triggers apoptotic pathways.

Within limits, all the changes of cell injury described previously can be offset, and cells can return to normal after injury abates *(reversible injury)*. However, persistent or excessive injury causes cells to pass a threshold into *irreversible injury* associated with extensive cell membrane damage, lysosomal swelling, and mitochondrial vacuolization with deficient ATP synthesis. Extracellular calcium enters the cell and intracellular calcium stores are released, leading to activation of enzymes that catabolize membranes, proteins, ATP, and nucleic acids. Proteins, essential coenzymes, and RNAs are lost from hyperpermeable plasma membranes, and cells leak metabolites vital for the reconstitution of ATP.

The transition from reversible to irreversible injury is difficult to identify, although two phenomena consistently characterize irreversibility:

- *Inability to reverse mitochondrial dysfunction* (lack of ATP generation) even after resolution of the original injury
- Development of profound disturbances in membrane function

Leakage of intracellular enzymes or proteins across abnormally permeable plasma membranes into the bloodstream provides important clinical markers of cell death. Cardiac muscle contains a specific isoform of the enzyme creatine kinase and of the contractile protein troponin; hepatocytes contain transaminases, and hepatic bile duct epithelium contains a temperature-resistant isoform of alkaline phosphatase. Irreversible injury in these tissues is consequently reflected by increased circulating levels of such proteins in the blood.

Examples of Cell Injury and Necrosis (p. 23)

Ischemic and Hypoxic Injury (p. 23)

Ischemia and hypoxic injury are the most common forms of cell injury in clinical medicine. *Hypoxia* is reduced O_2-carrying capacity; *ischemia*, which also clearly causes hypoxia, is due to reduced blood flow. Hypoxia alone allows continued delivery of substrates for glycolysis and removal of accumulated wastes (e.g., lactic acid); ischemia does neither and therefore tends to injure tissues faster than hypoxia alone.

Hypoxia leads to loss of ATP generation by mitochondria; ATP depletion has multiple, initially *reversible* effects (Fig. 1-3):

- Failure of Na^+/K^+-ATPase membrane transport causes sodium to enter the cell and potassium to exit; there is also increased Ca^{2+} influx as well as release of Ca^{2+} from intracellular stores. The net gain of solute is accompanied by isosmotic gain of water, *cell swelling*, and ER dilation. Cell swelling is also increased owing to the *osmotic load* from accumulation of metabolic breakdown products.
- *Cellular energy metabolism* is altered. With hypoxia, cells use *anaerobic glycolysis* for energy production (metabolism of glucose derived from glycogen). Consequently, *glycogen stores are rapidly depleted* along with lactic acid accumulation and *reduced intracellular pH*.
- Reduced protein synthesis results from detachment of ribosomes from rough ER.

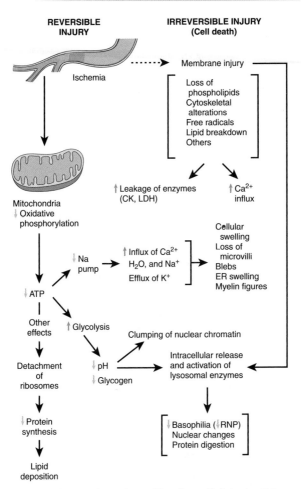

FIGURE 1-3 Sequence of events in reversible and irreversible ischemic cell injury. Although reduced adenosine triphosphate *(ATP)* levels play a central role, ischemia can also cause direct membrane damage. *CK,* Creatine kinase; *ER,* endoplasmic reticulum; *LDH,* lactate dehydrogenase; *RNP,* ribonucleoprotein.

All the aforementioned changes are reversible if oxygenation is restored. If ischemia persists, *irreversible* injury ensues, a transition largely dependent upon the extent of *ATP depletion* and *membrane dysfunction,* particularly mitochondrial membranes.

- ATP depletion induces the pore transition change in the mitochondrial membrane; pore formation results in reduced membrane potential and diffusion of solutes.
- ATP depletion also *releases cytochrome c,* a soluble component of the electron transport chain that is a key regulator in driving apoptosis (see later discussion).
- Increased cytosolic calcium activates membrane phospholipases, leading to progressive loss of phospholipids and membrane damage; decreased ATP also leads to diminished phospholipid synthesis.

- Increased cytosolic calcium *activates intracellular proteases*, causing degradation of intermediate cytoskeletal elements, rendering the cell membrane susceptible to stretching and rupture, particularly in the setting of cell swelling.
- Free fatty acids and lysophospholipids accumulate in ischemic cells as a result of phospholipid degradation; these are directly toxic to membranes.

Ischemia-Reperfusion Injury (p. 24)

Restoration of blood flow to ischemic tissues can result in recovery of reversibly injured cells or may not affect the outcome if irreversible damage has occurred. However, depending on the intensity and duration of the ischemic insult, additional cells may die *after* blood flow resumes, involving either necrosis or apoptosis. The process is characteristically associated with neutrophilic infiltrates. The additional damage is designated *reperfusion injury* and is clinically important in myocardial infarction, acute renal failure, and stroke. Several mechanisms potentially underlie reperfusion injury:

- New damage may occur during reoxygenation by increased generation of ROS from parenchymal and endothelial cells, as well as from infiltrating leukocytes. Superoxide anions produced in reperfused tissue result from incomplete reduction of O_2 by damaged mitochondria or because of the normal action of oxidases from tissue cells or invading inflammatory cells. Antioxidant defense mechanisms may also be compromised, favoring radical accumulation.
- Ischemic injury recruits circulating inflammatory cells (Chapter 2) through enhanced cytokine and adhesion molecule expression by hypoxic parenchymal and endothelial cells. The ensuing inflammation causes additional injury. By restoring blood flow, reperfusion may actually *increase* local inflammatory cell infiltration.
- *Complement* activation (normally involved in host defense; Chapter 2) may also contribute. Immunoglobulin M (IgM) antibodies can deposit in ischemic tissues; when blood flow is resumed, complement proteins are activated by binding to the antibodies, resulting in further cell injury and inflammation.

Chemical (Toxic) Injury (p. 24)

Chemical injury occurs by two general mechanisms:

- *Directly,* by binding to some critical molecular component (e.g., mercuric chloride binds to cell membrane protein sulfhydryl groups, inhibiting ATPase-dependent transport and causing increased permeability)
- *Indirectly,* by conversion to reactive toxic metabolites (e.g., carbon tetrachloride and acetaminophen); toxic metabolites, in turn, cause cellular injury either by direct covalent binding to membrane protein and lipids or, more commonly, by the formation of reactive free radicals

Apoptosis (p. 25)

Programmed cell death *(apoptosis)* occurs when a cell dies through activation of a tightly regulated internal suicide program. The function of apoptosis is to eliminate unwanted cells selectively, with minimal disturbance to surrounding cells and the host. The cell's plasma membrane remains intact, but its structure is altered so that the apoptotic cell fragments and becomes an avid target for phagocytosis. The dead cell is rapidly cleared before its contents have leaked out; therefore cell death by this pathway does not elicit an inflammatory reaction in the host. Thus, apoptosis is fundamentally different from necrosis, which is characterized by loss of membrane integrity, enzymatic digestion of cells, and frequently a host reaction (see Table 1-2). Nevertheless, apoptosis and necrosis sometimes coexist and may share some common features and mechanisms.

Causes of Apoptosis (p. 25)

Apoptosis can be physiologic or pathologic.

Physiologic Causes

- Programmed destruction of cells during embryogenesis
- Hormone-dependent involution of tissues (e.g., endometrium, prostate) in the adult
- Cell deletion in proliferating cell populations (e.g., intestinal epithelium) to maintain a constant cell number
- Death of cells that have served their useful purpose (e.g., neutrophils following an acute inflammatory response)
- Deletion of potentially harmful self-reactive lymphocytes

Pathologic Causes

- DNA damage (e.g., due to hypoxia, radiation, or cytotoxic drugs). If repair mechanisms cannot cope with the damage caused, cells will undergo apoptosis rather than risk mutations that could result in malignant transformation. Relatively mild injury may induce apoptosis, whereas larger doses of the same stimuli result in necrosis.
- Accumulation of misfolded proteins (e.g., due to inherited defects or due to free radical damage). This may be the basis of cell loss in a number of neurodegenerative disorders.
- Cell death in certain viral infections (e.g., hepatitis), either caused directly by the infection or by cytotoxic T cells.
- Cytotoxic T cells may also be a cause of apoptotic cell death in tumors and in the rejection of transplanted tissues.
- Pathologic atrophy in parenchymal organs after duct obstruction (e.g., pancreas).

Morphologic and Biochemical Changes in Apoptosis (p. 26)

Morphologic features of apoptosis (see Table 1-2) include cell shrinkage, chromatin condensation and fragmentation, cellular blebbing and fragmentation into apoptotic bodies, and phagocytosis of apoptotic bodies by adjacent healthy cells or macrophages. Lack of inflammation makes it difficult to detect apoptosis histologically.

- Protein breakdown occurs through a family of proteases called *caspases* (so named because they have an active site *c*ysteine and cleave at *asp*artate residues).
- Internucleosomal cleavage of DNA into fragments 180 to 200 base pairs in size gives rise to a characteristic ladder pattern of DNA bands on agarose gel electrophoresis.
- Plasma membrane alterations (e.g., flipping of phosphatidylserine from the inner to the outer leaf of the plasma membrane) allow recognition of apoptotic cells for phagocytosis.

Mechanisms of Apoptosis (p. 27) (Fig. 1-4)

Apoptosis is a cascade of molecular events that can be initiated by a variety of triggers. The process of apoptosis is divided into an *initiation phase*, when caspases become active, and an *execution phase*, when the enzymes cause cell death. Initiation of apoptosis occurs through two distinct but convergent pathways: the *intrinsic* mitochondrial pathway and the *extrinsic* death receptor–mediated pathway.

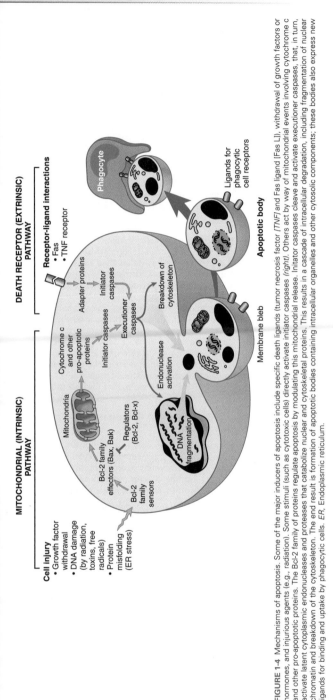

FIGURE 1-4 Mechanisms of apoptosis. Some of the major inducers of apoptosis include specific death ligands (tumor necrosis factor [*TNF*] and Fas ligand [Fas L]), withdrawal of growth factors or hormones, and injurious agents (e.g., radiation). Some stimuli (such as cytotoxic cells) directly activate initiator caspases (*right*). Others act by way of mitochondrial events involving cytochrome c and other pro-apoptotic proteins. The Bcl-2 family of proteins regulate apoptosis by modulating this mitochondrial release. Initiator caspases cleave and activate executioner caspases, that, in turn, activate latent cytoplasmic endonucleases and proteases that catabolize nuclear and cytoskeletal proteins. This results in a cascade of intracellular degradation, including fragmentation of nuclear chromatin and breakdown of the cytoskeleton. The end result is formation of apoptotic bodies containing intracellular organelles and other cytosolic components; these bodies also express new ligands for binding and uptake by phagocytic cells. *ER*, Endoplasmic reticulum.

Intrinsic (Mitochondrial) Pathway *(p. 28)*

When mitochondrial permeability is increased, *cytochrome c*, as well as other pro-apoptotic molecules, is released into the cytoplasm; death receptors are not involved. Mitochondrial permeability is regulated by more than 20 proteins of the Bcl family. Bcl-2 and Bcl-x are the two predominant *anti-apoptotic proteins* responsible for reducing mitochondrial leakiness. On the other hand, cellular stress (e.g., misfolded proteins, DNA damage) or loss of survival signals is sensed by other Bcl members (e.g., Bim, Bid, and Bad). These molecules then activate two critical pro-apoptotic proteins—Bax and Bak—that form oligomers that insert into the mitochondrial membrane and create permeability channels. With concomitantly decreasing Bcl-2/Bcl-x levels, mitochondrial membrane permeability increases, leaking out several proteins that can activate caspases. Thus, released *cytochrome c* binds to apoptosis activating factor-1 (Apaf-1) to form a large multimeric *apoptosome* complex that triggers caspase-9 (an initiator caspase) activation. *The essence of the intrinsic pathway is a balance between pro-apoptotic and anti-apoptotic molecules that regulate mitochondrial permeability.*

Extrinsic (Death Receptor–Initiated) Pathway *(p. 29)*

Death receptors are members of the tumor necrosis factor (TNF) receptor family (e.g., type 1 TNF receptor and Fas). They have a cytoplasmic *death domain* involved in protein-protein interactions. Cross-linking these receptors by external ligands, such as TNF or Fas ligand (FasL), causes them to trimerize to form binding sites for adapter proteins that serve to bring multiple inactive caspase-8 molecules into close proximity. Low-level enzymatic activity of these pro-caspases eventually cleaves and activates one of the assembled group, rapidly leading to a downstream cascade of caspase activation. This enzymatic pathway can be inhibited by a blocking protein called *FLIP;* viruses and normal cells can produce FLIP to protect themselves against Fas-mediated death.

Execution Phase *(p. 30)*

Caspases occur as inactive pro-enzymes that are activated through proteolytic cleavage; the cleavage sites can be hydrolyzed by other caspases or autocatalytically. *Initiator caspases* (e.g., caspase-8 and -9) are activated early in the sequence and induce the cleavage of the *executioner caspases* (e.g., caspase-3 and -6) that do the bulk of the intracellular proteolytic degradation. Once an initiator caspase is activated, the death program is set in motion by rapid and sequential activation of other caspases. Executioner caspases act on many cell components; they cleave cytoskeletal and nuclear matrix proteins, disrupting the cytoskeleton and leading to nuclear breakdown. In the nucleus, caspases cleave proteins involved in transcription, DNA replication, and DNA repair; in particular, caspase-3 activates a cytoplasmic DNAase resulting in the characteristic internucleosomal cleavage.

Apoptosis in Health and Disease *(p. 30)*

Growth Factor Deprivation

Examples include hormone-sensitive cells deprived of the relevant hormone, lymphocytes not stimulated by antigens or cytokines, and neurons deprived of nerve growth factor. Apoptosis is triggered by the intrinsic (mitochondrial) pathway due to a relative excess of pro-apoptotic versus anti-apoptotic members of the Bcl family.

DNA Damage

DNA damage by any means (e.g., radiation or chemotherapeutic agents) induces apoptosis through accumulation of the tumor-suppressor protein p53. This results in cell cycle arrest at G_1 putatively to allow time for DNA repair (Chapter 7). If repair cannot take place, p53 then induces apoptosis by increasing the transcription of several pro-apoptotic members of the Bcl family. Absent or mutated p53 (i.e., in certain cancers) reduces apoptosis and favors cell survival even in the presence significant DNA damage.

Protein Misfolding

Accumulation of misfolded proteins—due to oxidative stress, hypoxia, or genetic mutations—leads to the *unfolded protein response*, increasingly recognized as a feature of several neurodegenerative disorders. This response induces increased production of chaperones and increased proteasomal degradation with decreased protein synthesis. If the adaptive responses cannot keep pace with the accumulating misfolded proteins, caspases are activated and apoptosis results (Fig. 1-5).

TNF Family Receptors

Apoptosis induced by Fas-FasL interactions (see preceding discussion) are important for eliminating lymphocytes that recognize self-antigens; mutations in Fas or FasL result in autoimmune diseases (Chapter 6).

TNF is an important mediator of the inflammatory reaction (Chapter 2), but can also induce apoptosis (see preceding discussion). The major physiologic functions of TNF are mediated through activation of the transcription factor nuclear factor-κB (NF-κB), which in turn promotes cell survival by increasing anti-apoptotic members of the Bcl family. Whether TNF induces cell death, promotes cell survival, or drives inflammatory responses depends on which of two TNF receptors it binds, as well as which adapter protein attaches to the receptor.

Cytotoxic T Lymphocytes

Cytotoxic T lymphocytes (CTLs) recognize foreign antigens on the surface of infected host cells (Chapter 6) and secrete perforin, a transmembrane pore-forming molecule. This allows entry of the CTL-derived serine protease granzyme B that in turn activates multiple caspases, thereby directly inducing the effector phase of apoptosis. CTLs also express FasL on their surfaces and can kill target cells by Fas ligation (via FasL).

Disorders Associated with Dysregulated Apoptosis (p. 32)

Dysregulated ("too little or too much") apoptosis underlies multiple disorders:

- *Disorders with defective apoptosis and increased cell survival.* Insufficient apoptosis may prolong the survival or reduce the turnover of abnormal cells. Such accumulated cells may lead to (1) *cancers,* especially tumors with *p53* mutations, or hormone-dependent tumors, such as breast, prostate, or ovarian cancers (Chapter 7), and (2) *autoimmune disorders,* when autoreactive lymphocytes are not eliminated (Chapter 6).
- *Disorders with increased apoptosis and excessive cell death.* Increased cell loss can cause (1) *neurodegenerative diseases,* with drop out of specific sets of neurons (Chapter 28); (2) *ischemic injury* (e.g., myocardial infarction, Chapter 12; stroke, Chapter 28); and (3) *death of virus-infected cells* (Chapter 8).

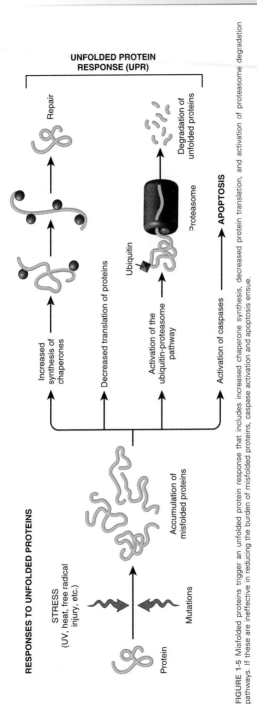

FIGURE 1-5 Misfolded proteins trigger an unfolded protein response that includes increased chaperone synthesis, decreased protein translation, and activation of proteasome degradation pathways. If these are ineffective in reducing the burden of misfolded proteins, caspase activation and apoptosis ensue.

Intracellular Accumulations (p. 32)

Cells may accumulate abnormal amounts of various substances.

- A *normal* endogenous substance (water, protein, carbohydrate, lipid) is produced at a normal (or even increased) rate, with the metabolic rate inadequate to remove it (e.g., fat accumulation in liver cells).
- An abnormal endogenous substance (product of a mutated gene) accumulates because of defective folding or transport, and inadequate degradation (e.g., α_1-antitrypsin disease, Chapter 18).
- A *normal* substance accumulates because of genetic or acquired defects in its *metabolism* (e.g., lysososmal storage diseases, Chapter 5).
- *Abnormal exogenous substances* may accumulate in normal cells because they lack the machinery to degrade such substances (e.g., macrophages laden with environmental carbon).

Lipids (p. 33)

Triglycerides (the most common), cholesterol and cholesterol esters, and phospholipids can accumulate in cells.

Steatosis (Fatty Change) (p. 33)

The terms describe an abnormal accumulation of triglycerides within parenchymal cells either due to excessive entry or defective metabolism and export. It can occur in heart, muscle, and kidney, but it is most common in the liver. Fatty change is typically reversible, but it can lead to inflammation and fibrosis.

Hepatic causes include alcohol abuse (most common in the United States), protein malnutrition, diabetes mellitus, obesity, toxins, and anoxia. Grossly, fatty livers are enlarged, yellow, and greasy; microscopically, there are small, intracytoplasmic droplets or large vacuoles of fat. The condition is caused by excessive entry or defective metabolism or export of lipids (Fig. 1-6):

- Increased fatty acids entering the liver (starvation, corticosteroids)
- Decreased fatty acid oxidation (hypoxia)
- Increased triglyceride formation (alcohol)
- Decreased apoprotein synthesis (carbon tetrachloride poisoning, starvation)
- Impaired lipoprotein secretion from the liver (alcohol)

Cholesterol and Cholesterol Esters (p. 34)

Cholesterol is normally required for cell membrane or lipid-soluble hormone synthesis; production is tightly regulated, but accumulation (seen as intracellular cytoplasmic vacuoles) can be present in a variety of pathologic states:

- *Atherosclerosis:* Cholesterol and cholesterol esters accumulate in arterial wall smooth muscle cells and macrophages (Chapter 11). Extracellular accumulations appear microscopically as cleftlike cavities formed when cholesterol crystals are dissolved during normal histologic processing.
- *Xanthomas:* In acquired and hereditary *hyperlipidemias*, lipids accumulate in clusters of "foamy" macrophages and mesenchymal cells.
- *Cholesterolosis:* Focal accumulations of cholesterol-laden macrophages occur in the lamina propria of gallbladders.
- *Niemann-Pick disease, type C:* This type of lysosomal storage disease is due to mutation of an enzyme involved in cholesterol catabolism.

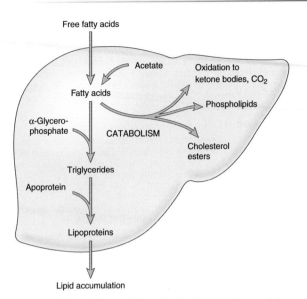

Free fatty acids

Acetate

Fatty acids

Oxidation to
ketone bodies, CO_2

Phospholipids

α-Glycero-
phosphate

CATABOLISM

Cholesterol
esters

Triglycerides

Apoprotein

Lipoproteins

Lipid accumulation

FIGURE 1-6 Schematic diagram of the mechanisms leading to fat accumulation in hepatic steatosis. Defects in any of uptake, catabolism, or secretion can result in lipid overload.

Proteins (p. 35)

Intracellular protein accumulation may be due to excessive synthesis, absorption, or defects in cellular transport. Morphologically visible accumulations appear as rounded, eosinophilic cytoplasmic droplets. In some disorders (e.g., *amyloidosis*, Chapter 6), abnormal proteins deposit primarily in the *extracellular* space.

- *Reabsorption droplets* of proteins accumulate in proximal renal tubules in the setting of chronic proteinuria. The process is reversible; the droplets are metabolized and clear if the proteinuria resolves.
- *Normally secreted proteins* can accumulate if produced in excessive amounts, e.g., immunoglobulin within plasma cells. In that case, the ER becomes grossly distended with eosinophilic inclusions called *Russell bodies*.
- *Defective intracellular transport and secretion*, e.g., α_1-*antitrypsin deficiency*, where partially folded intermediates of mutated proteins accumulate in hepatocyte ER. In many cases, pathology results not only from the unfolded protein response and apoptosis (see preceding discussion) but also from loss of protein function. Thus reduction in secreted α_1-antitrypsin also leads to emphysema (Chapter 15).
- *Accumulated cytoskeletal proteins.* Excess intermediate filaments (e.g., keratin or certain neurofilaments) are hallmarks of cell injury; thus, keratin intermediate filaments coalesce into cytoplasmic eosinophilic inclusions called *alcoholic hyaline* (Chapter 18), and the *neurofibrillary tangle* in Alzheimer's disease contains neurofilaments (Chapter 28).
- *Aggregates of abnormal proteins.* Aggregation of abnormally folded proteins (e.g., genetic mutations, aging, and so on), either intracellular and/or extracellular, can cause pathologic change; extracellular amyloid is an example.

Hyaline Change (p. 36)

Hyaline change refers to any deposit that imparts a homogeneous, glassy pink appearance in H&E-stained histologic sections. Examples of *intracellular hyaline change* include proximal tubule epithelial protein droplets, Russell bodies, viral inclusions, and alcoholic hyaline. *Extracellular hyaline change* occurs, for example, in damaged arterioles (e.g., due to chronic hypertension), presumably due to extravasated proteins.

Glycogen (p. 36)

Glycogen is commonly stored within cells as a ready energy source. *Excessive* intracellular deposits (seen as clear vacuoles) are seen with abnormalities of glycogen storage (so-called *glycogenoses*, Chapter 5) and glucose metabolism *(diabetes mellitus)*.

Pigments (p. 36)

Pigments are colored substances that can be exogenous (e.g., coal dust) or endogenous, such as melanin or hemosiderin.

- Exogenous pigments include carbon or coal dust (most common); when visibly accumulated within pulmonary macrophages and lymph nodes, these deposits are called *anthracosis*. Pigments from *tattooing* are taken up by macrophages and persist for the life of the cell.
- Endogenous pigments include:

    Lipofuscin, the so-called wear-and-tear pigment, is usually associated with cellular and tissue atrophy *(brown atrophy)*. This is seen microscopically as fine, yellow-brown intracytoplasmic granules. The pigment is composed of complex lipids, phospholipids, and protein, probably derived from cell membrane peroxidation.

    Melanin is a normal, endogenous, brown-black pigment formed by enzymatic oxidation of tyrosine to dihydroxyphenylalanine in melanocytes.

    Homogentisic acid is a black pigment formed in patients with alkaptonuria (lacking homogentisic oxidase) that deposits in skin and connective tissue; the pigmentation is called ochronosis.

    Hemosiderin is a hemoglobin-derived, golden–yellow-brown, granular intracellular pigment composed of aggregated ferritin. Accumulation can be localized (e.g., macrophage-mediated breakdown of blood in a bruise) or systemic, that is, resulting from increased dietary iron absorption (primary hemochromatosis), impaired utilization (e.g., thalassemia), hemolysis, or chronic transfusions (Chapter 18).

Pathologic Calcification (p. 38)

Pathologic calcification—the abnormal tissue deposition of calcium salts—occurs in two forms: *dystrophic calcification* arises in nonviable tissues in the presence of normal calcium serum levels, and *metastatic calcification* happens in viable tissues in the setting of hypercalcemia.

Dystrophic Calcification (p. 38)

Although frequently only a marker of prior injury, it can also be a source of significant pathology. Dystrophic calcification occurs in arteries in atherosclerosis, in damaged heart valves, and in areas of necrosis (e.g., coagulative, caseous, and liquefactive). Calcium can be intracellular and extracellular. Deposition ultimately involves precipitation of a crystalline calcium phosphate similar to bone hydroxyapatite:

- *Initiation (nucleation)* occurs extracellularly or intracellularly. *Extracellular* initiation occurs on membrane-bound vesicles from dead or dying cells that concentrate calcium due to their content of charged phospholipids; membrane-bound phosphatases that generate phosphates that form calcium-phosphate complexes; the cycle of calcium and phosphate binding is repeated, eventually producing a deposit. Initiation of *intracellular* calcification occurs in mitochondria of dead or dying cells.
- *Propagation* of crystal formation depends on the concentration of calcium and phosphates, the presence of inhibitors, and structural components of the extracellular matrix.

Metastatic Calcification (p. 38)

These calcium deposits occur as amorphous basophilic densities that can be present widely throughout the body. Typically, they have no clinical sequelae, although massive deposition can cause renal and lung deficits. Metastatic calcification results from hypercalcemia, which has four principal causes:

- *Elevated parathyroid hormone* (e.g., hyperparathyroidism due to parathyroid tumors or ectopic parathyroid hormone secreted by other neoplasms)
- *Bone destruction,* as in primary marrow malignancies (e.g., multiple myeloma) or by diffuse skeletal metastasis (e.g., breast cancer), by accelerated bone turnover *(Paget's disease),* or immobilization
- *Vitamin D–related disorders,* including vitamin D intoxication and systemic sarcoidosis
- *Renal failure,* causing secondary hyperparathyroidism due to phosphate retention and the resulting hypocalcemia

Cellular Aging (p. 39)

With increasing age, degenerative changes impact the structure and physiologic function of all organ systems. The tempo and severity of such changes in any given individual are influenced by genetic factors, diet, social conditions, and the impact of other comorbidities, such as atherosclerosis, diabetes, and osteoarthritis. *Cellular* aging—reflecting the progressive accumulation of sublethal cellular and molecular damage due to both genetic and exogenous influences—leads to cell death and diminished capacity to respond to injury; it is a critical component of the aging of the entire organism (Fig. 1-7).

Aging—at least in model systems—appears to be a regulated process influenced by a limited number of genes; this, in turn, implies that aging can potentially be parsed into definable mechanistic alterations:

- *Cellular senescence* refers to the concept that cells have a limited capacity for replication. Cells from children can have more rounds of replication than cells from geriatrics; in turn, cells from geriatrics replicate more than cells from patients with accelerated aging disorders (e.g., Werner syndrome, due to a DNA helicase mutation). Many changes in gene expression accompany cellular senescence, including those that inhibit cell cycle progression (e.g., increased p16INK4a). In particular, *telomere shortening* (i.e., incomplete replication of chromosome ends) is a major mechanism underlying cell senescence. Telomeres are short, repeated sequences of DNA that comprise the termini of chromosomes; they are important to ensure complete replication

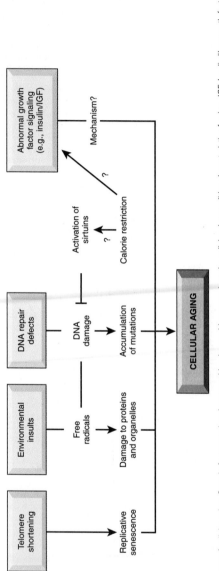

FIGURE 1-7 Mechanisms of cellular aging. Genetic factors and environmental insults combine to produce the cellular abnormalities characteristic of aging. *IGF*, Insulin-like growth factor.

of chromosomes and protect chromosomal ends from fusion and degradation. When cells replicate, a small section of the telomere is not replicated. As cells repeatedly divide, telomeres become progressively shortened, ultimately signaling a growth checkpoint where cells become senescent. *Telomerase* is an RNA–protein enzyme complex that maintains telomere length by using its own RNA as a template to add nucleotides to the ends of chromosomes; it is present in germ cells and stem cells, but is usually undetectable in somatic cells. In cancer cells, telomerase is often reactivated, consistent with the notion that telomere elongation (or at least preservation) may confer cell immortality.

• *Accumulated metabolic and genetic damage* clearly contribute to cellular aging. Ideally, any harm accruing from metabolic events or exogenous injury is counterbalanced by injury repair mechanisms. However, too much injury or too little compensatory response will lead to damage that can affect cell function and viability.

For example, ROS (discussed previously) covalently modify proteins, lipids, and nucleic acids and lead to a variety of breaks; the cumulative amount of oxidative damage increases with age. Increased ROS production (e.g., exposure to ionizing radiation or mitochondrial dysfunction) or diminished antioxidant defenses (glutathione peroxidase, superoxide dismutase) contributes to cellular senescence and correlates with a shortened life span of the organism.

The recognition and repair of damaged DNA is also a critical counterbalance. Thus, in patients with *Werner syndrome*, there is premature aging due to defective *DNA helicase* with accelerated accumulation of chromosomal damage; this mimics the injury that normally accompanies aging. Genetic instability is also characteristic of other disorders associated with premature aging (e.g., *ataxia-telangiectasia*, due to defective repair of DNA double-strand breaks).

Damaged organelles may also accumulate with age and contribute to cellular senescence; this is attributable in part to diminished function of the proteasome.

The most effective way to prolong the life span is *caloric restriction*, likely related to its ability to promote the activity of *sirtuins*, a family of proteins with histone deacetylase activity. Sirtuins increase the production of proteins that reduce apoptosis, stimulate protein folding, increase metabolic activity and insulin sensitivity, and reduce ROS. Signaling through the insulin or insulin-like growth factor-1 (IGF-1) receptors can also influence life span; inactivating insulin receptor mutations increase longevity.

2

Acute and Chronic Inflammation

Overview of Inflammation (p. 44)

Inflammation is the response of vascularized living tissue to injury. It may be evoked by microbial infections, physical agents, chemicals, necrotic tissue, or immune reactions. Inflammation is intended to contain and isolate injury, to destroy invading microorganisms and inactivate toxins, and to prepare the tissue for healing and repair (Chapter 3). Inflammation is characterized by:

- Two main components—a vascular wall response and an inflammatory cell response
- Effects mediated by circulating plasma proteins and by factors produced locally by the vessel wall or inflammatory cells
- Termination when the offending agent is eliminated and the secreted mediators are removed; active anti-inflammatory mechanisms are also involved
- Tight association with healing; even as inflammation destroys, dilutes, or otherwise contains injury it sets into motion events that ultimately lead to repair of the damage
- A fundamentally protective response; however, inflammation can also be harmful, for example, by causing life-threatening hypersensitivity reactions or relentless and progressive organ damage from chronic inflammation and subsequent fibrosis (e.g., rheumatoid arthritis, atherosclerosis)
- *Acute* and *chronic* patterns:

  Acute inflammation: Early onset (i.e., seconds to minutes), short duration (i.e., minutes to days), involving fluid exudation *(edema)* and polymorphonuclear cell (neutrophil) emigration
  Chronic inflammation: Later onset (i.e., days) and longer duration (i.e., weeks to years), involving lymphocytes and macrophages, with blood vessel proliferation and fibrosis (scarring)

There are five classic clinical signs of inflammation (most prominent in acute inflammation):

- Warmth (Latin: *calor*) due to vascular dilation
- Erythema (Latin: *rubor*) due to vascular dilation and congestion
- Edema (Latin: *tumor*) due to increased vascular permeability
- Pain (Latin: *dolor*) due to mediator release
- *Loss of function* (Latin: *functio laesa*) due to pain, edema, tissue injury, and/or scar

Acute Inflammation (p. 45)

Acute inflammation has three major components:

- Alterations in vascular caliber, leading to increased blood flow
- Structural changes in the microvasculature, permitting plasma proteins and leukocytes to leave the circulation to produce inflammatory *exudates*
- Leukocyte emigration from blood vessels and accumulation at the site of injury with activation

Reactions of Blood Vessels in Acute Inflammation (p. 46)

Normal fluid exchange in vascular beds depends on an intact endothelium and is modulated by two opposing forces:

- Hydrostatic pressure causes fluid to move out of the circulation.
- Plasma colloid osmotic pressure causes fluid to move into the capillaries.

DEFINITIONS

Edema is excess fluid in interstitial tissue or body cavities and can be either an exudate or a transudate.

Exudate is an inflammatory, extravascular fluid with cellular debris and high protein concentration (specific gravity of 1.020 or more).

Transudate is excess, extravascular fluid with low protein content (specific gravity of 1.012 or less); it is essentially an ultrafiltrate of blood plasma resulting from elevated fluid pressures or diminished plasma osmotic forces.

Pus is a purulent inflammatory exudate rich in neutrophils and cell debris.

Changes in Vascular Flow and Caliber (p. 46)

Beginning immediately after injury, the vascular wall develops changes in caliber and permeability that affect flow. The changes develop at various rates depending on the nature of the injury and its severity.

- *Vasodilation* causes increased flow into areas of injury, thereby *increasing hydrostatic pressure.*
- Increased vascular permeability causes *exudation* of protein-rich fluid (see later discussion).
- The combination of vascular dilation and fluid loss leads to increased blood viscosity and increased concentration of red blood cells (RBCs). Slow movement of erythrocytes *(stasis)* grossly manifests as vascular congestion *(erythema).*
- With stasis, leukocytes—mostly neutrophils—accumulate along the endothelium *(marginate)* and are activated by mediators to increase adhesion molecule expression and migrate through the vessel wall.

Increased Vascular Permeability (p. 47)

Increased vascular permeability can be induced by several different pathways:

- *Contraction of venule endothelium to form intercellular gaps:*
  - Most common mechanism of increased permeability
  - Elicited by chemical mediators (e.g., histamine, bradykinin, leukotrienes, etc.)
  - Occurs rapidly after injury and is reversible and transient (i.e., 15 to 30 minutes), hence the term *immediate-transient response*
  - A similar response can occur with mild injury (e.g., sunburn) or inflammatory *cytokines* but is delayed (i.e., 2 to 12 hours) and protracted (i.e., 24 hours or more)

- *Direct endothelial injury:*
  - Severe necrotizing injury (e.g., burns) causes endothelial cell necrosis and detachment that affects venules, capillaries, and arterioles
  - Recruited neutrophils may contribute to the injury (e.g., through reactive oxygen species)
  - Immediate and sustained endothelial leakage

- *Increased transcytosis:*
  - Transendothelial channels form by interconnection of vesicles derived from the *vesiculovacuolar organelle*
  - Vascular endothelial growth factor (VEGF) and other factors can induce vascular leakage by increasing the number of these channels

- *Leakage from new blood vessels:*
  - Endothelial proliferation and capillary sprouting *(angiogenesis)* result in leaky vessels
  - Increased permeability persists until the endothelium matures and intercellular junctions form

Responses of Lymphatic Vessels (p. 47)

Lymphatics and lymph nodes filter and "police" extravascular fluids. With the mononuclear phagocyte system, they represent a secondary line of defense when local inflammatory responses cannot contain an infection.

- In inflammation, lymphatic flow is increased to drain edema fluid, leukocytes, and cell debris from the extravascular space.
- In severe injuries, drainage may also transport the offending agent; lymphatics may become inflamed (*lymphangitis*, manifest grossly as red streaks), as may the draining lymph nodes (*lymphadenitis*, manifest as enlarged, painful nodes). The nodal enlargement is usually due to lymphoid follicle and sinusoidal phagocyte hyperplasia (termed *reactive lymphadenitis*, Chapter 13).

Reactions of Leukocytes in Inflammation (p. 48)

A critical function of inflammation is to deliver leukocytes to sites of injury, especially those cells capable of phagocytosing microbes and necrotic debris (e.g., neutrophils and macrophages). After recruitment, the cells must recognize microbes and dead material and effect their removal.

The type of leukocyte that ultimately migrates into a site of injury depends on the age of the inflammatory response and the original stimulus. In most forms of acute inflammation, *neutrophils predominate during the first 6 to 24 hours and are then replaced by monocytes after 24 to 48 hours.* There are several reasons for this sequence: neutrophils are more numerous in blood than monocytes, they respond more rapidly to chemokines, and they attach more firmly to the particular adhesion molecules that are induced on endothelial cells at early time points. After migration, neutrophils are also short-lived; they undergo apoptosis after 24 to 48 hours, whereas monocytes survive longer.

The process of getting cells from vessel lumen to tissue interstitium is called *extravasation* and is divided into three steps (Fig. 2-1):

- Margination, rolling, and adhesion of leukocytes to the endothelium
- Transmigration across the endothelium
- Migration in interstitial tissues toward a chemotactic stimulus

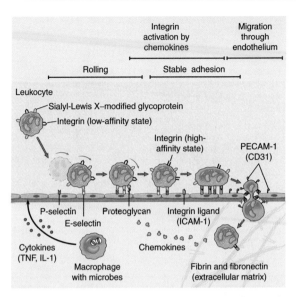

FIGURE 2-1 The multistep process of leukocyte migration through blood vessels, shown here for neutrophils. The leukocytes first roll (are loosely adherent with intermittent attachment and detachment of receptors), then (in sequence) become activated and firmly adhere to endothelium, transmigrate across the endothelium, pierce the basement membrane, and migrate toward chemoattractants emanating from the source of injury. Different molecules play predominant roles in different steps of this process—selectins in rolling, chemokines in activating the neutrophils to increase avidity of integrins, integrins in firm adhesion, and CD31 (PECAM-1) in transmigration. *ICAM-1,* Intercellular adhesion molecule-1; *IL-1,* interleukin-1; *PECAM-1,* platelet-endothelial cell adhesion molecule-1; *TNF,* tumor necrosis factor.

Leukocyte Adhesion to Endothelium (p. 48)

With progressive stasis of blood flow, leukocytes become increasingly distributed along the vessel periphery *(margination)*, followed by *rolling* and then *firm adhesion*, before finally crossing the vascular wall. Rolling, adhesion, and transmigration occur by interactions between complementary adhesion molecules on leukocytes and endothelium. Expression of these adhesion molecules is enhanced by secreted proteins called *cytokines*. The major adhesion molecule pairs are listed in Table 2-1:

- *Selectins (E, P, and L)* bind via lectin (sugar-binding) domains to oligosaccharides (e.g., sialylated Lewis X) on cell surface glycoproteins. These interactions mediate rolling.
- *Immunoglobulin family molecules* on endothelial cells include *intercellular adhesion molecule 1 (ICAM-1)* and *vascular cell adhesion molecule 1 (VCAM-1)*; these bind *integrins* on leukocytes and mediate firm adhesion.
- *Integrins* are α-β heterodimers (protein pairs) on leukocyte surfaces that bind to members of the immunoglobulin family molecules and to the extracellular matrix. The principal integrins that bind ICAM-1 are β_2 integrins *LFA-1* and *Mac-1* (also called *CD11a/CD18* and *CD11b/CD18);* the principal integrin that binds to VCAM-1 is the β_1 integrin VLA4.

Chemoattractants *(chemokines)* and cytokines affect adhesion and transmigration by modulating the surface expression or

TABLE 2-1	Endothelial-Leukocyte Adhesion Molecules	
Endothelial Molecule	Leukocyte Molecule	Major Role
P-selectin	Sialyl-Lewis X–modified proteins	Rolling (neutrophils, monocytes, T lymphocytes)
E-selectin	Sialyl-Lewis X–modified proteins	Rolling and adhesion (neutrophils, monocytes, T lymphocytes)
GlyCam-1, CD34	L-selectin*	Rolling (neutrophils, monocytes)
ICAM-1 (immunoglobulin family)	CD11/CD18 (β_2) integrins (LFA-1, Mac-1)	Adhesion, arrest, transmigration (neutrophils, monocytes, lymphocytes)
VCAM-1 (immunoglobulin family)	VLA-4 (β_1) integrin	Adhesion (eosinophils, monocytes, lymphocytes)
CD31 (PECAM)	CD31	Leukocyte migration through endothelium

*L-selectin is expressed weakly on neutrophils. It is involved in the binding of circulating T-lymphocytes to the high endothelial venules in lymph nodes and mucosal lymphoid tissues, and subsequent "homing" of lymphocytes to these tissues.

avidity of the adhesion molecules. These modulating molecules induce leukocyte adhesion in inflammation by three general mechanisms:

- *Redistribution of preformed adhesion molecules to the cell surface.* After histamine exposure, P-selectin is rapidly translocated from the endothelial Weibel-Palade body membranes to the cell surface, where it can bind leukocytes.
- *Induction of adhesion molecules on endothelium.* Interleukin-1 (IL-1) and tumor necrosis factor (TNF) increase endothelial expression of E-selectin, ICAM-1, and VCAM-1; such *activated* endothelial cells have increased leukocyte adherence.
- *Increased avidity of binding.* This is most important for *integrin* binding. Integrins are normally present on leukocytes in a low-affinity form; they are converted to high-affinity forms by a variety of chemokines. Such activation causes firm adhesion of the leukocytes to the endothelium and is required for subsequent transmigration.

Leukocyte Migration through Endothelium (p. 50)

Transmigration (also called *diapedesis*) is mediated by homotypic (like-like) interactions between platelet-endothelial cell adhesion molecule-1 = CD31 (PECAM-1) on leukocytes and endothelial cells. Once across the endothelium and into the underlying connective tissue, leukocytes adhere to the extracellular matrix via integrin binding to CD44.

Chemotaxis of Leukocytes (p. 50)

After emigrating through interendothelial junctions and traversing the basement membrane, leukocytes move toward sites of injury along gradients of chemotactic agents *(chemotaxis)*. For neutrophils, these agents include exogenous bacterial products and endogenous mediators (detailed later), such as complement fragments, arachidonic acid metabolites, and chemokines.

Chemotaxis involves binding of chemotactic agents to specific leukocyte surface G protein–coupled receptors; these trigger the production of phosphoinositol second messengers, in turn causing increased cytosolic calcium and guanosine triphosphatase (GTPase) activities that polymerize actin and facilitate cell movement. Leukocytes move by extending pseudopods that bind the extracellular matrix and then pull the cell forward (front-wheel drive).

Recognition of Microbes and Dead Tissues (p. 51)

Having arrived at the appropriate site, leukocytes distinguish offending agents and then destroy them. To accomplish this, inflammatory cells express a variety of receptors that recognize pathogenic stimuli, and deliver activating signals (Fig. 2-2).

* *Receptors for microbial products:* These include *toll-like receptors (TLRs),* one of 10 different mammalian proteins that recognize distinct components in different classes of microbial pathogens. Thus, some TLRs participate in cellular responses to bacterial lipopolysaccharide (LPS) or unmethylated CpG nucleotide fragments, whereas others respond to double-stranded RNA made by some viral infections. TLRs can be on the cell surface or within endosomal vesicles depending on the likely location of the pathogen (extracellular versus ingested). They function through receptor-associated kinases that in turn induce production of cytokines and microbicidal substances.
* *G protein–coupled receptors:* These receptors typically recognize bacterial peptides containing *N-formyl methionine* residues, or they are stimulated by the binding of various chemokines (see preceding discussion), complement fragments, or arachidonic acid metabolites (e.g., prostaglandins and leukotrienes). Ligand binding triggers migration and production of microbicidal substances.
* *Receptors for opsonins:* Molecules that bind to microbes and render them more "attractive" for ingestion are called *opsonins;* these include antibodies, complement fragments, and certain lectins (sugar-binding proteins). Binding of opsonized (coated) particles to their leukocyte receptor leads to cell activation and phagocytosis (see later).
* *Cytokine receptors:* Inflammatory mediators (cytokines) bind to cell surface receptors and induce cellular activation. One of the most important is interferon-γ, produced by activated T cells and natural killer cells, and the major macrophage-activating cytokine.

Removal of the Offending Agents (p. 52)

Recognition through any of the preceding receptors induces *leukocyte activation* (see Fig. 2-2). The most essential functional consequences of activation are enhanced phagocytosis and intracellular killing, although the release of cytokines, growth factors, and inflammatory mediators (e.g., prostaglandins) is also important.

Phagocytosis (p. 52)

Phagocytosis begins with leukocyte binding to the microbe; this is facilitated by opsonins, the most important being the immunoglobulin Fc fragment and the complement fragment C3b. Macrophage integrins, and the *macrophage mannose* and *scavenger receptors* (mannose is expressed as a terminal sugar on many microbes), are also important recognition proteins for phagocytosis.

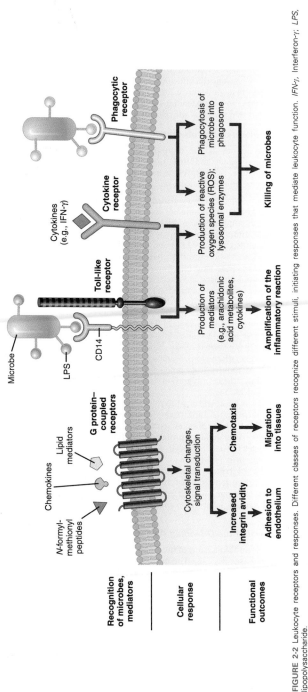

FIGURE 2-2 Leukocyte receptors and responses. Different classes of receptors recognize different stimuli, initiating responses that mediate leukocyte function. *IFN-γ*, Interferon-γ; *LPS*, lipopolysaccharide.

Engulfment (p. 53)

After binding to receptors, cytoplasmic pseudopods enclose the particle and eventually pinch off to make a *phagosome* vesicle. Subsequent fusion of phagosomes and lysosomes (forming a *phagolysosome*) discharges lysosomal contents into the space around the microbe but can also occasionally dump lysosomal granules into the extracellular space.

Killing and Degradation (p. 53)

Killing of phagocytosed particles is most efficient in activated leukocytes, and is accomplished largely by *reactive oxygen species (ROS)*. Phagocytosis stimulates an *oxidative burst*—a surge of oxygen consumption with production of reactive oxygen metabolites through activation of nicotinamide-adenine dinucleotide phosphate (NADPH) oxidase. The enzyme converts oxygen to superoxide anion ($O_2^{\bar{}}$), eventually resulting in hydrogen peroxide (H_2O_2). Lysosomal *myeloperoxidase (MPO)* then converts H_2O_2 and Cl^- into the highly bactericidal HOCl (hypochlorite—the active ingredient in bleach). Although the MPO system is the most efficient mechanism, other reactive oxygen species of the oxidative burst can also kill bacteria. Notably *reactive nitrogen species* such as peroxynitrite radical ($ONOO^{\bullet}$) derived from nitric oxide (NO) and superoxide are also highly microbicidal.

Microbial killing can also occur via oxygen-independent molecules found in leukocyte granules. These largely work by increasing membrane permeability and include *bactericidal permeability increasing protein, cathelicidins, lysozyme, lactoferrin, major basic protein of eosinophils*, and *defensins*.

Release of Leukocyte Products and Leukocyte-Mediated Tissue Injury (p. 54)

During activation and phagocytosis, leukocytes release products not only within the phagolysosome but also potentially into the extracellular space, where they can cause tissue injury. This may occur:

- As part of the normal response to a pathogen; such "collateral damage" may cause more pathology than the original infection
- Directed inappropriately against host tissues (*autoimmune disease;* Chapter 6)
- As an over-exuberant response against usually harmless substances (e.g., in *allergic reactions*)

The mechanisms underlying the damage inflicted are the same as those involved in anti-microbial defense. The most relevant mediators include:

- *Lysosomal enzymes*, regurgitated during *frustrated phagocytosis* (large indigestible materials), premature fusion of lysosomes with forming phagosomes, or when lysosomes are damaged by ingested material (e.g., urate crystals)
- Oxygen- and nitrogen-derived reactive metabolites

Defects in Leukocyte Function (p. 55)

Defects in leukocyte function (at any stage from endothelial adherence to microbicidal activity) interfere with inflammation and dramatically increase infection susceptibility. Defects, either genetic or acquired, include:

- *Genetic deficiencies in adhesion molecules: Leukocyte adhesion deficiency type I* is due to defective synthesis of β_2 integrins (LFA-1 and Mac-1); *type II deficiency* is due to a defect in fucose metabolism causing loss of sialyl-Lewis X (ligand for E- and P-selectin).

- *Genetic defects in phagolysosome formation:* In *Chédiak-Higashi syndrome,* neutrophils have aberrant organellar fusion with defective lysosomal enzyme delivery to phagosomes.
- *Genetic defects in microbicidal activity:* In *chronic granulomatous disease,* there are inherited defects in NADPH oxidase, leading to a defect in the respiratory burst, superoxide and H_2O_2 production, and the MPO bactericidal mechanism.
- *Acquired deficiencies of neutrophils:* Called *neutropenia,* this is the most common clinical cause of leukocyte defects; it may be caused by cancer chemotherapy or by metastatic tumor replacing normal bone marrow.

Termination of the Acute Inflammatory Response (p. 56)

Inflammation declines, in part, because mediators are produced only transiently and typically have short half-lives; however, because of its inherent capacity to damage tissues, inflammation must also be tightly and actively regulated. Thus, even as inflammation is developing, stop signals are also being triggered. These include a switch from pro-inflammatory arachidonate metabolites *(leukotrienes)* to anti-inflammatory forms *(lipoxins,* described later), production of anti-inflammatory cytokines such as transforming growth factor-β (TGF-β) and interleukin-10 (IL-10), synthesis of fatty acid–derived anti-inflammatory mediators *(resolvins and protectins),* and neural impulses that inhibit macrophage TNF production.

Mediators of Inflammation (p. 56)

- The vascular and cellular events of inflammation are mediated by numerous molecules derived either from plasma or from cells (Table 2-2). Plasma-derived mediators are typically synthesized in the liver and circulate as inactive precursors that are activated by proteolysis. Cell-derived mediators are either preformed and released by granule exocytosis (leading to immediate activity) or synthesized *de novo* following a stimulus (with some intrinsic lag time).
- Mediators are produced in response to either microbial products or factors released by necrotic tissues, thus insuring that inflammation is normally triggered only when and where it is required.
- Most mediators act by binding to specific receptors, although some have direct enzymatic activity (e.g., proteases) or mediate oxidative damage (e.g., ROS).
- Mediators can act in amplifying or regulatory cascades to stimulate the release of other downstream factors.
- Once generated, most mediators are short-lived, being degraded by enzymes, subdued by specific inhibitors, scavenged by antioxidants, or just decaying spontaneously.

Cell-Derived Mediators

Vasoactive Amines: Histamine and Serotonin (p. 57)

Released from preformed cellular stores, these are among the first mediators in inflammation. *They cause arteriolar dilation and increased permeability of venules.*

Mast cells are the major source of histamine, though basophils and platelets also contribute. Mast cell release is caused by physical

TABLE 2-2 The Actions of the Principal Mediators of Inflammation

Mediator	Principal Sources	Actions
Cell-Derived		
Histamine	Mast cells, basophils, platelets	Vasodilation, increased vascular permeability, endothelial activation
Serotonin	Platelets	Vasodilation, increased vascular permeability
Prostaglandins	Mast cells, leukocytes	Vasodilation, pain, fever
Leukotrienes	Mast cells, leukocytes	Increased vascular permeability, chemotaxis, leukocyte adhesion and activation
Platelet-activating factor	Leukocytes, mast cells	Vasodilation, increased vascular permeability, leukocyte adhesion, chemotaxis, degranulation, oxidative burst
Reactive oxygen species	Leukocytes	Killing of microbes, tissue damage
Nitric oxide	Endothelium, macrophages	Vascular smooth muscle relaxation, killing of microbes
Cytokines (TNF, IL-1)	Macrophages, endothelial cells, mast cells	Local endothelial activation (expression of adhesion molecules), fever/pain/anorexia/hypotension, decreased vascular resistance (shock)
Chemokines	Leukocytes, activated macrophages	Chemotaxis, leukocyte activation
Plasma Protein-Derived		
Complement products (C5a, C3a, C4a)	Plasma (produced in liver)	Leukocyte chemotaxis and activation, vasodilation (mast cell stimulation)
Kinins	Plasma (produced in liver)	Increased vascular permeability, smooth muscle contraction, vasodilation, pain
Protease activated during coagulation	Plasma (produced in liver)	Endothelial activation, leukocyte recruitment

IL-1, Interleukin-1; *MAC,* membrane attack complex; *TNF,* tumor necrosis factor.

agents (e.g., trauma, heat), allergic immune reactions involving IgE (Chapter 6), complement fragments C3a and C5a (*anaphylatoxins*), cytokines (e.g., IL-1 and IL-8), neuropeptides (e.g., *substance P*), and leukocyte-derived histamine-releasing factors.

Serotonin (5-hydroxytryptamine) has activities similar to histamine; major sources are platelets and neuroendocrine cells (not mast cells). Platelet release of both histamine and serotonin is stimulated by contact with collagen, thrombin, adenosine diphosphate (ADP), and antigen-antibody complexes, one of several links between clotting and inflammation.

Arachidonic Acid Metabolites: Prostaglandins, Leukotrienes, and Lipoxins (p. 58)

Activated cells release membrane-bound arachidonic acid (AA) through the enzymatic activity of phospholipase A_2. The 20-carbon polyunsaturated AA is then catabolized to generate short-range lipid mediators *(eicosanoids)* through the activities of two major enzyme classes (Fig. 2-3). Eicosanoids bind to membrane G protein–coupled receptors and can mediate almost every aspect of inflammation (Table 2-3):

- Cyclooxygenases (COX-1 is constitutively expressed; COX-2 is inducible) generate *prostaglandins* and *thromboxanes.* These enzymes are irreversibly inhibited by aspirin and reversibly inhibited by other non-steroidal anti-inflammatory drugs (NSAIDs). Corticosteroid anti-inflammatory effects include blockade of the transcription of phospholipase A_2 and COX-2.
- Lipoxygenases produce *leukotrienes* (pro-inflammatory mediators) and *lipoxins* (anti-inflammatory mediators). *Cell-cell interactions* are important in both leukotriene and lipoxin biosynthesis. AA products can diffuse from one cell to another, thereby allowing cells unable to otherwise synthesize specific eicosanoids to produce them from intermediates generated in other cells. Compounds that block 5-lipoxygenase activity have anti-inflammatory activity.

Platelet-Activating Factor (p. 60)

Platelet-activating factor (PAF) is a phospholipid-derived mediator produced by mast cells, platelets, leukocytes, and endothelium. Besides platelet aggregation and granule release (hence its name), PAF can elicit most of the vascular and cellular reactions of inflammation: vasodilation and increased vascular permeability (i.e., 100 to 10,000 times more potent than histamine), bronchoconstriction, increased leukocyte adhesion, chemotaxis, and the oxidative burst.

Reactive Oxygen Species (p. 60)

Oxygen-derived free radicals (including O_2^-, H_2O_2, and hydroxyl radical) are released extracellularly from leukocytes after phagocytosis and after exposure to chemokines, immune complexes, or microbial products. ROS can also combine with NO to form other reactive nitrogen intermediates. ROS effects include:

- Endothelial cell damage causing increased vascular permeability
- Injury to multiple cell types (e.g., tumor cells, red cells, parenchymal cells)
- Inactivation of anti-proteases (e.g., α_1-anti-trypsin), resulting in unopposed protease activity

Tissues are normally protected from the damaging effects of ROS by multiple pathways (Chapter 1), including serum proteins that scavenge free radicals (e.g., ceruloplasmin and transferrin) and enzymes that degrade them (e.g., superoxide dismutase, catalase, and glutathione peroxidase). The net effect of ROS on tissues depends on the balance between production and inactivation.

Nitric Oxide (p. 60)

Originally characterized as an endothelial-derived factor that caused vascular dilation by relaxing smooth muscle, NO is increasingly appreciated as an inhibitor of cellular inflammatory responses.

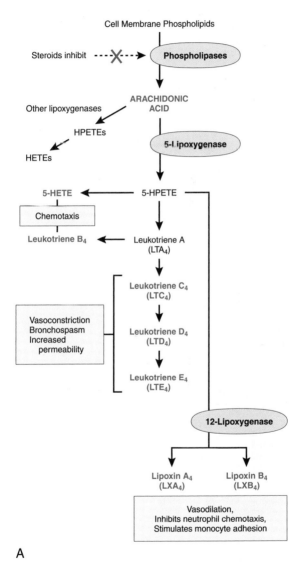

A

FIGURE 2-3 Generation of arachidonic acid metabolites and their roles in inflammation. The molecular targets of action of some anti-inflammatory drugs are indicated by an X. **A**, Lipoxygenase pathways. **B**, Cyclooxygenase pathways. *COX*, Cyclooxygenase; *HETE*, hydroxyeicosatetraenoic acid; *HPETE*, hydroperoxyeicosatetraenoic acid.

Continued

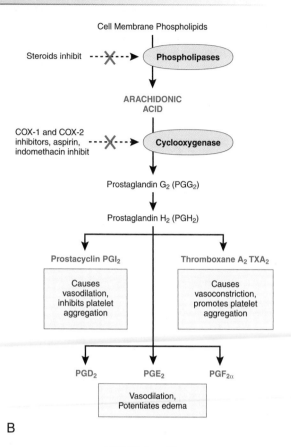

FIGURE 2-3, cont'd

TABLE 2-3 Principal Inflammatory Actions of Arachidonic Acid Metabolites (Eicosanoids)	
Action	**Eicosanoid**
Vasodilation	PGI$_2$ (prostacyclin), PGE$_1$, PGE$_2$, PGD$_2$
Vasoconstriction	Thromboxane A$_2$, leukotrienes C$_4$, D$_4$, E$_4$
Increased vascular permeability	Leukotrienes C$_4$, D$_4$, E$_4$
Chemotaxis, leukocyte adhesion	Leukotriene B$_4$, HETE

HETE, Hydroxyeicosatetraenoic acid; *PGI$_2$,* prostaglandin I$_2$.

- NO regulates inflammatory responses by inhibiting platelet aggregation and adhesion, inhibiting leukocyte recruitment, and blocking some features of mast cell-mediated inflammation.
- NO and its free radical derivatives are microbicidal and can also kill tumor cells.

NO is synthesized from arginine, molecular oxygen, NADPH, and other cofactors by *nitric oxide synthase (NOS)*. Three types of NOS—endothelial (eNOS), neuronal (nNOS), and cytokine inducible (iNOS)—exist, each with distinct expression patterns: (1) eNOS and nNOS are constitutively expressed but are activated only after increased cytoplasmic calcium and (2) iNOS is synthesized by macrophages after exposure to certain cytokines (e.g., IFN-γ).

Cytokines and Chemokines (p. 61) (See Chapter 6)

Cytokines are proteins produced principally by activated lymphocytes and macrophages (but also endothelium, epithelium, and connective tissue cells) that modulate the function of other cell types. *Chemokines* are cytokines that also stimulate leukocyte movement (chemotaxis).

Tumor Necrosis Factor and Interleukin-1 (p. 61)

Produced primarily by activated macrophages, these are two of the most important cytokines mediating inflammation. They affect endothelium, leukocyte, and fibroblast activation, as well as induce systemic responses (Fig. 2-4).

- Secretion is stimulated by endotoxin, immune complexes, toxins, physical injury, and a variety of inflammatory products.
- Endothelial activation increases the expression of adhesion molecules and chemical mediators (e.g., cytokines, chemokines, growth factors, eicosanoids, and NO), enzymes associated with matrix remodeling, and endothelial thrombogenicity.
- IL-1 and TNF induce systemic *acute-phase responses* associated with infection or injury including fever, anorexia, lethargy, neutrophilia, and release of corticotropin and corticosteroids.
- TNF also *regulates body mass* by promoting lipid and protein mobilization and by suppressing appetite. Sustained elevations in TNF (e.g., due to neoplasm or chronic infections) thus contribute to *cachexia*, a pathologic state characterized by weight loss and anorexia.
- IL-1 production is controlled by a multi-protein, intracellular complex dubbed the *inflammasome;* it is responsive to various microbial and necrotic cell triggers. Inflammasomes activate caspase family members to cleave inactive IL-1 precursors into the biologically active cytokine. Mutations in the inflammasome complex lead to constitutive caspase activation and thus unregulated IL-1 production; diseases associated with such mutations are called *inherited autoinflammatory syndromes* (e.g., *familial Mediterranean fever*). Affected individuals have fever and inflammatory symptoms without overt provocation, and they may also develop *amyloidosis* (Chapter 6) due to chronic inflammation. Urate acid crystals may also directly activate the inflammasome pathway, leading to the inflammation associated with *gout* (Chapter 26).

Chemokines (p. 62)

Chemokines are a family ($\sim$40 known) of small proteins expressed by multiple cell types that act primarily as leukocyte chemoattractants and activators. Chemokines are classified into four major classes, according to the arrangement of conserved cysteine (C) residues:

- *CXC chemokines* have one amino acid residue separating the first two conserved cysteine residues; their major activity involves neutrophil recruitment. IL-8 is typical of this group; it is produced by macrophages and endothelial cells after activation by TNF and IL-1 or microbial products.

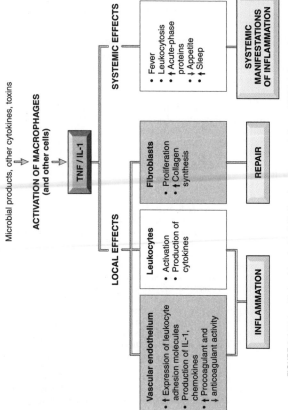

FIGURE 2-4 Major effects of interleukin-1 *(IL-1)* and tumor necrosis factor *(TNF)* in inflammation.

- *CC chemokines* have the first two conserved cysteine residues adjacent. CC chemokines (e.g., *monocyte chemoattractant protein-1*) generally recruit monocytes, eosinophils, basophils, and lymphocytes but not neutrophils. Although many chemokines in this class have overlapping properties, *eotaxin* selectively recruits eosinophils.
- *C chemokines* lack two of the four conserved cysteines; these are relatively specific for lymphocytes (e.g., *lymphotactin*).
- The only known *CX$_3$C chemokine* is *fractalkine*. It exists in two forms: an endothelial surface-bound protein (promotes firm mononuclear cell adhesion) or a soluble form—derived by proteolysis of the membrane-bound form (chemoattractant for mononuclear cells).

Chemokines mediate their activities by binding to G protein-linked receptors (~20 known), designated CXCR for the CXC chemokines, and CCR for the CC chemokines. Cells typically express more than one receptor type. There is also receptor-ligand "promiscuity"; thus, many different chemokine ligands can bind to the same receptor, and multiple receptors can frequently bind the same ligand.

Other Cytokines in Acute Inflammation (p. 63)

The list is long and growing; however, two of note are:

- IL-6: made by macrophages (mostly) and involved in multiple local and systemic inflammatory responses (e.g., acute phase responses)
- IL-17: made by T lymphocytes and involved in neutrophil recruitment

Lysosomal Constituents of Leukocytes (p. 63)

Release of lysosome granule content by neutrophils and monocytes contributes to the inflammatory response as well as to tissue injury.

- *Neutrophils* have two types of granules; smaller *specific (or secondary) granules* contain lysozyme, collagenase, gelatinase, lactoferrin, plasminogen activator, and histaminase; larger *azurophil (or primary) granules* contain myeloperoxidase, bactericidal factors (lysozyme, defensins), acid hydrolases, and a variety of neutral proteases (elastase, cathepsin G, collagenases).
- Specific and azurophil granules can prematurely empty into phagocytic vacuoles not yet completely surrounding engulfed material; alternatively, the contents can be directly secreted extracellularly or released after cell death. Acid proteases normally degrade proteins, bacteria, and debris only within the acidic phagolysosome, whereas neutral proteases can degrade extracellular components at neutral pH. Monocytes and macrophages also contain hydrolases (collagenase, elastase, phospholipase, and plasminogen activator) that are particularly important in chronic inflammatory reactions.
- The potentially harmful effects of proteases are modulated by multiple serum and tissue *antiproteases* (e.g., α_1-anti-trypsin inhibits neutrophil elastase), and inhibitor deficiencies can result in disease (e.g., α_1-anti-trypsin deficiency, Chapter 15).

Neuropeptides (p. 63)

Neuropeptides secreted by sensory nerves and leukocytes can initiate and propagate inflammatory responses. *Substance P,* for example, is a powerful mediator of vascular permeability, transmits pain signals, regulates blood pressure, and stimulates immune and endocrine cell secretion.

Plasma Protein–Derived Mediators (p. 63)

Three interrelated plasma-derived mediators play key roles in inflammation: complement, kinin, and clotting systems.

Complement System (p. 63) (Fig. 2-5)

- The complement system comprises more than 20 proteins; the most important are numbered C1 through C9. Synthesized by the liver, they circulate in plasma as inactive precursors that are activated by proteolysis. Activated complement fragments are themselves proteases that cleave other complement proteins in an amplifying cascade.
- The most important step for complement's biological activities is activation of the C3 component. C3 cleavage can occur through three possible mechanisms: the *classical pathway* triggered by C1 binding to antigen-antibody complexes; the *alternative pathway,* triggered—in the absence of antibody—by microbial surface molecules (e.g., endotoxin), complex polysaccharides, or cobra venom; and the *lectin pathway,* where C1 is activated by microbe carbohydrates interacting with circulating mannose-binding lectins.
- C3 cleavage results in functionally distinct fragments, C3a and C3b. C3a is released while C3b becomes covalently attached to the site where complement is being activated. C3b and other complement fragments combine to cleave C5 into C5a and C5b pieces.
- The biologic functions of complement fall into three general categories: *cell lysis, inflammation,* and *opsonization.*

  Cell lysis: C5b binds the late components (C6-C9), culminating in the formation of the *membrane attack complex (MAC,* composed of multiple C9 molecules). The MAC punches holes in cell membranes.
  Inflammation:
  - C3a and C5a (so-called *anaphylatoxins*) stimulate histamine release from mast cells and thereby increase vascular permeability and vasodilation.
  - C5a activates the arachidonate metabolism, causing additional inflammatory mediator release.
  - C5a is a powerful leukocyte chemoattractant.

  Opsonization: Binding of C3b—or its "inactive" degradation product iC3b—promotes phagocytosis by neutrophils and macrophages through specific C3b receptors.

- Complement activation is tightly regulated by cell-associated and circulating proteins that either stifle complement activation or remove activated fragments from cell walls.

Coagulation and Kinin System (p. 64)

Inflammation and blood clotting pathways are functionally interlinked (Fig. 2-6). The clotting system is divided into two interrelated systems—the *intrinsic* and *extrinsic pathways*—that converge to activate *thrombin* and ultimately form *fibrin* clots (detailed in Chapter 4). The intrinsic pathway, in particular, is a cascade of plasma proenzymes that can be set into motion by the proteolytic activity of activated *factor XII* (also called *Hageman factor).*

- Inflammation promotes clotting by increasing local and systemic production of several coagulation factors, making endothelium more pro-coagulant, and reducing anti-coagulant regulatory mechanisms.
- Thrombin promotes inflammation by binding to *protease-activated receptors (PARs),* G protein–coupled receptors present on platelets,

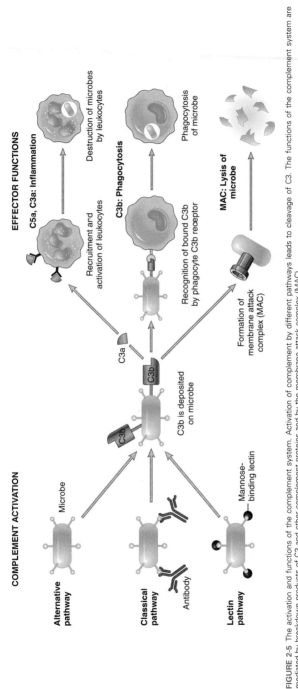

FIGURE 2-5 The activation and functions of the complement system. Activation of complement by different pathways leads to cleavage of C3. The functions of the complement system are mediated by breakdown products of C3 and other complement proteins and by the membrane attack complex (MAC).

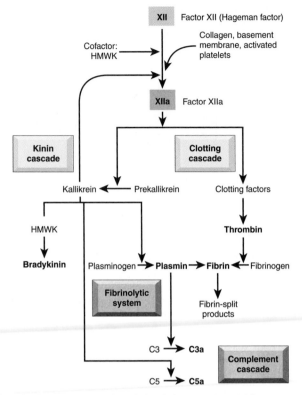

FIGURE 2-6 Interrelationships of the clotting cascade and inflammatory mediators. As shown, activated Factor XII (Hageman factor) is upstream of these pathways, but there are autocatalytic loops involving, for example, kallikrein (shown) and plasmin (not shown). Note that thrombin induces inflammation by binding to protease-activated receptors (PAR-1, in particular). *HMWK,* High-molecular-weight kininogen.

endothelium, and smooth muscle cells. PAR-1 engagement mobilizes P-selectin, induces cytokine and chemokine production; augments endothelial cell adhesion molecule expression; and increases synthesis of PAF, NO, and prostaglandins.

- *Activated factor XII* (called *XIIa*) also cleaves plasma *prekallikrein* to form the active enzyme *kallikrein*. Kallikrein, in turn, converts circulating *high-molecular-weight kininogen (HMWK)* into *bradykinin*, a peptide that causes blood vessel dilation, increased vascular permeability, and pain. Kallikrein is also a potent activator of factor XII (forming an autocatalytic loop), has direct chemotactic activity, and converts C5 to the chemoattractant C5a.
- Besides inducing the coagulation cascade, factor XIIa also activates the fibrinolytic system, thereby limiting the total clot size. In particular, kallikrein cleaves plasminogen to form *plasmin*, which degrades fibrin clots. Plasmin contributes to inflammation by cleaving C3 to produce C3 fragments, by forming *fibrin split* products that increase vascular permeability, and by activating factor XII (another autocatalytic loop).

TABLE 2-4   Role of Mediators in Different Reactions of Inflammation

Role in Inflammation	Mediators
Vasodilation	Prostaglandins Nitric oxide Histamine
Increased vascular permeability	Histamine and serotonin C3a and C5a (by liberating vasoactive amines from mast cells, other cells) Bradykinin Leukotrienes C_4, D_4, E_4 PAF Substance P
Chemotaxis, leukocyte recruitment and activation	TNF, IL-1 Chemokines C3a, C5a Leukotriene B_4 (Bacterial products, e.g., N formyl methyl peptides)
Fever	IL-1, TNF Prostaglandins
Pain	Prostaglandins Bradykinin
Tissue damage	Lysosomal enzymes of leukocytes Reactive oxygen species Nitric oxide

IL-1, Interleukin-1; *PAF,* platelet-activating factor; *TNF,* tumor necrosis factor.

Although there are a plethora of inflammatory mediators, a relative few may be most relevant clinically (Table 2-4).

Outcomes of Acute Inflammation (p. 66)

Acute inflammation will be affected by the nature and intensity of injury, the tissue involved and by host responsiveness; the process has one of three general outcomes:

- *Complete resolution* occurs with regeneration of native cells and restoration to normalcy
- *Healing by connective tissue replacement (fibrosis)* occurs after substantial tissue destruction, when inflammation occurs in non-regenerating tissues, or in the setting of abundant *fibrin exudation* (also called *organization*).
- *Progresses to chronic inflammation,* outlined in greater detail later.

Morphologic Patterns of Acute Inflammation (p. 66)

Although all acute inflammatory reactions are characterized by vascular changes and leukocyte infiltration, distinctive morphologic changes can be superimposed that suggest a specific underlying cause.

Serous Inflammation (p. 67)

Serous inflammation is marked by fluid transudates reflecting moderately increased vascular permeability. Such accumulations in the peritoneal, pleural, and pericardial cavities are called *effusions;* serous fluid can also accumulate elsewhere (e.g., burn blisters in skin).

Fibrinous Inflammation (p. 67)

Fibrinous inflammation is a more marked increase in vascular permeability, with exudates containing large amounts of fibrinogen. The fibrinogen is converted to fibrin through coagulation system activation. Involvement of serosal surfaces (e.g., pericardium or pleura) is referred to as *fibrinous pericarditis* or *pleuritis.* Fibrinous exudates can be resolved by fibrinolysis and macrophage clearance of debris. Larger exudates that cannot be cleared will be converted to fibrous scar *(organization)* by the ingrowth of vessels and fibroblasts.

Suppurative or Purulent Inflammation; Abscess (p. 68)

This pattern is characterized by purulent exudates *(pus)* consisting of neutrophils, necrotic cells, and edema. An *abscess* is a localized collection of purulent inflammation accompanied by liquefactive necrosis, often in the setting of bacterial seeding. With time, these may be walled off and then organized into fibrous scar.

Ulcers (p. 68)

Ulcers are local erosions of epithelial surfaces produced by sloughing of inflamed necrotic tissue (e.g., gastric ulcers).

Summary of Acute Inflammation (p. 68)

When encountering an injurious agent (e.g., microbe or dead cells), phagocytes attempt to eliminate these agents and secrete cytokines, eicosanoids, and other mediators. These mediators, in turn, act on vascular wall cells to induce vasodilation and on endothelial cells specifically to promote plasma efflux and further leukocyte recruitment. Recruited leukocytes are activated and will phagocytize offending agents, as well as produce additional mediators. As the injurious agent is eliminated, anti-inflammatory counterregulatory mechanisms quench the process, and the host returns to a normal state of health. If the injurious agent cannot be effectively eliminated, the result may be chronic inflammation.

Chronic Inflammation (p. 70)

Chronic inflammation is a prolonged process (i.e., weeks or months) in which active inflammation, tissue destruction, and healing all proceed simultaneously. It occurs:

• Following acute inflammation, as part of the normal healing process
• Due to persistence of an inciting stimulus or repeated bouts of acute inflammation
• As a low-grade, smoldering response *without* prior acute inflammation

Causes of Chronic Inflammation (p. 70)

• Persistent infection by intracellular microbes (e.g., tubercle bacilli, viruses) of low direct toxicity but nevertheless capable of evoking immunologic responses
• Immune reactions, particularly those against one's own tissues (e.g., autoimmune diseases), or abnormally regulated responses to normal host flora (inflammatory bowel disease) or benign environmental substances (allergy) (Chapter 6)

- Prolonged exposure to potentially toxic exogenous substances (e.g., silica, causing pulmonary silicosis) or endogenous substances (e.g., lipids, causing atherosclerosis)

Morphologic Features (p.70)

In contrast to acute inflammation—characterized by vascular changes, edema, and neutrophilic infiltration—chronic inflammation is typified by:

- *Infiltration with mononuclear inflammatory cells*, including macrophages, lymphocytes, and plasma cells
- *Tissue destruction,* induced by persistent injury and/or inflammation
- Attempts at *healing by connective tissue replacement*, accomplished by vascular proliferation *(angiogenesis)* and fibrosis

Role of Macrophages in Chronic Inflammation (p. 71)

Macrophages are the dominant cellular players in chronic inflammation.

- Macrophages derive from circulating monocytes induced to emigrate across the endothelium by chemokines. After reaching the extravascular tissue, monocytes transform into the phagocytic macrophage (Fig. 2-7).
- Macrophages are activated through cytokines produced by immune-activated T cells (especially IFN-γ) or by nonimmune factors (e.g., endotoxin). Depending on the nature of the stimulus (e.g., IFN-γ versus interleukin-4), macrophages produce pro-inflammatory mediators intended to increase their microbicidal capacity, or drive the process of wound repair, through production of mediators that cause fibroblast proliferation, connective tissue production, and angiogenesis (see Fig. 2-7).
- Although macrophage products are important for host defense, some mediators induce tissue damage. These include reactive oxygen and nitric oxide metabolites that are toxic to cells and proteases that degrade extracellular matrix.
- In short-lived inflammation with clearance of the initial stimulus, macrophages relatively quickly die off or exit via lymphatics. In chronic inflammation, macrophage accumulation persists by continued recruitment of monocytes and local proliferation.

Other Cells in Chronic Inflammation (p. 72)

- *Lymphocytes* are mobilized in both antibody- and cell-mediated immune reactions. Lymphocytes and macrophages interact in a bi-directional way—activated macrophages present antigen to T cells and also influence T cell activation through surface molecules and cytokines; in turn, activated T lymphocytes (particularly via IFN-γ) activate macrophages (Chapter 6).
- *Plasma cells* are terminally differentiated B cells that produce antibodies directed against either foreign antigen or altered tissue components.
- *Eosinophils* are characteristic of immune reactions mediated by IgE and in parasitic infections. Eosinophil recruitment depends on *eotaxin,* a CC chemokine. Eosinophils have granules containing *major basic protein (MBP)*, a cationic molecule that is toxic to parasites but also lyses mammalian epithelium (Chapter 6).
- *Mast cells* are widely distributed in connective tissues and participate in both acute and chronic inflammation. They express surface receptors that bind the Fc portion of IgE. In acute reactions, binding of specific antigens to these IgE antibodies leads to mast cell degranulation and mediator release (e.g., histamine). This type of response occurs during anaphylactic reactions to foods,

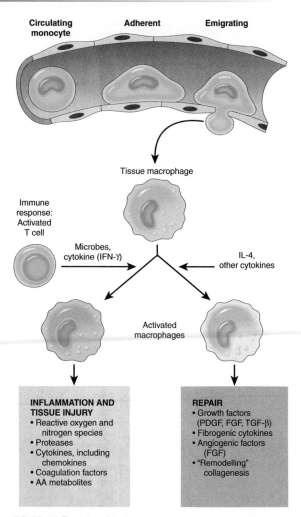

FIGURE 2-7 The roles of activated macrophages in chronic inflammation. Macrophages are activated by cytokines from immune-activated T cells or by nonimmune stimuli such as endotoxin. Depending on the nature of the activating stimuli, macrophages can make products that are microbicidal—but also cause tissue injury or can induce repair pathways that culminate in fibrosis. *AA,* Arachidonic acid; *IL-4,* interleukin-4; *PDGF,* platelet-derived growth factor; *FGF,* fibroblast growth factor; *TGF-β,* transforming growth factor-β.

insect venom, or drugs (Chapter 6). Activated mast cells also secrete a wealth of cytokines that can have either pro- or anti-inflammatory activities.

Granulomatous Inflammation (p. 73)

This distinctive form of chronic inflammation is characterized by focal accumulations of activated macrophages *(granulomas);* macrophage activation is reflected by enlargement and flattening of the cells (so-called *epithelioid* macrophages).

- Nodules of epithelioid macrophages in granulomatous inflammation are surrounded by a collar of lymphocytes elaborating factors necessary to induce macrophage activation. Activated macrophages may fuse to form multi-nucleate *giant cells*, and central necrosis may be present in some granulomas (particularly from infectious causes). Older granulomas can be surrounded by a rim of fibrosis.
- *Foreign body granulomas* are incited by particles that cannot be readily phagocytosed by a single macrophage but do not elicit a specific immune response (e.g., suture or talc).
- *Immune granulomas* are formed by immune T cell–mediated responses to persistent, poorly degradable antigens. IFN-γ from activated T cells causes the macrophage transformation to epithelioid cells and the formation of multinucleate giant cells. The prototypical immune granuloma is caused by the tuberculosis bacillus; in that setting, the granuloma is called a *tubercle* and classically exhibits *central caseous necrosis.*
- *Granulomatous inflammation* is a distinctive inflammatory reaction with relatively few (albeit important) possible causes.

  Infectious etiologies: Tuberculosis, leprosy, syphilis, cat-scratch disease, schistosomiasis, certain fungal infections
  Inflammatory causes: Temporal arteritis, Crohn disease, sarcoidosis
  Inorganic particulates: Silicosis, berylliosis

Systemic Effects of Inflammation (p. 74)

Systemic changes associated with inflammation are collectively called the *acute phase response,* or—in severe cases—the systemic inflammatory response syndrome (SIRS). These represent responses to cytokines produced either by bacterial products (e.g., endotoxin) or by other inflammatory stimuli. The acute phase response consists of several clinical and pathologic changes:

- *Fever* occurring when temperature elevation (i.e., $1°$ to $4°$ C) is produced in response to *pyrogens*, substances that stimulate prostaglandin synthesis in the hypothalamus. For example, endotoxin stimulates leukocyte release of IL-1 and TNF to increase cyclooxygenase production of prostaglandins. In the hypothalamus, PGE_2 stimulates intracellular second signals (e.g., cyclic AMP) that reset the temperature set point. Thus, aspirin reduces fever by inhibiting cyclooxygenase activity to block prostaglandin synthesis.
- *Acute-phase proteins* are plasma proteins, mostly synthesized in the liver, whose synthesis increases several hundred-fold in response to inflammatory stimuli (e.g., cytokines such as IL-6 and TNF). Three of the best-known examples are C-reactive protein (CRP), fibrinogen, and serum amyloid A protein (SAA). CRP and SAA bind to microbial cell walls and may act as opsonins and fix complement. They may also help clear necrotic cell nuclei and mobilize metabolic stores. Elevated fibrinogen leads to increased erythrocyte aggregation, leading to an increased *erythrocyte sedimentation rate* on *ex vivo* testing. *Hepcidin* is another acute phase reactant responsible for regulating release of intracellular iron stores; chronically elevated hepcidin is responsible for the iron-deficiency anemia associated with chronic inflammation (Chapter 14).
- *Leukocytosis* (increased white cell number in peripheral blood) is a common feature of inflammatory reactions. It occurs by accelerated release of bone marrow cells, typically with increased numbers of immature neutrophils in the blood *(shift to the left).* Prolonged infection also induces proliferation of bone marrow

precursors due to increased colony-stimulating factor (CSF) production. The leukocyte count usually climbs to 15,000 to 20,000 cells/μL, but may reach extraordinarily high levels of 40,000 to 100,000 cells/μL (referred to as *leukemoid reactions*). Bacterial infections typically increase neutrophil numbers *(neutrophilia)*; viral infections increase lymphocyte numbers *(lymphocytosis)*; parasitic infestations and allergic disorders are associated with increased eosinophils *(eosinophilia)*.

- *Other manifestations of the acute phase response* include increased pulse and blood pressure; decreased sweating (due to blood flow diverted from cutaneous to deep vascular beds to limit heat loss); rigors (shivering), chills, anorexia, somnolence, and mal-aise, probably due to effects of cytokines on the central nervous system (CNS).
- In severe bacterial infections *(sepsis)*, the large amounts of organisms and endotoxin in the blood stimulate the production of enormous quantities of several cytokines, notably TNF and IL-1. High levels of these cytokines can result in a clinical triad of disseminated intravascular coagulation (DIC), metabolic disturbances, and cardiovascular failure described as *septic shock* (Chapter 4).

Consequences of Defective or Excessive Inflammation (p. 75)

- *Defective inflammation* typically results in increased susceptibility to infections and delayed healing of wounds and tissue damage. Delayed repair occurs because inflammation is essential for clearing damaged tissues and debris, in addition to providing the necessary stimulus to get the repair process started.
- *Excessive inflammation* is the basis of many categories of human disease (e.g., allergies and autoimmune diseases) (Chapter 6). Inflammation also plays a critical role in cancer, atherosclerosis and ischemic heart disease, and some neurodegenerative diseases (e.g., Alzheimer disease). Prolonged inflammation and the accompanying fibrosis also cause pathologic changes in chronic infectious, metabolic, and other diseases.

3

Tissue Renewal, Regeneration, and Repair

Cell and tissue injury sets into motion events that will eliminate the offending agent, contain the damage, and prepare surviving cells for replication. The healing process is broadly separated into *regeneration* and *repair*.

DEFINITIONS

Regeneration implies complete reconstitution. Tissues with high proliferative capacity (e.g., hematopoietic system, gastrointestinal epithelium, etc.) can continuously renew themselves and regenerate after injury, provided their stem cells are not destroyed and provided they have an intact connective tissue scaffolding.

Repair may restore some normal structure, and therefore function, but may also leave some deficits. Healing in this setting involves some combination of regeneration and scar formation *(fibrosis)*. The relative contribution of the two processes depends on the capacity of the injured tissue to regenerate, the extent of injury (i.e., how much matrix is damaged), and the extent of fibrosis driven by the mediators of chronic inflammation.

Control of Normal Cell Proliferation and Tissue Growth (p. 80)

Cell populations in adult tissues are regulated by the relative rates of cell proliferation, differentiation, and apoptotic death.

- Increased cell proliferation can be accomplished by shortening the cell cycle or by recruiting quiescent cells into the cell cycle.
- Increased baseline cell numbers may reflect increased proliferation, decreased cell death, or decreased differentiation.
- Differentiated cells that cannot proliferate are called *terminally differentiated cells*. In some tissues, differentiated cells are not replaced (e.g., cardiac myocytes); in others, they die but are continuously replaced by new cells generated from stem cells (e.g., skin epithelium).
- Cell proliferation can involve physiologic (e.g., hormonal) or pathologic stimuli (e.g., injury, mechanical forces, or cell death).
- Proliferation and differentiation are controlled by soluble and/or contact-mediated signals, and these signals may be stimulatory or inhibitory.

Tissue Proliferative Activity (p. 81)

Tissues are divided into three groups according to their proliferative capacity:

- *Continuously dividing (labile) cells* proliferate throughout life, replacing those that are destroyed (e.g., surface epithelia and marrow hematopoietic cells). Typically, mature cells derive from *stem cells* (see later discussion) with unlimited capacity to proliferate. The progeny of mature cells have the capacity to differentiate into several cell types.
- *Quiescent (stable) cells* are normally involved in low-level replication but are capable of rapid division in response to stimuli (e.g., liver, kidney, fibroblasts, smooth muscle, and endothelial cells).
- *Nondividing (permanent) cells* (e.g., neurons and cardiac myocytes) cannot undergo division in postnatal life. Destruction of such cells typically leads to either glial proliferation (brain) or scar (heart), although limited re-population from a small group of stem cells has been demonstrated. Mature skeletal muscle does not divide but has regenerative capacity through the differentiation of intrinsic *satellite cells.*

Stem Cells (p. 82)

Stem cells are characterized by their *self-renewal capacity* and by their capacity to generate differentiated lineages. This is accomplished by either:

- *Asymmetric replication:* With each cell division, one cell retains self-renewing property while the other enters a differentiation pathway.
- *Stochastic differentiation:* The stem cell pool is maintained by balancing divisions that generate two stem cells with those that create two cells that differentiate.

Embryonic Stem Cells (p. 83)

Isolated from the inner cell mass of normal blastocysts, embryonic stem (ES) cells are *pluripotent*, that is, they have the capacity to generate all cell lineages. These pluripotent cells can give rise to *multipotent stem cells*, which have more restricted developmental potential and eventually produce differentiated cells that form adult tissues. ES cells can be maintained *in vitro* as undifferentiated cell lines or induced to differentiate along a variety of cell lineages, and they have been used as follows:

- ES cells identify signals required for normal tissue differentiation.
- ES cells generate animals congenitally deficient in specific genes *(knockouts)* by inactivating or deleting a gene in an ES cell and then incorporating the modified ES cell into a developing blastocyst. Similarly, replacement of a wild-type gene with a specific mutation *(knock-in)* can be performed. The power of the methodology has been further expanded by the ability to express gene deficiencies in only selected cell or tissue types, and by the ability to turn genes "on" and "off" at will in adult animals *(conditional gene deficiency)*.
- ES cells potentially repopulate damaged organs.

Induced Pluripotent Stem Cells (p. 84)

Functionally similar to ES cells, induced pluripotent stem (iPS) cells have been generated by "reprogramming" adult differentiated cells through transduction of genes encoding ES cell transcription factors. This is to be distinguished from generating pluripotent stem cells from adult differentiated cells by transferring their nucleus to an enucleated oocyte. Such *nuclear transfer techniques* are inefficient, and the resulting stem cells do not have high fidelity for gene expression, probably due to vagaries in histone demethylation in the transferred nuclei. The iPS cells, on the other hand, faithfully generate cells of all three germ layers and can be genetically manipulated. This suggests that they may become a source of patient-specific stem cells that can not only repair damaged tissues but also potentially replace congenitally defective cells.

Adult (Somatic) Stem Cells (p. 84)

Adult (somatic) stem cells have been identified in many mature tissues (e.g., bone marrow, gastrointestinal tract, skin, liver, pancreas, and adipose tissue). Typically they have a more limited capacity to differentiate.

- These cells reside within special *niche* microenvironments (e.g., bulge area of hair follicles) composed of stromal and other cell types that regulate the stem cell self-renewal and progeny generation.
- Somatic stem cells give rise to rapidly proliferating *transit amplifying cells* that lose the capacity for asymmetric division and become *progenitor cells* with a limited developmental potential.
- Somatic stem cells are typically responsible for generating the mature cells of the organ in which they reside, thereby maintaining normal tissue homeostasis; they also have variable potential to differentiate more broadly and to repopulate tissues following injury.
- *Transdifferentiation* is the term applied when a cell differentiates from one type to another; the capacity to transdifferentiate into multiple lineages is called *developmental plasticity*. Thus, hematopoietic stem cells (HSCs) that would normally only contribute to blood cell elements are capable of transdifferentiating *in vitro* into neurons, cardiomyocytes, hepatocytes, and other adult cell lineages.
- The extent that transdifferentiation actually occurs *in vivo* is uncertain, since stem cells can fuse with host cells, transferring genetic material and giving the (false) impression of transdifferentiation. Moreover, HSCs do not apparently contribute significantly to normal tissue homeostasis or to replacement of injured tissues. Instead, their role may be to migrate to sites of injury, where they produce innate immune cells or growth factors to promote healing.

Stem Cells in Tissue Homeostasis (p. 85)

- *Bone marrow* contains pluripotent HSCs capable of regenerating all blood cell elements, as well as multipotential *marrow stromal cells (MSCs)* capable of differentiating into bone, cartilage, fat, muscle, or endothelium, depending on the tissue to which they migrate.
- *Liver* stem cells residing in the canals of Hering (junction between hepatocytes and the biliary system) give rise to bipotent progenitors called *oval cells,* with the capacity to form hepatocytes or biliary epithelium. Liver stem cells are active only if direct hepatocyte proliferation is not possible (e.g., in fulminant hepatic failure).
- The *brain* contains *neural stem cells* capable of generating neurons, astrocytes, and oligodendroglial cells, although the extent to which these are integrated into neural circuits is unclear. They are found in the dentate gyrus of the hippocampus and the subventricular zone.
- *Skin* stem cells occur in the hair follicle bulge (contributing to follicular lineages), the epidermal interfollicular regions (generating

differentiated epidermis with a turnover of 4 weeks), and the sebaceous glands. Bulge stem cells can replenish epidermis after wounding, but they do not participate in normal epidermal homeostasis.

- *Small intestinal crypt epithelium* is monoclonal, deriving from a single stem cell located immediately above the Paneth cells (3 to 5 day turnover); *intestinal villus epithelium* represents differentiated epithelium derived from multiple crypts.
- Regarding the *skeletal and cardiac muscle,* skeletal and cardiac myocytes cannot proliferate. Regeneration of injured skeletal muscle is accomplished by proliferation of *satellite cells,* a stem cell pool in adult muscle. Similar cardiac progenitor cells appear to be present in heart but have limited capacity to contribute to myocardial regeneration (e.g., after infarction).
- *Limbal stem cells in the cornea* (i.e., between the epithelium of the cornea and conjunctiva) maintain the outermost layers of the corneal epithelium.

Cell Cycle and the Regulation of Cell Replication (p. 86)

The details of cell cycle regulation are covered in Chapter 7 within the context of cancer since defects in cell cycle control are important in the pathogenesis of malignancy. A general overview is presented here:

- Cell proliferation is stimulated by a combination of soluble growth factors and extracellular matrix (ECM) signals transmitted via integrins.
- The cell cycle comprises G_1 (pre-synthetic), S (DNA synthesis), G_2 (pre-mitotic), and M (mitotic) phases; quiescent cells are in a physiologic state called G_0 (Fig. 3-1).
- Cells can enter G_1 after completing a round of mitosis (continuously replicating cells), or they can enter from G_0.
- The cell cycle has multiple controls and redundancies, particularly between G_1 and the commitment to synthesize DNA in the S phase. Controls include activators, inhibitors, and sensors of molecular damage or transcriptional accuracy that operate as critical gatekeepers at various checkpoints in the cycle.
- Cell cycle progression is driven by protein phosphorylation events involving *cyclins* and *cyclin-dependent kinases (CDKs)*. Cyclins are regulatory proteins whose concentrations rise and fall during the cell cycle. CDKs are constitutively expressed protein kinases that become active after complexing with specific cyclins. Different combinations of cyclins and CDKs are associated with each of the important transitions in the cell cycle.
- Cyclin-CDK complexes are regulated by catabolism or by binding of *CDK inhibitors*.
- *Checkpoints* provide a *surveillance mechanism* for ensuring that critical transitions in the cell cycle occur in the correct order and that important events are completed with fidelity. For example, the tumor-suppressor gene *p53* is activated in response to DNA damage and inhibits further progression through the cell cycle by increasing expression of a CDK inhibitor.

Growth Factors (p. 87)

A veritable glut of growth factors are known. These are ligands that bind to specific receptors; some bind to multiple cell types, while some bind to a receptor with a very limited cellular distribution. Depending on the target cell, the activities induced by even the same growth factor can be quite different (they are said to be *pleiotropic*).

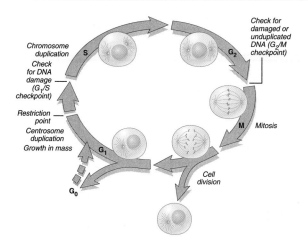

FIGURE 3-1 Shown are the cell cycle phases *(G₀, G₁, S, G₂, and M)*, the *G₁* restriction point, and the *G₁/S* and *G₂/M checkpoints*. In labile tissues (e.g., skin and the gastrointestinal tract) cells can cycle continuously; in stable tissues (e.g., liver) cells are quiescent *(in G₀)* but can enter the cell cycle at *G₁;* permanent, terminally differentiated cells (e.g., neurons and cardiac myocytes) have exited the cell cycle and lost the capacity to regenerate. *(Modified from Pollard TD, Earnshaw WC:* Cell biology, *Philadelphia, WB Saunders, 2002.)*

Besides stimulating proliferation, growth factors can influence cell movement, contractility, differentiation, and angiogenesis. Macrophages, platelets, and mesenchymal cells are typical sources, although epithelium, endothelial cells, mast cells, and T cells can also contribute. Major growth factors in regeneration and wound healing are summarized in Table 3-1:

- *Epidermal growth factor (EGF)* and *transforming growth factor-α (TGF-α)* have extensive homology and exert similar effects; they are mitogenic for fibroblasts, hepatocytes, and a variety of epithelial cells. The *EGF receptor* is actually a family of four different transmembrane proteins each with intrinsic tyrosine kinase activity. *EGFR1* (also called *ERB B1)* is the best characterized; mutations and amplification of this receptor are associated with a number of malignancies. The *ERB B2 receptor* (also called *HER-2* or *Ner2/Neu)*, whose main ligand is not yet identified, is overexpressed in a subset of breast cancers.
- *Hepatocyte growth factor (HGF)* is produced by fibroblasts, endothelial cells, and hepatocytes. In addition, HGF has mitogenic effects on most epithelial cells and promotes embryonic development. HGF is synthesized as an inactive form that is activated by serine proteases released at sites of injury. The HGF receptor (product of the *c-MET* proto-oncogene) is overexpressed in many tumors.
- *Platelet-derived growth factor (PDGF)* is actually a family of dimeric proteins found in platelet α-granules, but it is also made by endothelial cells (ECs), macrophages, and smooth muscle cells. By binding to distinct α- or β-receptors (with different ligand specificity), PDGF causes migration and proliferation of fibroblasts, monocytes, and smooth muscle cells.
- *Vascular endothelial growth factor (VEGF)* is a family of homodimeric proteins that promotes blood vessel formation in early development *(vasculogenesis)* and plays a central role in

TABLE 3-1   Growth Factors and Cytokines Involved in Regeneration and Wound Healing

Growth Factor	Symbol	Functions
Epidermal growth factor	EGF	Mitogenic for keratinocytes and fibroblasts; stimulates keratinocyte migration and granulation tissue formation
Transforming growth factor-α	TGF-α	Similar to EGF; stimulates replication of hepatocytes and most epithelial cells
Heparin binding EGF	HB-EGF	Keratinocyte replication
Hepatocyte growth factor/scatter factor	HGF	Enhances proliferation of hepatocytes, epithelial cells, and endothelial cells; increases cell motility, keratinocyte replication
Vascular endothelial cell growth factor (isoforms A, B, C, D)	VEGF	Increases vascular permeability; mitogenic for endothelial cells; angiogenesis
Platelet-derived growth factor (isoforms A, B, C, D)	PDGF	Chemotactic for PMNs, macrophages, fibroblasts, and smooth muscle cells; activates PMNs, macrophages, and fibroblasts; mitogenic for fibroblasts, endothelial cells, and smooth muscle cells; stimulates production of MMPs, fibronectin, and HA; stimulates angiogenesis and wound contraction
Fibroblast growth factor-1 (acidic),-2 (basic), and family	FGF	Chemotactic for fibroblasts; mitogenic for fibroblasts and keratinocytes; stimulates keratinocyte migration, angiogenesis, wound contraction, and matrix deposition
Transforming growth factor-β (isoforms 1, 2, 3); other members of the family are BMPs and activin	TGF-β	Chemotactic for PMNs, macrophages, lymphocytes, fibroblasts, and smooth muscle cells; stimulates TIMP synthesis, angiogenesis, and fibroplasia; inhibits production of MMPs and keratinocyte proliferation
Keratinocyte growth factor (also called *FGF-7*)	KGF	Stimulates keratinocyte migration, proliferation, and differentiation
Tumor necrosis factor	TNF	Activates macrophages; regulates other cytokines; multiple functions

BMP, Bone morphogenetic proteins; *HA*, hyaluronic acid; *MMPs*, matrix metalloproteinases; *PMNs*, polymorphonuclear leukocytes; *TIMP*, tissue inhibitor of MMP.
Modified from Schwartz SI: *Principles of surgery*, New York, McGraw-Hill, 1999.

new blood vessel growth in adults *(angiogenesis)*; it is particularly important in the angiogenesis associated with chronic inflammatory states, healing wounds, and tumor growth. VEGF members (VEGF-A through D and placental growth factor) bind to receptors with intrinsic tyrosine kinase activity (VEGFR1-3); VEGFR-2 is expressed by ECs and is the main receptor for vasculogenesis/angiogenesis. VEGF-C and -D bind to VEGFR-3 to induce lymphatic endothelial proliferation *(lymphangiogenesis)*.

- *Fibroblast growth factor (FGF)* is a family with more than 20 members; acidic (aFGF) and basic (bFGF) FGF are the best characterized. FGFs are secreted by a wide variety of cells and bind to extracellular matrix heparan sulfate to form reservoirs of inactive factors. Basic FGF, in particular, has the ability to induce all the steps necessary for angiogenesis (see later); FGF members are centrally involved in wound repair, tissue development, and hematopoiesis.

- *Transforming growth factor-β (TGF-β)* belongs to a large family (more than 30) of growth factors with wide-ranging functions. Produced by a variety of cell types (especially macrophages), TGF-β is a dimeric protein secreted in inactive form and activated by proteolysis; it binds cell surface receptors (types I and II) with serine/threonine kinase activity. Ligand binding leads to phosphorylation of cytoplasmic transcription factors called *Smads*. After phosphorylation, the various Smad isoforms complex with Smad 4, allowing entry to the nucleus and activation or inhibition of selected gene transcription. TGF-β is a growth inhibitor for most epithelial cells and has potent anti-inflammatory effects. It also promotes fibrosis by stimulating fibroblast chemotaxis, proliferation, and extracellular matrix synthesis, and by inhibiting collagen degradation.

- *Cytokines* are primarily important as mediators of immune and inflammatory responses (Chapter 6); however, many also have growth-promoting activities.

Signaling Mechanisms in Cell Growth (p. 89)

Growth factor binding to cell surface receptor triggers intracellular signals that induce gene transcription and promote cell cycle entry. The intercellular signaling occurs through three general modes:

- *Autocrine:* Cells respond to signaling substances that they produced themselves. This occurs for liver regeneration, the proliferation of antigen-stimulated lymphocytes, and commonly in tumors.

- *Paracrine:* A cell produces substances that affect target cells in close proximity. This is common in wound repair, inflammatory responses driven by cytokines, embryonic development, and liver regeneration.

- *Endocrine:* Cells synthesize *hormones* that circulate in the blood to act on distant targets. Growth factors and cytokines can also act in an endocrine fashion.

Receptors and Signal Transduction Pathways (p. 89)

The pathways by which ligand and receptor interactions transduce intracellular signals are schematized in Figure 3-2. Simplistically, signaling (i.e., conversion of extracellular stimuli to intracellular events) most commonly occurs by generating cascades of sequential protein kinases that commit entry into the cell cycle.

- *Receptor-ligand interactions:* Receptor-ligand interactions typically induce receptor clustering (usually dimerization) that then transduces a signal; single receptor molecules can also transduce

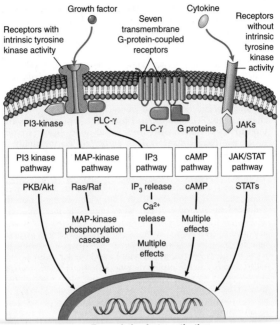

Transcription factor activation

FIGURE 3-2 Examples of signal transduction systems that require cell surface receptors. Shown are receptors with and without intrinsic kinase activity and seven transmembrane G protein–coupled receptors. *cAMP*, Cyclic adenosine monophosphate; *IP$_3$*, inositol triphosphate; *JAK*, Janus kinase; *MAP-kinase*, mitogen activated protein-kinase; *PI3-kinase*, phosphatidyl inositol 3-kinase; *PLC-γ*, phospholipase C-γ; *STAT*, signal transducer and activator of transcription.

signals but usually only after recruitment of secondary cytosolic adapter proteins.

• *Receptors with intrinsic kinase activity:* Most growth factor receptors (e.g., PDGFR, EGFR, and FGFR) have intrinsic tyrosine kinase activities that are activated following ligand binding and dimerization of receptor subunits. The active kinases then phosphorylate downstream effector molecules leading, in turn, to *their* activation. Phosphorylated receptor tyrosines also permit docking and activation of various cytosolic proteins, including those in the Ras signaling pathway, the phosphoinositide-3 (PI-3)–kinase pathway, phospholipase C-γ (PLC-γ) in the protein kinase C pathway, and members of the *Src* family of kinases.

  Activated Ras binds to Raf, which phosphorylates a family of mitogen-activated protein (MAP) kinases.

  The PI-3 pathway activates a series of kinases including Akt, promoting cell survival.

  PLC-γ activation leads to inositol 1,4,5-triphosphate (IP3) production followed by calcium release from endoplasmic reticulum, and diacylglycerol formation with protein kinase C activation (and additional protein phosphorylations).

• *Receptors without intrinsic kinase activity:* These receptors are typical among the cytokine receptors; they associate with and activate cytosolic protein kinases. For example, cytoplasmic Janus kinases (JAKs) link activated receptors with downstream signal transducers and activators of transcription (STAT) that shuttle into the nucleus and activate gene transcription.

- *G protein–coupled receptors:* These receptors (more than 1500 described) all contain seven transmembrane spans; they include the chemokine receptors as well as receptors for epinephrine and glucagon. Ligand binding induces a conformational change that allows activation of G protein complexes to generate intracellular second messengers including $3',5'$-cyclic adenosine monophosphate (cAMP). Activated G protein–coupled receptors can also signal through production of IP_3 and subsequent Ca^{2+} release from intracellular stores.

- *Steroid hormone receptors:* Ligands for these receptors are lipophilic and therefore directly diffuse through plasma membranes; receptors are typically intranuclear transcription factors that are activated by ligand binding.

Transcription Factors (p. 91)

Transcription factors include products of growth-promoting genes (e.g., c-*MYC* and c-*JUN*) as well as cell cycle–inhibiting genes (e.g., *p53*); they have a modular design with separate domains for binding to specific DNA sequence motifs and transcriptional regulation of the gene adjacent to the binding sequence. The end result of most signal transduction is altered gene transcription driven by changes in transcription factor activity. In general, the rapid responses demanded by cell signaling do not permit new synthesis of transcription factors, rather they rely on post-translational modifications that allow transcription factor migration into the nucleus. Modifications include dimerization, phosphorylation, release of constitutively bound inhibitors, or release from membranes by proteolysis.

Mechanisms of Tissue and Organ Regeneration (p. 92)

Amphibians have impressive regenenerative capabilities because quiescent cells (even cardiac myocytes) can readily reenter the cell cycle and because stem cells can efficiently repopulate sites of injury. Unfortunately, mammals lack this capacity; regeneration in damaged tissues is largely compensatory growth through cell hypertrophy and hyperplasia. While this can restore some functional capacity, it does not necessarily reconstitute the original anatomy. The inadequacy of true regeneration in mammals is ascribed to a rapid fibroproliferative response and scar formation after wounding. Although some adult human tissues have impressive restorative capacity (e.g., liver), other organs (e.g., kidney, pancreas, adrenal glands, thyroid, and lungs) are much more limited beyond the first few years of life. In the case of liver, regeneration after partial hepatectomy is in fact only *compensatory hyperplasia*, involving the replication of mature cells throughout the liver without stem cell participation (triggered and synchronized by HGF and IL-6 produced by hepatic non-parenchymal cells). In other organs, even that response is not possible; since adult kidneys cannot produce new nephrons, growth of the remaining kidney after unilateral nephrectomy involves nephron hypertrophy and limited tubular epithelial replication. Regeneration of pancreatic β cells involves limited proliferation of existing β cells, transdifferentiation of pancreatic ductal cells, or stem cell differentiation.

Extracellular Matrix and Cell-Matrix Interactions (p. 94)

ECM consists of:

- *Fibrous structural proteins* (e.g., collagens and elastin) that provide tensile strength and recoil
- *Adhesive glycoproteins* that connect ECM elements to each other and to cells
- A gel of *proteoglycans* and *hyaluronan* that provide resilience and lubrication

These macromolecules either assemble into an *interstitial matrix*, present in the spaces between cells, or into a *basement membrane*, apposed to cell plasma membranes. They provide mechanical support for cell migration and anchorage; act as a depot for growth factors; and maintain cell polarity, cell differentiation, and normal cell growth. Tissue repair depends not only on soluble factors but also on an intact ECM.

Collagen (p. 94)

These ECM elements provide tensile strength. At least 27 types of collagen are known (Table 3-2). A portion of each collagen molecule is composed of a triple helix braid of three polypeptide chains, each with a primary glycine-X-Y repeating sequence (X and Y are any amino acid except cysteine or tryptophan). Types I, II, III, V, and XI are fibrillar collagens (i.e., collagens with long, uninterrupted triple helical domains) and are most abundant. The collagen of skin and bone is mostly type I, while cartilage collagen is mostly type II. Type IV collagen has interrupted triple helices and forms sheets instead of fibrils; it is the major collagen of basement membrane (BM). Type VII forms anchoring fibrils between epithelium and also forms underlying mesenchymal support structures.

Procollagens are synthesized as individual α chains, followed by enzymatic hydroxylation of prolines and lysines. Three chains align to form a triple helix, and the product is secreted. In the extracellular space, the globular C- and N-terminal fragments are proteolytically cleaved, and lysine oxidase (whose enzymatic activity depends on vitamin C) oxidizes lysines and hydroxylysines to permit interchain cross-linking and stabilize the fibrils.

Elastin, Fibrillin, and Elastic Fibers (p. 96)

Elastin provides ECM with elasticity (stretch and recoil). Elastic fibers consist of an *elastin* central core with an associated scaffolding network of fibrillin, a 350-kD glycoprotein. Inherited defects in fibrillin (e.g., in *Marfan syndrome*) result in abnormal elastic fibers and influence the availability of active TGF-β in the ECM.

Cell Adhesion Proteins (p. 96)

For the most part, these proteins are transmembrane receptors. They are classified into four main families: *immunoglobulin family, cadherins, integrins,* and *selectins.*

- Members of all these receptor families can form *cell-cell connections* through homotypic interactions (i.e., same protein on two different cells) or heterotypic interactions (i.e., different proteins on two different cells).
- Cadherins and integrins also connect on their cytoplasmic face to the actin and intermediate filament cytoskeleton, thus mechanically linking cell surface forces to intracellular events.

TABLE 3-2 Main Types of Collagens, Tissue Distribution, and Genetic Disorders

Collagen Type	Tissue Distribution	Genetic Disorders
Fibrillar Collagens		
I	Ubiquitous in hard and soft tissues	Osteogenesis imperfecta Ehlers-Danlos syndrome— arthrochalasias type
II	Cartilage, intervertebral disc, vitreous	Achondrogenesis type II, spondyloepiphyseal dysplasia syndrome
III	Hollow organs, soft tissues	Vascular Ehlers-Danlos syndrome
V	Soft tissues, blood vessels	Classical Ehlers-Danlos syndrome
XI	Cartilage, vitreous	Sticklor syndrome
Basement Membrane Collagens		
IV	Basement membranes	Alport syndrome
Other Collagens		
VI	Ubiquitous in microfibrils	Bethlem myopathy
VII	Anchoring fibrils at dermal-epidermal junctions	Dystrophic epidermolysis bullosa
IX	Cartilage, intervertebral disks	Multiple epiphyseal dysplasias
XVII	Transmembrane collagen in epidermal cells	Benign atrophic generalized epidemolysis bullosa
XV and XVIII	Endostatin-forming collagens, endothelial cells	Knobloch syndrome (type XVIII collagen)

Courtesy of Dr. Peter H. Byers, Department of Pathology, University of Washington, Seattle, WA.

- *Integrins* form *cell-ECM connections* that attach cells to their surrounding matrix by binding to fibronectin and laminin.
- *Fibronectin* binds to many molecules (e.g., collagen, fibrin, proteoglycans, and cell surface receptors). Alternate splicing of fibronectin mRNA produces either tissue fibronectin (i.e., forming fibrillar aggregates at sites of wound healing) or plasma fibronectin (i.e., forming provisional blood clots in wounds preceding ECM deposition).
- *Laminin* is the most abundant glycoprotein in the BM; it has binding domains for both ECM and cell surface receptors.
- Ligand binding to integrins causes them to cluster on the cell surface to form *focal adhesion complexes* that recruit additional proteins and trigger signal transduction cascades including MAP kinase, protein kinase C, and PI3-kinase pathways (many of the same ones used by soluble growth factors in Figure 3-2). There is functional overlap between integrin and growth factor receptor signaling; both transmit environmental cues that the cell integrates to regulate proliferation, apoptosis, or differentiation.
- *Cadherins* (more than 90 types!) mediate calcium-dependent interactions with cadherins on adjacent cells; these form bands

of adhesion between adjacent cells, called *zonula adherens*, as well as spot welds, called *desmosomes*. Cadherins link to the actin cytoskeleton via *catenins*; cadherins bind β-catenins that link to α-catenins that connect to actin. Cell-cell interactions mediated through cadherins, and catenins play major roles in cell motility and differentiation; they also account for the phenomenon of "contact inhibition" of cell proliferation; β-catenin mutations are involved in carcinogenesis (Chapter 7).

- Other significant secreted adhesion molecules are:

    Secreted protein acidic and rich in cysteine (SPARC), also known as *osteonectin*, contributes to tissue remodeling after injury and is an angiogenesis inhibitor.
    Thrombospondins are a family of large multifunctional proteins; some inhibit angiogenesis.
    Osteopontin regulates calcification and mediates leukocyte migration.
    Tenacins are large multimeric proteins involved in morphogenesis and cell adhesion.

Glycosaminoglycans and Proteoglycans (p. 97)

These ECM components (also called *ground substance* or *mucopolysaccharides*) play a major role in regulating connective tissue structure, permeability, and growth factor activity. Glycosaminoglycans (GAGs) are long, repeating polymers of specific disaccharides; with the exception of *hyaluronan (HA),* they are linked to a core protein to form molecules called *proteoglycans*. Proteoglycans can also be integral membrane proteins (e.g., the *syndecans*). *HA* is a huge molecule with many disaccharide repeats; it serves as a ligand for cell surface receptors and other core proteins. HA also binds large amounts of water, thereby giving ECM its turgor and ability to resist compression.

Healing by Repair, Scar Formation, and Fibrosis (p. 98)

Although some tissues can be completely reconstituted after injury (e.g., bone after a fracture, or epithelium after a superficial skin wound), severe tissue injury that results in damage of parenchyma and stromal elements cannot heal by regeneration. In that situation, healing will instead be accomplished through a fibroproliferative response that deposits collagen and other ECM components *(scar)* that "patches" rather than restores a tissue. In most cases, healing is some combination of regeneration and scar; the outcome will be affected by (1) proliferative capacity of the damaged tissue, (2) integrity of the ECM, and (3) the chronicity of the associated inflammation. If damage is ongoing, inflammation becomes chronic, leading to excess ECM deposition called *fibrosis*.

The sequence of healing involves:

- Inflammation to eliminate the initial stimulus and remove injured tissue (Note that the subsequent steps of repair begin early during the inflammatory response and, in fact, are driven by mediators released by the recruited inflammatory cells.)
- Formation of new blood vessels *(angiogenesis)*
- Migration and proliferation of parenchymal and connective tissue cells *(fibroblasts)*
- Synthesis and deposition of ECM proteins *(scar formation)*
- Connective tissue remodeling

The principal factors involved in each step are listed in Table 3-3.

TABLE 3-3	Growth Factors and Cytokines Affecting Various Steps in Wound Healing
Activity in Wound Healing	**Factors Involved**
Monocyte chemotaxis	Chemokines, TNF, PDGF, FGF, TGF-β
Fibroblast migration/replication	PDGF, EGF, FGF, TGF-β, TNF, IL-1
Keratinocyte replication	HB-EGF, FGF-7, HGF
Angiogenesis	VEGF, angiopoietins, FGF
Collagen synthesis	TGF-β, PDGF
Collagenase secretion	PDGF, FGF, TNF; TGF-β inhibits

HB-EGF, Heparin-binding EGF; *IL-1,* interleukin-1; *TNF,* tumor necrosis factor; other abbreviations are given in Table 3-1.

Mechanisms of Angiogenesis (p. 99)

Angiogenesis is critical to wound healing, tumor growth, and the vascularization of ischemic tissues. During embryonic development, vessels arise by *vasculogenesis,* a primitive vascular network assembled from EC precursor *angioblasts.* In adult tissues, vessel formation is called *angiogenesis* (or *neovascularization*); it occurs by branching of preexisting vessels and by recruitment of endothelial precursor cells (EPCs) from bone marrow.

Angiogenesis from Preexisting Vessels (p. 99)

This occurs with vasodilation and increased vascular permeability:

- Nitric oxide dilates preexisting vessels.
- VEGF induces increased permeability.
- Metalloproteinases degrade the BM.
- Plasminogen activator disrupts EC cell-cell contact.
- ECs proliferate and migrate toward the angiogenic stimulus.
- EC maturation occurs, including growth inhibition and remodeling into capillary tubes.
- Periendothelial cells (i.e., pericytes for small capillaries and vascular smooth muscle cells for larger vessels) are recruited.

Angiogenesis from Endothelial Precursor Cells (p. 100)

In embryonic development, a common precursor *hemangioblast* generates both hematopoietic stem cells and angioblasts; the latter proliferate, migrate to peripheral sites, and can differentiate into ECs, pericytes, and vascular smooth muscle cells. Angioblast-like EPCs are also present in adult bone marrow, are increased in number in patients with ischemic conditions, and can initiate angiogenesis. They can replace lost ECs, endothelialize vascular implant, and promote the neovascularization of ischemic organs, cutaneous wounds, and tumors.

Growth Factors and Receptors Involved in Angiogenesis (p. 100)

VEGF is the most important factor, although FGF-2 can also enhance EC proliferation, differentiation, and migration. The VEGFR-2 tyrosine kinase receptor (largely restricted to ECs and EC precursors) is the most important receptor for angiogenesis. VEGF/VEGFR-2 interactions promote:

- EPC mobilization from bone marrow and enhance their proliferation and differentiation at sites of angiogenesis.
- EC proliferation and motility, promoting capillary sprouting.

Proper vascular branching is achieved and excessive angiogenesis is prevented by VEGF damping pathways involving membrane-bound NOTCH pathway ligands and receptors.

Stabilization of new vessels requires the recruitment of pericytes and smooth muscle cells and the deposition of ECM proteins:

- *Angiopoietin 1* interacts with the EC receptor *Tie2* to recruit periendothelial cells. The interaction also mediates vessel maturation from simple tubes into more elaborate vascular structures and helps maintain EC quiescence. *Angiopoietin 2-Tie2* interactions have the opposite effect; ECs become more responsive to VEGF stimulation.
- *PDGF* recruits smooth muscle cells.
- *TGF-β* stabilizes newly formed vessels by enhancing ECM production.

Extracellular Matrix Proteins as Regulators of Angiogenesis (p. 101)

The directed migration of ECs during angiogenesis is regulated by:

- *Integrins,* especially $\alpha_v\beta_3$; these are critical for forming and maintaining newly formed vessels.
- *Matrix and cellular proteins,* including thrombospondin 1, SPARC, and tenascin C, destabilize cell-matrix interactions and thereby promote angiogenesis.
- *Proteases* (e.g., plasminogen activators and metalloproteinases) remodel tissue during EC invasion. They also release matrix-bound VEGF and FGF-2 to stimulate angiogenesis, as well as inhibitors of angiogenesis (e.g., *endostatin,* a small fragment of collagen XVIII).

Cutaneous Wound Healing (p. 102)

Wound healing in the skin is illustrative of repair principles for most tissues. After a single injurious event, the healing progresses through overlapping phases (Fig. 3-3):

- *Inflammation*: Injury that leads to platelet adhesion and activation with clot formation, along with inflammatory vascular changes followed by inflammatory cell recruitment

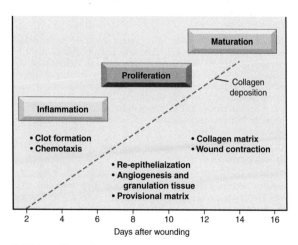

FIGURE 3-3 Phases of cutaneous wound healing. *(Modified from Broughton G et al: The basic science of wound healing, Plast Reconstr Surg 117:12S-34S, 2006.)*

- *Proliferation:* Migration and expansion of parenchymal cells (re-epithelialization), endothelial cells (angiogenesis), and connective tissue cells
- *Maturation:* ECM deposition and remodeling with wound contraction

Skin wounds are classically described as healing by *first* or *second intention.* The healing process is essentially the same in both; the distinction comes from the nature and extent of the wounds.

- Healing of a clean, uninfected surgical incision approximated by sutures is an example of healing by *primary union (first intention);* cell death and BM damage is minimal, and there is robust re-epithelialization with minimal fibrosis.
- A large cutaneous ulcer has substantially more associated inflammation, as well as parenchymal and stromal damage. It will heal by *secondary union (second intention)* with much greater angiogenesis, fibroblast ingrowth with abundant collagen deposition, and denser scar formation that will eventually contract.

Formation of Blood Clot (p. 102)

After wounding, a blood clot (Chapter 4) acts to stanch bleeding but also provides a matrix rich in growth factors and chemokines that acts as a scaffold for migrating leukocytes and stromal cells. Within 24 hours, neutrophils appear at the margins and begin the process of wound sterilization and debris degradation.

Formation of Granulation Tissue (p. 102)

Within 1 to 2 days of wounding (and peaking at 5 to 7 days), proliferating fibroblasts and endothelium form *granulation tissue,* a highly vascularized loose connective tissue and a hallmark of early tissue repair. The vessels are leaky (increasing protein and fluid deposition in the tissues), thereby causing local edema. Granulation tissue provides a framework for subsequent scar formation.

Cell Proliferation and Collagen Deposition (p. 102)

Within 2 to 4 days after wounding, neutrophils are largely replaced by macrophages, which then become the key cellular elements in clearing debris and directing the subsequent angiogenesis and ECM deposition. Eventually, the granulation tissue scaffolding is converted into a scar composed of fibroblasts and collagen. Macrophages are the main source in healing wounds of many of the factors (see Table 3-3) that drive fibroblast migration, proliferation, and ECM production. Of these, TGF-β is the most important fibrogenic agent.

Scar Formation (p. 104)

Two weeks after injury, the dominant feature is collagen deposition with regression of the vasculature; the granulation tissue is ultimately converted into a relatively avascular scar that is depleted of inflammation and covered by intact epithelium.

Wound Contraction (p. 104)

This is a feature of larger wounds, accomplished by *myofibroblasts* with the synthetic features of fibroblasts and the contractile capacity of smooth muscle cells. They will cause the surface area of the wound to be reduced.

Connective Tissue Remodeling (p. 105)

The replacement of granulation tissue with a scar involves changes in ECM composition. Besides driving ECM synthesis, the various growth factors also modulate the synthesis and activation of *matrix metalloproteinases (MMPs)*, a family of more than 20 enzymes that degrade ECM; these should be distinguished from neutrophil elastase, cathepsins, kinins, and plasmin, which also degrade ECM but are *serine* proteases and not MMPs. MMPs are secreted as proenzymes and activated extracellularly; they require zinc for their activity. MMP production is inhibited by TGF-β, contributing to the net fibrotic effect of TGF-β. MMPs include:

> *Interstitial collagenases* that cleave fibrillar collagen types I, II, and III
> *Gelatinases* that degrade amorphous collagen as well as fibronectin
> *Stromelysins* that act on a variety of ECM components, including proteoglycans, laminin, fibronectin, and amorphous collagens
> *ADAMs (a disintegrin and metalloproteinase-domain)*, membrane-bound MMPs that release extracellular domains of cell surface proteins (e.g., precursor forms of TNF and TGF-α)

Activated MMPs are inhibited by a number of *tissue inhibitors of metalloproteinases (TIMPs)*. Accumulation of ECM or subsequent remodeling of the connective tissue framework at sites of injury is a combination of increased synthesis and decreased degradation.

Recovery of Tensile Strength (p. 105)

Wound strength is initially dependent on suturing. When the sutures are removed (typically at 1 week), wound strength is only about 10% of normal. Tensile strength eventually plateaus at 70% to 80% of normal within 3 months; this is associated with increased collagen synthesis exceeding collagen degradation followed by cross-linking and increased collagen fiber size.

Local and Systemic Factors that Influence Wound Healing (p. 106)

Systemic factors include:

- Nutritional status of the host (e.g., protein nutrition and vitamin C intake)
- Metabolic status (diabetes mellitus delays healing)
- Circulatory status or vascular adequacy
- Hormones (e.g., glucocorticoids) (can impede the inflammatory and reparative process)

Local factors include:

- Size, location (well-vascularized tissues heal faster), and type of the wound (e.g., infectious versus necrosis versus trauma)
- *Local factors that delay healing* include infections, mechanical forces (e.g., motion or wound tension), and foreign bodies

Pathologic Aspects of Repair (p. 106)

- *Deficient scar formation:* Inadequate granulation tissue or collagen deposition and remodeling can lead to either *wound dehiscence or ulceration.*
- *Excessive repair:* Excessive granulation tissue *(proud flesh)* can protrude above the surrounding skin and block re-epithelialization. Excessive collagen accumulation forms a raised *hypertrophic scar;* progression beyond the original area of injury without subsequent regression is termed a *keloid.*
- *Formation of contractures:* Although wound contraction is a normal part of healing, an exaggerated process is designated a *contracture.* It will cause wound deformity (e.g., producing hand *claw* deformities, or limit joint mobility).

Fibrosis (p. 107)

The cell proliferation, cell-cell and cell-matrix interactions, and ECM deposition involved in wound healing also underlie the fibrosis associated with chronic inflammatory diseases such as rheumatoid arthritis and cirrhosis. Chronic inflammatory diseases are marked by recurrent injury or persistence of the inflammatory response (e.g., radiation injury or autoimmunity). In most cases, lymphocyte-macrophage interactions sustain the synthesis and secretion of growth factors and fibrogenic cytokines (TGF-β in particular), proteases, and other biologically active molecules; consequently, the ongoing inflammation drives progressive tissue injury and fibrosis. Osteopontin expression in tissues, possibly through effects on myofibroblast differentiation, is also associated with fibrosis.

Notably, fetal cutaneous wounds heal without scarring, variably attributed to non-fibrogenic forms of TGF-β, lack of osteopontin production, or absence of a Th_2 cytokine response that drives macrophage production of pro-fibrogenic mediators (Chapter 2).

4

Hemodynamic Disorders, Thromboembolic Disease, and Shock

Disturbances in normal blood flow are major sources of human morbidity and death (35% to 40% of deaths in Western society). These include hemorrhage, clotting, and *embolization* (migration of clots to other sites), as well as extravasation of fluid into the interstitium *(edema)* and blood pressure that is either too low or too high.

Edema (p. 111)

The movement of water and solutes between intravascular and interstitial spaces is balanced by the opposing forces of vascular hydrostatic pressure and plasma colloid osmotic pressure. Increased capillary pressure or diminished colloid osmotic pressure result in increased interstitial fluid. If the net movement of water into tissues exceeds lymphatic drainage, fluid will accumulate.

Increased interstitial fluid is called *edema*, while fluid in the various body cavities is called *hydrothorax, hydropericardium,* or *hydroperitoneum;* the last is more commonly called *ascites.* Edema may be localized (e.g., secondary to isolated venous or lymphatic obstruction) or systemic (as in heart failure); severe systemic edema is called *anasarca.*

Table 4-1 lists the causes of edema broadly grouped into *noninflammatory* (yields protein-poor *transudates*) and *inflammatory* (yields protein-rich *exudates,* discussed in Chapter 2).

Noninflammatory causes of edema:

- *Increased hydrostatic pressure* forces fluid out of the vessels. This can be regional (e.g., due to deep venous thrombosis in an extremity). *Systemic* edema is most commonly due to *congestive heart failure (CHF)* (Chapter 12) where compromised right heart function leads to venous blood pooling.
- *Reduced plasma osmotic pressure* occurs with albumin loss (e.g., due to proteinuria in *nephrotic syndrome*) (Chapter 20) or reduced albumin synthesis (e.g., due to cirrhosis [Chapter 18] or protein malnutrition). Reduced osmotic pressure leads to a net fluid movement into the interstitium with plasma volume contraction. The reduced plasma volume leads to diminished renal perfusion and resultant renin production (and downstream effects on angiotensin and aldosterone), but the subsequent salt and water retention cannot correct the plasma volume due to the underlying protein deficit.

TABLE 4-1 Pathophysiologic Categories of Edema

Increased Hydrostatic Pressure

Impaired venous return
  Congestive heart failure
  Constrictive pericarditis
  Ascites (liver cirrhosis)
  Venous obstruction or compression
    Thrombosis
    External pressure (e.g., mass)
    Lower extremity inactivity with prolonged dependency
Arteriolar dilation
  Heat
  Neurohumoral dysregulation

Reduced Plasma Osmotic Pressure (Hypoproteinemia)

Protein-losing glomerulopathies (nephrotic syndrome)
Liver cirrhosis (ascites)
Malnutrition
Protein-losing gastroenteropathy

Lymphatic Obstruction

Inflammatory
Neoplastic
Postsurgical
Postirradiation

Sodium Retention

Excessive salt intake with renal insufficiency
Increased tubular reabsorption of sodium
Renal hypoperfusion
Increased renin-angiotensin-aldosterone secretion

Inflammation

Acute inflammation
Chronic inflammation
Angiogenesis

Data from Leaf A, Cotran RS: *Renal pathophysiology*, ed 3, New York, 1985, Oxford University Press, p. 146. Used by permission of Oxford Press, Inc.

- *Sodium and water retention.* Primary salt retention, with obligatory associated water retention, causes *both* increased hydrostatic pressure and reduced osmotic pressure. Sodium retention can occur with any renal dysfunction (Chapter 20). Primary water retention can occur with release of antidiuretic hormone (ADH) either due to increased plasma osmolarity, diminished plasma volume, or inappropriately in the setting of malignancy; lung or pituitary pathology can also cause inappropriate ADH secretion.
- *Lymphatic obstruction* blocks removal of interstitial fluid. Obstruction is usually localized and related to inflammation or neoplastic processes.

Morphology (p. 113)

Edema is most easily appreciated grossly. Microscopically, it manifests only as subtle cell swelling and separation of the extracellular matrix.

- *Subcutaneous edema* may be diffuse or occur where hydrostatic pressures are greatest (e.g., influenced by gravity, called *dependent edema* [legs when standing, sacrum when recumbent]).

Finger pressure over substantial subcutaneous edema typically leaves an imprint, called *pitting edema.*

- Edema resulting from hypoproteinemia is generally more severe and diffuse. It is most evident in loose connective tissue (e.g., eyelids, causing *periorbital edema*).
- *Pulmonary edema* can result in lungs that are two to three times their normal weight. Sectioning reveals a frothy, blood-tinged mixture of air, edema fluid, and erythrocytes.
- *Brain edema* may be localized to sites of injury (e.g., abscess or neoplasm) or may be generalized (e.g., encephalitis, hypertensive crises, or obstruction to venous outflow). When generalized, the brain is grossly swollen with narrowed sulci and distended gyri flattened against the skull.

Clinical Consequences (p. 113)

- Subcutaneous edema can impair wound healing or infection clearance.
- Pulmonary edema impedes gas exchange and increases the risk of infection.
- Brain edema within the confined space of the skull can impede cerebral blood flow or cause *herniation*, compromising critical medullary centers.

Hyperemia and Congestion (p. 113)

Both terms mean increased blood volume at a particular site.

- *Hyperemia* is an *active process* due to augmented blood inflow from arteriolar dilation (e.g., skeletal muscle during exercise or at sites of inflammation). Tissues are red *(erythema)* owing to engorgement with oxygenated blood.
- *Congestion* is a *passive process* caused by impaired outflow from a tissue; it can be systemic (e.g., CHF) or local (e.g., an isolated venous obstruction). Tissues are blue-red *(cyanosis)* as worsening congestion leads to an accumulation of deoxyhemoglobin.
- Long-standing stasis of deoxygenated blood can result in hypoxia severe enough to cause ischemic tissue injury and fibrosis.

Morphology (p. 114)

In *acute congestion,* vessels are distended, and organs are grossly hyperemic. Capillary bed congestion is also commonly associated with interstitial edema. In *chronic congestion,* capillary rupture may cause focal hemorrhage. Subsequent erythrocyte breakdown results in hemosiderin-laden macrophages. Parenchymal cell atrophy or death (with fibrosis) may also be present. Grossly, tissues appear brown, contracted, and fibrotic. Lungs and liver are commonly affected.

- In *lungs,* capillary engorgement is associated with interstitial edema and airspace transudates. Chronic manifestations include hemosiderin-laden macrophages *(heart failure cells)* and fibrotic septa.
- In *liver,* acute congestion manifests as central vein and sinusoidal distention and occasionally with central hepatocyte degeneration. In chronic congestion, the central regions of the hepatic lobules are grossly red-brown and slightly depressed (loss of cells) relative to the surrounding uncongested tan liver (called *nutmeg liver*). Microscopically there is *centrilobular necrosis* with hepatocyte dropout and hemorrhage, including hemosiderin-laden macrophages. Since the centrilobular area is at the distal end of the hepatic blood supply, it is most subject to necrosis whenever liver perfusion is compromised.

Hemorrhage (p. 114)

Hemorrhage is a release of blood into the extravascular space. Rupture of a large artery or vein is usually due to vascular injury (e.g., trauma, atherosclerosis, inflammation, or neoplastic erosion of the vessel). Capillary bleeding can occur with chronic congestion. A tendency to hemorrhage from insignificant injury is seen in a variety of disorders, called *hemorrhagic diatheses.*

- Hemorrhage can be external or enclosed within a tissue (called a *hematoma*). Hematomas can be trivial (e.g., a bruise) or massive enough to cause death.
- *Petechiae* are minute, 1 to 2 mm hemorrhages in skin, mucous membranes, or serosal surfaces. These occur with increased intravascular pressure, low platelet counts *(thrombocytopenia),* or defective platelet function.
- *Purpura* are ≥ 3 mm hemorrhages. These occur for the same reasons as petechiae, as well as with trauma, local vascular inflammation *(vasculitis),* or increased vascular fragility (e.g., amyloidosis).
- *Ecchymoses* are ≥ 1 to 2 cm subcutaneous hematomas (i.e., *bruises*). They are typically associated with trauma but are also exacerbated by other bleeding disorders. The characteristic color changes in a bruise are due to progressive metabolism of extravasated hemoglobin by tissue macrophages.
- Large accumulations of blood in body cavities are called *hemothorax, hemopericardium, hemoperitoneum,* or *hemarthrosis* (joint), depending upon the location. Patients with extensive hemorrhage occasionally develop jaundice from massive erythrocyte breakdown and systemic bilirubin release.

The clinical significance of hemorrhage depends on the volume and rate of blood loss. Rapid loss of less than 20%, or slow losses of even larger amounts, may have little impact. Greater losses result in *hemorrhagic (hypovolemic) shock.* Location is also important, for example, bleeding that would be inconsequential when located in subcutaneous tissues may cause death when located in the brain. Chronic blood loss (e.g., peptic ulcer or menstrual bleeding) can result in iron deficiency anemia.

Hemostasis and Thrombosis (p. 115)

Hemostasis is a normal, physiologic process maintaining blood in a fluid, clot-free state within normal vessels while inducing a rapid, localized hemostatic plug at sites of vascular injury. *Thrombosis represents a pathologic state*; it is the inappropriate activation of hemostatic mechanisms in uninjured vessels or thrombotic occlusion after relatively minor injury. Hemostasis and thrombosis are closely related processes that depend upon three components: *endothelium, platelets,* and *coagulation cascade.*

Normal Hemostasis (p. 115)

After injury, there is a characteristic hemostatic response (Fig. 4-1):

- Transient reflex neurogenic arteriolar vasoconstriction augmented by endothelin (a potent endothelial-derived vasoconstrictor).
- Platelet adhesion and activation (i.e., shape change and secretory granule release) by binding to exposed subendothelial extracellular matrix (ECM). Secreted products recruit other platelets to form a temporary hemostatic plug (primary hemostasis).
- Activation of the coagulation cascade by release of tissue factor (also known as *thromboplastin* or *factor III*), a membrane-bound lipoprotein procoagulant factor synthesized by endothelium.

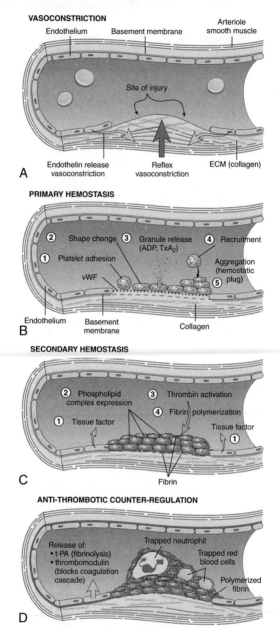

FIGURE 4-1 Diagrammatic representation of normal hemostasis. **A,** Vascular injury triggers transient vasoconstriction through local neurohumoral factors. **B,** Platelets adhere to exposed extracellular matrix *(ECM)* via von Willebrand factor *(vWF)* and are activated, undergoing a shape change and granule release; released adenosine diphosphate *(ADP)* and thromboxane A_2 *(TxA_2)* lead to further platelet aggregation to form the primary hemostatic plug. **C,** Local activation of the coagulation cascade (involving tissue factor and platelet phospholipids) results in fibrin polymerization, thereby "cementing" the platelets into a definitive secondary hemostatic plug. **D,** Counter-regulatory mechanisms (e.g., release of tissue plasminogen activator *[t-PA]* and thrombomodulin) limit the hemostatic process to the site of injury.

Coagulation culminates in thrombin generation and conversion of circulating fibrinogen to insoluble fibrin (see later). Thrombin also induces additional platelet recruitment and granule release. Polymerized fibrin and platelet aggregates together form a solid, permanent plug (secondary hemostasis).

- Activation of counter-regulatory mechanisms (e.g., tissue plasminogen activator [t-PA]) restricts the hemostatic plug to the site of injury.

Endothelium (p. 115)

Endothelial cells (ECs) regulate several, frequently opposing aspects of hemostasis. ECs normally exhibit antiplatelet, anticoagulant, and fibrinolytic properties; however, after injury or activation, ECs exhibit *procoagulant function* (Fig. 4-2). The balance between EC anti- and prothrombotic activities determines whether thrombus formation, propagation, or dissolution occurs.

- EC antithrombotic properties

  Intact endothelium blocks platelet access to thrombogenic subendothelial ECM
  Prostacyclin (PGI$_2$) and nitric oxide (NO) inhibit platelet binding.
  Adenosinediphosphatase degrades adenosine diphosphate (ADP), an inducer of platelet aggregation.
  Membrane-associated thrombomodulin converts thrombin to an anticoagulant protein.
  Tissue factor pathway inhibitor (TFPI) blocks intermediates in the coagulation cascade.
  Heparin-like surface molecules facilitate plasma antithrombin III inactivation of thrombin.
  t-PA cleaves plasminogen to form plasmin, which, in turn, degrades fibrin.

- EC prothrombotic properties

  EC produce *von Willebrand factor (vWF)*; EC damage allows platelets to bind the underlying ECM through interaction with vWF.
  Tissue factor production is the major activator of the extrinsic clotting cascade (see later).
  Plasminogen activator inhibitors (PAIs) limit fibrinolysis and favor thrombosis.

Platelets (p. 117)

After vascular injury, platelets encounter ECM constituents (collagen, proteoglycans, fibronectin, and other adhesive glycoproteins), which are normally sequestered beneath an intact endothelium. Then, platelets undergo *activation* involving adhesion and shape change, secretion (release reaction), and aggregation.

- *Platelet-ECM adhesion* is mediated through vWF, thereby acting as a bridge between platelet receptors (mostly glycoprotein Ib) and exposed collagen. Genetic deficiencies of *vWF* or glycoprotein-Ib (i.e., *Bernard-Soulier syndrome*) result in bleeding disorders.
- *Platelet granule secretion (release reaction)* occurs shortly after adhesion. *Alpha granules* express P-selectin adhesion molecules and contain coagulation and growth factors; *dense bodies* or *delta granules* contain ADP, calcium, and vasoactive amines (e.g., histamine). ADP is a potent mediator of *platelet aggregation,* and calcium is important for the coagulation cascade. The release reaction also results in surface expression of *phospholipid complex,* providing a locus for calcium and coagulation factor interactions in the *clotting cascade.*

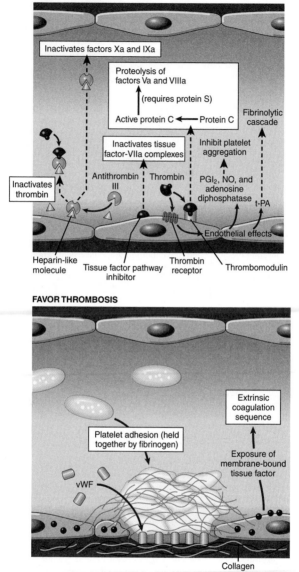

INHIBIT THROMBOSIS

Inactivates factors Xa and IXa

Proteolysis of factors Va and VIIIa

(requires protein S)

Active protein C ← Protein C

Fibrinolytic cascade

Inactivates tissue factor-VIIa complexes

Inhibit platelet aggregation

Inactivates thrombin

Antithrombin III

Thrombin

PGI_2, NO, and adenosine diphosphatase

t-PA

Endothelial effects

Heparin-like molecule

Tissue factor pathway inhibitor

Thrombin receptor

Thrombomodulin

FAVOR THROMBOSIS

Extrinsic coagulation sequence

Exposure of membrane-bound tissue factor

Platelet adhesion (held together by fibrinogen)

vWF

Collagen

FIGURE 4-2 Schematic illustration of some of the pro- and anticoagulant activities of EC. Not shown are the pro- and antifibrinolytic properties. *NO*, nitric oxide; *PGI_2*, prostacyclin; *t-PA*, tissue plasminogen activator; *vWF*, von Willebrand factor.

- *Platelet aggregation* (platelets adhering to other platelets) is promoted by ADP and thromboxane A_2 (TxA_2).

  ADP activation changes platelet GpIIb-IIIa receptor conformation to allow fibrinogen binding. Fibrinogen bridges multiple platelets, forming large aggregates (GpIIb-IIIa deficiencies result in *Glanzmann thrombasthenia* bleeding disorder).

Platelet-derived TxA_2 activates platelet aggregation and is a potent vasoconstrictor (recall that EC-derived PGI_2 inhibits platelet aggregation and is a potent vasodilator).

- Erythrocytes and leukocytes also aggregate in hemostatic plugs; leukocytes adhere to platelets via P-selectin and contribute to the inflammatory response accompanying thrombosis.

Coagulation Cascade (p. 118)

A sequence of inactive proenzymes are converted into activated enzymes, culminating in the generation of insoluble *fibrin* from the soluble plasma protein *fibrinogen*. Traditionally, coagulation has been divided into *extrinsic* and *intrinsic* pathways that converge at the stage of factor X activation (Fig. 4-3).

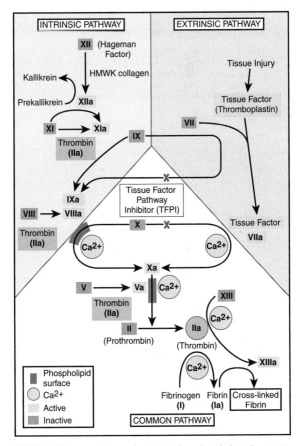

FIGURE 4-3 The coagulation cascade. Intrinsic and extrinsic pathways are interlinked at the level of factor IX activation. Note the multiple points where thrombin (factor IIa, *darker blue shading*) contributes to coagulation through positive feedback loops. The Xs denote points where TFPI inhibit factors IX and X activation by factor VIIa. Activated factors are indicated with a lowercase "a." *HMWK,* High-molecular-weight kininogen; *PL,* phospholipid surface.

- The intrinsic cascade is classically initiated by activation of Hageman factor (factor XII); the extrinsic cascade is activated by *tissue factor* (see preceding). There is a rather broad overlap between the two pathways and the division is largely an artifact of *in vitro* testing.

  Prothrombin time (PT) screens for the function of the proteins in the extrinsic pathway (VII, X, II, V, and fibrinogen)

  Partial thromboplastin time (PTT) screens for the function of the proteins in the intrinsic pathway (XII, XI, IX, VIII, X, V, II, and fibrinogen)

- Each reaction in the various pathways results from assembly of a complex held together by *calcium ions* on a *phospholipid complex* and composed of:

  Enzyme (activated coagulation factor)
  Substrate (proenzyme form of coagulation factor)
  Cofactor (reaction accelerator)

  Thus, clotting tends to remain localized to sites where assembly can occur (e.g., surfaces of activated platelets or endothelium).

- Besides catalyzing the cleavage of fibrinogen to fibrin, thrombin also exerts numerous effects on local vessel wall and inflammatory cells; it even *limits* the extent of hemostasis (see later). Most such effects are mediated through *protease-activated receptors (PARs)*, seven-transmembrane spanner proteins.

Control Mechanisms

Once activated, coagulation (and thrombolysis) must be restricted to sites of vascular injury to prevent clotting (or inappropriate clot lysis) of the entire vascular tree (see Fig. 4-2):

- Factor activation can only occur at sites of exposed phospholipids. Also, activated clotting factors are diluted by flow and are cleared by the liver and tissue macrophages.
- Antithrombins (e.g., *antithrombin III*), complexed with heparin-like cofactors on endothelium, inhibit thrombin and other serine proteases—factors IXa, Xa, XIa, and XIIa.
- Endothelial *thrombomodulin* modifies thrombin so that it can cleave *proteins C and S;* these, in turn, inactivate factors Va and VIIIa.
- TFPI inactivates tissue factor–factor VIIa complexes.
- Thrombin induces endothelial t-PA release; t-PA generates active *plasmin* from circulating *plasminogen*. Plasmin can also be generated by a factor XII–dependent pathway. Plasmin cleaves fibrin and interferes with its polymerization; the resulting *fibrin split products* also act as weak anticoagulants.
- Functional plasmin activity is restricted to sites of thrombosis:

  t-PA activates plasminogen most effectively when bound to fibrin meshwork.
  Free plasmin is rapidly neutralized by serum α_2-plasmin inhibitor.

- Endothelium modulates anticoagulation by releasing *plasminogen activator inhibitors (PAIs)*, which inhibit t-PA binding to fibrin. Thrombin and certain cytokines increase PAI production; cytokines released in the setting of severe inflammation can therefore cause intravascular thrombosis.

Thrombosis (p. 121)

Thrombosis is inappropriate activation of blood clotting in uninjured vasculature or thrombotic occlusion of a vessel after relatively minor injury. There are three primary influences on thrombus formation, called *Virchow's triad:*

1. *Endothelial injury* (p. 121) is dominant and can independently cause thrombosis (e.g., endocarditis or ulcerated atherosclerotic plaque). Injury can be due to hemodynamic stresses (e.g., hypertension or turbulent), endotoxin, radiation, or noxious agents (e.g., homocystinuria, hypercholesterolemia, or cigarette smoke). Thrombosis results from exposed subendothelial ECM, increased platelet adhesion or procoagulant production (i.e., tissue factor, PAI), or reduced anticoagulant activity (i.e., PGI_2, thrombomodulin, t-PA).

2. *Alterations in normal blood flow* (p. 121) can promote thrombosis. Normal blood flow is *laminar* (i.e., cellular elements flow centrally in the vessel lumen, separated from endothelium by a plasma clear zone). Stasis and turbulence (the latter forms eddy currents with local pockets of stasis):

   • Disrupt laminar flow and bring platelets into contact with the endothelium.
   • Prevent dilution of activated clotting factors by flowing blood.
   • Retard the inflow of clotting inhibitors.
   • Promote endothelial cell activation.

Stasis causes thrombosis in the venous circulation, cardiac chambers, and arterial aneurysms; turbulence causes thrombosis in the arterial circulation as well as endothelial injury. Hyperviscosity syndromes (e.g., polycythemia) or deformed erythrocytes (e.g., sickle cell anemia) result in small vessel stasis and also predispose to thrombosis.

3. *Hypercoagulability* (p. 122) is loosely defined as any alteration of the coagulation pathways that predisposes to thrombosis. It contributes less frequently to thrombosis but is critical in certain conditions (Table 4-2).

   • Heritable hypercoagulable states:

     Factor V gene mutations are the most common; 2% to 15% of caucasians (and 60% of patients with recurrent deep vein thrombosis) carry the so-called *Leiden mutation,* thereby rendering factor V resistant to protein C inactivation.
     Deficiencies of antithrombin III, protein C, or protein S also typically present with venous thrombosis and recurrent thromboembolism.

   • Acquired hypercoagulable states:

     Oral contraceptives or the hyperestrogenic state of pregnancy may cause hypercoagulability by increasing hepatic synthesis of coagulation factors and reduced synthesis of antithrombin III.
     Certain malignancies can release procoagulant tumor products.

   • *Heparin-induced thrombocytopenia syndrome* occurs when heparin products (unfractionated more commonly than low molecular weight heparin) induces circulating antibodies that activate platelets and injure ECs.
   • *Antiphospholipid antibody syndrome* occurs in patients with antibodies against anionic phospholipids that activate platelets or interfere with protein C activity.

Morphology (p. 123)

• Venous thrombi characteristically occur in sites of stasis and are *occlusive.*

TABLE 4-2 Hypercoagulable States

Primary (Genetic)

Common
Factor V mutation (G1691A mutation; factor V Leiden)
Prothrombin mutation (G20210A variant)
5,10-Methylenetetrahydrofolate reductase (homozygous C677T mutation)
Increased levels of factors VIII, IX, XI, or fibrinogen

Rare
Antithrombin III deficiency
Protein C deficiency
Protein S deficiency

Very Rare
Fibrinolysis defects
Homozygous homocystinuria (deficiency of cystathione β-synthetase)

Secondary (Acquired)

High Risk for Thrombosis
Prolonged bedrest or immobilization
Myocardial infarction
Atrial fibrillation
Tissue injury (surgery, fracture, burn)
Cancer
Prosthetic mechanical cardiac valves
Disseminated intravascular coagulation
Heparin-induced thrombocytopenia
Antiphospholipid antibody syndrome

Lower Risk for Thrombosis
Cardiomyopathy
Nephrotic syndrome
Hyperestrogenic states (pregnancy and postpartum)
Oral contraceptive use
Sickle cell anemia
Smoking

- Arterial or cardiac thrombi usually begin at sites of endothelial injury (e.g., atherosclerotic plaque, endocarditis) or turbulence (vessel bifurcation).

  Aortic or cardiac thrombi are typically *nonocclusive (mural)* as a result of rapid and high-volume flow.
  Smaller arterial thrombi can be *occlusive.*

- Thrombi are generally firmly attached at their site of origin and typically *propagate towards the heart.* Thus, arterial thrombi extend retrograde from the attachment point, whereas venous thrombi extend in the direction of blood flow. The propagating tail may not be well attached and may fragment to create an *embolus.*
- *Arterial and cardiac mural thrombi* have gross and microscopic laminations *(lines of Zahn)* produced by pale layers of platelets and fibrin alternating with darker erythrocyte-rich layers.
- *Venous thrombi (phlebothrombosis)* typically occur in a relatively static environment, resulting in a fairly uniform cast containing abundant erythrocytes among sparse fibrin strands *(red or stasis thrombi).* Phlebothrombosis most commonly affects the veins of the lower extremities (more than 90% of cases).
- *Valve thrombosis:*

  Infective endocarditis: Organisms form large, infected thrombotic masses *(vegetations)* with associated valve damage and systemic infection.

Nonbacterial thrombotic endocarditis: Non-infected, sterile vegetations develop in hypercoagulable states, typically without valve damage.

Verrucous (Libman-Sacks) endocarditis (sterile vegetations): This occurs in systemic lupus erythematosus due to immune complex deposition; inflammation can cause valve scarring.

Fate of the Thrombus (p. 124)

If a patient survives the immediate effects of a thrombus, some combination of the following occurs:

• *Propagation* (discussed earlier)
• *Embolization:* Thrombi dislodge and travel to other sites
• *Dissolution:* Dissolution by fibrinolytic activity
• *Organization and recanalization:* Ingrowth of endothelial cells, smooth muscle cells, and fibroblasts to create vascular channels, or incorporate the thrombus into the vessel wall
• *Mycotic aneurysm:* Rarely, microbial seeding of a thrombus leads to a mycotic aneurysm

Clinical Consequences (p. 125)

Thrombi are significant because they (1) *can obstruct vessels* and (2) *can embolize;* the relative importance depends on the site. Thus, although venous thrombi can cause distal congestion and edema, embolization is more clinically significant (e.g., from deep leg vein to lung). Conversely, although arterial thrombi can embolize, vascular obstruction (e.g., causing myocardial or cerebral infarctions) is much more important.

Venous Thrombosis (Phlebothrombosis). Venous thrombosis occurs most commonly in deep or superficial leg veins.

• Superficial thrombi usually occur in varicose saphenous veins, causing local congestion and pain but rarely embolizing. Local edema and impaired venous drainage predispose to skin infections and *varicose ulcers.*
• *Deep thrombi* in larger leg veins above the knee (e.g., popliteal, femoral, and iliac veins) can result in pain and edema, as well as increased risk for embolization. Venous obstruction is usually offset by collateral flow, and deep vein thromboses are asymptomatic in *approximately 50% of patients,* being recognized only after embolization.
• Deep venous thrombosis (DVT) occurs in multiple clinical settings:

Advanced age, bed rest, or immobilization, thereby diminishing the milking action of muscles in the lower leg and slowing venous return
Congestive heart failure (CHF)
Trauma, surgery, and burns result in reduced physical activity, injury to vessels, release of procoagulant substances from tissues, and reduced tPA
The puerperal and postpartum states are associated with amniotic fluid embolization (see later) and hypercoagulability
Tumor-associated procoagulant release *(migratory thrombophlebitis* or *Trousseau syndrome)*

Arterial and Cardiac Thrombosis. *Atherosclerosis* (Chapter 11) is the major cause of arterial thrombi due to abnormal flow and endothelial damage. *Myocardial infarction* with dyskinesis and endocardial damage can cause mural thrombi. *Rheumatic valvular disease* resulting in mitral valve scarring and stenosis, with left atrial dilation, predisposes to atrial thrombus formation; concurrent atrial fibrillation augments the blood stasis and propensity to thrombose. Cardiac and aortic mural thrombi can embolize peripherally; brain, kidneys, and spleen are prime targets.

Disseminated Intravascular Coagulation (p. 125)

Disseminated intravascular coagulation (DIC) is reflected by widespread fibrin microthrombi in the microcirculation. This is caused by disorders ranging from obstetric complications to advanced malignancy. DIC is not a primary disease, but rather it is a complication of any diffuse thrombin activation. Microthrombi can cause diffuse circulatory insufficiency, particularly in the brain, lungs, heart, and kidneys; there is also concurrent consumption of platelets and coagulation factors *(consumption coagulopathy)* with fibrinolytic pathway activation, thereby leading to uncontrollable bleeding. DIC is discussed in greater detail in Chapter 14.

Embolism (p. 125)

Embolism refers to any intravascular solid, liquid, or gaseous mass carried by blood flow to a site distant from its origin. Most (i.e., 99%) arise from thrombi, hence the term *thromboembolism*. Rare forms include fat droplets, gas bubbles, atherosclerotic debris *(atheroemboli)*, tumor fragments, bone marrow, or foreign bodies (e.g., bullets). Emboli lodge in vessels too small to permit further passage, resulting in partial or complete vascular occlusion and ischemic necrosis *(infarction)*.

Pulmonary Embolism (p. 126) (See Chapter 15)

Pulmonary emboli (PE) occur in 0.2% to 0.4% of hospitalized patients and cause about 200,000 deaths annually in the United States. Greater than 95% of PE originate from DVT, although DVT occur roughly 3-fold more commonly than PE. PE can occlude the main pulmonary artery, impact across the bifurcation *(saddle embolus)*, or pass into smaller arterioles. Multiple emboli can occur, either sequentially or as a shower of small emboli from a single large mass; in general, *one PE puts a patient at risk for more.* Rarely, emboli pass through atrial or ventricular defects into the systemic circulation *(paradoxical embolism)*.

- Most PE (60% to 80%) are small and clinically silent. They eventually organize and get incorporated into the vessel wall or leave a delicate, bridging fibrous *web.*
- Sudden death, right-sided heart failure *(cor pulmonale)*, or cardiovascular collapse occurs when 60% or more of the pulmonary circulation is obstructed with emboli.
- PE in medium-sized arteries can cause pulmonary hemorrhage but usually do not pulmonary infarction due to collateral bronchial artery flow; however, with left-sided cardiac failure (and diminished bronchial circulation), infarcts can result.
- PE in small end-arteriolar vessels typically cause hemorrhage or infarction.
- Multiple emboli over time can cause pulmonary hypertension and right ventricular failure.

Systemic Thromboembolism (p. 126)

Systemic thromboembolism refers to emboli in the arterial circulation. Approximately 80% arise from intracardiac mural thrombi; two thirds are secondary to myocardial infarcts, and 25% arise in the setting of dilated left atria and fibrillation. Systemic emboli can also originate from aortic aneurysms, thrombi on ulcerated atherosclerotic plaques, or valvular vegetations; they rarely originate from *paradoxical emboli* (venous emboli that pass through an atrial or ventricular septal defect, including patent foramen ovale); 10% to 15% are of unknown origin. Major sites for arteriolar embolization are the lower extremities (75%) and brain (10%); intestines, kidneys, spleen, and upper extremities are less frequent. The consequences of arterial emboli depend on collateral vascular supply, tissue vulnerability to ischemia, and vessel caliber; most arterial emboli cause tissue infarction.

Fat and Marrow Embolism (p. 126)

Pulmonary embolization of microscopic fat globules (with or without hematopoietic marrow elements) occurs after fractures of long bones or, rarely, after burns or soft tissue trauma. Fat embolism occurs in 90% of severe skeletal injuries; less than 10% have any clinical findings.

Fat embolism syndrome, which is fatal in approximately 10% of cases, is heralded by sudden pulmonary insufficiency 1 to 3 days after injury; 20% to 50% of patients have a diffuse petechial rash and may have neurologic symptoms (irritability and restlessness) that progress to delirium or coma. Thrombocytopenia and anemia can also occur. The pathogenesis involves mechanical obstruction by neutral fat microemboli, followed by local platelet and erythrocyte aggregation. Subsequent fatty acid release causes toxic injury to endothelium; platelet activation and granulocyte recruitment contribute free radicals, proteases, and eicosanoids.

Edema and hemorrhage (and pulmonary hyaline membranes) can be seen microscopically.

Air Embolism (p. 127)

Air embolism refers to gas bubbles within the circulation that obstruct vascular flow and cause ischemia. Small amounts in the coronary or cerebral circulation (introduced following surgery) can be catastrophic. Generally, in the pulmonary circulation, more than 100 cc is required to have a clinical effect; such volumes can be introduced during obstetrical procedures or after chest wall injury.

Decompression sickness is a special form of air embolism caused by sudden changes in atmospheric pressure; deep-sea divers and individuals in unpressurized aircraft during rapid ascent are at risk. Air breathed at high pressure causes increasing amounts of gas (particularly nitrogen) to be dissolved in blood and tissues. Subsequent rapid ascent (depressurization) allows the dissolved gases to expand and bubble out of solution to form gas emboli.

- Formation of gas bubbles in skeletal muscles and joints causes painful *bends*. In lungs, edema, hemorrhage, and focal emphysema lead to respiratory distress, or *chokes*. Gas emboli may also cause focal ischemia in a number of tissues, including brain and heart.
- A more chronic form of decompression sickness is *caisson disease;* persistent gas emboli in poorly vascularized portions of the skeleton (heads of the femurs, tibia, and humeri) lead to ischemic necrosis.

Amniotic Fluid Embolism (p. 127)

Embolization of amniotic fluid into the maternal pulmonary circulation is a serious (mortality rate ~80%) but uncommon (1 in 40,000 deliveries) complication of labor and postpartum period. The syndrome is characterized by sudden severe dyspnea, cyanosis, and hypotensive shock, followed by seizures and coma. Pulmonary edema, *diffuse alveolar damage,* and DIC ensue from release of toxic (fatty acid) and thrombogenic substances in amniotic fluid. Classic histologic findings include fetal squamous cells, mucin, lanugo hair, and fat from vernix caseosa in the maternal pulmonary micro-circulation.

Infarction (p. 127)

An infarct is an area of ischemic necrosis caused by occlusion of either the arterial supply (97% of cases) or venous drainage in a particular tissue. Almost all infarcts result from thrombotic or embolic events; other causes include vasospasm; extrinsic compression of a vessel by tumor, edema, or entrapment in a hernia sac; and twisting of vessels, such as testicular torsion or bowel volvulus. Traumatic vessel rupture is a rare cause. Occluded venous drainage (e.g., venous thrombosis) most often induces congestion only since bypass channels rapidly open to provide outflow. Thus, infarcts due to venous thrombosis are more likely in organs with a single venous outflow (e.g., testis or ovary).

Morphology (p. 128)

Infarcts may be either *red (hemorrhagic)* or *white (pale, anemic)* and may be either *septic* or *bland.*

- Red infarcts occur in:

  Venous occlusions (e.g., ovarian torsion)
  Loose tissues (e.g., lung)
  Tissues with dual circulations (e.g., lung and small intestine)
  Tissues previously congested because of sluggish venous outflow
  Sites of previous occlusion and necrosis when flow is reestablished

- *White infarcts* occur in solid organs (e.g., heart, spleen, and kidney) with end-arterial circulations (i.e., few collaterals).
- All infarcts tend to be wedge-shaped; the occluded vessel marks the apex, and the organ periphery forms the base. Lateral margins may be irregular, reflecting the pattern of adjacent vascular supply.
- The dominant histologic feature of infarction in most tissues is *coagulative necrosis,* followed temporally by an inflammatory response (hours to days) and by a reparative response (days to weeks) beginning in the preserved margins. Most infarcts are ultimately replaced by scar tissue, although (depending on the tissue) some parenchymal regeneration may occur where the underlying stromal architecture is spared.
- Infarction in the central nervous system (CNS) results in *liquefactive necrosis.*
- Septic infarctions occur when infected heart valve vegetations embolize or when microbes seed an area of necrosis; the infarct becomes an *abscess.*

Factors that Influence Development of an Infarct (p. 129)

The outcomes of vascular occlusion can range from no effect to death of a tissue or person. Major determinants of outcome include:

- *Anatomic pattern of vascular supply* (i.e., availability of alternative supply): Dual circulations (i.e., lung, liver) or anastomosing circulations (i.e., radial and ulnar arteries, circle of Willis, small intestine) protect against infarction. Obstruction of end-arterial vessels generally causes infarction (i.e., spleen, kidneys).

- *Rate of occlusion development:* Slowly developing occlusions less often cause infarction by allowing time to develop alternative perfusion pathways (e.g., collateral coronary circulation).
- *Vulnerability to hypoxia:* Neurons undergo irreversible damage after 3 to 4 minutes of ischemia; myocardial cells die after only 20 to 30 minutes. In contrast, fibroblasts within ischemic myocardium are viable even after many hours.
- *Oxygen content of blood:* Anemia, cyanosis, or CHF (with hypoxia) can cause infarction in an otherwise inconsequential blockage.

Shock (p. 129)

Shock is systemic hypoperfusion resulting from reduction in either cardiac output or the effective circulating blood volume; the result is hypotension, followed by impaired tissue perfusion and cellular hypoxia. Shock is the final common pathway for many lethal events, including severe hemorrhage, extensive trauma, large myocardial infarction, massive PE, and sepsis.

Shock is grouped into three major categories:

- *Cardiogenic shock:* Low cardiac output due to outflow obstruction (i.e., PE) or myocardial pump failure (e.g., myocardial infarction, arrhythmia, or tamponade)
- *Hypovolemic shock:* Low cardiac output due to hemorrhage or fluid loss (e.g. burn)
- *Septic shock:* Results from vasodilation and peripheral blood pooling caused by microbial infection (and the host immune response); it has a complicated pathogenesis (see later)

Rarer causes of shock are *neurogenic,* with loss of vascular tone and peripheral pooling (anesthetic accident or spinal cord injury), and *anaphylactic,* with systemic vasodilation and increased vascular permeability (IgE-mediated hypersensitivity, Chapter 6).

Pathogenesis of Septic Shock (p. 129)

With a 20% mortality rate and 200,000 deaths annually in the United States, septic shock ranks first among the causes of death in intensive care units. The incidence is increasing as a result of improved life support for high-risk patients, increasing use of invasive procedures, and greater numbers of immunocompromised individuals.

- Septic shock can be caused by localized infection even without spread into the bloodstream. Most cases of septic shock are now caused by Gram-positive bacteria, followed by Gram-negative bacteria and fungi.
- Morbidity and mortality in sepsis are consequences of tissue hypoperfusion and multi-organ dysfunction despite initially preserved or even increased cardiac output. This is due to systemic vasodilation accompanied by widespread EC activation and injury, leading to a hypercoagulable state and DIC. There are also systemic metabolic changes that suppress normal cellular function.
- The pathogenesis of sepsis is a combination of direct microbial injury and activation, and host inflammatory responses:

  Inflammatory mediators: Microbial cell wall components activate leukocytes and EC via toll-like receptors and other receptors of innate immunity. Activation triggers release of inflammatory cytokines, prostaglandins, reactive oxygen species, and platelet activating factor. Coagulation and complement cascades are also directly activated, which can, in turn, drive additional inflammatory responses (Chapter 2).

Endothelial cell activation and injury: EC activation leads to an adhesive, procoagulant EC phenotype with markedly increased thrombotic tendencies (DIC in up to 50% of cases), as well as vasodilation and increased permeability.

Metabolic abnormalities: Insulin resistance and hyperglycemia are characteristic of the septic state, attributable to inflammatory cytokines and the early production of stress-induced hormones such as glucagon, growth hormone, and cortisol. With time, adrenal insufficiency may supervene.

Immune suppression: The hyperinflammatory state initiated by sepsis can activate potent counter-regulatory immunosuppressive mechanisms.

Organ dysfunction: Hypotension, edema, and small vessel thrombosis all reduce oxygen and nutrient delivery to tissues; the cellular metabolism in various tissues is also deranged due to insulin resistance. Myocardial contractility may be directly impacted, and endothelial damage underlies the development of *acute respiratory distress syndrome* (Chapter 15).

The severity and outcome of sepsis depends on the extent and virulence of the infection, the immune status of the host, other co-morbidities, and the pattern and level of host mediator production. Therapy involves antibiotics, insulin administration, fluid resuscitation, and adequate exogenous steroids to correct adrenal insufficiency; approaches blocking specific inflammatory mediators have not generally been successful.

Stages of Shock (p 132)

Shock is a progressive disorder often culminating in death. In *septic shock,* the patient's demise results from multi-organ failure (as outlined earlier). Unless the initial insult is massive and rapidly lethal (e.g., exsanguination), *hypovolemic* or *cardiogenic shock* tend to evolve through three phases:

• *Nonprogressive phase:* The phase during which reflex neurohumoral compensatory mechanisms are activated (catechols, sympathetic stimulation, ADH, renin-angiotensin axis, etc.) and perfusion of vital organs is maintained.

• *Progressive phase:* The phase characterized by tissue hypoperfusion and worsening circulatory and metabolic abnormalities including lactic acidosis due to anaerobic glycolysis. The acidosis also blunts the vasomotor response, causing vasodilation.

• *Irreversible phase:* The phase during which damage is so severe that, even if perfusion is restored, survival is not possible. Renal shutdown due to *acute tubular necrosis* (Chapter 20) and ischemic bowel leaking microbes into the bloodstream *(sepsis)* can be terminal events.

Morphology (p. 132)

Shock of any form causes nonspecific cell and tissue changes largely reflecting hypoxic injury; brain, heart, lungs, kidneys, adrenals, and gastrointestinal tract are particularly affected. The *kidneys* develop extensive tubular ischemic injury (*acute tubular necrosis,* Chapter 20), causing oliguria, anuria, and electrolyte disturbances. The *lungs* are seldom affected in pure hypovolemic shock; however, *diffuse alveolar damage* (*shock lung,* Chapter 15) can occur in septic or traumatic shock. Outside of neuron and myocyte loss, virtually all tissues can recover if the patient survives.

Clinical Consequences (p. 133)

Clinical consequences depend on the precipitating insult:

- In hypovolemic and cardiogenic shock, there is hypotension with a weak, rapid pulse; tachypnea; and cool, clammy, cyanotic skin. In septic shock, the skin may initially be warm and flushed owing to peripheral vasodilation.
- Cardiac, cerebral, and pulmonary changes secondary to the shock state worsen the situation.
- Patients surviving the initial complications enter *a second phase dominated by renal insufficiency* and marked by a progressive fall in urine output, as well as severe fluid and electrolyte imbalances.
- Prognosis varies with the origin and duration of shock. Thus, 90% of young, otherwise healthy patients with hypovolemic shock survive with appropriate management, whereas cardiogenic or septic shock carry markedly worse mortality rates.

5

Genetic Disorders

Human Genetic Architecture (p. 136)

Human genome sequencing has provided some startling insights:

- Coding sequences constitute less than 2% of the total genome, while greater than 50% of the genome represents blocks of repetitive nucleotides of uncertain function.
- The genome contains only 20,000 to 25,000 genes that code for proteins, although alternative splicing can generate more than 100,000 proteins.
- On average, any two individuals share 99.5% of their DNA sequences, so that the remarkable diversity of humanity (and the basis of genetic diseases) rests in less than 0.5% of the DNA (or roughly 15 million base pairs).
- The most common forms of genetic variation are *single nucleotide polymorphism (SNP)* and *copy number variation (CNV)*.

  SNPs represent variations at single nucleotides and are mostly biallelic (i.e., only one of two nucleotide choices). More than 6 million SNPs have been identified in the human genome, but less than 1% occur in coding regions. Thus, although SNPs may have significance in causing disease, most are probably only markers co-inherited with the *authentic* genetic disease locus.

  CNVs represent variations in the numbers of large contiguous stretches of DNA from 1000 base pairs to millions of base pairs. While some CNVs are biallelic, others have multiple different variants in the population. CNVs account for 5 to 24 million base pairs of sequence difference between any two individuals; roughly 50% involve gene-coding sequences and may thus form much of the basis of phenotypic diversity.

Instead of focusing narrowly on individual genes, the completed human genome sequence allows *genomic* analysis—the study of *all* genes and their interactions. Genomics promises to help unravel complex multigenic diseases; DNA microarray analysis of tumors (Chapter 7) is but one example. However, alterations in primary sequence cannot alone explain human genetic diversity. Thus *epigenetics*—heritable changes in gene expression that are not caused by specific DNA sequences—are involved in tissue-specific expression of genes and genetic *imprinting* (see later discussion).

Beyond genomics, *proteomics*—the analysis of all the proteins expressed in a cell—is providing additional pathogenic insights. The ability to analyze all the patterns of genetic and protein expression is the province of computer-based *bioinformatics*.

It is also increasingly appreciated that genes that do not code for proteins can have important regulatory functions. Thus small RNA molecules, called *microRNAs (miRNAs)*, inhibit gene expression;

there are approximately 1000 miRNA genes in the human genome (5% of the total genome). Transcripts from these miRNA genes are processed in the cytoplasm to yield mature oligomers that are 21 to 30 nucleotides in length. Subsequent interactions between the processed miRNA, target messenger RNA (mRNA), and the RNA-induced silencing complex (RISC) leads to mRNA cleavage or represses its translation. The same pathway can be exploited therapeutically by the introduction of exogenous *small, interfering RNAs (siRNAs)* targeted to specific mRNA species (e.g., oncogenes).

Genes and Human Diseases (p. 137)

Genetic disorders are extremely common, with an estimated lifetime frequency of 67%; this includes not only "classic" genetic disorders but also cancer and cardiovascular diseases with complex multigenic contributions. If one counts all conceptuses, the actual frequency is probably greater, since 50% of early spontaneous abortions have a demonstrable chromosomal abnormality; the vast majority of genetic disorders do not result in a viable birth. Even so, approximately 1% of newborns have a gross chromosomal abnormality, and 5% of individuals younger than 25 years have a serious disease with a significant genetic component.

Causes of genetic disorders can be classified as follows:

- *Mutations in single genes:* These are usually *highly penetrant* (i.e., mutation typically results in disease) and follow classical Mendelian inheritance patterns.
- *Chromosomal (cytogenetic) disorders:* These arise from structural (e.g., breaks) or numerical alterations in chromosomes; they are usually highly penetrant.
- *Multigenic disorders:* These are the most common cause of genetic disorders and are caused by the complex interactions of multiple *variant* (not mutant) forms of genes *(polymorphisms)* and environmental factors. Independently, each polymorphism has only a small effect and is of low penetrance. Progress in genomics and bioinformatics has allowed *genome-wide association studies (GWAS)* to begin to identify the various genetic risk factors and contributions.

Mutations (p. 138)

A mutation is a permanent change in the DNA. Mutations in germ cells are transmitted to progeny (and cause heritable disease) while mutations in somatic cells are not transmissible but can affect cell behavior (e.g., malignant transformation). Mutations can involve changes in coding or non-coding regions of the genome. In addition, mutations can affect just one or a few nucleotides, or they can cause complete deletion of a gene.

- Point mutations in coding sequences

  Missense mutation: Single nucleotide substitutions can change the triplet base code and yield a different amino acid in the final protein product. This can be a *conservative* mutation if the new amino acid is not significantly different from the original, with minimal (if any) consequences. However, *nonconservative* mutations (e.g., substituting amino acids of different size or charge) can lead to loss of function, misfolding and degradation of the protein, or gain of function.

  Nonsense mutation: Single nucleotide substitutions can potentially result in the formation of an inappropriate "stop" codon; the resulting protein may then be truncated with loss of normal activity.

- Mutations within noncoding regions

  Point mutations or deletions in enhancer or promoter regions can significantly affect the regulation or level of gene transcription. Point mutations can lead to defective splicing and thus failure to form mature mRNA species.

- Frameshift mutations

  Loss of one or more nucleotides can alter the reading frame of the DNA. Insertions or deletions of multiples of three nucleotides may have no effect other than adding or deleting an amino acid. Frameshifts of other numbers of nucleotides lead to defective protein products (missense or nonsense).

- Trinucleotide repeat mutations

  This special category of mutations is characterized by amplification of triple-nucleotide sequences (e.g., fragile X syndrome or Huntington disease). Trinucleotide repeats are a common feature of many normal genetic sequences; however, mutations involving these repeats can see a 10-fold to 200-fold amplification of the normal number, leading to abnormal gene expression. This type of mutation is also dynamic, with the length of the trinucleotide repeat sequences frequently expanding during gametogenesis.

Mendelian Disorders (p. 140)

Mendelian disorders result from mutations in single genes that have a large effect. Every individual is a carrier of between five and eight potentially deleterious mutations; 80% are inherited (*familial*) while the remainder represent *de novo* mutations.

- Whether a given mutation will have an adverse outcome is influenced by compensatory genes and environmental factors.
- Some autosomal mutations produce partial expression in heterozygotes and full expression only in homozygotes (e.g., sickle cell disease).
- Mendelian traits can be dominant, recessive, or *codominant*, the latter referring to full expression of both alleles in a heterozygote.
- *Penetrance* refers to the percentage of individuals who carry a particular gene and also express the trait.
- *Variable expressivity* refers to variation in the effect caused by a particular mutation; thus manifestations of neurofibromatosis type I range from brown macules to skin tumors to skeletal deformities.
- *Pleiotropism* refers to multiple possible end effects of a single mutant gene; thus, in sickle cell disease, the mutant hemoglobin causes hemolysis and anemia, as well as vascular occlusion leading to splenic infarction and bone necrosis.
- *Genetic heterogeneity* refers to multiple different mutations leading to the same outcome; thus, different autosomal recessive mutations can cause childhood deafness.

Transmission Patterns of Single-Gene Disorders (p. 140)

Autosomal Dominant Disorders (p. 140)

Autosomal dominant disorders manifest in the heterozygous state and have the following general features:

- Disease is usually also present in a parent. When both parents of an affected individual are normal, a *de novo* germ cell mutation is suggested; this happens more commonly in the sperm of older fathers.

- Clinical features are modified by penetrance and expressivity.
- Clinical onset is often later than in autosomal recessive disorders.
- Most autosomal dominant mutations are *loss-of-function*, that is, they result in either reduced production of a gene product or reduced activity of a protein.

  Mutations in a key structural protein (e.g., collagen), especially if the mutation is part of a multimer, can interfere with the function of the normal gene product (i.e., by affecting folding), thereby leading to *dominant negative* effects.
  Mutations of components in complex metabolic pathways subject to feedback inhibition (e.g., the low-density lipoprotein receptor) are often autosomal dominant.
  Mutations in enzymes are usually not autosomal dominant since even loss of 50% activity can be compensated.

- *Gain-of-function* autosomal dominant mutations are less common; they cause disease by endowing a gene product with toxic properties or by increasing a normal activity.

Autosomal Recessive Disorders (p. 141)

Autosomal recessive disorders include most inborn errors of metabolism. In contrast to autosomal dominant disorders, the following features generally apply:

- The expression of the disease features tends to be more uniform.
- Complete penetrance is common.
- Onset is frequently early in life.
- *De novo* mutations are rarely detected clinically until several generations have passed and a heterozygote-heterozygote mating has occurred.
- Enzymes, rather than structural proteins, are more commonly affected.

X-Linked Disorders (p. 142)

All sex-linked disorders are X-linked and most are recessive. They are fully expressed in males, because mutant genes on the X chromosome do not have a Y chromosome counterpart (affected males are *hemizygous* for the X-linked mutant gene). Heterozygote females usually do not express the disease due to a paired normal X allele; however, random X inactivation in a population of cells can lead to a variable phenotype. X-linked dominant conditions are rare; affected women express the disease and transmit it to 50% of their sons *and* daughters, while affected men express the disease and transmit it to 100% of their daughters and none of their sons.

Biochemical and Molecular Basis of Single-Gene (Mendelian) Disorders (p. 142)

Enzyme Defects and Their Consequences (p. 143)

Mutations can result in the synthesis of a defective enzyme (reduced activity) or reduced synthesis of a normal enzyme. The outcome is a metabolic block with:

- Accumulation of a substrate that is toxic (e.g., phenylalanine in *phenylketonuria*)
- Decreased amount of an end product necessary for normal function (e.g., melanin in *albinism*)
- Decreased metabolism of a tissue-damaging substrate (e.g., neutrophil elastase in α_1-*antitrypsin deficiency*)

Defects in Receptors and Transport Systems (p. 144)

Defects can affect the intracellular accumulation of an important precursor (e.g., low-density lipoprotein in *familial hypercholesterolemia*) or export of a metabolite necessary for normal tissue homeostasis (e.g., chloride in *cystic fibrosis*).

Alterations in Structure, Function, or Quantity of Nonenzyme Proteins (p. 144)

Examples include the hemoglobinopathies (e.g., sickle cell disease, thalassemia) or *osteogenesis imperfecta* due to defective collagen.

Genetically Determined Adverse Reactions to Drugs (p. 144)

These otherwise clinically silent mutations are unmasked when specific compounds and/or substrates are administered that lead to toxic intermediates or cannot be appropriately catabolized.

Disorders Associated with Defects in Structural Proteins (p. 144)

Marfan Syndrome (p. 144)

Marfan syndrome is an autosomal dominant disorder resulting from 1 of 600 different (mostly missense) mutations in the *fibrillin-1* gene mapping to 15q21.1. Fibrillin is a glycoprotein component of microfibrils that provides a scaffold for the deposition of elastin; it is especially abundant in the connective tissues of the aorta, ligaments, and ciliary zonules that support the eye lens. The disorder, therefore, mostly affects the *skeletal, ocular,* and *cardiovascular systems.* Abnormal fibrillin results in defective microfibril assembly, resulting in reduced elasticity, as well as reduced sequestration of transforming growth factor-β (TGF-β); excess TGF-β reduces normal vascular smooth muscle development and matrix production.

Morphology (p. 145)

Skeletal changes:

- Tall stature with exceptionally long extremities
- Long, tapering fingers and toes (*arachnodactyly*)
- Laxity of joint ligaments, producing hyperextensibility
- *Dolichocephaly* (long head) with frontal bossing and prominent supraorbital ridges
- Spinal deformities (e.g., kyphosis and scoliosis)

Ocular changes:

- Bilateral dislocation of lenses (ectopia lentis)
- Increased axial length of the globe, giving rise to retinal detachments

Cardiovascular lesions:

- Mitral valve prolapse
- Aortic cystic medial degeneration causing aortic ring dilation and valvular incompetence. This is likely exacerbated by the excess TGF-β signaling.

Cutaneous changes:

- Striae

Clinical Features (p. 145)

There is great variability in the clinical expression, so that clinical diagnosis requires major involvement of two out of four systems (cardiovascular, skeletal, ocular, and cutaneous) and minor involvement of one other. Mitral valve prolapse is most common, although not life-threatening; affected valves are floppy, associated with mitral regurgitation. Cystic medial degeneration of the aorta is less common but clinically more important; the medial degeneration predisposes to medial dissections, often resulting in aortic rupture, a cause of death in 30% to 45% of affected patients.

Ehlers-Danlos Syndromes *(p. 145)*

Ehlers-Danlos syndromes (EDS) are a clinically and genetically heterogeneous group of disorders caused by *defects in collagen synthesis.* Major manifestations involve:

* *Skin:* Hyperextensible, extremely fragile, and vulnerable to trauma; wound healing is markedly impaired owing to defective collagen synthesis
* *Joints:* Hypermobile and prone to dislocation
* *Visceral complications:* Manifestations include rupture of the colon and large arteries, ocular fragility with corneal rupture and retinal detachment, and diaphragmatic hernias

EDS is divided into six variants on the basis of the predominant clinical manifestations and patterns of inheritance (Table 5-1):

* Reduced activity of lysyl hydroxylase, an enzyme essential for collagen cross-linking (type VI), is autosomal recessive.
* Mutations in type III collagen: Since a structural rather than an enzyme protein is affected, the pattern of inheritance is autosomal dominant. Blood vessels and intestines are especially rich in collagen type III and are therefore most susceptible.

TABLE 5-1 Classification of Ehlers-Danlos Syndromes (EDS)

EDS Type*	Clinical Findings	Inheritance	Gene Defects
Classical (I/II)	Skin and joint hypermobility, atrophic scars, easy bruising	Autosomal dominant	*COL5A1, COL5A2*
Hypermobility (III)	Joint hypermobility, pain, dislocations	Autosomal dominant	Unknown
Vascular (IV)	Thin skin, arterial or uterine rupture, bruising, small joint hyperextensibility	Autosomal dominant	*COL3A1*
Kyphoscoliosis (VI)	Hypotonia, joint laxity, congenital scoliosis, ocular fragility	Autosomal recessive	Lysyl-hydroxylase
Arthrochalasia (VIIa,b)	Severe joint hypermobility, skin changes mild, scoliosis, bruising	Autosomal dominant	*COL1A1, COL1A2*
Dermatosparaxis (VIIc)	Severe skin fragility, cutis laxa, bruising	Autosomal recessive	Procollagen *N*-peptidase

*EDS were previously classified by Roman numerals. Parentheses show previous numerical equivalents.

- Mutant procollagen chains that resist cleavage of *N*-terminal peptides, and thus result in defective conversion of type I procollagen to mature collagen: This mutation has a *dominant-negative* effect.

Disorders Associated with Defects in Receptor Proteins (p. 147)

Familial Hypercholesterolemia *(p. 147)*

Familial hypercholesterolemia results from mutations in the gene encoding the receptor for low-density lipoprotein (LDL). Mutations affecting other aspects of LDL uptake, metabolism, and regulation can cause a similar phenotype.

Normal Cholesterol Transport and Metabolism
(p. 147) (Figure 5-1)

- LDL is the major transport form of cholesterol in plasma.
- Although most cells possess high-affinity receptors for LDL apoprotein B-100, 70% of plasma LDL is cleared by the liver; uptake by other cells, especially mononuclear phagocytes, can occur through distinct *scavenger* receptors for chemically altered LDL (e.g., acetylated or oxidized).

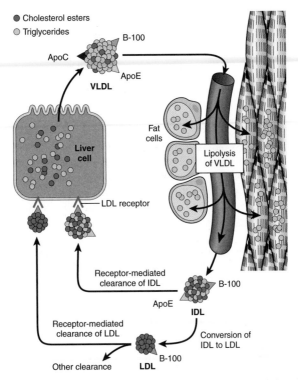

FIGURE 5-1 Schematic illustration of low-density lipoprotein *(LDL)* metabolism and the role of the liver in its synthesis and clearance. Lipolysis of very-low-density lipoprotein *(VLDL)* by lipoprotein lipase in the capillaries releases triglycerides that are then stored in fat cells and used as a source of energy in skeletal muscles. *ApoE,* Apoprotein E; *IDL,* intermediate density lipoprotein.

- The transport and metabolism of LDL in the liver involves:

  Binding to specific LDL plasma membrane receptors
  Internalization and subsequent dissociation from its receptor in the early endosome, followed by transport to lysosomes
  Lysosomal processing, leading to release of free cholesterol into cytoplasm through the action of NPC1 and 2 proteins (defects result in Niemann-Pick disease, type C [NPC])

- Free cholesterol affects three processes:

  Suppresses cholesterol synthesis by inhibiting the rate-limiting enzyme hydroxymethylglutaryl coenzyme A reductase
  Activates enzymes that esterify cholesterol
  Suppresses LDL receptor synthesis, thereby limiting further cholesterol uptake

Without intracellular cholesterol feedback inhibition of these processes, total circulating cholesterol levels increase. Heterozygotes occur at a frequency of roughly 1 in 500 in the general population and have two- to three-fold elevated cholesterol levels, homozygotes have five- to six-fold cholesterol elevations, with early onset of severe atherosclerosis and the possibility of cardiovascular events (e.g., myocardial infarction) before age 20 years. Xanthomas of the skin are also more prominent.

The various LDL receptor mutations fall into five general classes:

- *Class I:* Inadequate LDL receptor protein synthesis (rare)
- *Class II:* Abnormal LDL receptor folding leading to retention in the endoplasmic reticulum (common)
- *Class III:* Reduced binding capacity of LDL receptor protein
- *Class IV:* Inability of LDL receptor to internalize
- *Class V:* Inability of LDL and receptor to dissociate, with recycling to the cell surface

Disorders Associated with Defects in Enzymes (p. 149)

Lysosomal Storage Diseases (p. 149)

Lysosomal storage diseases result from a genetic deficiency of functional lysosomal enzymes or other proteins essential for their activity. Mutations can also affect the targeting of lysosomal enzymes after their synthesis in the endoplasmic reticulum (enzymes destined for the lysosome are tagged by appending a terminal mannose-6-phosphate residue during transit through the Golgi apparatus). In the absence of adequate lysosomal processing, catabolism of complex substrates is impaired, leading to accumulation of partially degraded metabolites within lysosomes. The lysosomes, enlarged with undigested macromolecules, can interfere with normal cell function; there is also deficient recycling of constituent nutrients.

Therapeutic approaches include:

- Enzyme replacement
- Substrate reduction
- Molecular "chaperones" to assist in the normal folding of mutant proteins

Lysosomal storage diseases are classified on the basis of the biochemical nature of the accumulated metabolite (Table 5-2). The tissues affected and the resultant clinical features depend on where the material to be degraded is normally located and in which sites it is typically catabolized. Since macrophages are particularly rich in lysosomes and are responsible for degradation of several

TABLE 5-2 Lysosomal Storage Diseases

Disease	Enzyme Deficiency	Major Accumulating Metabolites
Glycogenosis		
Type 2—Pompe disease	α-1,4-Glucosidase (lysosomal glucosidase)	Glycogen
Sphingolipidoses		
G_{M1} gangliosidosis Type 1—infantile, generalized Type 2—juvenile	G_{M1} ganglioside β-galactosidase	G_{M1} ganglioside, galactose-containing oligosaccharides
G_{M2} gangliosidosis Tay-Sachs disease Sandhoff disease G_{M2} gangliosidosis, variant AB	Hexosaminidase-α subunit Hexosaminidase-β subunit Ganglioside activator protein	G_{M2} ganglioside G_{M2} ganglioside, globoside G_{M2} ganglioside
Sulfatidoses		
Metachromatic leukodystrophy	Arylsulfatase A	Sulfatide
Multiple sulfatase deficiency	Arylsulfatases A, B, C; steroid sulfatase; iduronate sulfatase; heparan N-sulfatase	Sulfatide, steroid sulfate, heparan sulfate, dermatan sulfate
Krabbe disease	Galactosylceramidase	Galactocerebroside
Fabry disease	α-Galactosidase A	Ceramide trihexoside

Gaucher disease	Glucocerebrosidase	Glucocerebroside
Niemann-Pick disease: types A and B	Sphingomyelinase	Sphingomyelin
Mucopolysaccharidoses (MPS)		
MPS I H (Hurler)	α-L-Iduronidase	Dermatan sulfate, heparan sulfate
MPS II (Hunter)	L-Iduronosulfate sulfatase	
Mucolipidoses (ML)		
I-cell disease (ML II) and pseudo-Hurler polydystrophy	Deficiency of phosphorylating enzymes essential for the formation of mannose-6-phosphate recognition marker; acid hydrolases lacking the recognition marker cannot be targeted to the lysosomes but are secreted extracellularly	Mucopolysaccharide, glycolipid
Other Diseases of Complex Carbohydrates		
Fucosidosis	α-Fucosidase	Fucose-containing sphingolipids and glycoprotein fragments
Mannosidosis	α-Mannosidase	Mannose-containing oligosaccharides
Aspartylglycosaminuria	Aspartylglycosamine amide hydrolase	Aspartyl-2-deoxy-2-acetamido-glycosylamine
Other Lysosomal Storage Diseases		
Wolman disease	Acid lipase	Cholesterol esters, triglycerides
Acid phosphate deficiency	Lysosomal acid phosphatase	Phosphate esters

substrates, organs with abundant macrophages (e.g., liver and spleen) are often affected.

TAY-SACHS DISEASE (p. 150)

Tay-Sachs disease results from mutations in the α-subunit of the hexosaminidase enzyme complex; it is the most common of the three G_{M2}-gangliosidoses resulting from lysosomal G_{M2}-ganglioside accumulation (all have similar clinical outcomes). It is most common in Jews of Eastern European (i.e., Ashkenazic) origin. Antenatal diagnosis and carrier detection are possible by DNA probe analysis and enzyme assays on cells obtained from amniocentesis.

- Because neurons are rich in gangliosides, they are the cell type most severely affected; thus typical clinical features are motor and mental deterioration commencing at about 6 months of age and blindness and death by age 2 to 3 years.

Morphology (p. 151)

- Neuronal ballooning with lipid-filled cytoplasmic vacuoles
- Progressive neuronal destruction with microglial proliferation
- Accumulation of lipids in retinal ganglion cells, rendering them pale in color, thus accentuating the normal red color of the macular choroid (*cherry-red spot*)

NIEMANN-PICK DISEASES, TYPES A AND B (p. 152)

Niemann-Pick diseases, types A and B, are related disorders associated with sphingomyelinase deficiency (more than 100 mutations are described). Sphingomyelin accumulation is most prominent in mononuclear phagocytes, but it can also affect neurons. Like Tay-Sachs, these disorders are common in Ashkenazic Jews. Acid sphingomyelinase is an *imprinted* gene (see later) that is preferentially expressed from the maternal chromosome due to paternal gene epigenetic silencing.

Type A is more common. It is a severe infantile form of the disease that is clinically manifest at birth. Death typically occurs within 3 years. Affected cells are engorged with numerous small vacuoles that impart cytoplasmic foaminess.

- Diffuse neuronal involvement, leading eventually to cell death and central nervous system (CNS) atrophy; a retinal, cherry-red spot similar to that seen in Tay-Sachs occurs in roughly half the patients
- Extreme accumulation of lipids in mononuclear phagocytes, yielding massive hepatosplenomegaly and lymphadenopathy, with bone marrow infiltration
- Visceral involvement mainly affecting the gastrointestinal tract and lungs

Type B is associated with organomegaly but not CNS involvement, and patients typically survive into adulthood.

NIEMANN-PICK DISEASE, TYPE C (p. 153)

NPC is distinct from types A and B and is more common than both types combined. It is due to mutations in either *NPC1* (95% of cases) or *NPC2*, coding for proteins involved in cholesterol transport from lysosomes to the cytosol. Cholesterol and gangliosides are both accumulated, and patients can present with hydrops fetalis, neonatal hepatitis, or (most commonly) progressive neurologic degeneration beginning in childhood with ataxia, dystonia, and psychomotor regression.

GAUCHER DISEASE (p. 153)

Gaucher disease refers to a cluster of autosomal recessive disorders involving mutations leading to diminished glucocerebrosidase activity. Cleavage of ceramide (derived from cell membranes of senescent leukocytes and red blood cells as well as from turnover of brain gangliosides) is impaired. Glucocerebroside accumulation occurs in mononuclear phagocytes and, in some forms, the CNS. Disease manifestations are secondary to the burden of stored material, as well as macrophage activation and local cytokine production. Three variants are identified:

- *Type I* is the most common form (99% of cases) and occurs in adults with a higher incidence in European Jews; there are reduced, but detectable, levels of enzyme activity. This chronic, *non-neuronopathic* form is associated with glucocerebroside storage in mononuclear phagocytes. Although there is no brain involvement, patients have massive splenomegaly and lymphadenopathy, and marrow involvement leads to bone erosions that can cause pathologic fractures. Pancytopenia or thrombocytopenia results from hypersplenism; the life span is not markedly affected.
- *Type II* is the *acute neuronopathic form,* affecting infants but without a Jewish predilection. It is associated with hepatosplenomegaly, but progressive CNS deterioration predominates with death at a young age.
- *Type III* is intermediate with systemic involvement of macrophages, as well as progressive neurologic disease beginning in adolescence.

Morphology (p.153)

Affected cells (i.e., Gaucher cells) are distended with periodic acid–Schiff (PAS)-positive material with a fibrillary appearance resembling "crumpled tissue paper" (composed of elongated lysosomes containing stored lipid in bilayer stacks).

Clinical Features (p.154)

Prenatal diagnosis is possible by enzyme assay of amniotic fluid or by DNA probe analysis, although there are more than 150 known mutations. Replacement therapy with recombinant enzymes is effective but expensive; bone marrow transplant and/or gene transfer into bone marrow cells, as well as substrate reduction therapy, is being evaluated.

MUCOPOLYSACCHARIDOSES (p. 154)

Mucopolysaccharidoses (MPS) are a group of disorders resulting from inherited deficiencies of enzymes that degrade glycosaminoglycans (abundant in the extracellular matrix of connective tissues). Accumulated substrates include heparan sulfate, dermatan sulfate, keratan sulfate, and chondroitin sulfate.

Several MPS clinical variants (numbered I to VII) are known, each resulting from the deficiency of one specific enzyme. All are autosomal recessive except MPS II *(Hunter disease),* which is X-linked recessive. Severity relates to the degree of enzyme deficiency. In general, all forms are progressive and are characterized by:

- Coarse facial features
- Hepatosplenomegaly
- Corneal clouding
- Valve and subendothelial arterial thickening
- Joint stiffness
- Mental retardation

Morphology (p.154)

Affected cells are distended with clear cytoplasm (balloon cells) containing PAS-positive material. Accumulated mucopolysaccharides are found in many cell types, including mononuclear phagocytes, fibroblasts, endothelial cells, intimal smooth muscle cells, and neurons.

Clinical Features (p. 155)

The two most well-characterized syndromes are:

- *Hurler syndrome (MPS 1-H)* due to α-1-iduronidase deficiency is a severe form with onset at 6 to 24 months and death by the ages of 6 to 10 years, usually due to cardiovascular complications.
- *Hunter syndrome (MPS II)* is a syndrome lacking corneal opacification and with a generally milder course than Hurler syndrome.

Glycogen Storage Diseases (Glycogenoses) (p. 155)

Glycogen storage diseases result from hereditary deficiencies in the synthesis or catabolism of glycogen (Fig. 5-2); disorders may be restricted to specific tissues or can be systemic. On the basis of

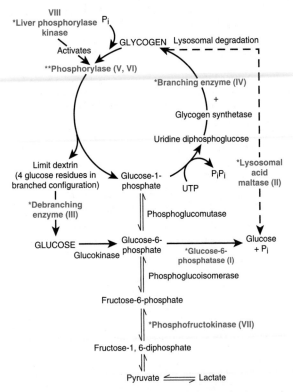

FIGURE 5-2 Glycogen metabolic pathways and the associated enzymatic deficiencies *(marked with *)* leading to glycogenoses; roman numerals indicate the type of glycogen storage disease. **Types V and VI result from muscle and liver phosphorylase deficiencies, respectively. P_i, Protease inhibitor; *UTP*, uridine triphosphate. *(Modified from Hers H, et al.: Glycogen storage diseases. In Scriver CR, et al. [eds]: The metabolic basis of inherited diseases, ed 6, New York, 1989, McGraw-Hill, p. 425.)*

specific enzymatic deficiencies and resultant clinical pictures, the glycogenoses are divided into three major groups:

- *Hepatic form* is due to deficiencies in enzymes that primarily influence liver glycogen catabolism; these are characterized by low blood glucose (hypoglycemia) and hepatic glycogen accumulation. The prototype is von Gierke disease (type I) due to glucose-6-phosphatase deficiency, which converts glucose 6-phosphate to glucose; others include deficiencies in liver phosphorylase or debranching enzyme (see Fig. 5-2).
- *Myopathic form* is characterized by deficiencies of enzymes that fuel glycolysis in striated muscles. These characteristically present with muscle weakness and cramping after exercise without exercise-induced rises in blood lactate; skeletal muscles show glycogen accumulation. McArdle disease (type V) is due to deficient muscle phosphorylase.
- *Miscellaneous forms* are associated with α-glucosidase deficiency (acid maltase) or lack of branching enzyme; typically these lead to glycogen overload in many organs and early death. Type II glycogenosis, or Pompe disease, results from deficiency of the lysosomal enzyme acid maltase (α-glucosidase). As in other lysosomal storage diseases, many organs are involved; however, cardiac involvement is most prominent in this disorder.

Alkaptonuria (Ochronosis) (p. 155)

In this autosomal recessive disease, lack of homogentisic oxidase blocks the metabolism of phenylalanine, leading to homogentisic acid accumulation. Excessive homogentisic acid leads to:

- Urinary excretion, imparting a black color if allowed to stand.
- *Ochronosis*, a blue-black pigmentation of the ears, nose, and cheeks resulting from binding of homogentisic acid to connective tissue.
- Arthropathy associated with deposition in articular cartilage; affected cartilage (typically vertebral column, knee, shoulders, and hips) loses resilience and is readily eroded.

Disorders Associated with Defects in Proteins that Regulate Cell Growth (p. 157)

Normal cellular growth and differentiation is regulated by proteins deriving from proto-oncogenes and tumor suppressor genes. Mutations in these genes are important in tumor pathogenesis (Chapter 7); nevertheless, only some 5% of all cancers are due to germ-line mutations (most are autosomal dominant), and the vast majority of cancer-associated mutations in these genes occur *de novo* in somatic cells.

Complex Multigenic Disorders (p. 157)

Such disorders result from the interplay of variant forms of genes and environmental factors. Genetic variants with at least two different alleles and an incidence in the population ≥ 1% are called *polymorphisms*. Complex genetic disorders occur when several polymorphisms—individually with modest effects and low penetrance—are inherited together. Not all polymorphisms are equally important; although 20 to 30 genes are implicated in type I diabetes, 6 to 7 are most important, and certain HLA alleles make up more than 50% of the risk. Some polymorphisms are disease specific, while others crop up in multiple mechanistically related diseases (i.e., immune-mediated disorders). Moreover, environmental influences significantly modify the risk of expression; hence the concordance rate—even in identical twins—is only 20% to 40%.

Chromosomal Disorders (p. 158)

Cytogenetic disorders may be due to alterations in the *number* or in the *structure* of chromosomes. Karyotypes are given as total number of chromosomes, followed by the sex chromosome complement, and then abnormalities in ascending numerical order (e.g., a male with trisomy 21 is designated: 47,XY,+21).

Numerical Disorders

* *Monosomy,* associated with one less normal chromosome
* *Trisomy,* associated with one extra chromosome
* *Mosaicism,* associated with one or more populations of cells, some with normal chromosomal complement, others with extra or missing chromosomes

Numerical disorders of chromosomes result from errors during cell division. Monosomy and trisomy usually result from chromosomal nondisjunction during gametogenesis (the first meiotic division), whereas mosaics are produced when mitotic errors occur in the zygote. Monosomy of autosomes usually results in early fetal death and spontaneous abortion, whereas trisomies can be better tolerated, and similar imbalances in sex chromosomes are usually compatible with life.

Structural Aberrations (Fig. 5-3)

* *Deletion:* Loss of a terminal or interstitial (midpiece) segment of a chromosome
* *Translocation:* Involves transfer of a segment of one chromosome to another:

    Balanced reciprocal involves exchange of chromosomal material between two chromosomes with no net gain or loss of genetic material.

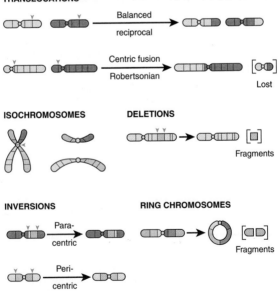

FIGURE 5-3 Types of chromosomal rearrangements.

Robertsonian (centric) fusion, or reciprocal translocation between two acrocentric chromosomes involves the short arm of one and the long arm of the other. The transfer of segments leads to formation of one abnormally large chromosome and one extremely small one. The latter is usually lost. This translocation predisposes to the formation of abnormal (unbalanced) gametes.

- *Isochromosome:* Formed when one arm (short or long) is lost and the remaining arm is duplicated, resulting in a chromosome of two short arms only or of two long arms; in live births, the most common isochromosome involves the X chromosome and is designated i(X)(q10) with resulting duplication (and thus trisomy) of genes on the long arm and deletion (with monosomy) for genes on the short arm
- *Inversion:* Rearrangement associated with two breaks in a chromosome, followed by inversion and reincorporation of the broken segment
- *Ring chromosome:* Deletion affecting both ends followed by fusion of the damaged ends

Cytogenetic Disorders Involving Autosomes (p. 161)

Trisomy 21 (Down Syndrome) (p. 161)

This is the most common chromosomal disorder (1 in 700 births) and a major cause of mental retardation.

- About 95% have a complete extra chromosome 21 (47,XY,+21). In 95% of these cases, the extra chromosome is maternal in origin. The incidence is strongly influenced by maternal age: 1 in 1550 births in women younger than 20 years; 1 in 25 births in women older than 45 years.
- Approximately 4% of all cases have extra chromosomal material derived from a parental chromosome bearing a translocation of the long arm of chromosome 21 to chromosome 22 or 14. Because the fertilized ovum already possesses two normal autosomes 21, the translocated chromosomal fragment provides the same triple-gene dosage as trisomy 21. Such cases are frequently (but not always) familial, because the parent is a carrier of a Robertsonian translocation. Maternal age has no impact.
- Mosaic variants make up about 1% of all cases; they have a mixture of cells with normal chromosome numbers and cells with an extra chromosome 21. Maternal age has no impact.
- Clinical features include:

  Flat facies with oblique palpebral fissures and epicanthic folds; simian hand creases

  Severe mental retardation

  40% have congenital heart disease, especially endocardial cushion defects, responsible for the majority of deaths in infancy and childhood

  10- to 20-fold increased risk of acute leukemia

  Abnormal immune responses leading to recurrent infections and thyroid autoimmunity

  Premature Alzheimer disease (AD)

  Duodenal Atresia, Anular Pancreas

Other Trisomies (p. 162)

Trisomy 18 *(Edwards syndrome)* and trisomy 13 *(Patau syndrome)* occur much less commonly than trisomy 21; both are associated with increased maternal age. Affected infants have severe malformations and usually die within the first year of life (Fig. 5-4).

Chromosome 22q11.2 Deletion Syndrome (p. 162)

Chromosome 22q11.2 deletion syndrome is fairly common (1 in 4000 births) and is due to a small deletion of band 11.2 on the long arm of chromosome 22. The clinical features associated with this deletion (below) constitute a spectrum that includes *DiGeorge syndrome* (Chapter 6) and *velocardiofacial syndrome*. T-cell immunodeficiency and hypocalcemia are more prominent in some cases (DiGeorge syndrome), whereas facial dysmorphology and cardiac malformations are more prominent in others (velocardiofacial syndrome):

- Congenital heart defects
- Abnormalities of palate
- Facial dysmorphism
- Developmental delay
- Increased incidence of psychiatric disorders (schizophrenia, bipolar, attention deficit hyperactivity disorder)
- Variable T-cell deficiency
- Hypoparathyroidism

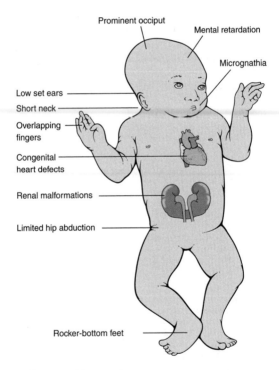

TRISOMY 18: EDWARDS SYNDROME

Incidence: 1 in 8000 births
  Karyotypes:
    Trisomy 18 type: 47,XX, +18
    Mosaic type: 46,XX/47,XX, +18

A

FIGURE 5-4 Clinical features and karyotypes of trisomy 18 (**A**) and trisomy 13 (**B**).

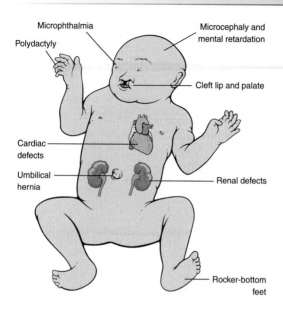

Microphthalmia

Polydactyly

Microcephaly and mental retardation

Cleft lip and palate

Cardiac defects

Umbilical hernia

Renal defects

Rocker-bottom feet

TRISOMY 13: PATAU SYNDROME

Incidence: 1 in 15,000 births
    Karyotypes:
        Trisomy 13 type: 47,XX, +13
        Translocation type: 46,XX,+13,der(13;14)(q10;q10)
        Mosaic type: 46,XX/47,XX, +13

B

FIGURE 5-4, cont'd

Cytogenetic Disorders Involving Sex Chromosomes (p. 164)

Imbalances in sex chromosomes are more common than autosomal imbalances, because they are typically better tolerated. The milder nature of X chromosome–associated aberrations, for example, is related to the fact that there is normally random inactivation of one X chromosome (Lyon hypothesis):

- Random inactivation of either paternal or maternal X chromosome occurs early in embryogenesis and leads to the formation of a Barr body.
- Normal females are functional mosaics with two cell populations, one with an inactivated paternal X chromosome and the other with an inactivated maternal X chromosome.
- With extra X chromosomes, all but one X chromosome is inactivated.

Because numerical aberrations of X chromosomes (extra or missing) are nevertheless associated with somatic and gonadal abnormalities, the Lyon hypothesis is modified as follows:

- Both X chromosomes are required for normal gametogenesis; the inactivated X is selectively reactivated in germ cells during gamete formation.

- X inactivation spares certain regions of the chromosome necessary for normal growth and development; up to 20% of the genes on the short arm of any "inactivated" X chromosome escape inactivation.

The Y chromosome is both necessary and sufficient for male development. Regardless of the number of X chromosomes, the presence of a single Y drives development toward the male sex.

Klinefelter Syndrome (p. 165)

Klinefelter syndrome is male hypogonadism associated with two or more X chromosomes and at least one Y chromosome. It has an incidence of roughly 1 in 660 live male births; 47,XXY is most common (i.e., 90% of cases) with the remainder being mosaics (e.g., 46,XY/47,XXY). Clinical features include:

- Male infertility
- Eunuchoid body habitus
- Minimal or no mental retardation
- Failure of male secondary sexual characteristics
- Gynecomastia with 20-fold increased risk of breast cancer relative to normal males; female distribution of hair
- Atrophic testes
- Plasma follicle-stimulating hormone and estrogen levels elevated; testosterone levels low

The hypogonadism and other clinical features are explained by the pattern of X inactivation. For example, the gene encoding the androgen receptor is on the X chromosome. It has highly polymorphous CAG trinucleotide repeats with longer CAG repeats leading to less receptor activity; fortuitously (or not) the X chromosome with the shorter CAG repeats is preferentially inactivated.

Turner Syndrome (p. 165)

Turner syndrome is hypogonadism in phenotypic females resulting from complete or partial monosomy of X chromosome; 45,X occurs in 57% of cases, with partial deletions of the X chromosome and mosaics (e.g., 45,X/46,XX) making up the rest. Sensitive techniques suggest that 75% of Turner syndrome patients may actually be mosaics. Isochromosomes of the long arm with deletion of the short arm (46,X,i[Xq]) and ring chromosomes with deletions of both long and short arms also yield a Turner phenotype. The karyotypic variability explains the hetrogeneity of the Turner phenotype (45,X is most severely affected). Clinical features include:

- Lymphedema of neck, hands, and feet
- Webbing of neck (due to lymphatic dilation during development)
- Short stature
- Broad chest and widely spaced nipples
- Primary amenorrhea
- Failure of the development of normal secondary sex characteristics
- Severely atrophic and fibrous ovaries (streak ovaries)
- Congenital heart disease, particularly aortic coarctation

Hypogonadism and the absence of secondary sexual maturation occurs because both X chromosomes are necessary for normal oogenesis and ovarian development. Thus affected patients have an accelerated loss of oocytes and essentially undergo menopause before they experience menarche. The short stature comes from the loss of both (expressed) copies of the *short stature homeobox gene (SHOX)* on the X chromosome, which affects height. The mechanisms of the cardiac malformations are unknown.

Hermaphroditism and Pseudohermaphroditism (p. 167)

- *True hermaphrodites* are extremely rare (ovaries and testes are both present, either combined as an ovotestis or with one gonad on each side). Fifty percent have 46,XX karyotype; most others are 46,XX/46,XY mosaics, with very few being 46,XY. Testes in a 46,XX individual implies cryptic chimerism of the *SRY* gene (dictates testicular differentiation), or possibly a Y-to-autosome translocation.
- *Female pseudohermaphrodites* have a 46,XX karyotype with normal ovaries and internal genitalia but ambiguous or virilized external genitalia. The most common cause is androgenic steroid exposure during gestation, for example, due to congenital adrenal hyperplasia or androgen-secreting maternal tumors.
- *Male pseudohermaphrodites* have Y chromosomes; the gonads are therefore exclusively testes, but external genitalia are either ambiguous or completely female. The condition results from defective virilization of the male embryo because of reduced androgen synthesis or resistance to action of androgens. The most common form is *complete testicular feminization*, an X-linked disorder associated with mutations in the androgen receptor gene located on Xq11-Xq12.

Single-Gene Disorders with Nonclassic Inheritance (p. 167)

Diseases Caused by Trinucleotide-Repeat Mutations (p. 167)

Approximately 40 disorders, including Huntington disease, myotonic dystrophy, Friedrich ataxia, fragile-X syndrome, and multiple types of spinocerebellar ataxia, are associated with the expansion of stretches of trinucleotides; neurodegenerative changes dominate the clinical picture.

- Most of these repeats contain guanine (G) and cytosine (C) nucleotides, and they can occur in non-coding regions (fragile-X) or coding regions (Huntington disease).
- Expansions in coding regions (typically CAG trinucleotides) lead to the production of polyglutamine tracts in the proteins and subsequent aberrant folding with aggregation (with large intranuclear inclusions), mitochondrial dysfunction, an unfolded protein stress response, and apoptosis.
- Expansions in non-coding regions suppress the synthesis of the affected protein.
- The proclivity for trinucleotide expansion depends of the sex of the transmitting parent; in fragile-X, expansions occur in oogenesis, whereas in Huntington disease, they occur during spermatogenesis.

Fragile X Syndrome (p. 169)

Fragile X syndrome is prototypical of these disorders; it is a common cause of familial mental retardation. It is characterized cytogenetically by a "fragile site" on Xq27.3 visualized as a discontinuity of chromosomal staining when cells are grown in folate-deficient medium.

- The site on Xq has multiple CGG nucleotide repeats in the 5′ untranslated region of the *familial mental retardation-1 (FMR-1)* gene. In normal individuals, the average number of repeats is 29 (range of 6 to 55), whereas affected individuals have 200 to 4000 repeats; patients with *premutations* (clinically silent) have 55 to 200 CGG repeats.
- In carrier females, the premutations undergo amplification during oogenesis, resulting in full mutations that are then passed on

to progeny. The worsening of clinical presentation with succeeding generations is called *anticipation*.

- Because the mutations are carried on the X chromosome, this is an X-linked recessive disorder; however, because premutations are amplified only during oogenesis, the transmission pattern differs from classic X-linked disorders. Consequently, carrier males with premutations do not typically have any symptoms and do not transmit the disease. Conversely, almost all sons and approximately 50% of daughters of carrier females are affected. Carrier females are also affected (i.e., mentally retarded) at a 30% to 50% frequency, which is much higher than in typical X-linked disorders.
- Expansion of the trinucleotide repeats in *FMR-1* beyond 230 copies leads to abnormal gene methylation and transcriptional suppression.
- The molecular basis of fragile X syndrome is related to loss of function of the FMR protein (FMRP), a cytoplasmic protein abundant in brain and testis. FMRP is an RNA-binding protein associated with polyribosomes; it suppresses the translation of certain transcripts at synaptic junctions. Loss of FMRP leads to increased protein translation, and the resulting imbalance adversely impacts neuronal function with permanent changes in synaptic activity.
- Affected males have severe mental retardation, and 80% have enlarged testes. Other physical features, such as an elongated face and large mandible, are inconsistent.
- Carriers of premutations also develop premature ovarian failure (females) and progressive neurodegeneration (males).

Mutations in Mitochondrial Genes—Leber Hereditary Optic Neuropathy (p. 171)

Ova contain multiple mitochondria, whereas spermatozoa contain few; hence the mitochondrial content of zygotes is derived almost entirely from the ovum (sperm mitochondria also tend to be selectively degraded after formation of the fertilized zygote). Thus, mitochondrial DNA (mtDNA) is transmitted entirely by females, and diseases resulting from mutations in mitochondrial genes are *maternally inherited*.

- Affected females transmit the disease to all their male and female offspring; daughters and not sons pass the disease further along to progeny.
- Expression of disorders resulting from mutations in mitochondrial genes is unpredictable. When a cell carrying normal and mutant mtDNA divides, the proportion of normal and mutant DNA in the daughter cells is random and quite variable (a situation called *heteroplasmy*). There is also a threshold effect related to a minimum number of mutant mtDNA required to see oxidative dysfunction.
- mtDNA encodes 22 tRNAs, 2 rRNAs, and 13 genes for proteins involved in oxidative phosphorylation. Consequently, mtDNA mutations predominantly affect organs heavily dependent on mitochondrial energy metabolism, such as the neuromuscular system, liver, heart, and kidney. Prototypical is Leber hereditary optic neuropathy, resulting in progressive blindness, neurologic dysfunction, and cardiac conduction defects.

Genomic Imprinting (p.171)

This is an epigenetic process resulting in differential inactivation of either maternal or paternal alleles of certain genes. *Maternal imprinting* refers to transcriptional silencing of the maternal allele, whereas *paternal imprinting* refers to inactivation of the paternal allele. Imprinting occurs in the ovum or sperm before fertilization and then is stably transmitted to all somatic cells. The process involves differential DNA methylation or histone H4 deacetylation, leading to selective gene inactivation; 200 to 600 genes are estimated to be imprinted, and although some may occur in isolation, most are clustered in groups regulated by common *cis*-acting elements.

Prader-Willi Syndrome and Angelman Syndrome *(p. 172)*

Prader-Willi syndrome and Angelman syndrome are uncommon genetic disorders caused by deletion of neighboring regions on chromosome 15 (15q12). In this region there are both maternally and paternally imprinted genes. Prader-Willi syndrome occurs when the paternal 15q12 is deleted, leaving only the "silenced" maternal gene product. Angelman syndrome involves deletion of the maternal 15q12 region, leaving behind only the "silenced" paternal gene.

- *Prader-Willi syndrome* is characterized by mental retardation, short stature, hypotonia, obesity, and hypogonadism. In some cases, an entire paternal chromosome 15 is absent, replaced instead by two maternally derived (and therefore silenced) chromosomes 15 (uniparental disomy).
- *Angelman syndrome* patients exhibit mental retardation, ataxia, seizures, and inappropriate laughter. These can also occur through uniparental disomy (receipt of two paternal chromosomes 15).

In Angelman syndrome, the affected paternally imprinted gene is *UBE3A*, coding for a ubiquitin protein-ligase with a role in directing proteasomal degradation of a variety of intracellular proteins in particular regions of the brain. The converse gene(s) in Prader-Willi syndrome are not known, although a gene encoding small nuclear riboprotein N—involved in gene splicing—has been implicated.

Gonadal Mosaicism *(p. 173)*

Gonadal mosaicism results from mutations that selectively affect cells embryologically destined to form gonads. Because germ cells are affected, one or more offspring can manifest disease even though somatic cells are uninvolved and the affected individual is phenotypically normal.

Molecular Diagnosis of Genetic Diseases *(p. 173)*

Molecular techniques to detect diseases at the nucleic acid level have the advantages of exquisite sensitivity (PCR allows amplification and analysis of minute amounts of material) and the fact that DNA-based tests are not dependent on gene products expressed in only selected cells.

Indications for Analysis of Germ Line Genetic Alterations *(p. 173)*

Diagnosis of germ line genetic diseases involves cytogenetics, fluorescence *in situ* hybridization (FISH), or molecular analyses.

- Prenatal evaluation, which is performed on fetal cells obtained by amniocentesis, by chorionic villus biopsy, or from cord blood, is indicated for:

    Advanced maternal age (35 years or more)
    Parent with a structural chromosomal abnormality (e.g., Robertsonian translocation)

Previous child with chromosomal abnormality
Carrier of an X-linked disease (to determine fetal gender)

- Postnatal evaluation, performed on peripheral blood lymphocytes, is indicated for:

Multiple congenital anomalies
Unexplained mental retardation
Suspected chromosomal abnormalities (e.g., Downs or Prader-Willi)
Suspected fragile X syndrome
Infertility, to rule out sex chromosomal abnormality
Recurrent abortion (both parents must be evaluated to rule out carriers of balanced translocation)

Indications for Analysis of Acquired Genetic Alterations (p.174)

- Diagnosis and management of malignancy:

Specific mutations or cytogenetic alterations that are hallmarks of certain tumors (e.g., *BCR-ABL* in chronic myelogenous leukemia)
Determination of clonality as an indicator of maligancy
Identification of genetic alterations that can influence therapy (e.g., EGF-receptor mutations in lung cancer)
Determination of treatment efficacy (presence of residual disease)
Detection of therapy-resistant mutants of a given tumor

- Diagnosis and management of infectious disease:

Detection of specific microorganism (e.g., HIV, mycobacteria, etc.)
Identification of specifically drug-resistant microbes
Determination of treatment efficacy (e.g., residual viral loads in hepatitis C)

Polymerase Chain Reaction and Detection of DNA Sequence Alterations (p. 174)

Diagnosis of genetic diseases by recombinant DNA technology can be accomplished by:

- *Direct* methods involving sequencing of mutant genes
- *Indirect* methods without direct sequencing and involving association with other markers, such as restriction fragment length.

Direct Detection of DNA Sequence Alterations by DNA Sequencing (p. 174)

When a causal gene is known or suspected, direct sequencing may be the most efficacious approach; it has identified mutations in multiple genetic disorders. Recessive diseases usually have only a small number of recurrent mutations, while dominant disorders can have mutations across the entire coding region. Speed and cost have previously limited genome-wide sequencing, although newer techniques may soon enable routine sequencing of entire individual genomes.

Detection of DNA Mutations by Indirect Methods (p.174)

Detection of DNA mutations by indirect methods has the benefits of lower cost and higher throughput.

- Altered DNA restriction sites result in different-sized products (visualized on gel electrophoresis) when DNA from normal or affected individuals is digested by specific restriction enzymes.

- Analyses with fluorescently tagged oligonucleotides that differentially hybridize with normal or specific mutant genes can also be extended to fluorescently tagged nucleotides that differentially incorporate into PCR-amplified normal or mutant sequences. This approach allows the detection of mutant DNA even in heterogeneous mixtures.
- Real-time polymerase chain reaction (PCR) with oligonucleotide probes induce differential elongation of mutant versus normal sequences.
- Mutations affect the length of DNA (e.g., deletions or expansions); these can be detected by restriction fragment digestion or by PCR analysis (e.g., expanded trinucleotide repeats in fragile X syndrome).

Polymorphic Markers and Molecular Diagnosis (p. 176)

When the specific gene related to a particular disease is not known, or if multiple genes contribute to a phenotype, *surrogate* markers in the genome can be used instead to identify risk. Such *linkage analysis* assumes that marker loci near disease alleles will be transmitted through pedigrees *(linkage disequilibrium)*. Eventually a disease "haplotype" can be defined by a panel of marker loci that co-segregate with the putative diseases allele(s). The approach assumes a large enough pedigree of normal and affected family members to allow statistical linkage of markers to disease.

Marker loci in linkage studies are naturally-occurring *polymorphisms*, that is, normal variants in DNA sequences. These include:

- *Single nucleotide polymorphisms (SNPs)* occur at a frequency of roughly 1 in 1000 base pairs, in both exons and introns. They serve as a physical landmark in the genome and are stably transmitted through generations.
- *Repeat-length polymorphisms* are represented by *microsatellite repeats* (repeats of 2 to 6 base pairs, usually less than 1 kb in length) and *minisatellite repeats* (15 to 70 base pair repeat motifs, 1 to 3 kb long). The lengths of such repeats is variable in the population but are stably transmitted across generations, so they can be linked to putative disease alleles. Moreover, they are easy to analyse by gel electrophoresis with PCR primers that flank the repeat sequences.

Polymorphisms and Genome-Wide Analyses (p. 177)

Classical linkage analysis is limited when a disease allele has low penetrance or is only one of several genes that contribute to a multifactorial phenotype. This problem can be circumvented by GWAS that study the linkage of genetic variants (SNPs and repeat polymorphisms) among large cohorts in the general population with and without disease (rather than families). In GWAS, polymorphisms that are over-represented in a disease population are assumed to link to causal candidate genes. The approach has been made possible by:

- Haplotype maps (HapMaps) that provide linkage disequilibrium patterns for major ethnic groups, allowing small numbers of scattered polymorphisms to stand in as markers representing much larger portions of the genome
- High-density chip-based methods where up to a million SNPs can be sequenced at a time
- Sophisticated low-cost computing capacity

Molecular Analysis of Genomic Alterations (p. 178)

Genetic lesions with large deletions, duplications, or more complex rearrangments typically require other diagnostic approaches besides PCR and direct sequence analyses:

- *Southern blotting* (p.178): DNA is digested with restriction enzymes; after electrophoresis, the fragments are hybridized with a nucleotide probe against the genetic region of interest and compared with patterns from normal individuals.
- *FISH* (p. 179): Fluorescently labeled nucleotide probes are used to "paint" all or parts of chromosomes, enabling the detection of aneuploidy or complex genetic recombinations.
- *Array-based comparative genomic hybridization (array CGH;* p. 179): An approach used when the specific genetic abnormality is not known; test DNA and reference (normal) DNA are labeled with different fluorescent dyes (e.g., green and red) and then hybridized to chip-bound DNA probes that span the human genome (up to 100,000 probes per chip). If comparable amounts of each DNA are present, then the fluorescent pattern is merged (in this case, becomes yellow); if there are duplications or deletions, then one or the other colors predominate, and the signal is green or red.

Epigenetic Alterations (p. 180)

These are heritable chemical modifications of DNA or chromatin (e.g., methylation of DNA or acetylation of histones) that do not modify the primary DNA sequence but impact genetic expression. Examples include imprinting and X inactivation. Analysis requires treating DNA with chemicals (e.g., sodium bisulfite) that convert unmethylated or methylated nucleotides to a species that can be uniquely detected or by using antibodies to precipitate modified histones and then sequence the associated DNA.

RNA Analysis (p. 181)

Although mRNA is overall less stable than DNA, sequencing mRNA expression patterns can be useful for:

- Quantification of RNA viruses (e.g., hepatitis C and human immunodeficiency virus [HIV])
- Chromosomal translocations where the break-point is scattered over a large stretch of intronic sequence; rearrangements may be more readily detected after DNA splicing to make mRNA

6

Diseases of the Immune System

The immune system evolved primarily to defend against microbial invasion; it accomplishes this by distinguishing self from non-self (exogenous or foreign) molecules and marshaling a plethora of effector mechanisms to either eliminate or neutralize the perceived invader. The pathways to recognition and elimination involve both *innate* (nonspecific) and *adaptive* (antigen-specific) components and are well reviewed in pages 183 to 197 of *Robbins and Cotran Pathologic Basis of Disease,* eighth edition. Although the pathways of the immune system are exquisitely tuned and generally well regulated, overly exuberant responses to foreign invaders can lead to pathologic consequences. Moreover, the immune system occasionally loses tolerance for self components and can thereby incite effector responses to a variety of normal tissue components—the basis of autoimmune disease.

Hypersensitivity and Autoimmune Disorders (p. 197)

Pathology related to the immune system falls into four broad general categories:

- *Hypersensitivity* reactions (e.g., allergy, immune complex–mediated injury)
- *Autoimmunity* (immune responses to self; the same mechanisms are involved in rejection of transplanted tissues)
- *Deficiency* states, congenital or acquired
- *Amyloidosis,* a disorder of extracellular protein accumulation, frequently with an underlying immunologic association

Mechanisms of Hypersensitivity Reactions (p. 197)

Hypersensitivity reactions imply an excessive response to an antigenic stimulus. General concepts are:

- Both exogenous and endogenous antigens can elicit a hypersensitivity response.
- Diseases occurring as a result of hypersensitivity responses are often associated with particular susceptibility genes (e.g., *histocompatibility molecules,* also called *human leukocyte antigens [HLA]*).
- Hypersensitivity reactions represent an imbalance between immune effector mechanisms and control mechanisms that normally limit immune responses.

Hypersensitivity responses are divided into four general categories based on the underlying mechanisms of immune injury (Table 6-1).

TABLE 6-1 Mechanisms of Immunologically Mediated Hypersensitivity Reactions

Type of Reaction	Prototypic Disorder	Immune Mechanisms	Pathologic Lesions
Immediate (type I) hypersensitivity	Anaphylaxis; allergies; bronchial asthma (atopic forms)	Production of IgE antibody → immediate release of vasoactive amines and other mediators from mast cells; later recruitment of inflammatory cells	Vascular dilation, edema, smooth muscle contraction, mucus production, tissue injury, inflammation
Antibody-mediated (type II) hypersensitivity	Autoimmune hemolytic anemia; Goodpasture syndrome	Production of IgG, IgM → binds to antigen on target cell or tissue → phagocytosis or lysis of target cell by activated complement or Fc receptors; recruitment of leukocytes	Phagocytosis and lysis of cells; inflammation; in some diseases, functional derangements without cell or tissue injury
Immune complex–mediated (type III) hypersensitivity	Systemic lupus erythematosus; some forms of glomerulonephritis; serum sickness; Arthus reaction	Deposition of antigen-antibody complexes → complement activation → recruitment of leukocytes by complement products and Fc receptors → release of enzymes and other toxic molecules	Inflammation, necrotizing vasculitis (fibrinoid necrosis)
Cell-mediated (type IV) hypersensitivity	Contact dermatitis; multiple sclerosis; type I diabetes; rheumatoid arthritis; inflammatory bowel disease; tuberculosis	Activated T lymphocytes → (i) release of cytokines → inflammation and macrophage activation; (ii) T cell–mediated cytotoxicity	Perivascular cellular infiltrates; edema; granuloma formation; cell destruction

Immediate (Type I) Hypersensitivity (p. 198)

Immediate (type I) hypersensitivity is classically mediated by immunoglobulin E (IgE) antibodies directed against specific antigens (allergens). These can occur as local reactions or involve systemic responses. Susceptibility to immediate hypersensitivity reactions *(atopy)* is genetically determined, with linkage studies showing association with HLA and a number of cytokines that contribute to T_H2 immune responses (mapping to 5q31).

IgE synthesis requires T_H2 CD4+ helper T cell responses; in particular, interleukin-4 (IL-4) and IL-13 induce and enhance B cell IgE synthesis. T_H2 cells also produce other cytokines that contribute to the type I hypersensitivity response; thus, IL-4 promotes the development of additional T_H2 cells, and IL-5 is involved in the development and activation of *eosinophils*—important effector cells in type I hypersensitivity responses.

IgE antibodies synthesized after prior exposure to an allergen are bound to mast cells and basophils via specific surface Fc receptors (FcεR1). On re-exposure, allergen binds to and cross-links the IgE-FcεR1 and results in an immediate reaction (minutes), followed by late-phase reactions (hours) due to:

- Release *(degranulation)* of preformed vesicles containing *primary mediators*
- *De novo* synthesis and release of *secondary mediators*

Mast cells can also be activated by other stimuli (yielding responses similar to those elicited by allergens):

- Complement fragments C3a and C5a *(anaphylatoxins)* binding to surface receptors
- Chemokines (chemotactic peptides, e.g., IL-8) and adenosine
- Drugs (e.g., codeine and morphine)
- Mellitin (in bee venom)
- Physical stimuli such as sunlight, trauma, and heat or cold

The consequences of mast cell and basophil activation are schematized in Figure 6-1:

- An *initial rapid response* (i.e., 5 to 30 minutes) is characterized by vasodilation, increased vascular permeability, bronchial smooth muscle contraction, and glandular secretions. This is driven by pre-formed mediators stored in secretory vacuoles and typically resolves within 60 minutes:

  Biogenic amines (e.g., histamine): Bronchial smooth muscle contraction, increased vascular permeability and dilation, and increased mucus secretion
  Enzymes contained in granule matrix (e.g., chymase, tryptase): Generate kinins and activated complement by cleaving precursor proteins
  Proteoglycans (e.g., heparin)

- A *second (delayed) phase,* with onset 2 to 24 hours after initial allergen exposure, is characterized by inflammatory cell infiltrates and tissue damage (especially epithelium). It can persist for days and is driven by lipid mediators and cytokines produced by the activated mast cells:

  Lipid mediators: Produced from precursors released from mast cell membranes by phospholipase A_2
  Leukotriene B4: Highly chemotactic for neutrophils, monocytes, and eosinophils
  Leukotrienes C4, D4, and *E4:* Thousands-fold more potent than histamine for increasing vascular permeability and bronchial smooth muscle contraction

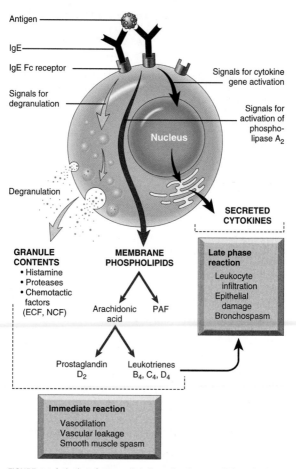

FIGURE 6-1 Activation of mast cells in immediate hypersensitivity and release of their mediators. *ECF,* Eosinophil chemotactic factor; *IgE,* immunoglobulin E; *NCF,* neutrophil chemotactic factor; *PAF,* platelet-activating factor.

Prostaglandin D2: Intense bronchospasm and mucus secretion

Platelet-activating factor (PAF): Platelet aggregation, histamine release, bronchoconstriction, vasodilation, and increased vascular permeability; chemotactic for neutrophils and eosinophils and can cause activation with degranulation

Cytokine mediators: Recruit and activate inflammatory cells; include TNF-α, IL-1, and chemokines; IL-4 released from mast cells amplifies the T_H2 response

SYSTEMIC ANAPHYLAXIS (p. 201)

Systemic anaphylaxis typically follows parenteral or oral administration of foreign proteins, drugs (e.g., penicillin), food (e.g., peanuts), or insect toxins (e.g., bee venom). The severity reflects the level of sensitization; even minuscule doses can induce anaphylactic shock in a sensitized host. Pruritus, urticaria, and erythema occur minutes after exposure, followed by bronchoconstriction and laryngeal edema; this can escalate into laryngeal obstruction, hypotensive shock, and death within minutes to hours.

LOCAL IMMEDIATE HYPERSENSITIVITY REACTIONS (p. 201)

About 10% to 20% of the U.S. population suffers from localized allergic symptoms (e.g., urticaria, angioedema, rhinitis, and asthma) to common inhaled or ingested allergens (pollens, house dust, animal dander, etc).

Antibody-Mediated (Type II) Hypersensitivity (p. 201)

Antibody-mediated (type II) hypersensitivity is mediated by antibodies against extrinsic or endogenous antigens present on cell surfaces or in the extracellular matrix; complement activation also plays a significant role. Subsequent pathology is a consequence of three mechanisms (Fig. 6-2); examples are listed in Table 6-2:

* *Opsonization and phagocytosis*: Cells can be directly lysed by the C5-C9 complement membrane attack complex (MAC) or can be *opsonized* (enhanced phagocytosis) as a result of fixation of antibody or C3b fragments. Bound antibody can also cause cell lysis (without phagocytosis) by cells bearing Fc receptors (e.g., natural killer [NK] cells), so-called *antibody-dependent cell-mediated cytotoxicity (ADCC)*.
* *Inflammation*: Antibodies (and subsequent complement activation) lead to recruitment and activation of antigen non-specific inflammatory cells (neutrophils and macrophages). These release injurious proteases and reactive oxygen species that lead to tissue pathology.
* *Cellular dysfunction*: Certain antibodies can inappropriately activate or block normal cellular or hormonal function without causing tissue damage.

Immune Complex–Mediated (Type III) Hypersensitivity (p. 204)

Immune complex–mediated (type III) hypersensitivity is mediated by antigen-antibody complexes—immune complexes—forming either in the circulation or at sites of antigen deposition. Antigens can be exogenous (e.g., infectious agents) or endogenous; immune complex–mediated disease can be either systemic or local. Examples are given in Table 6-3.

* *Systemic disease* (p. 204) results from the deposition of circulating immune complexes; it can occur as a response to inoculation of a large volume of exogenous antigen *(acute serum sickness)* or can result from antibody responses to endogenous antigens *(lupus erythematosus)* or infectious agents *(polyarteritis nodosa)*. The process is divided into three phases:

  Formation of immune complexes: Newly synthesized antibodies typically arise about a week after antigen inoculation; the antibodies then bind to the foreign molecules to form circulating immune complexes.

  Deposition of immune complexes: Propensity for deposition depends on the physicochemical nature of the complexes (e.g., charge, size) and local vascular characteristics (e.g., fenestration, permeability). Deposition is greatest with medium-sized complexes (e.g., slight antigen excess) and in vascular beds that filter (e.g., glomerulus and synovium).

  Injury caused by immune complexes: Immune complex deposition activates the complement cascade; subsequent tissue injury derives from complement-mediated inflammation and cells bearing Fc receptors.

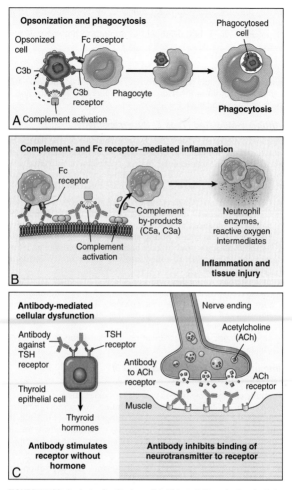

FIGURE 6-2 Mechanisms of antibody-mediated injury. **A**, Opsonization of cells by antibodies and complement components and ingestion by phagocytes. **B**, Inflammation induced by antibody binding to leukocyte Fc receptors and by activated complement fragments. **C**, Anti-receptor antibodies disturb receptor function (e.g., anti-acetylcholine [ACh] receptor antibodies impair neuromuscular synaptic transmission in myasthenia gravis or anti–thyroid-stimulating hormone [TSH] receptor antibodies activate thyroid epithelial cells in Graves disease).

Single large antigen exposures tend to induce acute, self-limited disease that resolves as the inciting antigen is eliminated (e.g., poststreptococcal glomerulonephritis); repeated or prolonged exposure leads to chronic, recurrent tissue injury (e.g., lupus).

Morphology (p. 205)

The classic lesion is *acute necrotizing vasculitis* with vessel wall necrosis and intense neutrophil accumulation. Necrotic tissue and protein accumulations composed of immune complexes, complement, and exuded serum proteins contribute to a smudgy

TABLE 6-2   Examples of Antibody-Mediated Diseases (Type II Hypersensitivity)

Disease	Target Antigen	Mechanisms of Disease	Clinicopathologic Manifestations
Autoimmune hemolytic anemia	Erythrocyte membrane proteins (Rh blood group antigens, blood group antigen)	Opsonization and phagocytosis of erythrocytes	Hemolysis, anemia
Autoimmune thrombocytopenic purpura	Platelet membrane proteins (GpIIb:IIIa or GpIb/IX)	Opsonization and phagocytosis of platelets	Bleeding
Pemphigus vulgaris	Proteins in intercellular junctions of epidermal cells (cadherin)	Antibody-mediated activation of proteases, disruption of intercellular adhesions	Skin vesicles (bullae)
Vasculitis caused by ANCA	Neutrophil granule proteins, presumably released from activated neutrophils	Neutrophil degranulation and inflammation	Vasculitis
Goodpasture syndrome	Noncollagenous protein in basement membranes of kidney glomeruli and lung alveoli	Complement- and Fc receptor-mediated inflammation	Nephritis, lung hemorrhage
Acute rheumatic fever	Streptococcal cell wall antigen; antibody cross-reacts with myocardial antigen	Inflammation, macrophage activation	Myocarditis, arthritis
Myasthenia gravis	Acetylcholine receptor	Antibody inhibits acetylcholine binding, down-modulates receptors	Muscle weakness, paralysis
Graves disease (hyperthyroidism)	TSH receptor	Antibody-mediated stimulation of TSH receptors	Hyperthyroidism
Insulin-resistant diabetes	Insulin receptor	Antibody inhibits binding of insulin	Hyperglycemia, ketoacidosis
Pernicious anemia	Intrinsic factor of gastric parietal cells	Neutralization of intrinsic factor, decreased absorption of vitamin B_{12}	Abnormal erythropoiesis, anemia

ANCA, Antineutrophil cytoplasmic antibodies; *TSH,* thyroid-stimulating hormone.
From Abbas AK, Lichtman H: *Cellular and molecular immunology,* ed 5, Philadelphia, 2003, WB Saunders.

TABLE 6-3 Examples of Immune Complex–Mediated Diseases

Disease	Antigen Involved	Clinicopathologic Manifestations
Systemic lupus erythematosus	DNA, nucleoproteins, others	Nephritis, arthritis, vasculitis
Polyarteritis nodosa	Hepatitis B virus surface antigen (in some cases)	Vasculitis
Poststreptococcal glomerulonephritis	Streptococcal cell wall antigen(s); may be "planted" in glomerular basement membrane	Nephritis
Acute glomerulonephritis	Bacterial antigens (Treponema); parasite antigens (malaria, schistosomes); tumor antigens	Nephritis
Reactive arthritis	Bacterial antigens (Yersinia)	Acute arthritis
Arthus reaction	Various foreign proteins	Cutaneous vasculitis
Serum sickness	Various proteins, e.g., foreign serum (anti-thymocyte globulin)	Arthritis, vasculitis, nephritis

eosinophilic deposition, called *fibrinoid necrosis.* Superimposed thrombosis and downstream tissue necrosis may also be present. Immune complexes and complement can be visualized by immunofluorescence or by electron microscopy (electron-dense deposits). In chronic lesions there is intimal thickening and vascular and/or parenchymal scarring.

LOCAL IMMUNE COMPLEX DISEASE (ARTHUS REACTION) (p. 205)

Local immune complex disease is characterized by a localized tissue vasculitis and necrosis; it occurs when the formation or deposition of immune complexes is extremely localized (e.g., *intracutaneous* antigen injection in previously sensitized hosts carrying the appropriate circulating antibody).

T Cell–Mediated (Type IV) Hypersensitivity *(p. 205)*

T cell–mediated (type IV) hypersensitivity is mediated by antigen-specific T lymphocytes and includes delayed-type hypersensitivity (CD4+ T) cells and T cell–mediated cytotoxicity (CD8+ T) cells (Fig. 6-3).

REACTIONS OF CD4+ T CELLS: DELAYED-TYPE HYPERSENSITIVITY AND IMMUNE INFLAMMATION (p. 205)

This response is largely mediated by helper CD4+ T cells and can be of two major types; responses associated with T_H1 CD4+ T cells are predominated by macrophages, while those driven by T_H17 cells are characterized by a greater neutrophil infiltration.

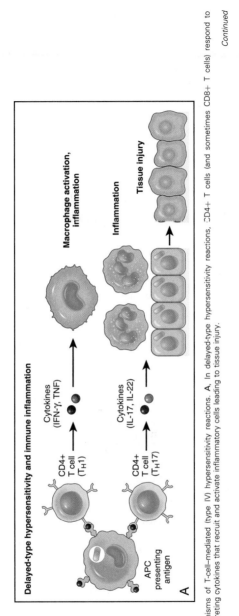

FIGURE 6-3 Mechanisms of T-cell–mediated (type IV) hypersensitivity reactions. **A.** In delayed-type hypersensitivity reactions, CD4+ T cells (and sometimes CD8+ T cells) respond to local antigens by secreting cytokines that recruit and activate inflammatory cells leading to tissue injury.

Continued

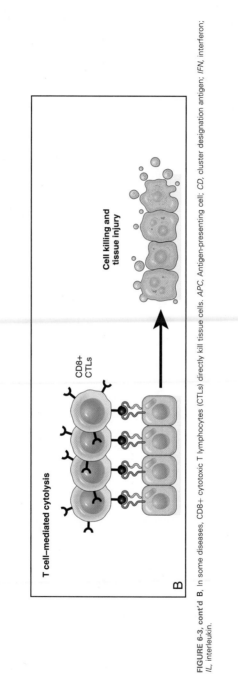

FIGURE 6-3, cont'd B, In some diseases, CD8+ cytotoxic T lymphocytes (CTLs) directly kill tissue cells. *APC,* Antigen-presenting cell; *CD,* cluster designation antigen; *IFN,* interferon; *IL,* interleukin.

- *Stimulation and differentiation*: Recognition of processed peptide antigens on antigen presenting cells leads to production of IL-2, an autocrine proliferation factor. Whether proliferating CD4+ T cells differentiate into T_H1 or T_H17 lineages depends on the cytokine environment at the time of initial T cell activation. IL-12 production by antigen presenting cells induces T_H1 cells, which—in turn—produce interferon-γ (IFN-γ) that promotes further T_H1 development and thus amplifies the reaction. Conversely, IL-1, IL-6, IL-23, and transforming growth factor-β (TGF-β) will stimulate differentiation to T_H17 cells.

- *Responses of differentiated effector T cells:*

    The major effector cytokine of activated T_H1 cells is IFN-γ; it activates macrophages, increases class II histocompatibility molecule expression (improving antigen presentation capacity), induces TNF-α and IL-1 production (promoting inflammation), and increases IL-12 secretion (amplifying the T_H1 process). Activated macrophages then clear the offending agent; sustained activation (or the inability to clear the stimulus) can result in greater inflammation and tissue injury.

    Stimulated T_H17 cells secrete IL-17, IL-22, and other cytokines that recruit and activate neutrophils and monocytes—and IL-21, which amplifies the T_H17 response.

    The classic delayed-type hypersensitivity (DTH) response is the *tuberculin reaction* to intracutaneous injection of purified protein derivative (PPD) derived from the tubercle bacillus. Prior tuberculosis infection results in circulating PPD-responsive memory CD4+ T cells; subsequent PPD injection into such an individual leads to the recruitment and activation of these cells beginning at 6 to 8 hours and peaking at 24 to 72 hours (the *delayed* in DTH). Histologically, there is a perivascular mononuclear cell infiltrate (CD4+ T cells and macrophages) with evidence of endothelial activation.

    Granulomatous inflammation occurs when persistent or nondegradable antigens (e.g., foreign bodies) lead to chronic macrophage activation manifesting as large *epithelioid* cells; nodules of these activated cells are called *granulomas*.

    Contact dermatitis is another example of a DTH response, in this case to modified self. An example is poison ivy; its active constituent, urushiol, binds to host proteins and alters their antigenicity.

REACTIONS OF CD8+ T CELLS: CELL-MEDIATED CYTOTOXICITY (p. 207)

Generation of CD8+ cytotoxic T lymphocytes (CTLs) is the principal pattern of response to many viral infections and to tumor cells; CTLs also contribute to allograft rejection. CTL-induced injury is mediated by perforin-granzyme and Fas-FasL pathways that ultimately induce apoptosis.

Autoimmune Diseases (p. 208)

Immune reactions against self-antigens—autoimmunity—result from breakdown in *self-tolerance*, the normal state of nonresponsiveness to one's own antigens.

Immunologic Tolerance (p. 209)

The mechanisms of self-tolerance can be either central or peripheral:

Central Tolerance (p. 209)

This refers to the process by which T and B cells that recognize self antigens are either killed (*negative selection*) or rendered harmless. Many self antigens are expressed in the thymus and presented by thymic APC; when developing T cells with high-affinity T cell receptors for these self antigens encounter thymic APC they are deleted. A protein called *autoimmune regulator (AIRE)* is responsible for inducing the self antigen expression, and interestingly, mutations in AIRE result in an autoimmune polyendocrinopathy (Chapter 24). Additionally, some autoreactive T cells are not deleted, but rather develop into regulatory T cells.

When developing B cells strongly recognize self antigens, they frequently reactivate the machinery for immunoglobulin rearrangement, thereby generating new non-reactive B cell receptors *(receptor editing)*. If receptor editing does not occur, self-reactive B cells also undergo apoptosis.

Clonal deletion is not perfect, however, and numerous "normal" T and B cells can be found with receptors that recognize self antigens. Unless muzzled by the elements of peripheral tolerance, they can cause autoimmune disease.

Peripheral Tolerance (p. 209)

Autoreactive cells that escape central regulatory mechanisms can be removed or inactivated in the periphery through one of the following pathways:

- *Anergy:* Irreversible functional inactivation may occur when T cells recognize self antigen in the absence of necessary co-stimulatory signals (e.g., via B7-CD28 interactions). Alternatively, APC can inhibit T cell activation by signals transmitted through T-cell CTLA-4 or PD-1 receptors. If self-reactive B cells encounter antigen in peripheral tissues in the absence of T-cell help, they lose the capacity for any subsequent antigenic stimulation.
- *Suppression by regulatory T cells:* Regulatory T cells—CD4+ cells expressing CD25 (the α-chain of the IL-2 receptor) and the Foxp3 transcription factor—may inhibit lymphocyte activation and effector functions by secreting cytokines such as IL-10 and TGF-β. Mutations in *Foxp3* cause a severe autoimmune disease called *immune dysregulation, polyendocrinopathy, enteropathy, X-linked (IPEX)*.
- *Deletion by activation-induced cell death:* Self antigens that are abundant in the peripheral tissue may cause persistent activation of self-reactive T cells, leading to either increased relative expression of pro-apoptotic molecules (e.g., Bim), or expression of FasL on these cells. Increased FasL expression induces apoptosis of the T cells by engaging Fas co-expressed on these cells; self-reactive B cells expressing Fas can also be deleted by the FasL-positive T cells. Mutations in the *FAS* gene leads to *autoimmune lymphoproliferative syndrome*.
- *Antigen sequestration:* Immune-privileged sites such as testis, eye, and brain may sequester tissue antigens across a relatively impermeant blood-tissue barrier. Release of such previously "privileged" antigens (e.g., due to physical injury) is the postulated mechanism for post-traumatic orchitis and uveitis.

Mechanisms of Autoimmunity: General Principles (p. 211)

Autoimmunity arises through some combination of susceptibility genes (causing loss of self tolerance) and environmental triggers (especially infections).

Role of Susceptibility Genes (p. 212)

Most autoimmune disorders are complex multigenic disorders. Although many are associated with specific histocompability molecule HLA alleles (potentially related to affects on negative selection or regulatory T-cell development), the expression of particular HLA molecules is not—by itself—the cause of autoimmunity. As previously described, defects in pathways that normally regulate either peripheral or central tolerance have also been demonstrated (e.g., AIRE, Fas-FasL, CTLA-4, IL-2 receptor, and Foxp3). Polymorphisms in other genes have also been implicated:

- *PTPN-22* encodes a tyrosine phosphatase and is associated with multiple autoimmune disorders (e.g., type I diabetes and rheumatoid arthritis); a defective phosphatase would not adequately counter the activity of lymphocyte tyrosine kinases and could thus lead to excessive activation.
- *NOD-2* is part of the sensing mechanism for intracellular microbes and is associated with inflammatory bowel disease; defective NOD-2 could result in exaggerated inflammation to otherwise well-tolerated commensal GI organisms.
- *IL-2 and IL-7 receptor polymorphisms* are associated with multiple sclerosis; polymorphisms may affect regulatory T-cell development and maintenance.

Role of Infections (p. 212)

Autoimmune disease onset is often temporally associated with infection. This may occur secondary to co-stimulator up-regulation, which overwhelms peripheral tolerance mechanisms. Infection might also break tolerance by *molecular mimicry*; if a microbe shares epitopes with self antigens, immune responses directed against the pathogen could cross-react with and damage normal tissues. Tissue injury occurring in the course of response to infection can also structurally alter self antigens, or release normal self antigens; these molecules would then activate T cells that are not tolerant to the altered or previously cryptic antigens.

General Features of Autoimmune Diseases (p. 212)

Once induced, autoimmune diseases tend to be progressive, albeit with occasional relapses and remissions. This is, in part, due to intrinsic amplification loops that the immune system employs to allow initially small numbers of responsive cells to eventually overcome infection. In addition, immune responses are subject to the phenomenon of *epitope spreading*; many possible epitopes within self antigens are not normally presented to developing T cells, and thus there is no opportunity to develop tolerance to such *cryptic* peptides. However, if such epitopes become recognizable in postnatal life as a result of molecular alteration of self antigens, T cells reactive to them can cause persistent autoimmunity. The phenomenon is called *epitope spreading* because the immune response "spreads" to determinants that were not initially recognized.

The clinical and pathologic consequences of a specific autoimmune disease will be influenced by the nature of the response; thus T_H1 responses will have a macrophage-rich inflammation and substantial antibody-mediated elements, whereas neutrophil-mediated injury will predominate in T_H17 responses. Different autoimmune diseases also show substantial clinical and pathologic overlaps, so that precise classification may not be possible.

Systemic Lupus Erythematosus (p. 213)

Systemic lupus erythematosus (SLE) is the prototypical systemic autoimmune disorder, characterized by numerous autoantibodies, especially *antinuclear antibodies (ANAs)*. Incidence approaches 1 in 2500 in some general populations; the female to male ratio is 9:1 with 1 in 700 women of child-bearing age affected.

Spectrum of Autoantibodies in SLE (p. 213)

ANAs are typically detected by indirect immunofluorescence. The patterns of immunofluorescence (e.g., homogeneous, peripheral, speckled, nucleolar), though nonspecific, can suggest the type of circulating autoantibody. ANAs also occur in other autoimmune disorders, and in up to 10% of normal individuals (Table 6-4), but *anti-double-stranded DNA and anti-Smith antigen antibodies strongly suggest SLE.*

Besides ANAs, SLE patients produce other autoantibodies, some directed against blood elements (i.e., red blood cells, platelets, leukocytes). Moreover, 40% to 50% of SLE patients have antibodies to phospholipid-associated proteins *(antiphospholipid antibodies).* Some bind to cardiolipin antigen, giving rise to false-positive results for syphilis. Others interfere with (prolong) *in vitro* coagulation assays; these so-called *lupus anticoagulants* actually exert a *pro*coagulant effect *in vivo*, causing recurrent vascular thromboses, miscarriages, and cerebral ischemia *(secondary antiphospholipid antibody syndrome).*

Etiology and Pathogenesis of SLE (p. 215)

- *Genetic factors:* Monozygotic twin concordance (more than 20%) and familial and HLA clustering strongly implicate a genetic predisposition. Although the cause is unknown, the presence of a plethora of autoantibodies suggests a basic defect in the maintenance of B-cell tolerance. Congenital deficiencies in certain complement components (i.e., C2, C4, or C1q) may also impair immune complex clearance and favor tissue deposition.
- *Immunologic factors:* Defective elimination of self-reactive B cells, and ineffective peripheral tolerance mechanisms are most important; inappropriate B-cell activation by nuclear RNA and DNA via toll-like receptors (TLR), or activation via abnormal elaboration of type I interferons or other cytokines may contribute. Finally, CD4 T cells specific for nucleosomal antigens may escape tolerance induction.
- *Environmental factors:* Ultraviolet (UV) light exacerbates SLE by driving apoptosis, increasing IL-1 production by keratinocytes, and potentially by altering DNA to increase its immunogenicity. Estrogen is also implicated because of the gender- and age-predilection of the disease, and certain drugs (e.g., hydralazine and procainamide) can directly induce SLE-like responses. Interestingly, although up to 80% of patients receiving procainamide have ANAs (primarily anti-histone and not anti-dsDNA), only a third have clinical symptoms, and those usually remit after cessation of the offending agent.

A Model for the Pathogenesis of SLE (p. 216)

Cell injury (e.g., UV and other environmental insults) leads to apoptosis and an increased burden of nuclear antigens. Defective B- and T-cell tolerance leads to autoantibodies directed against the nuclear antigens, with the resulting immune complexes being ingested by B cells and dendritic cells; subsequent TLR engagement causes further cellular activation, cytokine production, and augmented autoantibody synthesis, which causes more apoptosis in a self-amplifying loop.

Mechanisms of Tissue Injury (p. 217)

Tissue damage occurs primarily through formation of immune complexes (type III hypersensitivity) or by antibody-mediated injury to blood cells (type II hypersensitivity). Although ANAs cannot penetrate cells, these circulating autoantibodies may

TABLE 6-4 Antinuclear Antibodies in Various Autoimmune Diseases

Nature of Antigen	Antibody System	Disease, % Positive					
		SLE	Drug-Induced LE	Systemic Sclerosis—Diffuse	Limited Scleroderma—CREST	Sjögren Syndrome	Inflammatory Myopathies
Many nuclear antigens (DNA, RNA, proteins)	Generic ANA (indirect IF)	>95	>95	70-90	70-90	50-80	40-60
Native DNA	Anti–double-stranded DNA	40-60	<5	<5	<5	<5	<5
Histones	Antihistone	50-70	>95	<5	<5	<5	<5
Core proteins of small nuclear ribonucleoprotein particles (Smith antigen)	Anti-Sm	20-30	<5	<5	<5	<5	<5
Ribonucleoprotein (U1RNP)	Nuclear RNP	30-40	<5	15	10	<5	<5
RNP	SS-A(Ro)	30-50	<5	<5	<5	70-95	10
RNP	SS-B(La)	10-15	<5	<5	<5	60-90	<5
DNA topoisomerase I	Scl-70	<5	<5	28-70	10-18	<5	<5
Centromeric proteins	Anticentromere	<5	<5	22-36	90	<5	<5
Histidyl-t-RNA synthetase	Jo-1	<5	<5	<5	<5	<5	25

Boxed entries indicate high correlation.
ANA, Antinuclear antibody; *RNP,* ribonucleoprotein; *SLE,* systemic lupus erythematosus; *LE,* lupus erythematosus.

nevertheless form immune complexes with intracellular contents released from otherwise damaged cells.

Morphology (p. 217)

Although any organ can be involved, the most characteristic tissues affected are skin, blood vessels, kidneys, and connective tissue. *Classically, there is a type III hypersensitivity response with acute necrotizing vasculitis and fibrinoid deposits involving small arteries and arterioles.* Immunoglobulin, dsDNA, and C3 can be found in vessel walls, and a perivascular lymphocytic infiltrate is frequently present. In chronic cases, vessels show a fibrous thickening and luminal narrowing.

- *Kidney:* The kidney is involved in virtually all cases of SLE; the principal mechanism of injury is immune complex deposition. Five patterns of *lupus nephritis* are recognized with increasing degrees of cellular infiltration, microvascular thrombosis, and vascular wall deposition; in turn, these are associated with increasing degrees of hematuria, proteinuria, hypertension, and renal insufficiency.
- *Skin:* Malar erythema is the classic lesion *(butterfly rash),* along with variable cutaneous lesions ranging from erythema to bullae occurring elsewhere. Sunlight exacerbates the lesions. Microscopically, there is basal layer degeneration with dermal-epidermal junction immunoglobulin and complement deposits. The dermis shows variable fibrosis, perivascular mononuclear cell infiltrates, and vascular fibrinoid change.
- *Joints:* There is a *nonspecific, nonerosive synovitis* with minimal joint deformity.
- *Central nervous system:* Neuropsychiatric manifestations are probably secondary to endothelial injury and occlusion (antiphospholipid antibodies) or impaired neuronal function as a result of autoantibodies to a synaptic membrane antigen.
- *Pericarditis and other serosal cavity involvement:* Serositis is initially fibrinous with focal vasculitis, fibrinoid necrosis, and edema; this progresses to adhesions, possibly obliterating serosal cavities (i.e., the pericardial sac).
- *Cardiovascular system:* Principal involvement is pericarditis; myocarditis is much less common, and—although a classic finding—*nonbacterial verrucous (Libman-Sacks) endocarditis* happens infrequently. The latter features numerous small, warty vegetations (1 to 3 mm) on the inflow or outflow surfaces (or both) of the mitral and tricuspid valves. There may also be diffuse leaflet thickening of the mitral or aortic valves with functional stenosis or insufficiency. There is an increasing incidence of accelerated coronary atherosclerosis, potentially attributable to exacerbation of traditional risk factors (e.g., hypertension, hypercholesterolemia), to immune complex, and to antiphospholipid antibody–mediated vascular injury.
- *Spleen:* Splenomegaly with capsular thickening and follicular hyperplasia are common. Penicilliary artery perivascular fibrosis is characteristic, producing an *onion-skin* appearance.
- *Lungs:* Pleuritis and/or effusions occur in 50% of patients; there is also chronic interstitial fibrosis and secondary pulmonary hypertension.

Clinical Features (p. 220)

The clinical manifestations of SLE are protean. It typically presents insidiously as a systemic, chronic, recurrent, febrile illness with symptoms referable to virtually any tissue but especially joints, skin, kidneys, and serosal membranes. Autoantibodies to hematologic components may induce thrombocytopenia, leukopenia, and anemia. The course of the disease is highly variable; rarely, it is fulminant with death in weeks to months.

- Occasionally, it may cause minimal symptoms (hematuria, rash) and remit even without treatment.
- More often, the disease is characterized by recurrent flares and remissions over many years and is held in check by immunosuppressive regimens.
- Five-year survival is 90%; 10-year survival is 80%; death is most commonly caused by renal failure or intercurrent infections.

Chronic Discoid Lupus Erythematosus (p. 221)

This disease is limited to cutaneous lesions that grossly and microscopically mimic SLE. Only 35% of patients have a positive ANA. As in SLE, there is deposition of immunoglobulin and C3 at the dermal-epidermal junction. After many years, 5% to 10% of affected individuals develop systemic manifestations.

Rheumatoid Arthritis (p. 221) (See Chapter 26)
Sjögren Syndrome (p. 221)

Sjögren syndrome is characterized by dry eyes *(keratoconjunctivitis sicca)* and dry mouth *(xerostomia)* resulting from immune-mediated lacrimal and salivary gland destruction. About 40% of cases occur in isolation (the primary form or *sicca syndrome*); the remainder is associated with other autoimmune diseases (e.g., rheumatoid arthritis, which is most common), SLE, or scleroderma; 90% of patients are women between ages 35 and 45 years.

- Most patients have rheumatoid factor (an IgM autoantibody that binds self IgG) without having rheumatoid arthritis; ANAs against ribonucleoproteins SS-A (Ro) and SS-B (La) are especially common (see Table 6-4).
- Injury is probably a consequence of both cellular and humoral mechanisms; it is most likely initiated by CD4+ T cells reacting to an unknown self-antigen after an initiating infectious injury. Epstein-Barr virus and hepatitis C have been implicated, and patients infected with human T-cell lymphotropic virus (HTLV)-1 develop similar lesions.

Morphology (p. 222)

The lacrimal and salivary glands (other exocrine glands may also be involved) initially show a periductal lymphocytic infiltrate with ductal epithelial hyperplasia and luminal obstruction. This is followed by acinar atrophy, fibrosis, and eventual fatty replacement, with an expanding lymphocytic infiltrate that can develop lymphoid follicles and germinal centers. Changes secondary to loss of glandular secretion include corneal inflammation, erosion, and ulceration, and atrophy of oral mucosa with inflammatory fissuring and ulceration; patients frequently develop nasal drying and crusting and, rarely, septal perforation. Laryngitis, bronchitis, or pneumonitis can result from respiratory involvement.

Clinical Features (p. 222)

Xerostomia makes swallowing foods difficult, and the keratoconjunctivitis can markedly affect vision. Extraglandular involvement occurs in a third of patients with synovitis, pulmonary fibrosis, and peripheral neuropathy; although glomerular lesions are rare, renal tubular dysfunction (e.g., renal tubular acidosis and phosphaturia) occur commonly in association with tubulointerstitial nephritis. Adenopathy may occur with pleomorphic lymph node infiltrates and there is a 40-fold increased risk of developing B-cell lymphoma. *Mikulicz syndrome* is a term for lacrimal and salivary gland enlargement from any cause; distinguishing Sjögren syndrome from other etiologies (e.g., sarcoidosis, leukemia, lymphoma) requires lip biopsy (to examine minor salivary glands).

Systemic Sclerosis (Scleroderma) (p. 223)

Scleroderma is a chronic autoimmune inflammatory disorder characterized by widespread vascular injury and progressive perivascular and interstitial fibrosis of multiple organs. Cutaneous involvement is greatest (where it may be confined for years), although the fibrosis frequently involves the gastrointestinal tract, kidneys, heart, muscles, and lung. The female to male ratio is 3:1, with peak incidence in the 50- to 60-year age group. There are two major clinical categories:

- *Diffuse scleroderma* with widespread skin involvement and rapid progression with early visceral involvement
- *Limited scleroderma* with limited cutaneous involvement, late visceral involvement, and a relatively benign course

Patients with limited disease can also develop *c*alcinosis, Raynaud phenomenon, *e*sophageal dysmotility, *s*clerodactyly, and *t*elangiectasia, or *CREST syndrome*

Etiology and Pathogenesis (p. 223)

- *Abnormal immune responses:* Current speculation is that CD4+ T cells respond to yet unidentified antigens and release cytokines (e.g., TGF-β and IL-13) that activate additional inflammatory cells and fibroblasts. Inappropriate humoral immunity is also triggered, producing a number of autoantibodies including ANAs (see Table 6-4); these are good markers of disease but may not necessarily cause injury:

  Antitopoisomerase I (anti-Scl-70) is highly specific and is associated with diffuse scleroderma and pulmonary fibrosis.
  Anticentromere antibody is found more commonly in patients with limited disease and CREST syndrome.

- *Vascular damage:* Microvascular injury is a hallmark feature of systemic sclerosis and indeed may be the primary inciting pathology. Although the cause of the injury is unknown, it is speculated to be either a consequence of direct autoimmune attack or a by-product of chronic perivascular inflammation. Regardless, repeated cycles of endothelial injury followed by platelet aggregation lead to the release of a number of growth factors and cytokines (e.g., PDGF, TGF-β) that ultimately induce vascular smooth muscle and fibroblast proliferation, as well as matrix synthesis, that narrow the vascular lumen.
- *Fibrosis*: This results not only from scarring in the setting of ischemic injury but also as a consequence of fibrogenic cytokine elaboration and hyperresponsiveness of fibroblasts to the various growth factors.

Morphology (p. 224)

Vessels throughout the body exhibit perivascular lymphocytic infiltrates with focal vascular occlusion and edema; this is temporally followed by progressive perivascular fibrosis and vascular hyaline thickening. The manifestation of these vascular changes varies with the tissue type:

- *Skin:* Skin grossly exhibits diffuse sclerosis with atrophy. Affected areas are initially edematous with a doughy consistency. Eventually, fibrotic fingers become tapered and claw-like with diminished mobility, and the face a drawn mask. Focal vascular obliteration causes ulceration, and fingertips may undergo auto-amputation.

- *Alimentary tract:* The alimentary tract shows progressive atrophy and fibrosis of the muscularis, most prominently in the esophagus, where it assumes a rubber-hose consistency. Throughout the GI tract, there is mucosal thinning, ulceration, and scarring.
- *Musculoskeletal system:* Inflammatory synovitis progressing to fibrosis is common; joint destruction is uncommon. Muscle involvement begins proximally with edema and mononuclear perivascular infiltrates, progressing to interstitial fibrosis with myofiber degeneration.
- *Kidneys:* The kidneys are affected in two thirds of patients; *renal failure accounts for 50% of deaths in systemic sclerosis.* The most prominent changes are in vessel walls (especially interlobular arteries) with intimal proliferation and deposition of mucinous or collagenous material. Hypertension is present in 30% of cases, 10% of which have a malignant course. Hypertension further accentuates the vascular changes, often resulting in fibrinoid necrosis with thrombosis and necrosis.
- *Lungs:* Lungs show variable fibrosis of small pulmonary vessels with diffuse interstitial and alveolar fibrosis progressing in some cases to honeycombing.
- *Heart:* Perivascular infiltrates with interstitial fibrosis occasionally evolve into a restrictive cardiomyopathy. There may also be conduction system involvement with resultant arrhythmias.

Clinical Features (p. 225)

Although sharing features with SLE, rheumatoid arthritis, and polymyositis, the striking feature of systemic sclerosis is the cutaneous fibrosis. Other associated clinical findings include the following:

- *Raynaud's phenomenon* (episodic arteriolar constriction in the extremities) occurs in virtually all patients and precedes other symptoms in more than 70% of patients.
- Dysphagia results from esophageal fibrosis (i.e., 50% of patients).
- Gastrointestinal involvement leads to malabsorption, intestinal pain, or obstruction.
- Pulmonary fibrosis causes respiratory and/or right-sided heart failure.
- Direct cardiac involvement can induce arrhythmias or heart failure secondary to microvascular infarction.
- Malignant hypertension develops that potentially culminates in fatal renal failure.

Inflammatory Myopathies (p. 225) (See Chapter 27)

Mixed Connective Tissue Disease (p. 226)

This may not be a distinct entity but rather a heterogeneous subgroup of other autoimmune disorders (i.e., SLE, polymyositis, and systemic sclerosis) and can, with time, evolve into classic SLE or scleroderma. It is characterized by:

- High antibody titers to U1 ribonucleoprotein (see Table 6-4)
- Modest initial renal involvement
- Good initial response to steroids
- Serious complications are pulmonary hypertension and progressive renal disease

Polyarteritis Nodosa and Other Vasculitides (p. 226) (See Chapter 11)

Rejection of Tissue Transplants (p. 226)

Transplant rejection involves several mechanisms of immune-mediated injury discussed previously; foreign allografts are subject to antibody-mediated injury, as well as CTL and DTH responses.

Mechanisms of Recognition and Rejection of Allografts (p. 226)

The host immune system is triggered by the presence of foreign HLA histocompatibility molecules on the endothelium and parenchymal cells of the transplanted tissue (Fig. 6-4). HLA molecules occur in two forms—class I and class II—that drive distinct aspects of the specific immune response (see also pp. 190-193 of *Robbins and Cotran Pathologic Basis of Disease,* ed 8).

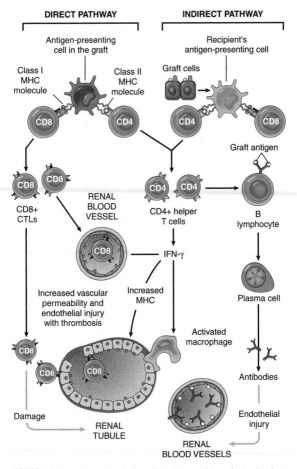

FIGURE 6-4 Recognition and rejection of histoincompatible grafts. In the direct pathway, class I and class II antigens on donor antigen-presenting cells (APCs) are recognized by host CD8+ cytotoxic T cells and CD4+ helper T cells, respectively. CD4+ cells proliferate and produce cytokines that induce tissue damage by a local delayed-type hypersensitivity (DTH) response, stimulating B cells and CD8+ T cells. CD8+ T cells responding to graft antigens differentiate into cytotoxic T lymphocyte (CTL) that directly kill graft cells. In the indirect pathway, graft antigens are displayed by host APCs and primarily activate CD4+ T cells; these, in turn, damage the graft by DTH mechanisms, including the induction of antibodies. *IFN-γ,* Interferon-γ; *MHC,* major histocompatibility complex.

- *Class I molecules* are expressed on all nucleated cells; they are heterodimers composed of a polymorphic heavy-chain glycoprotein (coded on one of three closely linked loci: HLA-A, HLA-B, and HLA-C) and a non-polymorphic β_2-microglobulin. Class I molecules bind peptide fragments derived from *endogenous proteins* (e.g., viral products in a virally infected cell) and present these processed antigens to CD8+ CTL, resulting in their activation.

- *Class II molecules* are confined to APC, including dendritic cells, macrophages, B cells, and activated T cells; they are heterodimers composed of non-covalently associated α and β chains coded in the HLA-D region (with three serologically defined sub-loci DP, DQ, and DR). Class II molecules bind peptide fragments derived from *exogenous proteins* and present these processed antigens to CD4+ helper T lymphocytes, resulting in their activation.

Host T cells recognize allograft HLA by two pathways—*direct* and *indirect*:

- *Direct pathway*. Host T cells recognize donor HLA on APC derived from the donor; the most important cells in this process are donor dendritic cells. Host CD8+ T cells recognize donor class I HLA molecules and mature into CTL; host CD4+ T cells recognize donor class II HLA molecules; they proliferate and differentiate to form T_H1 (and possibly T_H17) effector cell populations.

- *Indirect pathway*. Host T cells recognize donor HLA after processing and presentation on host APC (analogous to any other exogenous processed antigen). The principal response is therefore a DTH mediated by CD4+ T lymphocytes.

Rejection of Solid Organs (p. 228) (see Fig. 6-4)

Following lymphocyte activation, rejection is mediated by the following:

- Direct CTL-mediated parenchymal and endothelial cytolysis
- Macrophage-mediated damage
- Cytokine-mediated vascular and parenchymal dysfunction
- Microvascular injury also causes downstream tissue ischemia
- *Antibody-mediated responses* can also be important; these tend to induce injury to endothelial cells rather than parenchymal cells

Hyperacute Rejection (p. 228)

Hyperacute rejection occurs when the recipient has been previously sensitized to graft antigens (e.g., by blood transfusion or pregnancy). Preformed, circulating antibody binds to graft endothelial HLA with an immediate (minutes to days) complement- and ADCC-mediated injury. Grossly, the organ is cyanotic, mottled, and flaccid. Microscopically, the lesions resemble immune complex–mediated disease; immunoglobulin and complement are deposited in the vessel walls with endothelial injury, fibrin-platelet microthombi, neutrophil infiltrates, and arteriolar fibrinoid necrosis followed by distal parenchymal infarction.

Acute Rejection (p. 228)

Acute rejection typically occurs within days or months of transplantation or after cessation of immunosuppressive therapy. Both cellular and humoral mechanisms can contribute.

- *Acute cellular rejection* is characterized by an interstitial mononuclear cell infiltrate (macrophages, and both CD4+ and CD8+ T cells).
- *Acute humoral rejection (rejection vasculitis)* is mediated by newly synthesized (not preformed) anti-donor antibodies that cause a

necrotizing vasculitis with consequent thrombosis. Complement activation contributes, and complement C4d deposition in vascular beds is used as a diagnostic feature of humoral rejection. A subacute vasculitis may also occur, with intimal thickening (by proliferating fibroblasts, smooth muscle cells, and macrophages); resultant vascular narrowing can cause infarction.

Chronic Rejection (p. 229)

Chronic rejection occurs over months to years and is characterized by progressive organ dysfunction. *Morphologically,* arteries show dense obliterative intimal fibrosis, causing allograft ischemia.

Based on the mechanisms of allograft rejection, *means to increase graft survival* (p. 229) include:

- HLA matching between donor and recipient
- Immunosuppressive therapy that blocks T cell activation or co-stimulation, IL-2 production (e.g., cyclosporine) or signaling (e.g., rapamycin), T lymphocyte proliferation (e.g., mycophenolate and azothioprine), and inflammation (e.g., glucocorticoids)
- T cell destruction (anti–T cell antibodies)
- Plasmapheresis or anti–B cell therapy

Immunosuppression carries the risk of increased susceptibility to opportunistic infections and certain malignancies (e.g., Epstein-Barr virus–induced lymphomas).

Transplantation of Hematopoietic Cells (p. 230)

Bone marrow transplantation—used for treating hematologic malignancies (e.g., leukemia), aplastic anemia, or immunodeficiency states—requires lethal levels of irradiation (and/or chemotherapy) to eradicate any malignant cells, create a satisfactory graft bed, and minimize host rejection of the grafted marrow. Besides the significant toxicity of the "conditioning regimen," complications include:

- *Recipient NK cells or radiation-resistant T cells:* These cells can mediate donor marrow cell rejection.
- *Graft-versus-host disease (GVHD):* Immunocompetent donor lymphocytes in an HLA-non-identical recipient recognize host cells as foreign and induce CD8+ and CD4+ T cell–mediated injury. Any tissues can be affected but host immune cells (immunosuppression) and biliary epithelium (jaundice), skin (desquamative rash), or gastrointestinal mucosa (bloody diarrhea) bear the brunt of the attack. In *chronic GVHD,* ongoing cutaneous and GI injury can resemble that seen in systemic sclerosis. Reactivation of cytomegalovirus infection, particularly in the lung, can be fatal.

GVHD and the infectious complications of bone marrow transplantation can be lethal; HLA matching and selective donor marrow T-cell depletion (and/or immunosuppression) can minimize the severity. Unfortunately, T-cell–depleted marrow engrafts poorly, and in leukemic patients the malignancy relapse rate is increased when T-cell–depleted marrow is used (donor T cells can exert a potent *graft-versus-leukemia* effect).

Immunodeficiency Syndromes (p. 230)

- *Primary immunodeficiencies* are usually hereditary and manifest between 6 months and 2 years of life as maternal antibody protection is lost.
- *Secondary immunodeficiencies* result from altered immune function due to infections, malnutrition, aging, immunosuppression, irradiation, chemotherapy, or autoimmunity.

Primary Immunodeficiencies (p. 231) (Fig. 6-5)

X-Linked Agammaglobulinemia (Bruton's Agammaglobulinemia) (p. 231)

X-linked agammaglobulinemia (Bruton's agammaglobulinemia) is one of the most common primary immunodeficiency syndromes. It manifests as *recurrent bacterial infections* (*Haemophilus influenzae, Streptococcus pneumoniae,* or *Staphylococcus aureus*—bacteria that require antibody opsonization for clearance) beginning at about 6 months of age. There is virtually no serum immunoglobulin, but cell-mediated immune function is normal. Consequently, viral and fungal infections are not usually problematic, although enterovirus, echovirus (causing a fatal encephalitis), and vaccine-associated poliovirus (causing paralysis) can cause disease since the causal pathogens are normally neutralized by circulating antibodies. *Giardia lamblia,* an intestinal parasite normally neutralized by secreted IgA, can also cause persistent infections.

- Affected individuals lack mature B cells due to mutations in the *B-cell tyrosine kinase gene (BTK);* BTK is normally expressed in early B cells and is critical for transduction of signals from the antigen receptor complex that drive B-cell maturation. Pre-B cells are present in normal numbers in marrow, but lymph nodes and spleen lack germinal centers, and plasma cells are absent from all tissues.
- T-cell numbers and function are entirely normal.
- Increased incidence (up to 35%) of autoimmune connective tissue diseases, chronic infections, and/or a break-down in self tolerance are implicated.
- Therapy involves immunoglobulin replacement therapy with normal donor serum.

Common Variable Immunodeficiency (p. 233)

Common variable immunodeficiency comprises a heterogeneous group of disorders, congenital and acquired, sporadic and familial. The common feature is hypogammaglobulinemia in the absence of other well-defined causes; generally all immunoglobulin classes are affected, but occasionally only IgG is. The pathogenesis may involve intrinsic B cell defects in maturation or survival or, more commonly, defective B cell development secondary to T cell shortcomings. Clinical features include:

- Initial presentation similar to X-linked agammaglobulinemia, that is, recurrent sinopulmonary infections, serious enterovirus infections, and persistent *G. lamblia* infections.
- Comparable numbers of both sexes with onset in late childhood or adolescence.
- Adenopathy with hyperplastic B cell zones, reflecting intact B-cell proliferation but lack of IgG-mediated feedback inhibition.
- Increased incidence of autoimmune diseases (20% of patients) and lymphoid malignancies.

Isolated IgA Deficiency (p. 233)

Isolated IgA deficiency is a common immunodeficiency (1 in 600 people of European descent in the United States) with *virtually absent serum and secretory IgA* (also occasionally IgG_2 and IgG_4 subclasses). It can be familial or acquired after toxoplasmosis, measles, or other viral infection. The basic defect is failure of IgA-positive B cells to mature; immature forms are present in normal numbers. Features include the following:

- Mucosal immunity is most affected. Although usually asymptomatic, patients can have recurrent sinopulmonary and gastrointestinal infections.

- Increased incidence of respiratory tract allergies and autoimmune diseases (i.e., SLE, rheumatoid arthritis).
- Patients can have antibodies directed against IgA, and transfusion of IgA-containing blood products can induce anaphylaxis.

Hyper-IgM Syndrome (p. 233)

Hyper-IgM syndrome is characterized by the production of IgM without IgG, IgA, or IgE antibodies; it results from failure of T cells to support B-cell immunoglobulin *isotype switching*. Such

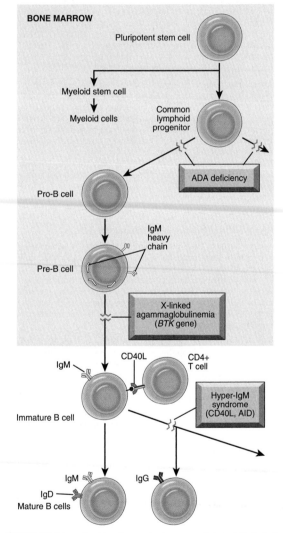

FIGURE 6-5 Schematic of lymphocyte development and sites of blockade for some of the primary immunodeficiency disorders; affected genes are indicated in parentheses. *ADA,* Adenosine deaminase; *AID,* activation-induced deaminase; *BTK,* B-cell tyrosine kinase; *CD40L,* CD40 ligand; *IgA,* immunoglobulin A; *IgM,* immunoglobulin M; *SCID,* severe combined immunodeficiency disease.

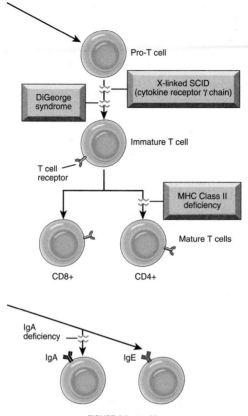

FIGURE 6-3, cont'd

switching depends on interaction of T cell CD40 ligand (CD40L) with B cell CD40. In 70% of patients, the disease is X-linked due to mutation of the *CD40L* gene encoded on the X chromosome (Xq26). In the remainder, there are mutations in CD40 or in *activation-induced deaminase (AID)*; the latter is a DNA-editing enzyme required for isotype switching. Features include the following:

- Lack of opsonizing IgG leads to recurrent bacterial infections.
- Patients are also susceptible to *Pneumocystis jiroveci* since T-cell/macrophage interactions in cell-mediated immune responses involve CD40-CD40L binding.
- Many of the IgM antibodies react with blood cells, resulting in autoimmune hemolytic anemia, thrombocytopenia, or neutropenia.

DiGeorge Syndrome (Thymic Hypoplasia) *(p. 234)*

DiGeorge syndrome (thymic hypoplasia) is a multiorgan disorder resulting from congenital failure of development of the third and fourth pharyngeal pouches and absence of the organs that normally arise from them; deletion of a gene mapping to 22q11 is seen in 90% of cases. Features include:

- *Thymic hypoplasia or aplasia:* T-cell deficiency with lack of cell-mediated responses (especially to fungi and viruses); immuno-globulin levels are normal or reduced depending on the severity of the T cell deficiency
- *Parathyroid hypoplasia:* Abnormal calcium regulation with hypo-calcemic tetany
- *Congenital defects of heart and great vessels*
- *Dysmorphic facies*

Severe Combined Immunodeficiency (p. 234)

Severe combined immunodeficiency disease (SCID) is a heterogeneous group of autosomal or X-linked recessive disorders characterized by *defects in both T- and B-cell function.* With impairment of both cellular and humoral immunity, lymphoid tissues are diffusely hypoplastic, and patients are susceptible to recurrent severe infections from a wide range of bacterial, viral, and fungal organisms. Without marrow transplantation, SCID is usually fatal within 1 year; X-linked SCID is also the first human disease in which gene therapy to replace a defective gene in a stem cell has been successfully applied. Mechanisms causing SCID include:

- An X-linked disorder (causing 50% to 60% of SCID) resulting from mutation in the signal-transducing γ chain (γc) subunit common to several cytokine receptors (IL-2, IL-4, IL-7, IL-9, IL-11, IL-15, and IL-21). The defect in the IL-7 stimulatory pathways is most profound because IL-7 is required for the proliferation of lymphoid progenitors, especially in the T-cell lineage. With inadequate T-cell help, B-cell antibody production is severely reduced. Ineffective IL-15 receptor signaling also results in deficiency of NK cells.
- Autosomal recessive disorders, the most common of which is *adenosine deaminase deficiency,* leading to accumulation of lymphocyte-toxic metabolites (e.g., deoxyadenosine and deoxy-ATP).

Immunodeficiency with Thrombocytopenia and Eczema (Wiskott-Aldrich Syndrome) (p. 235)

Immunodeficiency with thrombocytopenia and eczema (Wiskott-Aldrich syndrome) is an X-linked disorder characterized by recurrent infections. It is caused by mutations in the gene for Wiskott-Aldrich syndrome protein (WASP) located at Xp11.23; WASP links cell surface receptors and intracellular cytoskeleton and may be important for cell migration and signal transduction. Features include:

- Relatively normal thymus, but peripheral lymphoid T cell depletion with subsequent defective cellular immunity.
- No antibody production to polysaccharides and poor response to protein antigens.
- Increased incidence of non-Hodgkin B-cell lymphoma.

Genetic Deficiencies of the Complement System (p. 235)

Genetic deficiencies of the complement system have been described for virtually all complement components and for several complement regulatory proteins. C2 deficiency is most common but is not associated with serious infections, presumably because the alternative complement pathway is unaffected. However, inherited deficiencies of C2 (or C1q and C4) impair immune complex clearance and increase the risk of immune complex–mediated diseases (e.g., SLE). Deficiency of C3 impairs both complement pathways and hence leads to increased susceptibility to bacterial infections.

Defects in later-acting complement components (C5-C8) result in recurrent *Neisseria* infections.

C1 esterase inhibitor deficiency is associated with *hereditary angioedema*, resulting from defective regulation of complement activation, as well as the activation of coagulation factor XII and the kallikrein system. Patients have recurrent episodes of edema affecting skin, airways, and GI tract.

Deficiencies of other complement regulatory proteins (e.g., decay-accelerating factor and CD59) can lead to uncontrolled complement activation on red cells and endothelium leading to the constellation of findings in *paroxysmal nocturnal hemoglobinuria* (Chapter 14).

Secondary Immunodeficiencies (p. 235)

As a group, these are substantially more common than primary immune deficiencies and can result from various infections, malnutrition, aging, immunosuppression, irradiation, chemotherapy, or autoimmunity.

Acquired Immunodeficiency Syndrome (p. 235)

Acquired immunodeficiency syndrome (AIDS) is caused by the retrovirus human immunodeficiency virus (HIV); it is characterized by profound suppression of T-cell–mediated immunity leading to opportunistic infections, secondary neoplasms, and neurologic disorders.

Epidemiology (p. 236)

Transmission of HIV occurs through:

- *Sexual contact:* Seventy-five percent of all cases worldwide have this mode of transmission; virus is carried in semen and vaginal secretions (as free virus and within infected lymphocytes) and enters the host via mucosal abrasions (rectal, oral, vaginal) or direct mucosal cell contact. Transmission occurs by direct inoculation into the bloodstream, or infection of host mucosal dendritic cells or CD4+ T cells. Transmission is enhanced by concurrent sexually transmitted diseases, either by causing increased mucosal ulceration or by increasing the numbers of virus-containing inflammatory cells in genital fluids.
- *Parenteral inoculation:* Intravenous (IV) drug users constitute a significant population, with recipients of blood product concentrates (e.g., hemophiliacs) or blood transfusions now being substantially less common (fewer than 1 in 2 million blood transfusions in the United States). Risk of transmission from accidental needle stick is less than 0.3%, and anti-retroviral therapy post-exposure reduces the risk an additional eight-fold. Risk of transmission from insect bites is virtually impossible.
- *Vertical transmission from infected mothers to fetuses or newborns:* This may be transplacental *in utero*, during delivery through an infected birth canal, or through ingestion of breast milk. Ninety percent of children with AIDS have an HIV-infected mother and have had transplacental or perinatal transmission; the risk ranges from 7% to 49% with intra- and peripartum transmission being most common in the United States. Risk is increased with high viral load and chorioamnionitis.

In the United States, five major risk groups are identified:

- *Homosexual/bisexual men:* Roughly half of the reported cases of AIDS. This mode of transmission appears to be in decline.
- *IV drug users* (without a history of homosexual contact): This encompasses approximately 20% of all patients.

- *Hemophiliacs*: Approximately 0.5% of cases; mainly those patients receiving large amounts of pooled factor VIII or IX concentrates before 1985.
- *Blood or component recipients (excluding hemophiliacs)*: Approximately 1% of all patients. Ten percent of pediatric AIDS patients presumably developed their infection through blood or blood products received before 1985.
- *Heterosexual contact*: About 10% of patients acquire the disease through heterosexual contacts with other high-risk groups; roughly a third of new cases are attributable to this route. Outside the United States and Europe, male-to-female transmission (most through vaginal intercourse) is the most common mode of spread; female-to-male transmission is still uncommon in the United States (20-fold less common than male-to-female heterosexual transmission).

In approximately 5% of cases, no risk factors can be identified. HIV is *not* transmitted by casual (nonsexual) contact.

Etiology: The Properties of HIV (p. 237)

HIV is a non-transforming retrovirus in the lentivirus family; it causes immunodeficiency by destruction of target T cells. There are two different but genetically related forms; HIV-1 is most commonly associated with AIDS in the United States, Europe, and Central Africa, while HIV-2 causes a similar disease in India and West Africa.

- The HIV-1 lipid envelope, derived from the infected host membrane during budding, is studded with two viral glycoproteins, gp120 and gp41; both are critical for HIV infection.
- There is substantial variability in the envelope proteins, making vaccine targeting against specific antigenic structures extremely difficult.
- The virus core contains the capsid protein p24, nucleocapsid protein p7/p9, two copies of genomic RNA, and three viral enzymes: protease, integrase, and reverse transcriptase.
- p24 is the most readily detectable viral antigen and is the target in most diagnostic antibody assays.
- The viral genome contains typical retroviral *gag, pol*, and, *env* genes; the *gag* and *pol* gene products are synthesized as a larger precursor protein that must be proteolytically processed. Components of antiviral therapy are thus directed against the protease, as well as the retroviral polymerase.
- Besides the typical retroviral *gag, pol*, and, *env* genes, HIV has several genes (not present in other retroviruses) important for viral synthesis and assembly. These genes include *tat, vpu, vif, nef*, and *rev; tat* and *rev* for example, regulate HIV transcription and may be therapeutic targets.

Pathogenesis of HIV Infection and AIDS (p. 238)

Depletion of CD4+ helper T-cell (and impaired functioning of any surviving helper T cells) causes profound immunosuppression and constitutes the central pathogenic pathway of AIDS; the central nervous system (CNS) is another important target.

LIFE CYCLE OF HIV (p. 239)

- The CD4 antigen (also present at lower levels on monocytes, macrophages, and dendritic cells) is the high-affinity receptor for the HIV gp120 protein.
- HIV gp120 must also bind co-receptors on target cells to facilitate cell entry; the major co-receptors are chemokine receptors

CCR5 and CXCR4. CCR5 is found mainly on monocyte/macrophage lineages; consequently, HIV using this co-receptor are denoted M-tropic. Conversely, CXCR4 is mostly found on T lymphocytes, and viruses using that co-receptor are denoted T-tropic. M-tropic viruses typically constitute the majority of HIV in the blood of acutely infected individuals; over the course of an infection the more virulent T-tropic viruses accumulate. Individuals with mutations in the CCR5 co-receptor (roughly 1% of the Caucasian American population are homozygous) are resistant to infection by M-tropic HIV strains.

- After gp120 interacts with CD4 and one of the co-receptors, the non-covalently linked gp41 protein undergoes a conformational change that allows the virus to be internalized.
- The genome undergoes reverse transcription, generating double-stranded complementary (proviral) DNA. HIV causes productive infections only in memory and activated T cells; naïve T cells are "protected" by the activity of a cytidine deaminase that introduces cytosine-to-uracil mutations in the proviral DNA. This enzyme is inactivated by previous T cell activation.
- In quiescent T cells, the proviral DNA remains in the cytoplasm as a linear episomal form. However, in proliferating T cells (e.g., after antigenic stimulation), the proviral DNA circularizes, enters the nucleus, and is integrated into the host genome.
- After integration, proviral DNA may be silent (latent) for months to years; alternatively, proviral DNA can be transcribed in activated cells to generate viral particles. Cell activation results in nuclear translocation of the NF-κB transcription factor; it binds to the long-terminal-repeat sequences that flank the HIV genome, and it induces viral transcripts.

MECHANISMS OF T-CELL IMMUNODEFICIENCY IN HIV
INFECTION (p. 240)

Most T-cell loss is attributable to the direct cytopathic effect of replicating virus; this may be due to interference with normal host cell protein synthesis or to increased membrane permeability associated with viral budding. Other mechanisms that contribute to T-cell loss include:

- Progressive destruction of the architecture and cellular composition of the lymphoid organs, including cells important for maintaining a cytokine environment conducive to CD4+ maturation
- Chronic activation of uninfected cells (responding to HIV or opportunistic infections), leading eventually to *activation-induced cell death*
- Fusion of infected and noninfected cells via gp120 (forming syncytia or giant cells), leading to cell death
- Binding of soluble gp120 to noninfected CD4+ T cells leading to activation of apoptotic pathways or to CTL-mediated killing
- Besides cell death, HIV infection also causes qualitative defects in T cell function including diminished T_H1 responses (relative to T_H2), defective intracellular signaling, and reduced antigen-induced T cell proliferation

HIV INFECTION OF NON-T CELLS (p. 241)

- Infected monocytes and macrophages bud relatively small amounts of virus and are refractory to HIV cytopathic effects; these infected monocyte/macrophages can thus act as HIV reservoirs (potentially transferring virus to T cells during antigen presentation), as well as vehicles for viral transport, especially to the CNS.

- Mucosal dendritic cells transport virus to regional lymph nodes. Nodal follicular dendritic cells are important HIV reservoirs; viral particles coated with anti-HIV antibodies attach to the dendritic cell Fc receptors and can continually infect T cells as they come in close contact during passage through lymph nodes.
- Despite defects in T cell help, and therefore the inability to mount antibody responses to newly encountered antigen, there is also paradoxical polyclonal B-cell activation. This can occur through reactivation or re-infection with cytomegalovirus and/or EBV, direct activation by gp41, or increased IL-6 production by infected macrophages.

PATHOGENESIS OF CENTRAL NERVOUS SYSTEM
INVOLVEMENT (p. 242)

CNS involvement occurs predominantly through infected monocytes that circulate to the brain and either directly release toxic cytokines (IL-1, TNF, and so on), induce neuronal NO production via gp41, or cause neuron damage via soluble gp120.

Natural History of HIV Infection (p. 243)

HIV infection can be divided into three phases (Fig. 6-6):

- *Primary Infection, Virus Dissemination, and the Acute Retroviral Syndrome* (p. 243): Primary infection, virus dissemination, and the acute retroviral syndrome is characterized by transient viremia, widespread seeding of mucosal lymphoid tissue and infection of memory T cells (expressing CCR5), a temporary (but substantial) fall in CD4+ T cells, followed by antibody seroconversion and partial control of viral replication by the generation of CD8+ antiviral T cells. Clinically, a self-limited acute illness (the *acute retroviral syndrome*) occurs in 40% to 90% of infected individuals with sore throat, fatigue, myalgias, fever, rash, adenopathy, and/or weight loss. Clinical improvement and a partial recovery in CD4+ T-cell counts occur within 6 to 12 weeks; the level of circulating CD4+ T cells is the most reliable short-term indicator of disease progression. The viral load at the end of the acute phase also reflects the balance between HIV production and host defenses. This viral set-point is an important predictor of the rate of progression of HIV disease; high viral loads at the end of the acute phase portend rapid progression to AIDS.
- *Chronic Infection: Phase of Clinical Latency* (p. 244): Chronic infection is characterized by clinical latency (absence of symptoms) despite ongoing vigorous viral replication; lymph nodes and spleen are the major sites of viral production. There is initially a brisk regeneration of T cells, but eventually recurrent viral infection and associated T cell death leads to progressive depletion. Concomitant with T cell loss is a decline in immune function and an increasing viral burden, with a shift to T-tropic viruses. Patients may develop minor opportunistic infections such as oral candidiasis. The period of clinical latency is typically 7 to 10 years in untreated patients, although *rapid progressors* may see this period truncated to 2 to 3 years. 5% to 15% will be *long-term non-progressors* who remain symptom-free, with stable CD4 counts and low viral loads, for 10 or more years; 1% are *elite controllers* with a vigorous anti-HIV response and undetectable plasma virus.
- *AIDS* (p. 245): AIDS is heralded by a rapid decline in host defenses manifested by low CD4+ counts and a dramatic increase in viral burden; patients frequently present with prolonged fever, weight loss, and diarrhea, followed by serious opportunistic infections, secondary neoplasms, or neurologic disease (*AIDS indicator diseases*).

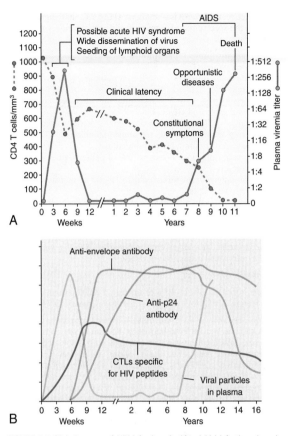

FIGURE 6-6 Clinical course of HIV infection. **A,** After initial infection, there is widespread viral dissemination and a sharp decrease in peripheral CD4+ T cell counts. With the ensuing immune response to HIV the viral load is diminished, followed by a prolonged period of clinical latency; during this period, viral replication continues. The CD4+ T-cell count gradually decreases during the following years, until it reaches a critical level below which constitutional symptoms and various opportunistic diseases supervene. **B,** Immune response to HIV infection. A cytotoxic T lymphocyte *(CTL)* response to HIV is detectable 2 to 3 weeks after the initial infection, peaking at 9 to 12 weeks. Marked expansion of virus-specific CD8+ T-cell clones occurs during this time; the humoral immune response peaks at about 12 weeks. *(A, Redrawn from Fauci AS, Lane HC: Human immunodeficiency virus disease: AIDS and related conditions. In Fauci AS, et al. (eds): Harrison's principles of internal medicine, ed 14, New York, 1997, McGraw-Hill, p. 1791.)*

Clinical Features of AIDS *(p. 245)*

These run the gamut from asymptomatic to the acute retroviral syndrome to life-threatening infection or malignancy. The clinical features of full-blown AIDS include:

OPPORTUNISTIC INFECTIONS *(p. 246)*

Opportunistic infections account for the majority of deaths in untreated patients with AIDS; most cases represent reactivation of latent infections rather than *de novo* infections. The advent of highly active anti-retroviral therapy (HAART) has significantly changed the spectrum and frequency of these secondary opportunistic infections.

- *Pneumocystis jiroveci* pneumonia occurs in 15% to 30% of untreated patients.
- *Candida* is the most common fungal pathogen (oral, vaginal, or esophageal).
- Cytomegalovirus may be systemic, but it more commonly involves the eye and GI tract.
- Tuberculosis and atypical mycobacterial infections occur late in the setting of severe immunosuppression; a third of AIDS deaths worldwide are attributable to tuberculosis.
- *Cryptococcus* infections occur in 10% of patients, predominantly as meningitis.
- *Toxoplasma gondii* causes encephalitis and is responsible for 50% of CNS mass lesions.
- JC papovavirus causes progressive multifocal leukoencephalopathy.
- Herpes simplex virus manifests as chronic mucocutaneous ulcerations.
- *Cryptosporidium, Isospora belli,* microsporidia, and atypical mycobacteria, as well as enteric bacteria *(Shigella and Salmonella)* can cause intractable diarrhea.

TUMORS (p. 246)

Tumors occur in 25% to 40% of untreated AIDS patients; a common feature is that they are all caused by oncogenic DNA viruses:

- *Kaposi sarcoma (KS)* is the most common neoplasm, although HAART has reduced the frequency. KS lesions are composed of spindle cells forming vascular channels with associated chronic inflammatory infiltrates; these lesions are caused by *human herpesvirus-8 (HHV-8),* also called *KS herpesvirus.* Latent HHV-8 infection results in the production of viral homologues of cyclin D, and several p53 inhibitors, thus promoting cell proliferation. In addition, infected cells make a pro-inflammatory viral homologue of IL-6, and a G-protein coupled receptor that induces the release of vascular endothelial growth factor. Besides infecting endothelial cells to produce KS, HHV-8-infected B cells may also be the source of *primary effusion lymphomas* in AIDS patients. AIDS-associated KS is quite distinct from the sporadic form of KS in non-HIV-infected individuals (Chapter 11).
- *Lymphomas* may be systemic, CNS, or body-cavity-based; 6% of AIDS patients develop such tumors. Aggressive B-cell non-Hodgkin lymphomas, especially involving extranodal sites, constitute 80% of these. Primary CNS lymphomas are 1000-fold more common in AIDS patients than in the general population. The etiology of the lymphomas is likely a sustained polyclonal B cell proliferation driven by EBV infection, followed by the emergence of an oligoclonal or monoclonal population; 50% of systemic lymphomas and 100% of central nervous system lymphomas carry the EBV genome.
- *Other tumors* include squamous cell carcinoma of the uterine cervix and anus, likely reflecting greater susceptibility to HPV infection.

CENTRAL NERVOUS SYSTEM DISEASE (p. 248)

CNS disease occurs in 40% to 60% of patients. In addition to opportunistic infections and tumors, patients can present with acute aseptic meningitis, vacuolar myelopathy, and peripheral neuropathy. Most common is a progressive encephalopathy, designated *AIDS-dementia complex* (Chapter 28).

EFFECT OF ANTIRETROVIRAL THERAPY ON THE CLINICAL
COURSE OF HIV INFECTION (p. 248)

- HAART involves more than 25 compounds in six distinct drug categories; triple drug regimens in compliant patients are effective in reducing viral burden to non-detectable levels indefinitely, with gradual recovery of T-cell counts. Morbidity and mortality has dropped commensurately.
- Treated patients still carry viral DNA in their lymphoid tissues and can spread the infection, or they can develop active infection if treatment is stopped.
- Long-term HAART can also cause toxicities including fat redistribution, insulin resistance, premature cardiovascular disease, and renal and hepatic dysfunction.
- *Immune reconstitution inflammatory syndrome* can occur as a consequence of a recovering immune system in the presence of a heavy burden of persistent microbes (e.g., atypical mycobacteria or *Pneumocystis*).

Morphology (p. 249)

With the exception of the CNS, the tissue changes in AIDS are neither specific nor diagnostic; the pathologic features are those of the various opportunistic infections and neoplasms (discussed elsewhere in the organ-specific chapters).

- *Lymph nodes:* Adenopathy in early HIV infection reflects the initial polyclonal B-cell proliferation (and hypergammaglobulinemia), showing nonspecific, predominantly follicular hyperplasia with mantle zone attenuation and intense medullary plasmacytosis. HIV particles can be demonstrated in germinal centers by *in situ* hybridization, localized mainly on the surface of follicular dendritic cells. With progression to full-blown AIDS, the lymphoid follicles become involuted *(burned out)*, with general lymphocyte depletion and follicular disruption. Similar lymphoid depletion occurs in the spleen and thymus.
- *Inflammatory responses to infections:* These responses may be sparse or atypical, and infectious organisms may not be apparent without special stains.

Amyloidosis (p. 249)

Amyloid is a heterogeneous group of fibrillar proteins that *share the ability to aggregate into an insoluble, cross-beta-pleated sheet tertiary conformation;* amyloid fibrils accumulate extracellularly in tissues due either to excess synthesis or resistance to catabolism. As amyloid accumulates, it produces pressure atrophy of adjacent parenchyma. Depending on tissue distribution and degree of involvement, the clinical effects of amyloid can range from life threatening to an asymptomatic incidental finding at autopsy.

Properties of Amyloid Proteins (p. 249)

By electron microscopy, amyloid is composed predominantly (95%) of non-branching fibrils 7.5 to 10 nm in diameter, associated with a minor (5%) *P component*—stacks of pentagonal, doughnut-shaped structures. Of more than 20 distinct forms thus identified, three are most common (Table 6-5):

- *Amyloid light chain (AL):* Immunoglobulin light chains (or amino-terminal fragments thereof) derived from plasma cells; lambda light chain amyloid occurs more often than kappa; associated with plasma cell tumors (e.g., multiple myeloma).

TABLE 6-5   Classification of Amyloidosis

Clinicopathologic	Associated Diseases	Major Fibril Protein	Chemically Related Precursor Protein
Systemic (Generalized) Amyloidosis			
Immunocyte discrasias with amyloidosis (primary amyloidosis)	Multiple myeloma and other monoclonal B-cell proliferations	AL	Immunoglobulin light chains, chiefly λ light chain
Reactive systemic amyloidosis (secondary amyloidosis)	Chronic inflammatory conditions	AA	SAA
Hemodialysis-associated amyloidosis	Chronic renal failure	Aβ$_2$m	β$_2$-microglobulin
Hereditary amyloidosis	—	AA	SAA
Familial amyloidotic neuropathies (several types)	—	ATTR	Transthyretin
Systemic senile amyloidosis	—	ATTR	Transthyretin
Localized Amyloidosis			
Senile cerebral	Alzheimer disease	Aβ	APP
Endocrine Medullary carcinoma of thyroid	—	A Cal	Calcitonin
Islet of Langerhans	Type II diabetes	AIAPP	Islet amyloid peptide
Isolated atrial amyloidosis	—	AANF	Atrial natriuretic factor
Prion diseases	Various prion diseases of the central nervous system	Misfolded prion protein (PrP^{SC})	Normal prion protein PrP

- *Amyloid-associated (AA):* An 8500-dalton non-immunoglobulin protein derived from a larger serum precursor called *serum amyloid–associated (SAA)* protein synthesized by hepatocytes as part of the "acute phase response"; AA amyloid is associated with chronic inflammatory states.
- *β-Amyloid (Aβ):* A 4000-dalton peptide that forms the core of cerebral plaques and deposits within cerebral vessel walls in Alzheimer disease; it derives from a transmembrane amyloid precursor protein (Chapter 28).

Other less-common forms of amyloid:

- *Transthyretin (TTR):* A normal serum protein that binds and transports thyroxine and retinol. Excess amounts of normal TTR can deposit in geriatric hearts (senile systemic amyloidosis) while mutant forms of the protein are deposited in a group of hereditary diseases called *familial amyloid polyneuropathy.*
- *β_2-microglobulin:* The smaller nonpolymorphic peptide component of class I HLA molecules and a normal serum protein; it is deposited in a form of amyloidosis that complicates long-term hemodialysis.

Pathogenesis of Amyloidosis *(p. 251)*

Proteins that form amyloid are either:

- Normal proteins that have a propensity to fold improperly and associate to form fibrils; over-production (or defective catabolism) thus leads to deposition.
- Mutant proteins that are prone to misfolding and aggregation; even "normal" levels of synthesis can cause deposition.

Classification of Amyloidosis *(p. 252)*

Amyloidosis is subdivided into *systemic* (generalized) and *localized* (tissue-specific) forms and is further classified on the basis of predisposing conditions (see Table 6-5).

Systemic amyloidosis is associated with the following conditions:

- *Primary amyloidosis: Immunocyte dyscrasias with amyloidosis* is due to AL-type amyloid; it occurs in 5% to 15% of patients with multiple myeloma (Chapter 13). Malignant plasma cells synthesize abnormal quantities of a single immunoglobulin (*M spike* on serum protein electrophoresis) or immunoglobulin light chain (*Bence Jones* protein). The vast majority of cases of AL-type systemic amyloidosis are *not* associated with *overt* B-cell neoplasms but nevertheless have elevated monoclonal immunoglobulins, light chains, or both.
- *Reactive secondary amyloidosis:* This is due to AA-type amyloid. Secondary amyloidosis is associated with chronic inflammatory states (infectious and noninfectious) (e.g., rheumatoid arthritis, scleroderma, dermatomyositis, bronchiectasis, chronic osteomyelitis), and non-immunocyte tumors (e.g., Hodgkin lymphoma and renal cell carcinoma).
- *Hemodialysis-associated amyloidosis:* This affects 60% to 80% of patients on chronic hemodialysis. This form is due to deposition (in joints, synovium, and tendon sheaths) of β_2-microglobulin not filtered by normal dialysis membranes.
- *Heredofamilial amyloidosis:* These include a number of rare entities, often confined to specific geographic locations. The most common and best characterized form is *familial Mediterranean fever,* a recurrent, febrile illness caused by over-production of IL-1; this is caused by mutations in the *pyrin* protein involved in regulating cytokine production. The amyloid is of AA type, suggesting that chronic inflammation plays a pivotal role.

Localized amyloidosis is amyloid confined to a single organ or tissue:

- Localized forms of AL immunocyte-derived amyloid with associated plasma cell infiltrates; nodular deposits can occur in lung, larynx, skin, bladder, and tongue and periorbitally.
- *Endocrine amyloid* occurs in tumors associated with hormone synthesis; for example, thyroid medullary carcinoma making procalcitonin that deposit as amyloid fibrils.
- *Amyloid of aging* occurs typically in the eighth and ninth decades and is most commonly due to deposition of non-mutant

transthyretin. Although amyloid distribution is systemic, the dominant involvement is of the heart, manifesting as a restrictive cardiomyopathy or arrhythmias. In addition to sporadic senile systemic amyloidosis, another form—more common in blacks—occurs due to mutant transthyretin.

Morphology (p. 253)

In general, there is no consistent or distinctive pattern of organ involvement for the systemic amloidoses, except perhaps hemodialysis-associated amyloid. Macroscopically, affected tissues are enlarged, waxy, and firm. Microscopically, routine stains reveal only amorphous, acellular, hyaline, eosinophilic extracellular material. With special stains (e.g., Congo red), amyloid is salmon-pink, and characteristic yellow-green birefringence may be seen using polarized light.

- *Kidneys:* Initial mesangial and subendothelial deposition progresses to complete glomerular hyalinization. Peritubular deposits begin in the tubular basement membrane and gradually extend into the interstitium. Hyaline thickening of arterial and arteriolar walls with narrowing lumen eventually causes ischemia with tubular atrophy and interstitial fibrosis.
- *Spleen:* Spleen may be enlarged (up to 800 g). Amyloid deposits begin between cells. With time, one of two patterns emerges:

  Sago spleen: Deposits are limited to the splenic follicles, giving rise to *tapioca-like* granules on gross inspection.
  Lardaceous spleen: Amyloid largely spares the follicles and is deposited in the red pulp. Fusion of deposits forms large geographic areas of amyloid.

- *Liver:* The liver shows hepatomegaly. Microscopically, amyloid first deposits in the space of Disse, gradually encroaching on parenchyma and sinusoids to produce pressure atrophy with massive hepatic replacement.
- *Heart:* Distinctive (although not always present) are minute, typically atrial, pink-gray subendocardial droplets representing focal amyloid accumulations. Vascular and subepicardial deposits may also occur. Microscopically, there are interstitial and perimyocyte deposits, progressively leading to pressure atrophy.
- *Other organs:* Nodular deposits in the tongue can cause macroglossia *(tumor-forming amyloid of the tongue).* Deposits on the carpal ligament of the wrist (e.g., in hemodialysis-associated amyloid) can cause carpal tunnel syndrome.

Clinical Features (p. 254)

- Renal involvement can give rise to proteinuria, and nephrotic syndrome (Chapter 20). Cardiac amyloid can present as insidious congestive heart failure or arrhythmias, and gastrointestinal amyloidosis can present with malabsorption.
- Diagnosis is made on the basis of biopsy and characteristic Congo red stain. Favored biopsy sites are the kidney (when renal manifestations are present) and the rectum or gingiva (in systemic disease). Abdominal fat pad aspirates can also yield diagnostic tissue but have low sensitivity.
- In amyloidosis associated with B-cell dyscrasias, serum and urine electrophoresis and bone marrow biopsy (for plasmacytosis) are indicated.
- In systemic amyloidosis, the prognosis is poor. Median survival after diagnosis in the setting of B-cell dyscrasias is about 2 years, and myeloma-associated amyloid is worse. Reactive amyloidosis may have a slightly better outlook, depending on the ability to control the underlying inflammatory condition.

7

Neoplasia

Nomenclature (p. 260)

The terms *neoplasm* (literally "new growth") and *tumor* are used interchangeably; these refer to abnormal masses of tissue, the growth of which is virtually autonomous and exceeds that of normal tissues. In contrast to non-neoplastic proliferations (Chapter 3), the growth of tumors persists after cessation of the initiating sti'mulus. Tumors are broadly classified based on clinical behaviors:

- *Benign:* These have an "innocent" behavior characterized by a localized lesion without spread to other sites and amenable to surgical resection; the patient typically survives, although there are exceptions
- *Malignant:* These are called *cancers,* with aggressive behavior including invasion and destruction of adjacent tissues and capacity for spread to other sites *(metastasis)*

All tumors have two basic components:

- Clonal expansions of neoplastic cells constituting the tumor parenchyma
- Supporting stroma composed of non-neoplastic connective tissue and blood vessels; abundant collagenous stroma is called *desmoplasia,* and such tumors are rock hard or *scirrhous.*

The type of neoplasm is based on the characteristics of its parenchyma. Tumor nomenclature is summarized in Table 7-1; while benign tumors frequently have an "-oma" suffix, it is worth emphasizing that some terms do not follow the rules (e.g., melanoma, lymphoma, and mesothelioma are all malignant).

Benign Tumors (p. 260)

Benign mesenchymal tumors include lipoma, fibroma, angioma, osteoma, and leiomyoma. The nomenclature for benign epithelial tumors is less straightforward, incorporating elements of histogenesis, macroscopic appearance, and microscopic architecture:

- *Adenomas:* Epithelial tumors arising in glands or forming glandular patterns
- *Cystadenomas:* Adenomas producing large cystic masses, common in ovary
- *Papillomas:* Epithelial tumors forming gross or microscopic finger-like projections
- *Polyp:* Tumor projecting macroscopically above the mucosa (e.g., a colon polyp)

TABLE 7-1 Nomenclature of Tumors		
Tissue of Origin	**Benign**	**Malignant**
Composed of One Parenchymal Cell Type		
Tumors of Mesenchymal Origin		
Connective tissue and derivatives	Fibroma	Fibrosarcoma
	Lipoma	Liposarcoma
	Chondoma	Chondrosarcoma
	Osteoma	Osteogenic sarcoma
Endothelial and Related Tissues		
Blood vessels	Hemangioma	Angiosarcoma
Lymph vessels	Lymphangioma	Lymphangiosarcoma
Synovium		Synovial sarcoma
Mesothelium		Mesothelioma
Brain coverings	Meningioma	Invasive meningioma
Blood Cells and Related Cells		
Hematopoietic cells		Leukemias
Lymphoid tissue		Lymphomas
Muscle		
Smooth	Leiomyoma	Leiomyosarcoma
Striated	Rhabdomyoma	Rhabdomyosarcoma
Tumors of Epithelial Origin		
Stratified squamous	Squamous cell papilloma	Squamous cell or epidermoid carcinoma
Basal cells of skin or adnexa		Basal cell carcinoma
Epithelial lining of glands or ducts	Adenoma	Adenocarcinoma
	Papilloma	Papillary carcinomas
	Cystadenoma	Cystadenocarcinoma
Respiratory passages	Bronchial adenoma	Bronchogenic carcinoma
Renal epithelium	Renal tubular adenoma	Renal cell carcinoma
Liver cells	Liver cell adenoma	Hepatocellular carcinoma
Urinary tract epithelium (transitional)	Transitional cell papilloma	Transitional cell carcinoma
Placental epithelium	Hydatidiform mole	Choriocarcinoma
Testicular epithelium (germ cells)		Seminoma
		Embryonal carcinoma
Tumors of Melanocytes	Nevus	Malignant melanoma
More Than One Neoplastic Cell Type—Mixed Tumors, Usually Derived from One Germ Cell Layer		
Salivary glands	Pleomorphic adenoma (mixed tumor of salivary origin)	Malignant mixed tumor of salivary gland origin
Renal anlage		Wilms tumor
More Than One Neoplastic Cell Type Derived from More Than One Germ Cell Layer		
Totipotential cells in gonads or in embryonic rests	Mature teratoma, dermoid cyst	Immature teratoma, teratocarcinoma

Malignant Tumors (p. 261)

Malignant tumors are divided into two general categories:

- *Carcinomas* derived from epithelial cells
- *Sarcomas* of mesenchymal cell origin

The nomenclature for specific malignant tumors is based on their appearance and/or presumed cell of origin (see Table 7-1). Malignant epithelial tumors resembling stratified squamous epithelium are denoted *squamous cell carcinoma*, while those with glandular growth patterns are called *adenocarcinomas*. Sarcomas are designated by the appropriate cell prefix (e.g., smooth muscle malignancies are *leiomyosarcomas*). Not infrequently, neoplasms composed of poorly differentiated unrecognizable cells can only be designated as undifferentiated malignant tumors.

Some tumors appear to have more than one parenchymal cell type:

- *Mixed tumors* derive from a neoplastic clone of a single germ cell layer that differentiates into more than one cell type (e.g., mixed salivary gland tumors containing epithelial cells and myxoid stroma)
- *Teratomas* are composed of various parenchymal cell types representative of more than one germ cell layer. They arise from totipotential cells capable of forming endodermal, ectodermal, and mesenchymal tissues and can have both benign and malignant forms. Such tumors typically occur in testis or ovary, or rarely midline embryonic rests

Two *non-neoplastic* lesions grossly resemble tumors, and have ominous names:

- *Choristomas:* These are ectopic rests of non-transformed tissues (e.g., pancreatic cells under the small bowel mucosa).
- *Hamartomas:* These are masses of disorganized tissue indigenous to a particular site (i.e., lung hamartomas exhibit cartilage, bronchi, and blood vessels); many have clonal, recurrent genetic translocations.

Characteristics of Benign and Malignant Neoplasms (p. 262)

Classification of a tumor as *benign* or *malignant* ultimately depends on its clinical behavior; however, morphologic evaluation (and, increasingly, molecular profiling) allows categorization based on degree of differentiation, growth rate, local invasion, and metastasis.

Differentiation and Anaplasia (p. 262)

Differentiation refers to how closely tumor cells histologically (and functionally) resemble their normal cell counterparts; lack of differentiation is called *anaplasia*. In general, neoplastic cells in benign lesions are well differentiated; cells in malignant neoplasms can range from well differentiated to completely undifferentiated. Well-differentiated tumors, whether benign or malignant, tend to retain the functional characteristics of their normal counterparts, for example, hormone production by endocrine tumors or keratin production by squamous epithelial tumors. Malignant cells can revert to embryologic phenotypes or express proteins not elaborated by the original cell of origin.

Histologic changes in tumors include:

- *Pleomorphism:* Variation in the shape and size of cells and/or nuclei
- *Abnormal nuclear morphology:* Darkly stained *(hyperchromatic)* nuclei with irregularly clumped chromatin, prominent nucleoli, and increased nuclear-to-cytoplasmic ratios (approaching 1:1 versus normal ratios of 1:4 or 1:6)

- *Abundant and/or atypical mitoses:* Reflect increased proliferative activity, and abnormal cell division (e.g., tripolar mitoses, so-called *Mercedes-Benz* sign)
- *Loss of polarity:* Disturbed orientation, and tendency for forming anarchic, disorganized masses
- *Tumor giant cells:* Cells with single polyploid nuclei or multiple nuclei
- *Ischemic necrosis:* Due to insufficient vascular supply

Dysplasia is the term used to describe the constellation of histologic changes seen in a neoplasm. Dysplasia (literally "disordered growth") refers to loss of cellular uniformity and architectural organization and can range from mild to severe. Dysplasia can occur adjacent to frank malignancy and, in many cases, antedates the development of cancer. However, *dysplasia does not equate to malignancy,* and moreover, *dysplastic cells do not necessarily progress to cancer;* removal of the inciting stimulus from dysplastic epithelium (e.g., chronic irritation) can result in reversion to complete normalcy. When dysplastic changes are marked and *involve the entire thickness of an epithelium,* the lesion is referred to as *carcinoma in situ.* This lesion can be forerunner to invasive carcinoma.

Rates of Growth (p. 265)

Most malignant tumors grow more rapidly than benign tumors. Nevertheless, some cancers grow slowly for years and only then enter a phase of rapid growth; others expand rapidly from the outset. Growth of cancers arising from hormone-sensitive tissues (e.g., the breast) may be affected by hormonal variations associated with pregnancy and menopause.

Ultimately, the progression of tumors and their growth rates are determined by an excess of cell production over cell loss; this is influenced by: doubling time, fraction of cells replicating at any time, and rate of cell death or shedding. Important concepts include the following:

- Fast-growing tumors can have a high cell *turnover,* that is, rates of proliferation and apoptosis are both high.
- The portion of tumor cells that is actively proliferating is called the *growth fraction.* In the early submicroscopic phase of tumor growth, the vast majority of cells are proliferating; by the time of clinical detection, most cells are not actively replicating. The growth fraction of tumor cells has a profound impact on susceptibility to therapeutic intervention, because most anticancer treatments typically act only on cells that are in cycle. Surgical debulking or radiation treatment induces surviving tumor cells to enter the cell cycle and thus increase the efficacy of subsequent chemotherapy.
- In general, but not always, the growth rate of tumors inversely correlates with the level of differentiation; better-differentiated tumors grow more slowly.

Cancer Stem Cells and Cancer Cell Lineages (p. 267)

A clinically detectable tumor (i.e., containing 10^9 cells) is a heterogeneous population of cells originating from the clonal expansion of a single cell. Tumor stem cells can be derived by mutation of normal stem cells or from differentiated precursors that acquire the asymmetric division properties of stemness. They have the capacity to sustain persistent growth of the larger tumor; tumor-initiating cells (T-ICs) have been functionally defined by their ability to indefinitely maintain tumor growth after transplant into immunodeficient murine hosts. Such tumor stem cells, as with their normal counterparts in adult tissues, would likely have an extremely low rate of replication; consequently, they may be resistant to typical tumor treatments. This concept is important because therapies that efficiently kill the rapidly replicating progeny may well leave behind stem cells that can regenerate the entire tumor.

Local Invasion (p. 268)

- Most benign tumors grow as cohesive, expansile masses that develop a surrounding rim of condensed connective tissue, or *capsule*. These tumors do not penetrate the capsule or the surrounding normal tissues, and the plane of cleavage between the capsule and the surrounding tissues facilitates surgical enucleation.
- Malignant neoplasms are typically invasive and infiltrative, destroying surrounding normal tissues. They commonly lack a well-defined capsule and cleavage plane, making simple excision impossible. Consequently, surgery requires removal of a considerable margin of healthy and apparently uninvolved tissue.

Metastasis (p. 269)

Metastasis involves invasion of lymphatics, blood vessels, or body cavities by tumor, followed by transport and growth of secondary tumor cell masses discontinuous from the primary tumor. *This is the single most important feature distinguishing benign from malignant.* With notable exceptions of central nervous system (CNS) tumors and cutaneous basal cell carcinomas, almost all malignant tumors have the capacity to metastasize.

Pathways of Spread (p. 269)

Cancer dissemination occurs by three routes:

- *Seeding of body cavities and surfaces* (p. 269) occurs by dispersion into peritoneal, pleural, pericardial, subarachnoid, or joint spaces. Ovarian carcinoma typically spreads transperitoneally to the surface of abdominal viscera, often without deeper invasion. Mucus-secreting appendiceal carcinomas can fill the peritoneum with a gelatinous neoplastic mass called *pseudomyxoma peritonei.*
- *Lymphatic spread* (p. 269) transports tumor cells to regional nodes and, ultimately, throughout the body. Although tumors do not contain functional lymphatics, lymphatic vessels at tumor margins appear sufficient. Lymph nodes draining tumors are frequently enlarged; this can result from metastatic tumor cell proliferation or from reactive hyperplasia to tumor antigens. Biopsy of the proximal *sentinel lymph node* draining a tumor can allow accurate prognostication regarding tumor metastasis.
- *Hematogenous spread* (p. 270) is typical of sarcomas but is also the favored route for certain carcinomas (e.g., renal). Because of their thinner walls, veins are more frequently invaded than arteries, and metastasis follows the pattern of venous flow; understandably, lung and liver are the most common sites of hematogenous metastases.

Epidemiology (p. 270)

Epidemiologic studies allow the identification of environmental, racial, gender, and cultural risk factors. In addition, such studies also shed light on pathogenic mechanisms.

Cancer Incidence (p. 271)

Cancers of the prostate, lung, and colon are the most common cancers in men; breast, lung, and colon cancers are the most common in women. Cancer is responsible for approximately 23% of all United States deaths annually with lung cancer being the dominant cause in both sexes. The good news is that cancer death rates have declined 18.4% in men and 10.4% in women since 1990.

Geographic and Environmental Factors (p. 272)

Environmental factors significantly influence the incidence and outcomes of cancers; thus, in Japan, the death rate from gastric cancer is seven-fold higher than the United States, while lung cancer mortality is more than two-fold greater in the United States. In Japanese immigrants to the United States, death rates fall between those of Japanese and American natives. Carcinogenic exposures may be environmental (e.g., ultraviolet [UV] radiation or air pollution), or may be from medications, occupation, or diet; obesity is associated with 14% to 20% of cancer deaths, and alcohol and smoking also significantly contribute to cancer risk.

Age (p. 273)

Most cancer occurs in individuals older than 55 years; it is the main cause of death in women aged 40 to 79 and in men aged 60 to 79. The rising incidence with increasing age is attributed to accumulation of somatic mutations and a decline in immune surveillance. Nevertheless, certain cancers are particularly common in children, and 10% of deaths in patients younger than 15 years are cancer related. These malignancies are not typically carcinomas but rather leukemia, lymphoma, CNS tumors, and sarcomas.

Genetic Predisposition to Cancer (p. 273)

Heredity can influence cancer development even in the setting of well-defined environmental causes. However, only 10% of malignancies are attributable to inherited mutations, and the frequency is much lower (i.e., 0.1%) for certain cancers. Nevertheless, genes that are causally associated with tumors with a strong hereditable component are also frequently involved in the more common sporadic forms of the same tumors. Genetic predisposition to cancer falls in three general categories (Table 7-2).

Autosomal Dominant Inherited Cancer Syndromes (p. 274)

Autosomal dominant inherited cancer syndromes are characterized by a single mutant gene that greatly increases cancer risk, although incomplete penetrance and variable expressivity occur. The heritable component is usually a point mutation in one allele of a tumor suppressor gene (e.g., *RB* in retinoblastoma or *APC* in familial adenomatous polyposis); the silencing of the second allele occurs somatically, typically due to chromosome deletion or recombination.

- With the exception of Li-Fraumeni syndrome (p53 mutations), there is no increased general predilection for cancers; rather, tumors develop only in selected tissues. Thus, in multiple endocrine neoplasia type 2 (MEN-2) (i.e., RET tyrosine kinase mutation) only thyroid, parathyroid, and adrenal glands are affected; in multiple endocrine neoplasia type 1 (MEN-1) (i.e., menin

TABLE 7-2	Examples of Inherited Predisposition to Cancer
Gene	**Inherited Predisposition**
Inherited Cancer Syndromes (Autosomal Dominant)	
RB	Retinoblastoma
p53	Li-Fraumeni syndrome (various tumors)
p16/INK4A	Melanoma
APC	Familial adenomatous polyposis/colon cancer
NF1, NF2	Neurofibromatosis 1 and 2
BRCA1, BRCA2	Breast and ovarian tumors
MEN1, RET	Multiple endocrine neoplasia 1 and 2
MSH2, MLH1, MSH6	Hereditary nonpolyposis colon cancer
PTCH	Nevoid basal cell carcinoma syndrome
PTEN	Cowden syndrome (epithelial cancers)
LKB1	Peutz-Jegher syndrome (epithelial cancers)
VHL	Renal cell carcinomas
Inherited Autosomal Recessive Syndromes of Defective DNA Repair	
Xeroderma pigmentosum	
Ataxia-telangiectasia	
Bloom syndrome	
Fanconi anemia	
Familial Cancers	

Familial clustering of cases, but role of inherited predisposition not clear for each individual
    Breast cancer
    Ovarian cancer
    Pancreatic cancer	

transcription factor mutation) only pituitary, parathyroids, and pancreas are involved.
- There is typically an associated *marker phenotype* (e.g., multiple benign colonic tumors in familial polyposis).

Defective DNA-Repair Syndromes (p. 275)

Defective DNA-repair syndromes are typically autosomal recessive and predispose to DNA instability in the face of environmental carcinogens; an autosomal dominant form is hereditary nonpolyposis colon cancer [HNPCC] resulting from inactivation of a DNA mismatch repair gene.

Familial Cancers (p. 275)

Familial cancers are characterized by familial clustering of specific forms of cancer, for example, familial forms of common cancers (e.g., breast, colon, brain, and ovary), but the transmission pattern is not clear in any individual case. Onset is often early with multiple or bilateral tumors, and typically there is a marker phenotype (e.g., familial colon cancers do not arise in preexisting polyps).

The predisposition is usually autosomal dominant, but susceptibility may also be due to multiple low-penetrance alleles.

Nonhereditary Predisposing Conditions (p. 276)

Proliferation—regenerative, metaplastic, hyperplastic, or dysplastic—all increase the risk of developing malignancy, since it is proliferating cells that accumulate the genetic lesions necessary for carcinogenesis.

Chronic Inflammation and Cancer (p. 276)

Inflammation:

- Increases the pool of stem cells that can be subject to the effects of mutagens
- Produces cytokines and growth factors to drive cell survival and proliferation
- Promotes genomic instability by the production of reactive oxygen species

Precancerous Conditions (p. 276)

The phrase *precancerous conditions* is a misnomer since, in the great majority, no malignant transformation occurs. Nevertheless, certain disorders (e.g., *leukoplakia* of oral mucosa, penis, or vulva) have a well-defined association with cancer, and some benign tumors are a focus of subsequent malignancy (e.g., colonic villous adenomas can develop into cancer as they enlarge). Although cancer can arise in previously benign tumors, this is uncommon, and most malignant tumors arise *de novo*.

Molecular Basis of Cancer (p. 276)

The molecular pathogenesis of cancer is schematized in Figure 7-1, and the following are fundamental principles:

- *Non-lethal genetic damage underlies carcinogenesis;* genetic injury can be inherited in the germ line or acquired in somatic cells through spontaneous mutation or environmental exposures.
- Tumors develop as clonal progeny of a single genetically damaged progenitor cell
- Four classes of normal regulatory genes are the targets of genetic damage:

  Growth-promoting proto-oncogenes
  Growth-inhibiting tumor-suppressor genes
  Genes that regulate apoptosis
  Genes that regulate DNA repair; defective DNA repair predisposes to genomic mutations *(mutator phenotype)*

- Carcinogenesis is a multistep process. The attributes of malignancy (e.g., invasiveness, excessive growth, escape from the immune system, etc.) are acquired incrementally, a process called *tumor progression*. At the genetic level, progression results from accumulation of successive mutations
- Although tumors begin as monoclonal proliferations, by the time they are clinically evident, they are extremely heterogeneous

Essential Alterations for Malignant Transformation (p. 278)

Certain fundamental changes in cell physiology contribute to development of the malignant phenotype:

- Self-sufficiency in growth signals (proliferation without external stimuli)
- Insensitivity to growth-inhibitory signals

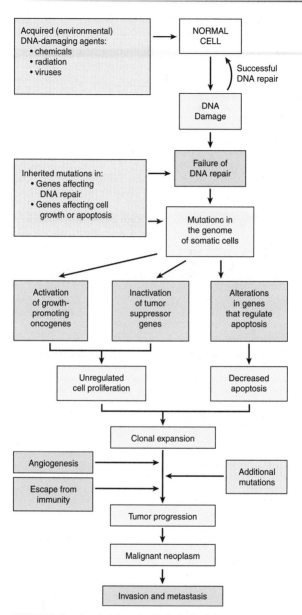

FIGURE 7-1 Flow chart depicting a simplified scheme of the molecular basis of cancer.

- Evasion of apoptosis
- Defects in DNA repair
- Limitless replicative potential (related to telomere maintenance)
- Sustained angiogenesis to provide adequate nutrition and waste removal

- Ability to invade and metastasize
- Ability to escape immune recognition and regulation

Self-Sufficiency in Growth Signals (p. 279)

Normal cell proliferation involves the following steps:

- Growth factor binding to cell surface receptor
- Transient and limited activation of the receptor and associated membrane or cytoplasmic signal-transduction proteins
- Nuclear transmission via second messengers
- Induction and activation of nuclear regulatory factors that initiate DNA transcription
- Entry into and progression through the cell cycle

Cancer is characterized by proliferation in the absence of growth-promoting signals. *Oncogenes* are genes that promote autonomous cell growth in cancer cells; their unmutated normal counterparts are *proto-oncogenes*. Proteins encoded by proto-oncogenes may function as growth factors or their receptors, transcription factors, or cell cycle components. *Oncoproteins* are the protein products of oncogenes; they resemble the normal products of proto-oncogenes except that they lack normal regulatory elements, and their synthesis may be independent of normal growth stimuli.

Proto-Oncogenes, Oncogenes, and Oncoproteins (p. 279)

Mutations convert proto-oncogenes into constitutively active oncogenes that endow the cell with growth self-sufficiency. These can be grouped in the following categories (Table 7-3):

Growth Factors (p. 280)

Tumors can acquire the ability to produce growth factors to which they are also responsive—leading to an autocrine stimulation loop; in most cases the growth factor gene is not mutated. Growth factor–driven division is not in itself sufficient for neoplastic transformation; rather, it increases the risk of acquiring mutations during increased proliferation.

Growth Factor Receptors (p. 280)

Several oncogenes encode growth factor receptors; these drive malignant transformation by being constitutively activated—either through mutations that cause activation in the absence of ligand binding or through over-expression, rendering cells more sensitive to smaller quantities of growth factors. Antibody blockade of over-expressed receptors or small molecule inhibition of constitutively active receptors allows *targeted therapy* of tumors.

Signal-Transducing Proteins (p. 281)

Such oncoproteins mimic the function of normal cytoplasmic signal-transducing proteins; most are sited at the inner leaflet of the plasma membrane. The best-studied is the *RAS* family of guanosine triphosphate (GTP)-binding proteins (*G proteins*).

The *RAS* Oncogene (p. 282). Mutated RAS proteins are present in 15% to 20% of all human tumors, although the frequency can be much higher (e.g., 90% of pancreatic and 50% of colonic adenocarcinomas); most differ from their normal counterparts by point mutations. Normal RAS proteins alternate between activated (i.e., GTP-bound) signal-transmitting and inactive (i.e., guanosine diphosphate [GDP]-bound) quiescent forms. Conversion from active to inactive RAS is mediated by intrinsic GTPase activity and can be augmented by GTPase-activating proteins (GAPs). Mutant RAS proteins lack GTPase activity and are therefore locked in the signal-transmitting GTP-bound form; activated RAS, in

TABLE 7-3   Selected Oncogenes, Their Modes of Activation, and Associated Human Tumors

Category	Protooncogene	Mode of Activation	Associated Human Tumor
Growth Factors			
PDGF-β chain	SIS	Overexpression	Astrocytoma Osteosarcoma
Fibroblast growth factors	HST-1 INT-2	Overexpression Amplification	Stomach cancer Bladder cancer Breast cancer Melanoma
TGF-α	TGF-α	Overexpression	Astrocytomas Hepatocellular carcinomas
HGF	HGF	Overexpression	Thyroid cancer
Growth Factor Receptors			
EGF-receptor family	ERB-B1 (ECFR) ERB-B2	Overexpression Amplification	Squamous cell carcinomas of lung, gliomas Breast and ovarian cancers
CSF-1 receptor	FMS	Point mutation	Leukemia
Receptor for neurotrophic factors	RET	Point mutation	Multiple endocrine neoplasia 2A and 2B, familial medullary thyroid carcinomas
PDGF receptor	PDGF-R	Overexpression	Gliomas
Receptor for stem cell (steel) factor	KIT	Point mutation	Gastrointestinal stromal tumors and other soft-tissue tumors

Continued

TABLE 7-3	Selected Oncogenes, Their Modes of Activation, and Associated Human Tumors—cont'd		
Category	Protooncogene	Mode of Activation	Associated Human Tumor
Proteins Involved in Signal Transduction			
GTP-binding	K-RAS	Point mutation	Colon, lung, and pancreatic tumors
	H-RAS	Point mutation	Bladder and kidney tumors
	N-RAS	Point mutation	Melanomas, hematologic
Nonreceptor tyrosine kinase	ABL	Translocation	Chronic myeloid leukemia
			Acute lymphoblastic leukemia
RAS signal transduction	BRAF	Point mutation	Melanomas
WNT signal transduction	β-catenin	Point mutation	Hepatoblastomas, hepatocellular carcinoma
		Overexpression	
Nuclear Regulatory Proteins			
Transcriptional activators	C-MYC	Translocation	Burkitt lymphoma
	N-MYC	Amplification	Neuroblastoma, small cell carcinoma of lung
	L-MYC	Amplification	Small cell carcinoma of lung
Cell-Cycle Regulators			
Cyclins	CYCLIN D	Translocation	Mantle cell lymphoma
		Amplification	Breast and esophageal cancers
	CYCLIN E	Overexpression	Breast cancer
Cyclin-dependent kinase	CDK4	Amplification or point mutation	Glioblastoma, melanoma, sarcomas

CSF-1, Colony-stimulating factor-1; *EGF,* epidermal growth factor; *GTP,* guanosine triphosphate; *HGF,* hepatocyte growth factor; *PDGF,* platelet-derived growth factor; *TGF-α,* transforming growth factor-α.

turn, activates the mitogen-activated protein (MAP) kinase pathway, leading to cell proliferation. Mutations in GAPs, or in downstream members of the *RAS* signaling cascade (e.g., RAF or MAP kinase), lead to a similar proliferative phenotype.

Alterations in Nonreceptor Tyrosine Kinases (p. 283)

The activity of these tyrosine kinases influences cell proliferation. Thus, c-*ABL* codes for a tyrosine kinase whose activity is normally tightly regulated; in chronic myeloid leukemia (CML) however, translocation of c-*ABL* with fusion to the *BCR* gene produces a hybrid protein that self associates through the BCR moiety and exhibits potent unregulated tyrosine kinase activity. Inhibitors of the BCR-ABL kinase (e.g., imatinib mesylate) have high therapeutic efficacy in treating CML. Other examples of mutations involving nonreceptor tyrosine kinases include activating point mutations in the JAK2 tyrosine kinase; these mutant forms constitutively activate STAT transcription factors and are associated with polycythemia vera and primary myelofibrosis.

Transcription Factors (p. 284)

Growth autonomy can also occur through mutations in nuclear transcription factors (e.g., *MYC, JUN, FOS, REL,* and *MYB* oncogenes) that regulate the expression of growth-related genes.

The *MYC* Oncogene (p. 284). The *MYC* oncogene is most commonly involved in human tumors; the proto-ongogene is rapidly induced when quiescent cells are signaled to divide and likely functions by activating genes involved in proliferation. MYC overexpression (e.g., due to gene amplification, gene translocations, or altered posttranslational regulation) leads to malignancy

Cyclins and Cyclin-Dependent Kinases (p. 284)

Loss of cell cycle control is central to malignant transformation. Autonomous growth can be driven by over-expression or mutation (with increased activity) of cyclins or cyclin-dependent kinases (CDKs), or by mutation (with loss of activity) of CDK inhibitors; indeed, dysregulation of cyclin D, CDK 4, RB, or the CDK inhibitor p16/INK4a is seen in the vast majority of human cancers (see also Chapter 3 regarding cell cycle regulation). The G_1/S transition (where DNA damage must be identified and repaired before replication) and the G_2/M transition (where fidelity of DNA synthesis must be verified before mitosis) are critical cell cycle checkpoints; mutations in the damage sensors or repair mechanisms are a major source of genetic instability in cancer cells.

Insensitivity to Growth Inhibition and Escape from Senescence: Tumor-Suppressor Genes (p. 286)

Besides activation of growth-promoting oncogenes, cancer can also arise by inactivation of *tumor suppressor genes* that normally inhibit cell proliferation. Generally both alleles of a tumor-suppressor gene must be mutated for carcinogenesis to occur; because heterozygous cells have adequate tumor suppressor activity, the mutation of the second normal tumor suppressor (leading to carcinogenesis) is also referred to as *loss of heterozygosity (LOH)*. The protein products of such tumor suppressors can be transcription factors, cell cycle inhibitors, signal transduction molecules, receptors, or factors involved in DNA damage repair (Table 7-4).

RB (p. 288). The *RB* gene is the prototypic tumor-suppressor gene. Among other activities, its gene product regulates the

TABLE 7-4 Selected Tumor Suppressor Genes Involved in Human Neoplasms

Subcellular Location	Gene	Function	Tumors Associated with Somatic Mutations	Tumors Associated with Inherited Mutations
Cell surface	TGF-β receptor	Growth inhibition	Carcinomas of colon	Unknown
	E-cadherin	Cell adhesion	Carcinoma of stomach	Familial gastric cancer
Inner aspect of plasma membrane	NF-1	Inhibition of RAS signal transduction and of p21 cell-cycle inhibitor	Neuroblastomas	Neurofibromatosis type 1 and sarcomas
Cytoskeleton	NF-2	Cytoskeletal stability	Schwannomas and meningiomas	Neurofibromatosis type 2, acoustic schwannomas and meningiomas
Cytosol	APC/β-catenin	Inhibition of signal transduction	Carcinomas of stomach, colon, pancreas; melanoma	Familial adenomatous polyposis coli/colon cancer
	PTEN	PI-3 kinase signal transduction	Endometrial and prostate cancers	Unknown
	SMAD 2 and SMAD 4	TGF-β signal transduction	Colon, pancreas tumors	Unknown
Nucleus	RB	Regulation of cell cycle	Retinoblastoma; osteosarcoma carcinomas of breast, colon, lung	Retinoblastomas, osteosarcoma
	p53	Cell-cycle arrest and apoptosis in response to DNA damage	Most human cancers	Li-Fraumeni syndrome; multiple carcinomas and sarcomas
	WT-1	Nuclear transcription	Wilms tumor	Wilms tumor
	p16 (INK4a)	Regulation of cell cycle by inhibition of cyclin-dependent kinases	Pancreatic, breast, and esophageal cancers	Malignant melanoma
	BRCA-1 and BRCA-2	DNA repair	Unknown	Carcinomas of female breast and ovary; carcinomas of male breast
	KLF6	Transcription factor	Prostate	Unknown

PI, Phosphatidylinositol; TGF, transforming growth factor.

advancement of cells through the G_1/S checkpoint. By sequestering E2F less efficiently, *RB* mutations lead to increased E2F transcription factor activity; thus cells can cycle in the absence of a growth stimulus. Several oncogenic DNA viruses (e.g., human papillomavirus [HPV]) synthesize proteins that bind to RB and displace the E2F transcription factors, thereby contributing to persistent cell cycling.

RB contributes to the pathogenesis of the childhood tumor *retinoblastoma* through a *two-hit* mechanism:

• Both normal *RB* alleles must be inactivated (i.e., two hits) for retinoblastoma to develop
• In familial cases (i.e., 40% of retinoblastomas), children inherit one defective germ line copy of *RB*; retinoblastoma develops when the remaining normal *RB* gene undergoes somatic mutation. In sporadic cases, both normal *RB* alleles are lost by somatic mutation in a retinoblast
• Patients with familial retinoblastoma have increased risk of developing other tumors such as osteosarcomas.

p53: Guardian of the Genome (p. 290). The p53 protein prevents the propagation of genetically defective cells (p63 and p73 are related family members with similar activities):

• When cells are "stressed" (e.g., by damage to DNA), p53 undergoes post-translational phosphorylation, releasing it from an associated MDM2 protein that normally targets it for degradation. The sensing of DNA damage is accomplished through two protein kinases, *ataxia-telangiectasia mutated (ATM)*, and *ataxia-telangiectasia and Rad3-related (ATR)*.
• The unshackled p53 then acts as a transcription factor for additional genes (including miRNAs) that arrest the cell cycle and promote DNA repair; G_1 cell cycle arrest, for example, is mediated largely through p53-dependent transcription of the CDK inhibitor p21.
• If DNA can be repaired during the cell cycle arrest, MDM2 transcription increases and p53 is subsequently degraded, allowing the cell to progress into S phase.
• If DNA damage cannot be repaired, p53 induces cellular senescence by altering E2F signaling pathways, or it can induce apoptosis by increasing transcription of pro-apoptotic genes.

p53 is mutated in more than 50% of all human cancers; patients with germ line p53 mutations *(Li-Fraumeni syndrome)* have a higher risk of malignancy (e.g., leukemias, sarcomas, breast cancer, and brain tumors) due to inactivation of the normal allele (i.e., LOH) in somatic cells. Similar to RB, p53 can also be functionally inactivated by products of DNA oncogenic viruses.

Adenomatous Polyposis Coli/β-Catenin Pathway (p. 292). Adenomatous polyposis coli (APC) genes are a class of tumor suppressors that down-regulate growth-promoting signals in the WNT signaling pathway. APC protein is a negative regulator of β-catenin activity; it binds and regulates the degradation of cytoplasmic β-catenin. During normal embryonic development, WNT binding to its surface receptor causes APC dissociation from β-catenin, allowing β-catenin to enter the nucleus and drive proliferation. In the absence of normal APC, cells respond as if under continuous WNT signaling; cytoplasmic β-catenin levels increase, resulting in increased nuclear translocation and ultimately increased transcription of c-*MYC, cyclin D1*, and other genes. Those born with one mutant *APC* allele develop thousands of adenomatous polyps in the colon, of which one or more will eventually develop into colonic cancers (Chapter 17). About 70% to 80% of sporadic colon cancers also exhibit *APC* LOH; β-catenin mutations are also seen in more than 50% of hepatoblastomas and more than 20% of hepato-cellular carcinomas. E-cadherins that facilitate cell-cell interactions also interact with β-catenin; loss of intercellular adhesion (due to injury or mutation) results in increased cytoplasmic β-catenin that can drive cellular proliferation.

Other Genes that Function as Tumor Suppressors (p. 294)

INK4a/ARF (p. 294). This locus encodes two proteins; p16/INK4a blocks RB phosphorylation and thus maintains the RB checkpoint, while p14/ARF prevents p53 destruction. Mutations occur in bladder, head, and neck tumors, as well as in certain leukemias; gene activity can also be silenced by epigenetic hypermethylation in cervical cancers.

The TGF-β Pathway (p. 294). TGF-β receptor ligation causes intracellular signaling (e.g., via SMAD 2 and SMAD 4) that up-regulates the expression of growth-inhibitory genes, including CDK inhibitors. Mutations affecting the TGF-β receptor or SMAD signaling are inactivated in 100% of pancreatic cancers and more than 80% of colon carcinomas.

PTEN (p. 294). PTEN is a *p*hosphatase and *ten*sin homologue that acts as a tumor suppressor brake on the pro-survival/pro-growth PI3 kinase/AKT pathway (Chapter 3).

NF1 (p. 294). NF1 is a tumor-suppressor gene coding for *neurofibromin*; the protein has a GTPase activity that regulates signal transduction through RAS. *NF-1* LOH impairs the conversion of active (i.e., GTP-bound) RAS to inactive (i.e., GDP-bound) RAS; thus cells are continuously stimulated to divide. Germline inheritance of one mutant allele of *NF-1* predisposes to the development of numerous benign neurofibromas when the second *NF-1* gene is lost or mutated (i.e., neurofibromatosis type I); some progress to malignancy.

VHL (p. 295). Germline mutation of the von Hippel-Lindau gene is associated with hereditary renal cell cancer, pheochromocytomas, hemangioblastomas of the CNS, and retinal angiomas. The VHL protein is part of a ubiquitin ligase complex involved in the degradation of hypoxia-inducible transcription factor 1α (HIF1α); mutations in VHL lead to increased cytoplasmic HIF1α and subsequent increased nuclear translocation that drives cell growth and angiogenic factor production.

WT1 (p. 295). Mutational inactivation of *WT1* (either germline or somatic) is associated with the development of Wilms tumors. The WT1 protein is a transcriptional activator of genes involved in renal and gonadal differentiation; the tumorigenic function of WT1 deficiency relates to its role in genitourinary differentiation.

Evasion of Apoptosis (p. 295)

Neoplastic cell accumulation requires not only oncogene activation and/or tumor suppressor inactivation but also mutations in pathways that would otherwise induce the aberrant cell to undergo apoptosis (e.g., due to DNA damage or loss of adhesion). The major apoptosis pathways are described in Chapter 1.

The prototypic anti-apoptotic protein is BCL2; it and related molecules (e.g., BCL-XL) prevent programmed cell death by limiting the exit of cytochrome c from mitochondria (recall that cytochrome *c* activates the proteolytic enzyme caspase 9 pathway). Over-expression of *BCL2* extends cell survival; if such cells are already genetically unstable, they will continue to accrue additional oncogene and tumor suppressor gene mutations. *BCL2* over-expression in follicular B-cell lymphomas is the classic example of this anti-apoptotic mechanism; 85% of these lymphomas have a t(14;18) translocation juxtaposing *BCL2* with a transcriptionally active immunoglobulin heavy chain locus; the result is *BCL2* over-expression. Other genes of the *BCL2* family (e.g., *BAX* and *BAK*) are pro-apoptotic, and so-called *BH3-only proteins* can sense intracellular damage signals and neutralize the activity of BCL2 and BCL-XL.

Genes not directly related to the *BCL2* family can also regulate apoptosis; thus p53 normally induces programmed cell death when DNA repair is ineffective.

Limitless Replicative Potential: Telomerase (p. 296)

Telomerase (normally expressed only in germ cells and stem cells) is not active in most somatic cells; as a consequence, chromosomal telomeres progressively shorten with each division until DNA replication can no longer proceed. Indeed, shortened telomeres are interpreted by DNA-repair machinery as double-stranded breaks, leading to cell cycle arrest via p53 and RB and *cellular senescence*. If p53 and RB mutations disable these check-points, non-homologous end-joining pathways swing into action, leading to the fusion of the shortened ends of two chromosomes. Such inappropriate repair system activation leads to dicentric chromosomes that are then torn asunder at anaphase, resulting in a new round of double-stranded breaks. The resulting genetic instability of multiple cycles of bridge-fusion-breakage leads to *mitotic catastrophe* and cell death. Cancer cells overcome these limitations by reactivating telomerase or occasionally through DNA recombination that also elongates telomeres; more than 90% of human tumors show increased telomerase activity.

Angiogenesis (p. 297)

Despite genetic mutations that drive proliferation and promote survival, tumors (like normal tissues) still require nutrients and waste removal; thus they cannot enlarge beyond a 1 to 2 mm size without inducing new blood vessel growth *(angiogenesis).* Neovascularization also stimulates tumor growth through the endothelial cell production of growth factors such as insulin-like growth factor and PDGF. In the absence of new vessels, tumor cannot access the vasculature so that angiogenesis also clearly influences metastatic potential. It is noteworthy that new tumor vessels differ from normal vasculature by being dilated and leaky with slow and abnormal flow.

Tumor growth is a balancing act between angiogenic and anti-angiogenic factors. Most tumors do not initially induce angiogenesis and thus remain small or *in situ.* The subsequent *angiogenic switch* involves either the production of angiogenesis factors or the loss on inhibitors such as thrombospondin-1 (normally induced by p53), angiostatin, or endostatin. Tumors and/or host stromal and inflammatory cells can all be sources of pro- or anti-angiogenic factors. Hypoxia is a major driving force for angiogenesis, primarily through the action of the HIF1α transcription factor. Endothelial growth proteins include *vascular endothelial growth factor (VEGF)* and *basic fibroblast growth factor (bFGF)* (Chapter 3); proteases can also release pre-formed angiogenic mediators (e.g., bFGF) from the ECM.

Invasion and Metastasis (p. 298)

The steps involved in invasion and metastasis are depicted in Figure 7-2. Cells within a primary tumor are heterogeneous with respect to the various requisite metastatic attributes; consequently, only a distinct minority can complete all the steps and form distant tumors.

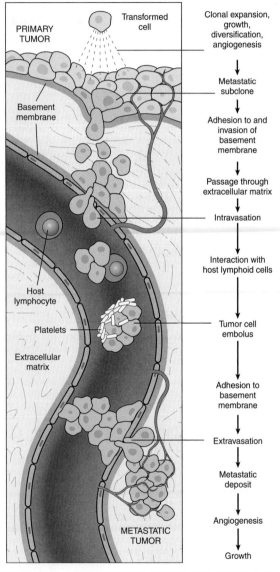

FIGURE 7-2 The metastatic cascade: sequential steps involved in the hematogenous spread of a tumor.

Invasion of Extracellular Matrix (p. 298)

To metastasize, tumor cells must dissociate from adjacent cells and then degrade, adhere, and migrate through ECM.

- *Detachment*: In normal epithelial cells, loss of attachment (e.g., through integrins) to the ECM typically induces programmed cell death; clearly, tumor cells become resistant to such apoptotic pathways. Epithelial cells also bind each other through adhesion molecules, including a family of glycoproteins called *cadherins*. In several carcinomas, there is down-regulation of epithelial (E)-cadherins (or their intracellular linkers called *catenins*), thereby reducing cellular cohesion.
- *ECM degradation*: Tumors directly elaborate proteases or can induce stromal cell to produce them. Although tumor cells can rapidly squeeze between fibers *(ameboid migration)*, matrix degradation creates ready passage for migration; additionally, ECM degradation releases a host of growth factors. Thus, matrix metalloproteinase 9 (MMP9) degrades epithelial and vascular basement membrane type IV collagen, in addition to releasing ECM-sequestered pools of VEGF.
- *ECM attachment*: Invading cells must express adhesion molecules that allow interaction with the ECM. Conversely, catabolism of the ECM (e.g., via MMP9) can create novel binding sites that promote tumor cell migration.
- *Migration*: Besides diminished adhesivity, tumor cells have increased locomotion, in part attributable to autocrine cytokines and motility factors; they also migrate in response to stromal cell chemotactic factors, degraded ECM components, and liberated stromal growth factors.

Vascular Dissemination and Homing of Tumor Cells (p. 300)

Tumor cells embolize in the bloodstream as self-aggregates and by adhering to circulating leukocytes and platelets; this may confer some protection from host anti-tumor effector mechanisms. Exactly where tumor cell emboli eventually lodge and begin growing is influenced by:

- Vascular and lymphatic drainage from the site of the primary tumor (discussed previously)
- Interaction with specific receptors; certain tumor cells express CD44 adhesion molecules that avidly bind high endothelial venules in lymph nodes; other tumors exhibit specific chemokine receptors that interact with ligands uniquely expressed in certain vascular beds (e.g., CXCR4 and CCR7 in breast cancer)
- The microenvironment of the organ or site (e.g., a tissue rich in protease inhibitors might be resistant to penetration by tumor cells)

Molecular Genetics of Metastasis Development (p. 301)

Relative to the number of cells in a tumor or the number of tumor cells present in the circulation at a given time, the overall frequency of metastases is remarkably small. This metastatic inefficiency has been classically ascribed to the multiple mutations that must accrue in any individual cell; however, some tumors show high frequencies of cells with the requisite "metastatic signature" but do not develop secondary spread because of host stromal and inflammatory counter-measures. Metastases may also require that any mutations occur specifically in tumor stem cells and not just the progeny cells. Finally, specific "metastasis suppressor genes" or "metastasis promoter genes" (e.g., miRNA) have been described that also impact the capacity of primary lesions to develop secondary tumor spread.

Genomic Instability—Enabler of Malignancy (p. 302)

DNA repair pathways do not directly influence cell proliferation, rather they act indirectly by correcting DNA errors that occur spontaneously during cell division or subsequent to mutagenic chemicals or irradiation. Thus *DNA repair genes are not directly oncogenic;* however, defective proteins permit mutations to occur in other genes. Inherited mutations in DNA repair proteins greatly increases the risk of carcinogenesis *(genomic instability syndromes),* and defects in DNA repair pathways also occur in sporadic malignancies. Defects can occur in three types of DNA repair systems:

• Mismatch repair
• Nucleotide excision repair
• Recombination repair

Hereditary Nonpolyposis Colon Cancer Syndrome (p. 302)

Patients inherit one defective copy of DNA repair genes involved in *mismatch repair* (e.g., *MSH2* and *MLH1*) with a second hit occurring in a colonic epithelial cell. Loss of the normal "spell checker" function of the mismatch repair enzymes leads to gradual accumulation of errors in multiple genes including proto-oncogenes and tumor suppressor genes. Mismatch repair mutations are heralded by *microsatellite instability.* Microsatellites are tandem repeats of one to six nucleotides scattered throughout the genome; in normal tissues, the length of these remains constant. Variation of microsatellite length is a hallmark of mismatch repair defects.

Xeroderma Pigmentosum (p. 302)

Nucleotide excision repair genes are specifically required for correcting UV light–induced pyrimidine dimer formation. Patients with defects in these genes develop skin cancers due to UV mutagenic effects.

Diseases with Defects in DNA Repair by Homologous Recombination (p. 302)

These autosomal recessive disorders (e.g., Bloom syndrome, Fanconi anemia, and ataxia-telangiectasia) are characterized by hypersensitivity to DNA-damaging agents (e.g., ionizing radiation or chemical cross-linking agents). In ataxia-telangiectasia, *ATM* gene mutations yield a protein kinase unable to sense DNA double-stranded breaks; while normal ATM protein phosphorylates p53 leading to cell cycle arrest or apoptosis, defective ATM allows DNA-damaged cells to proliferate and accumulate additional mutations. In Bloom syndrome, the mutated protein is a helicase normally involved in DNA repair by homologous recombination.

Mutations in *BRCA1* or *BRCA2* account for 25% of cases of familial breast cancer; patients who inherit defective copies of *BRCA1* also have an increased risk of developing ovarian or prostate cancers, while patients with defective germline *BRCA2* have increased risk for cancers of ovary, prostate, pancreas, stomach, bile ducts, and melanocytes. Both genes are involved in the repair of double-stranded DNA breaks by homologous recombination. Interestingly, these genes are rarely inactivated in sporadic breast cancers.

Stromal Microenvironment and Carcinogenesis (p. 303)

Cancers are heterogeneous collections, including malignant cells, as well as non-cancerous inflammatory and stromal cells. Increasingly it is recognized that while tumors clearly influence their surrounding stroma (e.g., by inducing neovascularization and desmoplastic matrix), the host stromal cells, ECM, and inflammation can also modulate (i.e, inhibit *and* augment) tumor growth.

Metabolic Alterations: The Warburg Effect (p. 303)

Cancer cells preferentially utilize glycolysis for energy generation rather than the more energy efficient mitochondrial oxidative phosphorylation pathways—even in the presence of adequate oxygen. The phenomenon was originally described by Otto Warburg in 1931 (hence the name), and current non-invasive tumor imaging (i.e., positron emission tomography [PET] scans) takes advantage of the metabolic hyperactivity by visualizing uptake of non-metabolizable glucose analogues. The phenomenon is most likely explained by the increased need of proliferating tumors to shunt important precursor molecules into new lipid and nucleotide synthesis rather than into energy generation. It may also explain the role of apparent oncogenes and tumor suppressor genes that affect intracellular energy sensing and/or metabolic pathways more than cell turnover.

Dysregulation of Cancer-Associated Genes (p. 304)

Besides oncogene activation or tumor suppressor inactivation, large chromosomal changes (visible by karyotyping) and epigenetic changes (e.g., DNA methylation) can induce malignancy.

Chromosomal Changes (p. 304)

Translocations (common in hematopoietic malignancies) and inversions can activate protooncogenes by:

- Shifting protooncogenes away from normal regulatory elements, resulting in overexpression. In the case of the t(8:14)(q24:q32) translocation in Burkitt lymphoma, the tightly regulated c-*myc* gene moves to the immunoglobulin heavy chain gene locus, resulting in its overexpression.
- Forming new hybrid genes that fortuitously encode growth-promoting chimeric molecules. In the reciprocal t(9:22) translocation *(Philadelphia chromosome)*, a truncated portion of the c-*abl* proto-oncogene is joined with the *BCR* (break-point cluster region) gene to form a fusion protein that has constitutive kinase activity. Transcription factors are often the partners in gene fusions occurring in cancer cells.
- *Deletions* (p. 306) are more common in non-hematopoietic solid tumors and are typically attributable to loss of a critical tumor suppressor gene, for example, 13q14 deletions contain the *RB gene*.

Gene Amplification (p. 306)

Reduplication and amplification of DNA sequences may underlie the protooncogene activation associated with overexpression. Examples include N-myc overexpression in 25% to 30% of neuroblastomas and ERB-B2 overexpression in 20% of breast cancers.

Epigenetic Changes (p. 306)

Post-translational modification of histones (e.g., acetylation) and DNA methylation—without changes in the primary DNA sequence—can influence gene expression including silencing tumor suppressor genes (e.g., *p14ARF* in gastrointestinal cancers and *p16INK4a* in various malignancies). Therapeutic strategies to demethylate selected DNA sequences may be efficacious in these cases.

miRNAs and Cancer (p. 307)

These small, non-coding, single-stranded RNAs are incorporated into silencing complexes and can mediate post-transcriptional gene silencing (Chapter 5). Deletions of miRNA sequences can drive oncogene expression, while overactivity can inhibit tumor suppressor gene function.

Molecular Basis of Multistep Carcinogenesis (p. 308)

No single genetic alteration is sufficient to induce cancers *in vivo*. A variety of controls influenced by multiple categories of genes—oncogenes, tumor suppressor genes, apoptosis-regulating genes, senescence-modulating genes—must be lost for the emergence of cancer cells. This situation is exemplified by the colon adenoma-to-carcinoma sequence (Fig. 7-3); the evolution of benign adenomas to carcinomas is marked by increasing and additive effects of mutations. The accumulation of mutations with increasing genetic instability can be promoted by loss of p53, DNA repair genes, or both. Over time tumors acquire additional changes that result in greater malignant potential, for example, accelerated growth,

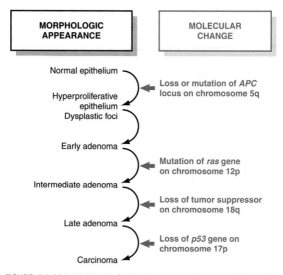

FIGURE 7-3 Molecular model for the evolution of colorectal cancers in the adenoma-carcinoma sequence. Although adenomatous polyposis coli *(APC)* mutation is an early event and loss of p53 occurs late in tumorigenesis, the timing for other changes can be quite variable. Note also that individual tumors may not have all the changes listed or may have other "passenger mutations" that occur as a result of genomic instability but are not necessarily causally related to oncogenesis. *(Adapted from Vogelstein B, Kinzler KW: Colorectal tumors. In Vogelstein B, Kinzler KW: The genetic basis of human cancer, New York, 2002, McGraw-Hill, p. 583.)*

invasiveness, angiogenesis, and the ability to form distant metastases. Despite the fact that tumors are initially *monoclonal in origin, by the time they become clinically evident, they are extremely heterogeneous.*

Carcinogenic Agents and Their Cellular Interactions (p. 309)

Environmental agents that cause genetic damage and induce neoplastic transformation include:

- Chemical carcinogens
- Radiant energy
- Oncogenic viruses and other microbes

Steps Involved in Chemical Carcinogenesis (p. 309)

Neoplastic transformation brought about by chemicals is broadly divided into two stages:

- *Initiation* refers to the induction of certain irreversible changes (mutations) in the genome. Initiated cells are not transformed cells; they do not have growth autonomy or unique phenotypic characteristics. In contrast to normal cells, however, they give rise to tumors when appropriately stimulated by promoting agents. Initiators fall in two categories:

  Direct-acting agents (p. 310) require no metabolic conversion to become carcinogenic (e.g., many alkylating agents used for chemotherapy)

  Indirect-acting agents (p. 310) require metabolic conversion most commonly through cytochrome P-450 mixed function oxidases (e.g., polycyclic hydrocarbons and benzo[*a*]pyrene). These enzymes have polymorphisms within the population that can influence their activity. Thus smokers with a certain highly inducible form of the P-450 gene *CYP1A1* have a seven-fold higher risk of developing lung cancer than smokers with a different genotype.

  Metabolic pathways can also inactivate carcinogens and the carcinogenic potential of any given molecule is therefore a balance of activation and inactivation.

- *Promotion* refers to the process of tumor induction in *previously initiated cells*. The effect of promoters is relatively short-lived and reversible; they do not affect DNA and are non-tumorigenic by themselves.

Molecular Targets of Chemical Carcinogens (p. 311)

Carcinogens are typically electrophilic compounds that are highly reactive with nucleophilic targets, DNA being the primary and most important. Interaction with DNA induces mutations by altering the primary sequence; although any gene can be mutated, oncogenes and tumor suppressors are especially important targets (e.g., *RAS* and *p53*). Because specific sequences are targeted by different chemicals, an analysis of the mutations found in human tumors can sometimes identify a culprit carcinogen.

Initiation and Promotion of Chemical Carcinogenesis (p. 311)

Unrepaired DNA alterations are essential first steps in *initiating* tumors; however, the damaged DNA template must also be replicated to make the changes permanent. Thus, in order for initiation to occur, carcinogen-altered cells must undergo at least one cycle of replication to "fix" the change in the DNA. Quiescent cells may never be affected by chemical carcinogens unless a mitotic stimulus is also provided.

Thus the initial mutagenic event in most instances requires subsequent exposure to *promoters* in order to induce cellular proliferation. These can include various hormones, drugs, phenols, and phorbol esters.

Radiation Carcinogenesis (p. 311)

Radiant energy, in the form of UV rays or ionizing radiation, is carcinogenic.

Ultraviolet Rays (p. 312)

Sun-derived UV radiation, especially UVB (280 to 320 nm), can cause skin cancer. Fair-skinned people who live in sunny climes or have less ozone protection are at greatest risk. Carcinomas and melanomas of exposed skin are particularly common in Australia and New Zealand. Risk of non-melanoma skin cancers is associated with cumulative exposure; melanoma risk is associated with intense intermittent exposures (e.g., sunbathing). Damage to DNA occurs through the formation of pyrimidine dimers; repair of these dimers requires nucleotide excision mechanisms that can be mutated in *xeroderma pigmentosum* or can be overwhelmed, leading to non-templated DNA-repair mechanisms that are error-prone.

Ionizing Radiation (p. 312)

Radiation from electromagnetic (e.g., x-rays) and particulate (e.g., α and β particles or neutrons) sources are all carcinogenic. The ability of ionizing radiation to cause cancer lies in its ability to induce DNA mutations; these can occur directly or indirectly by the generation of free radicals from water or oxygen.

In humans, there is a hierarchy of cellular vulnerability to radiation-induced neoplasms:

- Most common are myeloid leukemias, followed by thyroid cancer in children.
- Cancers of the breast and lung are less commonly radiation induced.
- Skin, bone, and gut are the least susceptible to radiation carcinogenesis.

Microbial Carcinogenesis (p. 312)

Helicobacter pylori is a bacterial cause of gastric malignancies. Although a variety of DNA and RNA viruses cause cancer in animals, relatively few are yet implicated in human cancer:

- Human T-cell lymphotropic virus type I (HTLV-1)
- Human papillomavirus (HPV)
- Epstein-Barr virus (EBV)
- Hepatitis B and C virus (HBV and HCV)
- Kaposi sarcoma herpesvirus (KSHV), also called *human herpesvirus type 8 (HHV-8)*
- Merkel cell polyomavirus

Oncogenic RNA Viruses (p. 312)

HTLV-1 is a retrovirus causing a T cell leukemia/lymphoma that is endemic in Japan and the Caribbean but occurs sporadically elsewhere. HTLV-1 has a CD4+ T cell tropism, and infection requires transmission of infected cells (e.g., via sexual intercourse, blood products, or breastfeeding). Leukemia develops in 3% to 5% of infected individuals after a 40- to 60-year latency. The transforming activity resides in a viral-encoded Tax protein that inactivates p16/INK4a and enhances cyclin D activation, thus leading to increased cell replication. Tax also interferes with DNA repair mechanisms, leading to genomic instability, and activates NF-κB, a transcription factor that regulates several pro- and anti-apotitic genes. The resulting T cell proliferation and genomic instability eventually results in the emergence of a monoclonal neoplastic population.

Oncogenic DNA Viruses (p. 313)

Oncogenic DNA viruses integrate into the host cell genome, forming a stable association. The virus cannot complete its replicative cycle because essential viral genes are interrupted during viral DNA integration; consequently, the virus may remain latent for years. Viral genes that are transcribed early in the viral life cycle are typically important for cellular transformation.

Human Papillomavirus (p. 313)

Approximately 70 genetically distinct types of HPV have been identified. Some types (e.g., 1, 2, 4, and 7) cause benign squamous papillomas (i.e., warts) in humans; the viral genome is typically not integrated, remaining as an episome. Integration appears to be a requisite step in oncogenesis.

- Genital warts with low malignant potential are caused by distinct HPV types (*low-risk* types, e.g., HPV-6 and HPV-11).
- Cervical squamous cell cancers contain HPV types 16 or 18 in more than 90% of cases.
- In HPV-associated cervical carcinomas there is random integration of the viral genomes into the host cell DNA; however, for any given tumor the integration is clonal. The key feature is that integration interrupts the viral DNA within the E1/E2 open reading frame, leading to loss of the E2 viral repressor and subsequent over-expression of the E6 and E7 viral proteins. These proteins transform cells by binding to and inhibiting the functions of Rb and p53 tumor suppressor proteins, as well as CDK inhibitors.
- HPV infection alone is typically not sufficient for carcinogenesis; interaction with cigarette smoking, other infections, dietary deficiencies, and hormones are also required.

Epstein-Barr Virus (p. 314)

This is a herpesvirus that infects B cells and oropharyngeal epithelium. B cells are latently infected, becoming immortalized, acquiring the ability for indefinite propagation. The immortalization is largely mediated through the action of the Epstein-Barr virus (EBV) latent membrane protein-1 (LMP-1) that constitutively activates NF-κB and JAK/STAT pathways to promote B cell proliferation and survival. A second gene, *EBNA-2*, encodes a nuclear protein that also constitutively activates a variety of host proteins such as *cyclin D* and *src* proto-oncogenes. In immunocompetent hosts, EBV-driven B cell proliferation is readily checked; immune system inactivation is the key to EBV-related oncogenesis. EBV is associated with four human cancers:

- *Burkitt lymphoma* is a B cell tumor associated with a t(8;14) translocation or with other translocations that inactivate c-MYC; it need not be associated with EBV, and indeed in non-endemic areas of the world, 80% of the tumors do not contain the EBV genome; however, in central Africa and New Guinea, where Burkitt lymphoma is the major childhood malignancy, 90% of tumors contain the EBV genome. Thus EBV alone does not cause Burkitt lymphoma. However, in patients with subtle or overt immune dysregulation (e.g., due to chronic malaria) unchecked B cell proliferation may lead to additional mutations (including the t[8;14] translocation) to replicate autonomously.

- *B-cell lymphomas in immunosuppressed patients* (e.g., AIDS patients, transplant recipients) can be associated with EBV. These patients have polyclonal B-cell proliferations that transform into monoclonal lymphomas. In transplant recipients, withdrawal of immunosuppressive drugs can cause regression of such EBV-induced proliferations.
- *Hodgkin lymphoma* is associated with EBV (Chapter 13).
- *Nasopharyngeal carcinoma* is endemic in southern China and some other locales; the EBV genome is found in all such tumors, and LMP-1 is implicated in driving cell proliferation. As in Burkitt lymphoma, EBV probably acts in concert with other factors to induce malignant transformation.

Hepatitis B and C Viruses (p. 315)

Approximately 70% to 85% of hepatocellular carcinomas worldwide are due to HBV or HCV infections. The mechanism is multifactorial but the dominant effect is immunologically mediated chronic inflammation.

- By causing hepatocellular injury and resulting regenerative hyperplasia, the pool of mitotically active cells subject to damage by carcinogenic agents is increased.
- Activated immune cells also produce a plethora of mediators (e.g., reactive oxygen species) that are mutagenic.
- HBV encodes a regulatory element called *HBx* that can inactivate p53, as well as cause transcriptional activation of several protooncogenes.

H. pylori (p. 315) causes no clinical consequences in the great majority of infected individuals; however, in 3% of cases, infection can lead to gastric carcinoma through pathways involving prolonged chronic inflammation. Strains associated with adenocarcinoma also express a cytotoxin-associated A (CagA) gene that induces unregulated proliferation.

H. pylori is also associated with gastric lymphomas. Prolonged infection induces *H. pylori*–reactive T cells that secrete cytokines that promote polyclonal B-cell proliferation. These proliferating cells eventually become monoclonal and T cell independent by accumulating mutations (e.g., t[11:18] translocations). The resultant tumor is called *marginal zone lymphoma* or *MALToma* (for *m*ucosa-*a*ssociated *l*ymphoid *t*issue lymphoma, Chapter 13).

Host Defense against Tumors—Tumor Immunity (p. 316)

Tumors are not entirely "self" and can be potentially controlled by the immune system *(immune surveillance);* this is supported by the fact that certain malignancies show an increased incidence in immunocompromised hosts. Moreover, cancers can elicit tumor-specific T cells and antibodies, and immune cells frequently accumulate in and around tumors. Since tumors clearly occur in immunocompetent hosts, immune surveillance in some cases may be inadequate. It is also likely that immune surveillance will promote *cancer immunoediting* that modulates tumor immunogenicity.

Tumor Antigens (p. 316)

These comprise tumor-specific antigens, present only on tumor cells, and tumor-associated antigens, present on tumor cells as well as some normal cells.

Tumor-specific antigens represent new proteins not previously encountered by the immune system. They are presented in association with cell surface major histocompatibility complex class I molecules and recognized by cytotoxic T cells:

- Products of mutated oncogenes and tumor suppressor genes (e.g., p53 or BCR-ABL)
- Products of other mutated genes resulting from intrinsic genetic instability and a mutator phenotype
- Overexpressed or aberrantly expressed cellular proteins; frequently, these represent proteins that are expressed at low levels in normal tissues but are markedly overexpressed in tumors (e.g., tyrosinase is expressed in normal melanocytes but overexpressed in melanomas, where it induces an immune response)
- Tumor antigens produced by oncogenic viruses
- Oncofetal antigens that may be normally expressed developmentally but are not normally seen on adult tissues; during malignant transformation, these proteins may elicit immune responses
- Altered cell surface glycolipids and glycoproteins; tumors frequently have dysregulated expression of the enzymes responsible for lipid and protein glycosylation and can lead to the appearance of tumor-specific epitopes on carbohydrate side chains, or on an aberrantly exposed polypeptide cores

Tumor-associated antigens include oncofetal antigens (e.g., carcinoembryonic antigen [CEA]) and lineage-specific antigens (e.g., CD10 on B cells). They do not typically evoke immune responses but are useful for tumor diagnosis and may be targets for immunotherapy.

Antitumor Effector Mechanisms (p. 318)

Cell-mediated and humoral immunity both participate, but CD8+ cytotoxic T lymphocyte (CTL)-mediated killing is the principal mechanism of antitumor immunity; natural killer (NK) cells and activated macrophages may also contribute.

Immune Surveillance and Escape (p. 319)

Tumors may escape immunosurveillance by:

- Selective outgrowth of antigen-negative variants
- Loss or reduced expression of histocompatibility antigens, thus becoming less susceptible to cytotoxic T-cell lysis (although NK cells have increased activity in that setting)
- Failure of tumors to express co-stimulatory molecules; this not only prevents sensitization but may actually render responding cells anergic or apoptotic
- Tumor-induced immunosuppression (e.g., due to TGF-β production)
- Antigen masking by increased glycocalyx production
- Apoptosis of cytotoxic T cells due to tumor cell FasL expression

Clinical Aspects of Neoplasia (p. 320)

Although malignant tumors are more threatening than benign, both can cause problems because of:

- Location and impingement on adjacent structures
- Functional activity such as hormone production
- Bleeding and infection
- Symptoms from tumor rupture or infarction
- Cachexia (wasting)

Local and Hormonal Effects (p. 320)

- *Location:* Intracranial tumors (e.g., pituitary adenoma) can expand and destroy the remaining pituitary gland, giving rise to an endocrine disorder; tumors of the gastrointestinal tract may cause obstruction of the bowel or may ulcerate and cause bleeding
- *Hormone production:* These may cause paraneoplastic syndromes such as hypoglycemia (insulin production) or hypercalcemia (parathyroid hormone-producing tumors)

Cancer Cachexia (p. 320)

Loss of body fat, lean body mass, and profound weakness are referred to as *cancer cachexia*. Its cause is multifactorial, but is largely driven by TNF and other cytokines elaborated by inflammatory cells in response to tumors:

- Loss of appetite
- Metabolic changes causing reduced synthesis and storage of fat and increased mobilization of fatty acids from adipocytes
- Increase catabolism of muscle and adipose tissue by ubiquitin-proteasome pathways

Paraneoplastic Syndromes (p. 321)

These are tumor-associated syndromes where the symptoms are not directly related to the spread of the tumor or to the elaboration of hormones indigenous to the tumor tissue. Paraneoplastic syndromes may be the earliest clinical manifestations of a neoplasm and can mimic distant spread (Table 7-5). The most common syndromes include:

- *Endocrinopathies:* Some non-endocrine cancers produce hormones or hormone-like factors (ectopic hormone production). Thus small-cell lung cancer causes *Cushing syndrome* by elaborating ACTH; 50% of patients with this endocrinopathy have lung carcinoma.
- *Hypercalcemia* is the most common paraneoplastic syndrome. It is caused by bone resorption resulting from the elaboration of parathyroid hormone (PTH)-like peptides. Cancer-associated hypercalcemia due to osteolysis induced by bone metastases is *not* considered a paraneoplastic syndrome.
- *Neuropathic paraneoplastic syndromes* include peripheral neuropathies, cortical cerebellar degeneration, and myasthenic syndromes. In most cases, the mechanisms are thought to involve autoantibodies against tumor antigens that cross-react with normal host tissues.
- *Thrombotic diatheses* result from production of thromboplastic substances by tumor cells and manifest as disseminated intravascular coagulation, migratory thrombophlebitis *(Trousseau syndrome),* or valvular vegetations *(nonbacterial thrombotic endocarditis).*

Grading and Staging of Tumor (p. 322)

This assessment provides a semiquantitative estimate of the clinical gravity of a tumor. Both histologic grading and clinical staging are valuable for prognostication and for planning therapy, although staging has proved to be of greater clinical value.

- *Grading* is based primarily on the degree of differentiation (how well the tumor resembles its normal counterpart), and, occasionally, architectural features or number of mitoses. In general, higher-grade tumors (more poorly differentiated) are more aggressive than lower-grade tumors.

TABLE 7-5	**Paraneoplastic Syndromes**	
Clinical Syndromes	**Major Forms of Underlying Cancer**	**Causal Mechanism**
Endocrinopathies		
Cushing syndrome	Small-cell carcinoma of lung Pancreatic carcinoma Neural tumors	ACTH or ACTH-like substance
Syndrome of inappropriate antidiuretic hormone secretion	Small-cell carcinoma of lung; intracranial neoplasms	Antidiuretic hormone or atrial natriuretic hormones
Hypercalcemia	Squamous cell carcinoma of lung Breast carcinoma Renal carcinoma Adult T-cell leukemia/lymphoma	Parathyroid hormone–related protein (PTHRP), TGF-α, TNF, IL-1
Hypoglycemia	Ovarian carcinoma Fibrosarcoma Other mesenchymal sarcomas	Insulin or insulin-like substance
Carcinoid syndrome	Hepatocellular carcinoma Bronchial adenoma (carcinoid) Pancreatic carcinoma	Serotonin, bradykinin
Polycythemia	Gastric carcinoma Renal carcinoma Cerebellar hemangioma Hepatocellular carcinoma	Erythropoietin
Nerve and Muscle Syndromes		
Myasthenia	Bronchogenic carcinoma	Immunological
Disorders of the central and peripheral nervous system	Breast carcinoma	
Dermatologic Disorders		
Acanthosis nigricans	Gastric carcinoma Lung carcinoma Uterine carcinoma	Immunological; secretion of epidermal growth factor
Dermatomyositis	Bronchogenic, breast carcinoma	
Osseous, Articular, and Soft-Tissue Changes		
Hypertrophic osteoarthropathy and clubbing of the fingers	Bronchogenic carcinoma	Unknown

Continued

TABLE 7-5	Paraneoplastic Syndromes—cont'd	
Clinical Syndromes	**Major Forms of Underlying Cancer**	**Causal Mechanism**
Vascular and Hematologic Changes		
Venous thrombosis (Trousseau phenomenon)	Pancreatic carcinoma Bronchogenic carcinoma Other cancers	Tumor products (mucins that activate clotting)
Nonbacterial thrombotic endocarditis	Advanced cancers	
Red cell aplasia	Thymic neoplasms	Unknown
Others		
Nephrotic sundrome	Various cancers	Tumor antigens, immune complexes

ACTH, Adrenocorticotropic hormone; *IL,* interleukin; *TGF,* transforming growth factor; *TNF,* tumor necrosis factor.

- *Staging* is based on the size of the primary tumor and the extent of local and distant spread. The major system currently used is the American Joint Committee on Cancer (AJCC) staging; the classification involves a TNM designation—T for tumor (i.e., size and local invasion), N for regional lymph node involvement, and M for distant metastases.

Laboratory Diagnosis of Cancer (p. 323)

Histologic and Cytologic Method (p. 323)

Histologic examination is the most important method of diagnosis. Besides traditional formalin-fixed and paraffin-embedded sections, quick-frozen sections provide rapid diagnoses during procedures. Proper histologic diagnosis requires complete clinical data (i.e., age, gender, site, previous therapy, etc.), good tissue preservation, and adequate specimen sampling.

Cytologic interpretation is based chiefly on changes in the appearance of individual cells. In the hands of experts, false-positive results are uncommon, but false-negative results do occur because of sampling errors. When possible, cytologic diagnosis must be confirmed by biopsy before therapeutic intervention.

- *Fine-needle aspiration* involves aspiration of cells and fluids from tumors or masses; improved imaging techniques allow the sampling of deep as well as more readily palpated lesions
- *Cytologic (Pap) smears* involve examination of shed cells; exfoliative cytologic examination is used most commonly in the diagnosis of cancer of the uterine cervix and tumors of the stomach, bronchus, endometrium, and urinary bladder.

Immunohistochemistry (p. 324)

Immunohistochemisty detects cell products or surface markers using specific antibodies. Antibody binding is visualized by fluorescent labels, or chemical reactions that generate a colored product. Immunohistochemistry is useful in the following settings:

- Diagnosis of undifferentiated tumors by the detection of tissue-specific intermediate filaments or other markers

- Determination of the site of origin of metastases by using reagents that identify specific cell types (e.g., prostate-specific antigen for prostate cancer)
- Detection of molecules that have prognostic or therapeutic significance (e.g., immunochemical detection of hormone receptors in breast cancer, or products of proto-oncogenes, e.g., ERB-B2, on breast cancers)

Flow Cytometry (p. 324)

Flow cytometry can be used to rapidly and quantitatively measure the presence of membrane antigens or DNA content of tumor cells. It is routinely used in the diagnosis and classification of leukemias and lymphomas.

Molecular Diagnosis (p. 324)

- *Diagnosis of malignancy:* In lymphocytic lesions, PCR can distinguish monoclonal (neoplastic) and polyclonal (reactive) proliferations. Fluorescence in situ hybridization (FISH)- or PCR-based detection of characteristic translocations can also diagnose specific malignancies, and unique translocations detected by PCR can distinguish among similar-appearing tumors (e.g., small round blue cell tumors in children). *Spectral karyotyping* can analyze all chromosomes from a single cell using a pallet of fluorochromes; it can detect even small translocations or insertions and determine the origin of chromosome fragments.
- *Prognosis of malignancy:* Certain genetic alterations are associated with poor prognosis; identification of these can stratify treatment. Thus N-*MYC* amplifications bode ill for neuroblastomas and HER-2/NEU over-expression in breast cancer is an indication for monoclonal antibody therapy against the ERBB2 receptor.
- *Detection of residual disease:* The ability to detect extremely small numbers of malignant cells can be useful for evaluating therapy efficacy or for assessing tumor recurrence. Thus the PCR-based detection of the *BCR-ABL* fusion gene product aids in determining whether tumor kill has been effective or if the tumor has recurred.
- *Diagnosis of hereditary predisposition to cancers:* Diagnosis of a predisposition to cancer (e.g., breast cancer and endocrine neoplasms) can be detected by mutational analysis of *BRCA-1*, *BRCA-2*, and *RET* genes, allowing family screening and risk stratification.

Molecular Profiles of Tumors (p. 325)

Microarray analysis of mRNA levels provides *gene expression signatures* or *molecular profiles* for tumors. Such analyses in association with tumor proteomics increasingly have relevance for identifying tumor subtypes and also have prognostic and therapeutic significance. The heterogeneity of tumors and the contribution of associated stromal and inflammatory elements can confound such analyses; this can be overcome by *laser capture microdissection* techniques that allow the specific analysis of selected cells as identified from histologic sections.

Tumor Markers (p. 326)

Tumor markers are tumor-derived or -associated molecules that are detected in blood or other body fluids. These are not primary methods of diagnosis, rather they are diagnostic adjuncts that can be used for screening large populations. They are also useful in determining therapeutic responses or tumor recurrence. In most cases, tumor markers are not specific for malignancy so that elevated levels must be interpreted in the context of other possible pathologies. Examples include:

- *Prostate specific antigen (PSA)* elaborated by prostate epithelium; elevated levels can reflect malignancy, or can also be seen with benign prostatic hypertrophy or prostatic inflammation.
- *Carcinoembryonic antigen (CEA)* that is normally produced by fetal gut, liver, and pancreas. This can be elaborated by cancers of the colon, pancreas, stomach, and breast, as well as in non-neoplastic conditions (e.g., alcoholic cirrhosis, hepatitis, and ulcerative colitis).
- *α-Fetoprotein (AFP)* that is normally produced by fetal yolk sac and liver; elevated levels occur in liver and testicular germ cell tumors but also occur in non-neoplastic conditions (e.g., cirrhosis and hepatitis).

8

Infectious Diseases

General Principles of Microbial Pathogenesis (p.332)

Despite vaccines and antibiotics, two of the top ten leading causes of death in the United States are infectious diseases (i.e., pneumonia/influenza and sepsis). These particularly contribute to the mortality in elderly individuals and those immunosuppressed by acquired immunodeficiency syndrome (AIDS), chronic disease, transplantation, or anticancer drugs. In developing countries, infectious diseases—abetted by malnutrition and unsanitary living conditions—contribute to more than 10 million deaths annually.

Categories of Infectious Agents (p. 332)
(Table 8-1)

Prions (p. 332)

Prions are composed only of a modified host protein called *prion protein (PrP)*; they lack RNA and DNA and are therefore not viruses.

- Disease occurs when the PrP undergoes a conformational change that confers resistance to proteases; the resistant form promotes conversion of normal PrP to the abnormal conformation, hence the infectious nature of the disease.
- Prions cause *spongiform encephalopathies* (e.g., Creutzfeldt-Jakob disease and "mad-cow disease"; Chapter 28).

Viruses (p. 332)

Viruses are obligate intracellular organisms, requiring host cell metabolism for replication.

- Viruses contain DNA or RNA (but not both) within a protein coat *(capsid)* that may be surrounded by a lipid bilayer *(envelope)*.
- They cause transient acute illness (e.g., colds, influenza), chronic disease (e.g., hepatitis B virus [HBV], human immunodeficiency virus [HIV]), or lifelong latent infection with potential for long-term reactivation (e.g., herpesviruses).

Bacteria (p. 334)

Bacteria lack nuclei and other membrane-bound organelles but have cell walls; cell walls are sandwiched between phospholipid bilayers *(Gram-negative bacteria)* or outside a single bilayer *(Gram-positive bacteria)*.

- Bacteria can be classified by:

  Gram staining (positive or negative)
  Morphology (spherical = cocci; rod = bacilli; corkscrew = spirochete)

TABLE 8-1 Clases of Human Pathogens and Their Lifestyles

Taxonomic	Size	Site of Propagation	Examples	Disease
Prions	30–50 kD	Intracellular	Prion protein	Creutzfeld-Jacob disease
Viruses	20–300 nm	Obligate intracellular	Poliovirus	Poliomyelitis
Bacteria	0.2–15 µm	Obligate intracellular Extracellular Facultative intracellular	*Chlamydia trachomatis* *Streptococcus pneumoniae* *Mycobacterium tuberculosis*	Trachoma, urethritis Pneumonia Tuberculosis
Fungi	2–200 µm	Extracellular Facultative intracellular	*Candida albicans* *Histoplasma capsulatum*	Thrush Histoplasmosis
Protozoa	1–50 µm	Extracellular Facultative intracellular Obligate intracellular	*Trypanosoma gambiense* *Trypanosoma cruzi* *Leishmania donovani*	Sleeping sickness Chagas disease Kala-azar
Helminths	3 mm–10 m	Extracellular Intracellular	*Wuchereria bancrofti* *Trichinella spiralis*	Filariasis Trichinosis

Oxygen requirements (aerobic or anaerobic)

- Growth may be extracellular, intracellular, or both (facultative intracellular).
- While bacteria are major causes of severe infectious diseases, most individuals happily coexist with 10^{10} oral bacteria, 10^{12} skin bacteria, and 10^{14} gastrointestinal bacteria (99.9% of the latter are anaerobic). Most have symbiotic, or at least commensal, relationships with their human host.
- Obligate intracellular bacteria include *Chlamydia* and *Rickettsia*; these replicate in intracellular membrane-bound vacuoles in epithelium and endothelium, respectively.

  Chlamydiae cause pathology by appropriating host adenosine triphosphate (ATP) synthetic capacity. They cause urogenital infections, conjunctivitis, trachoma, and respiratory infections.

  Rickettsiae are transmitted by arthropod vectors (ticks, mites, lice); by injuring endothelium, they cause vascular thrombosis (Rocky Mountain spotted fever and epidemic typhus)

- *Mycoplasma* lack cell walls and are the smallest of the free-living microbes. They cause atypical pneumonia or non-gonococcal urethritis.

Fungi (p. 335)

Fungi are eukaryotes with thick, chitin-containing cell walls and ergosterol-containing cell membranes; they grow in humans as rounded yeast forms or as slender hyphae (septated or aseptate).

- Fungi may cause superficial or deep infections (called *mycoses*):

  Superficial infections (skin, hair, nails) are caused by *dermatophytes* and are termed *tinea* (e.g., tinea pedis is athlete's foot)

  Invasion of subcutaneous tissues can cause abscesses (sporotrichosis), or granulomas.

  Deep fungal infections can spread systemically and invade a variety of tissues. In normal hosts, these typically heal or remain latent; in immunocompromised hosts substantial damage (and death) can result.

- Some fungal species have geographic predilections (e.g., *Coccidiodes* in the southwest United States and *Histoplasma* in the Ohio River valley); most opportunistic fungi (e.g., *Candida, Aspergillus,* and *Mucor*) are relatively ubiquitous.
- In immunodeficient hosts, opportunistic fungi cause life-threatening systemic infections with tissue necrosis, hemorrhage, and vascular occlusion, often with little inflammatory response.
- In AIDS patients, the opportunistic fungus *Pneumocystis jiroveci* causes pneumonia.

Protozoa (p. 335)

Protozoa are motile, single-celled eukaryotes.

- Protozoa can replicate intracellularly (e.g., *Plasmodium* in erythrocytes, *Leishmania* in macrophages) or extracellularly in the urogenital system, intestine, or blood.
- Infections may be transmitted sexually (e.g., *Trichomonas*), by ingestion of contaminated food or water (e.g., *Giardia,* or *Entamoeba*), or by blood-sucking insects (e.g., *Plasmodium* and *Leishmania*)

Helminths (p. 335)

Helminths are highly differentiated multicellular organisms with complex life cycles involving humans and intermediary hosts.

- Humans may harbor adult worms, immature stages, or asexual larval forms. Adult worms in residence do not typically multiply but rather produce eggs or larvae that are passed in the stool.
- Disease severity is proportional to the number of infecting organisms; inflammatory responses are typically generated against eggs or larvae and not adult forms.

Ectoparasites (p. 336)

Ectoparasites are insects (e.g., bedbugs, fleas) or arthropods (e.g., ticks, lice, mites, spiders) that attach to and live on the skin. They may directly injure their human host or be vectors for other pathogens.

Special Techniques for Diagnosing Infectious Agents (p. 336)

Some infectious agents can be directly observed in routine hematoxylin and eosin–stained sections (e.g., CMV inclusion bodies; *Candida* and *Mucor;* most protozoans; all helminths). Most microbes, however, are best visualized after special stains that take advantage of particular cell wall characteristics (Table 8-2). Cultures of fluids or lesional tissues may be performed to speciate organisms and to determine drug sensitivity. Antibody titers to specific pathogens can also be used to diagnose infection; immunoglobulin M (IgM) antibodies suggest an acute infection, whereas immunoglobulin G (IgG) antibodies suggest something more remote. Nucleic acid tests are used to diagnose *M. tuberculosis, N. gonnorrhoeae,* and *Chlamydia trachomatis* and to quantify HIV, HBV, and hepatitis C virus (HCV) to monitor response to treatment.

New and Emerging Infectious Diseases (p.336)

The list of disease-causing microorganisms is constantly expanding (see Table 8-3 in *Robbins and Cotran Pathologic Basis of Disease,* ed 8, p. 337).

- Some are recent discoveries due to difficulty in culturing, e.g., *Helicobacter* gastritis, HBV and HCV, and Legionnaires pneumonia.
- Some are genuinely new to humans, for example, HIV (causing AIDS), *Borrelia burgdorferi* (causing Lyme disease), and the coronavirus (causing severe acute respiratory syndrome [SARS]).

TABLE 8-2 Special Techniques for Diagnosing Infectious Agents	
Technique	**Organisms**
Gram stain	Most bacteria
Acid-fast stain	Mycobacteria, nocardiae (modified)
Silver stains	Fungi, legionellae, pneumocystis
Periodic acid–Schiff stain	Fungi, amebae
Mucicarmine stain	Cryptococci
Giemsa stain	Campylobacteria, leishmaniae, malaria, parasites
Antibody probes	Viruses, rickettsiae
Culture	All classes
DNA probes	Viruses, bacteria, protozoa

- Some have become more common as a result of therapeutic or AIDS-induced immunosuppression (e.g., cytomegalovirus [CMV], Kaposi sarcoma herpesvirus, *Mycobacterium avium-intracellulare, P. jiroveci,* and *Cryptosporidium parvum*).
- Some have been previously well recognized in one region, but are recently entering a new population or geographic locale (e.g., West Nile virus).
- Human demographics and behaviors are important variables in the emergence of new infectious diseases; thus, reforestation of the eastern United States led to the expansion of the populations of animal vectors (mice and deer) for Lyme disease. Antibiotic resistance has also led to the emergence of increasingly virulent microorganism (e.g., methicillin-resistant staphylococcus).

Agents of Bioterrorism (p. 337)

Such pathogens are those that pose the greatest danger due to efficient disease transmission, significant morbidity and mortality, relative ease of production and distribution, difficulty in defending against, or by provoking alarm and fear in the general public (see Table 8-4 in *Robbins and Cotran Pathologic Basis of Disease,* ed 8, p. 337).

Transmission and Dissemination of Microbes (p. 338)

Routes of Entry of Microbes (p. 338)

Barriers that prevent microbes from entering the body include intact skin and mucosal surfaces, their secretory products (lysozyme in tears, acid in stomach), and cells and proteins of host immunity. In the skin and gastrointestinal tract, a substantial population of normal flora also prevents new microbes from gaining admission by eliminating unfilled niches. Successful microorganisms either take advantage of barrier failure or have virulence factors that enable them to circumvent these barricades.

- *Skin defenses* (p. 338) include a keratinized outer layer, fatty acids, and low pH.

  These barriers can be breached directly (e.g., schistosomiasis), or by skin damage that allows access of otherwise less virulent microbes (e.g., macerated skin, cuts, burns, intravenous [IV] lines, or insect bites).

- *Gastrointestinal tract defenses* (p. 338) include gastric acid, pancreatic bile, lytic enzymes, a mucous layer, defensins, and secreted immunoglobulin A (IgA).

  These barriers are lost in the setting of low gastric acidity, antibiotics that alter the normal flora, loss of pancreatic function, or diminished bowel motility.

- *Respiratory tract defenses* (p. 339) include bronchial epithelium ciliary activity, a mucous layer, defensins, secreted IgA, and alveolar macrophages.

  These barriers are compromised when the mucociliary clearance mechanism is disrupted (e.g., by smoking) or when host macrophage clearance is ineffective (e.g., in tuberculosis)

- *Urogenital tract defenses* (p. 339) include frequent bladder flushing with urine; in the vagina, catabolism of glycogen by normal commensal lactobacilli lowers the pH and reduces fungal growth.

  These barriers are lost with bladder atonia, flow obstruction, or reflux; antibiotics kill the lactobacilli and render the vagina susceptible to candidal infection.

Spread and Dissemination of Microbes *(p. 339)*

Microbes can be transmitted person-to-person via respiratory, fecal-oral, sexual, or transplacental routes. Animal-to-human transmission can occur through direct contact or ingestion *(zoonotic infections);* alternatively, insect or arthropod vectors may passively spread infection or serve as required hosts for pathogen replication and development.

Some microbes proliferate locally; others penetrate the epithelial barrier and spread distally via lymphatics, blood, or nerves, so that disease manifestations occur at sites distant from microbial entry.

Release of Microbes from the Body *(p. 340)*

For purposes of microbial propagation, an exit strategy is as important as how an organisms enters its host. Mechanisms of passing from an infected host include skin shedding, coughing, sneezing, urinary or fecal voiding, sexual contact, or insect or animal vectors. Some microbes are hardy and can survive extended periods in dust, food, or water; others may need quick transmission and require direct person-to-person contact.

Sexually Transmitted Infections *(p. 341)*

Groups at greater risk for sexually transmitted infections (STIs) include adolescents, men who have sex with men, and IV drug users. Sexual practices such as oral or anal sex also influence the microbes transferred and mechanisms of infection. (See Table 8-5 in *Robbins and Cotran Pathologic Basis of Disease,* ed 8, p. 341, and Chapters 21 and 22.)

> Infection with one STI-associated organism increases the risk for additional STIs; this is because the risk factors are the same, and mucosal injury facilitates co-infection by multiple agents.
> STI in pregnancy can be spread to the fetus either *in utero* or at delivery, resulting in severe injury.

Healthcare-Associated Infections *(p. 342)*

Nosocomial (hospital-acquired) infections affect 1.7 million patients in the United States annually; because of broad-spectrum antibiotic use in hospitals, microbes mediating these infections are also more likely to be drug-resistant. Blood transfusion and organ transplant are rare mechanisms; transmission is most commonly via the hands of healthcare workers or through contaminated surfaces (e.g., bedrails).

Host Defenses against Infections *(p. 342)*

Besides host barrier function, the innate and adaptive immune systems are critical to preventing infection or in ultimately eradicating it (Chapter 6). In some cases, a stalemate between host and microorganism results in a state of microbial latency without much pathology. However, subsequent diminution of host immunity can result in aggressive reactivation and disease (e.g., latent Epstein-Barr virus [EBV] or tuberculosis infections).

How Microorganisms Cause Disease *(p. 342)*

Infectious disease results from the interaction of microbial virulence characteristics and host immune responses. Infectious agents cause damage by:

- Entering cells and directly causing cell death
- Releasing toxins that kill cells
- Releasing enzymes that degrade tissue components
- Damaging blood vessels, causing ischemic necrosis
- Inducing host inflammatory cell responses that directly or indirectly injure tissues

Mechanisms of Viral Injury (p. 342)

Viruses have a predilection for infecting specific cell types (*tropism*) that influences what tissue(s) will be injured. This occurs by:

- Binding to specific cell surface proteins (HIV binds to CD4 and the CXCR4 chemokine receptor on T cells)
- Cell-type-specific proteases may be necessary to enable binding (host protease activation of influenza virus hemagglutinin)
- Cell-type-specific transcription factors (JC virus can only proliferate in oligodendroglia)
- Physical barriers, local temperature, and pH (enteroviruses resist gut acid and enzymes)

Once inside cells, viruses damage or kill host cells by:

- Direct cytopathic effects
  Inhibiting host DNA, RNA, or protein synthesis
  Producing degradative enzymes or toxic proteins
  Inducing apoptosis
  Damaging the plasma membrane (e.g., HIV)
  Lysing cells (e.g., rhinoviruses and influenza viruses)

- Inducing an anti-viral host immune response
  Cytotoxic T cells or NK cells

- Transformation of infected cells (Chapter 7)

Mechanisms of Bacterial Injury (p. 343)

Bacterial Virulence (p. 343)

Microbial damage depends on the ability of infecting bacteria to adhere to host cells, invade cells and tissues, or deliver toxins.

- Virulence genes are frequently clustered together in the microbe genome as *pathogenicity islands.*
- Plasmids and bacteriophages are mobile genetic elements that can encode and transfer virulence factors between different bacteria (e.g., toxins or antibiotic resistance).
- In large populations, virulence factor expression may be coordinated by the secretion of autoinducer peptides that turn on specific genes in the population, a process called *quorum sensing.*
- Communities of bacteria—particularly in association with artificial surfaces (catheters and artificial joints)—can form *biofilms* where the organisms live within a viscous polysaccharide "slime" that facilitates adhesion and also frustrates attempts at immune cell clearance or antibiotic permeation.

Bacterial Adherence to Host Cells (p. 343)

Bacterial *adhesins* are surface molecules that bind to specific host cells or matrix; besides being the first step in infection, adhesin specificities can also influence tissue tropisms.

Pili are filamentous bacterial surface proteins that can also mediate adhesion. In addition, these can be targeted by immune responses; pilus variation is a mechanism used by *N. gonorrhea* to escape immune clearance.

Virulence of Intracellular Bacteria (p. 344)

Intracellular bacteria can kill host cells by rapid replication and lysis (*Shigella* and *E. coli*). Alternatively, they may permit continued host cell viability while evading intracellular defenses and proliferating within endosomes (*M. tuberculosis*) or cytoplasm (*Listeria monocytogenes*).

Bacterial Toxins (p. 344)

Bacterial toxins may be either endotoxins (intrinsic components of the cell wall) or exotoxins (secreted by the bacteria).

- *Endotoxin* (lipopolysaccharide [LPS]) is a cell wall component of Gram-negative bacteria composed of a common long-chain fatty acid (i.e., lipid A) and a variable carbohydrate chain (i.e., O antigen). Low doses of the lipid A component elicit protective inflammatory cell recruitment and cytokine production. However, higher doses contribute to septic shock, disseminated intravascular coagulation, and acute respiratory distress syndrome (Chapter 4).
- *Exotoxins* damage host tissues by several mechanisms:

    Enzymes destroy tissue integrity by digesting structural proteins.
    Exotoxins alter intracellular signaling; a number of exotoxins have a binding (B) subunit that delivers a toxic active (A) component into the cell cytoplasm, where it modifies signaling pathways to cause cell dysfunction or death (e.g., in diptheria, anthrax, or cholera).
    Neurotoxins block neurotransmitter release and cause paralysis (e.g., in botulism and tetanus).
    Superantigens stimulate large numbers of T cells by linking T-cell receptors with class II major histocompatibility complex (MHC) molecules on antigen presenting cells; the result is massive T-cell proliferation and cytokine release (e.g., toxic shock syndrome due to *S. aureus*).

Injurious Effects of Host Immunity (p. 344)

Host immune responses to microbes cause pathology in the following ways:

- Granulomatous responses can sequester pathogens but can cause secondary tissue damage and fibrosis (e.g., *M. tuberculosis*).
- Liver damage following HBV infection is due to the immune destruction of infected hepatocytes.
- Antibodies directed against bacterial antigens may cross-react with host molecules (e.g., rheumatic heart disease), or may form immune complexes that lodge in vascular beds (e.g., post-streptococcal glomerulonephritis).
- Chronic inflammation and epithelial injury may lead to malignancy (e.g., *H. pylori* and gastric cancer).

Immune Evasion by Microbes (p. 345)

Immune evasion is an important determinant of microbial virulence. Mechanisms include (Fig. 8-1):

- Replication in sites inaccessible to host immune response (*Clostridium difficile* replicates in the small bowel lumen) or rapid invasion of host cells before immune responses become effective (malaria sporozoites entering hepatocytes). Latent viral infections and parasitic cysts are other examples.
- Constantly changing surface antigens (*Borrelia*, African trypanosomes, and HIV)
- Escaping phagocytosis or complement-mediated lysis (the carbohydrate capsule of pneumococcus prevents phagocytsosis)
- Inhibiting innate immune mechanisms (viruses produce cytokine homologues that function as antagonists)
- Decreased recognition of infected cells by T cells (herpesviruses alter MHC expression and impair antigen presentation) or compromising lymphocyte function (i.e., HIV)

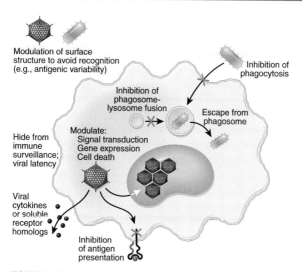

FIGURE 8-1 An overview of mechanisms used by viral and bacterial pathogens to evade innate and adaptive immunity. *(Modified with permission from Finlay B, McFadden G: Anti-immunology: evasion of the host immune system by bacterial and viral pathogens, Cell 124:767-782, 2006.)*

Infections in Immunosuppressed Hosts (p. 346)

The nature of such infections depends on which effector mechanisms are impaired.

- Genetic immunodeficiencies

    B cells: X-linked agammaglobulinemia is associated with *S. pneumoniae, Haemophilus influenzae, S. aureus,* rotavirus, and enterovirus infections

    T cells: Intracellular pathogens (e.g., viruses and some parasites)

    Complement proteins: *S. pneumoniae, H. influenzae,* and *Neisseria meningitidis* infections)

    Neutrophil function: *S. aureus* infections, Gram-negative bacteria, and fungi

- Acquired immunodeficiencies: HIV annihilation of T-helper cells is associated with a variety of infections; many were well-recognized pathogens before AIDS, while others (Kaposi sarcoma herpesvirus, cryptococcus, and *Pneumocystis*) were uncommon.

- Immunosuppression in organ transplantation or during bone marrow engraftment renders patients susceptible to virtually all organisms, including common environmental microbes *(Aspergillus* and *Pseudomonas)*.

- Diseases of organs other than the immune system also render patients susceptible to specific organisms. Lack of splenic function in sickle cell disease increases risk of infection by encapsulated bacteria *(S. pneumoniae)*, and patients with cystic fibrosis commonly get *Pseudomonas* infections.

Spectrum of Inflammatory Responses to Infection (p. 347)

Although microbes have impressive molecular diversity, tissue responses to them follow five basic histologic patterns (below). Important caveats:

- Similar patterns can occur secondary to physical or chemical injury, or in primary inflammatory disorders.
- Patterns may overlap due to concurrent infections.
- The same microbe can cause different patterns in different patients due to host idiosyncratic responses (e.g., granulomas in patients exhibiting *tuberculoid leprosy* and tissue necrosis in patients exhibiting *lepromatous leprosy*).
- Patterns should be consistent with the organisms cultured or identified by microscopy.

Suppurative (Purulent) Inflammation (p. 347)

Suppurative (purulent) inflammation is usually caused by pyogenic bacteria, mostly extracellular Gram-positive cocci and Gram-negative rods.

- These elicit increased vascular permeability and neutrophil recruitment through bacterial chemoattractants.
- Lesions vary from tiny microabscesses to consolidation of entire lung lobes; these may resolve without sequelae (pneumococcal pneumonia) or may scar *(Klebsiella)*.

Mononuclear and Granulomatous Inflammation (p. 347)

Mononuclear and granulomatous inflammation are patterns typical for viruses, intracellular bacteria, spirochetes, intracellular parasites, and helminths.

- The cell type that predominates depends on the host response to a particular pathogen: plasma cells in chancres of primary syphilis, lymphocytes in viral infections of the brain, or macrophages in *M. avium-intracellulare* infections of AIDS patients.
- Granulomatous inflammation, characterized by accumulation of activated macrophages, is usually evoked by resistant organisms that evoke a strong T-cell response *(M. tuberculosis)*.

Cytopathic-Cytoproliferative Reaction (p. 348)

Cytopathic-cytoproliferative reaction usually occurs in viral infections; there is cell proliferation and necrosis with sparse inflammation.

- Other features include inclusion bodies (herpesvirus), fused cells (measles viruses), blisters (herpesviruses), or warty excrescences (papillomaviruses).

Tissue Necrosis (p. 348)

Tissue necrosis is caused by rampant viral infections (e.g., fulminant HBV infection), secreted bacterial toxins (e.g., *Clostridium perfringens*), or direct protozoan cytolysis of host cells (e.g., *E. histolytica*); there is severe tissue necrosis often in the absence of inflammation.

Chronic Inflammation and Scarring (p. 348)

Outcomes range from complete healing to scarring; excessive scarring can cause dysfunction. Inflammation can be severe despite a paucity of organisms *(M. tuberculosis)*.

Viral Infections (p. 348)

Viral infections can be transient, chronic latent, or chronic productive, or they can promote cellular transformation and malignancy. (See Table 8-7 in *Robbins and Cotran Pathologic Basis of Disease*, ed 8, p. 349.)

Acute (Transient) Infections (p. 348)

Viruses that cause transient infections are structurally heterogenous, but each elicits an immune response that effectively eliminates the virus.

Measles (Rubeola) (p. 349)

Measles (rubeola) is an RNA paramyxovirus transmitted by respiratory droplets; it is a leading cause of vaccine-preventable morbidity and mortality worldwide.

- Initial replication is within upper respiratory epithelial cells, with subsequent spread to local lymphoid tissue and then systemically.
- Ulcerated oral mucosal lesions near Stensen ducts form pathognomonic *Koplik spots.* There is marked lymphoid follicular and germinal center hyperplasia, with pathognomonic multinucleated giant cells with eosinophilic inclusion bodies, called *Warthin-Finkeldey cells* (also seen in lungs and sputum).
- Infection can cause croup, pneumonia, diarrhea, keratitis (with scarring and blindness), and encephalitis.
- T cell–mediated responses control the initial infection; the characteristic measles rash is due to hypersensitivity to measles-infected cutaneous cells. Antibody-mediated immunity protects against re-infection.
- Subacute sclerosing panencephalitis and inclusion body encephalitis (in immunocompromised individuals) are rare late complications.

Mumps (p. 350)

Mumps is a paramyxovirus spread by respiratory droplets.

- Initial replication is in lymph nodes draining the upper respiratory tract, followed by hematogenous spread to salivary glands and other sites.
- Infection of salivary gland ductal epithelium leads to desquamation, edema, and inflammation, and thus, the classic salivary gland swelling and pain.
- Spread can also occur to testes, ovary, pancreas, and central nervous system; aseptic meningitis is the most common extrasalivary gland complication (10% of infections).
- In mumps orchitis, swelling contained within the tunica albuginea can compromise the vascular supply and cause infarction.

Poliovirus (p. 350)

Poliovirus is a spherical, unencapsulated RNA enterovirus transmitted by the fecal-oral route; other enteroviruses cause diarrhea and rashes (coxsackievirus A), conjunctivitis (enterovirus 70), meningitis (coxsackievirus and echovirus), and myopericarditis (coxsackievirus B).

- The virus infects via CD155, a surface molecule not present in other species; there are no non-human reservoirs.
- Multiplication in intestinal mucosa and lymph nodes is followed by a transient viremia and fever; nervous system involvement may occur by systemic viremia or retrograde transport via motor neurons. Antiviral antibodies control the disease.
- Although infection is usually asymptomatic, poliovirus invades the central nervous system (CNS) in 1 of 100 infected persons, replicating in motor neurons of the spinal cord (causing muscular paralysis) or brain stem *(bulbar poliomyelitis).*

West Nile Virus (p. 351)

West Nile virus is an arthropod-borne flavivirus *(arbovirus);* the group also includes the pathogens causing dengue and yellow fever.

It is transmitted by mosquitos (birds being the major viral reservoir), but it has also been transmitted by transfusion, by organ transplant, in breast milk, and transplacentally.

- Initial replication occurs in skin dendritic cells, which carry virus to lymph nodes for further expansion; subsequent hematogenous spread can lead to CNS neuronal infection. Rare complications include hepatitis, myocarditis, or pancreatitis. Immunosuppressed and elderly individuals are at greatest risk.
- CNS complications (e.g., meningitis, encephalitis, meningoencephalitis) develop in roughly 1 of 150 clinically apparent infections. Meningoencephalitis carries a 10% mortality rate; survivors can have long-term cognitive and neurologic impairment.

Viral Hemorrhagic Fevers (p. 351)

Viral hemorrhagic fevers (e.g., Ebola, Marburg, and Lassa) are systemic infections caused by enveloped RNA viruses from four different families (i.e., arenaviruses, filoviruses, bunyaviruses, and flaviviruses).

- Transmission occurs through infected insects or animals. Consequently the viruses are geographically restricted to their hosts' habitat; humans are not the natural reservoir but occasionally transmit infection to other humans.
- Manifestations range from mild acute disease (e.g., fever, headache, rash, myalgia, neutropenia, and thrombocytopenia) to severe life-threatening hemodynamic deterioration and shock.
- Most of these viruses infect endothelial cells and thus hemorrhagic manifestations can be secondary to endothelial or platelet dysfunction. However, macrophage and dendritic cell infection can also result in profound cytokine release.

Chronic Latent Infections (Herpesvirus Infections) (p. 351)

These large, encapsulated double-stranded DNA viruses cause acute infection followed by latent infections where viruses persist in a noninfectious form, with periodic reactivation and shedding of infectious virus.

Herpes Simplex Virus (p. 352)

Herpes simplex virus (HSV) replicates in skin and mucous membranes at the site of initial inoculation (usually orophraynx or genitals), causing vesicular lesions.

- Classic HSV lesions include large, pink-purple, virion-containing intranuclear inclusions *(Cowdry-type A inclusions)*, as well as inclusion-bearing multinucleated syncytia.
- After epithelial infection, viruses spread to associated sensory neurons and then by retrograde axonal transport to the sensory neuron ganglia to establish latent infections. During reactivation, virus spreads from regional ganglia back to skin or mucous membranes.
- HSV lesions range from self-limited cold sores and gingivostomatitis (HSV-1) to genital sores (mainly HSV-2) to life-threatening disseminated visceral infections (hepatitis and bronchopneumonitis) and encephalitis.
- HSV-1 is also the major infectious cause of corneal blindness in the United States. *Herpes epithelial keratitis* reflects virus-induced cytolysis of the superficial corneal epithelium. *Herpes stromal keratitis* results in mononuclear cell infiltrates around keratinocytes and endothelial cells; subsequent neovascularization, scarring, and corneal opacification leads to blindness.

Varicella-Zoster Virus (p. 353)

Varicella-zoster virus (VZV) is transmitted by aerosols, disseminates hematogenously, and causes widespread vesicular skin lesions. Acute VZV infection causes *chickenpox;* reactivation of latent VZV causes *shingles* (or *herpes zoster*).

- Skin lesions evolve rapidly from macules to vesicles, classically resembling "a dew drop on a rose petal." Histologically, vesicles contain epithelial cell blisters and intranuclear inclusions similar to HSV.
- Like HSV, VZV infects mucous membranes, skin and neurons, establishing a latent infection in sensory ganglia.
- Shingles occurs when latent VZV in dorsal root ganglia reactivates, infecting sensory nerves that carry viruses to the skin and causing painful vesicular lesions, typically in a dermatomal distribution.
- VZV can also cause interstitial pneumonia, encephalitis, transverse myelitis, and necrotizing visceral lesions, particularly in immunocompromised hosts.

Cytomegalovirus (p. 353)

CMV is carried in breast milk, respiratory droplets, blood, and saliva, and can have transplacental ("congenital"), venereal, fecal-oral, transfusion, or organ transplantation modes of transmission.

- CMV infection causes marked cellular enlargement with characteristic large intranuclear inclusions surrounded by a clear halo and smaller basophilic cytoplasmic inclusions.
- Infections are usually asymptomatic in immunocompetent hosts but can manifest as a mononucleosis-like syndrome (e.g., fever, atypical lymphocytosis, lymphadenopathy, and hepatosplenomegaly). CMV can infect dendritic cells and cause transient but severe immunosuprression; viruses remain latent in leukocytes.
- In immunosuppressed patients, CMV can cause life-threatening colitis or pneumonitis; hepatitis, chorioretinitis, and meningo-encephalitis are also significant morbidities. CMV is the most common opportunistic viral pathogen in AIDS.
- Although 95% of congenitally infected infants are asymptomatic, CMV can produce *cytomegalic inclusion disease (CID);* manifestations are similar to erythroblastosis fetalis and include intrauterine growth retardation, hemolytic anemia, jaundice, and encephalitis. Infants who survive usually have permanent deficits including deafness and mental retardation.

Chronic Productive Infections (p. 355)

In some infections, the immune system cannot eliminate the virus, resulting in persistent viremia. High mutation rates (e.g., in HIV and HBV) may be a mechanism to evade the immune system.

Hepatitis B Virus (p. 355) (see also Chapter 18)

HBV is a DNA virus member of the hepadnavirus family; it can be transmitted percutaneously (i.e., IV drug use or transfusion), perinatally, and sexually.

- HBV infects hepatocytes; cellular injury occurs mainly due to immune responses to infected liver cells and *not* cytopathic effects of the virus.
- The effectiveness of the cytotoxic T-cell immune response largely determines whether a person clears the virus or becomes a chronic *carrier.*
- Chronic hepatitis is associated with lymphocytic inflammation, apoptotic hepatocytes, and progressive destruction of the liver parenchyma; ongoing viral infection and subsequent host responses can result in cirrhosis and hepatocellular carcinoma.

Transforming Infections (p. 355)

These are viruses implicated in causing human cancer.

Epstein-Barr Virus (p. 355)

EBV infections occur through close contact, including saliva, blood, or venereal transmission.

- EBV infection begins in naso- and oropharyngeal epithelial cells, followed by infection of B cells in underlying lymphoid tissues; virus binds to CD21, the complement C3d receptor.
- In a minority of infected B cells, EBV has a productive lytic infection, releasing more virions. In most cells, EBV establishes a latent infection via genes that can induce B cell proliferation as well as production of non-specific antibodies (*heterophile antibodies*); these antibodies can agglutinate sheep or horse erythrocyes in the laboratory (allowing a presumptive EBV diagnosis) but do not react with EBV.
- EBV causes *infectious mononucleosis*, a benign, self-limited disease characterized by fever, fatigue, sore throat, lymphocytosis, generalized lymphadenopathy, and splenomegaly; hepatitis and rash can also occur. Symptoms are secondary to the host immune response:

  CD8+ cytotoxic T cells (the *atypical lymphocytes* seen in the blood) recognize and lyse EBV-infected B cells.
  Reactive proliferation of these T cells leads to lymphadenopathy and splenomegaly.

- Persistence of EBV in a small population of latently infected cells can result in late reactivation and B cell proliferation. In immunocompromised individuals, EBV is associated with B-cell lymphoma (Chapter 13); EBV also contributes to some cases of Burkitt lymphoma, where a 8:14 translocation of the c-*myc* oncogene is a characteristic oncogenic event (Chapter 7).

Bacterial Infections (p. 357) (See Table 8-8 in *Robbins and Cotran Pathologic Basis of Disease*, ed 8, p. 358)

Gram-Positive Bacterial Infections (p. 357)

Staphylococcal Infections (p. 357)

Staphylococcal infections are distinctive for local destructiveness; the organisms are pyogenic (pus-forming) cocci that grow in clusters.

- *S. aureus* causes a variety of skin infections (*boils, carbuncles, impetigo*), osteomyelitis, pneumonia, endocarditis, food poisoning, and toxic shock syndrome.
- Less virulent staphylococci cause opportunistic infections in IV drug abusers and in patients with catheters or prosthetic heart valves (*S. epidermidis*); *S. saprophyticus* is a common cause of urinary tract infections.
- Virulence factors include:

  Surface proteins that allow host cell adherence
  Enzymes that degrade host proteins, promoting invasion and tissue destruction
  Toxins that damage host cell membranes (*hemolysins*) or induce skin sloughing (exfoliative toxins), vomiting (enterotoxins), or shock (superantigens)

- Antibiotic resistance is a growing problem with *S. aureus* infections; methicillin-resistant *S. aureus* (MRSA) can now be a virulent community-acquired infection.

Streptococcal and Enterococcal Infections (p. 359)

Streptococcal and enterococcal infections are cocci that grow in pairs or chains. The streptococci are classified by their pattern of hemolysis on blood agar: β (complete or clear hemolysis), α (partial or green hemolysis), and γ (no hemolysis, rarely pathogenic).

- β-hemolytic streptococci are grouped by their carbohydrate (Lancefield) antigens:

  Group A *(S. pyogenes)* causes pharyngitis, scarlet fever, erysipelas, impetigo, rheumatic fever, toxic shock syndrome, necrotizing fasciitis, and glomerulonephritis.
  Group B *(S. agalactiae)* colonizes the female genital tract and causes chorioamnionitis in pregnancy, as well as neonatal sepsis and meningitis.

- α-Hemolytic streptococci include *S. pneumoniae*, a common cause of adult community-acquired pneumonia and meningitis.
- Viridans-group includes both α- and γ-hemolytic streptococci that are normal oral flora but are common causes of endocarditis; *S. mutans* is the major cause of dental caries (metabolizes sucrose to lactic acid, which demineralizes tooth enamel).
- *Enterococci* cause endocarditis and urinary tract infections; many are antibiotic resistant.
- Streptococcal virulence factors include:

  Capsules that resist phagocytosis *(S. pyogenes and S. pneumoniae)*.
  M-proteins that inhibit complement activation *(S. pyogenes)*.
  Exotoxins that cause fever and rash *(S. pyogenes)* in scarlet fever.
  Pneumolysin destroys host-cell membranes and damages tissue *(S. pneumoniae)*.

- Enterococci have an antiphagocytic capsule and produce enzymes that degrade host tissues
- Streptococcal infections are characterized by diffuse interstitial neutrophilic infiltrates with minimal host tissue destruction (except for some virulent strains of *S. pyogenes* that cause a rapidly progressive fasciitis and have been dubbed "flesh-eating bacteria").

Diphtheria (p. 360)

Diphtheria is caused by *Corynebacterium diptheriae,* a slender Gram-positive rod with clubbed ends; it is passed as an aerosol or through skin exudates.

- Diphtheria is a life-threatening disease characterized by an oropropharyngeal fibrinosuppurative exudate; *C. diphtheriae* growth in this membrane elaborates an exotoxin that injures heart, nerves, and other organs.
- Diphtheria toxin is a phage-encoded two-part (A-B) toxin that blocks host protein synthesis. The B fragment binds to the cell surface and facilitates entry of the A subunit; the A subunit blocks protein synthesis by ADP ribosylation (and inactivation) of elongation factor-2.

Listeriosis (p. 361)

L. monocytogenes is a Gram-positive, facultative intracellular bacillus causing severe food-borne infections.

- *Listeria* causes sepsis and meningitis in elderly and immunosuppressed people and placental infections in pregnant women with consequent neonatal infections.
- *L. monocytogenes* express leucine-rich proteins caused *internalins* that bind epithelial E-cadherin and promote internalization; the bacillus then uses listeriolysin O and two phospholipases to

degrade the phagolysosome membrane and escape into the cytoplasm.
- In the cytoplasm, a bacterial protein (ActA) induces actin polymerization to propel the bacteria into adjacent cells.
- Resting macrophages internalize but do not kill *Listeria;* macrophages activated by interferon-γ effectively phagocytize and kill the bacterium.
- *L. monocytogenes* evokes exudative inflammation with numerous neutrophils.

Anthrax (p. 361)

Bacillus anthracis is a spore-forming Gram-positive bacillus prevalent in animals having contact with spore-contaminated soil.

- Humans contract anthrax through exposure to contaminated animal products or powdered spores (a biologic weapon).
- Three major anthrax syndromes are known; in all cases, lesions are characterized by necrosis with neutrophil and macrophage exudates:

  Cutaneous: Painless, pruritic papules that become edematous vesicles followed by a black eschar
  Inhalation: Rapidly leads to sepsis, shock, and frequently death
  Gastrointestinal: Contracted by eating contaminated meat; causes severe, bloody diarrhea and often death

- Anthrax toxin is composed of a B subunit involved in toxin endocytosis and A subunits of two different types:

  Edema factor converts ATP to cyclic adenosine monophosphate (cAMP) that causes cellular water efflux.
  Lethal factor is a protease that causes cell death by destroying mitogen-activated protein kinase kinases.

Nocardia (p. 362)

Nocardia are aerobic Gram-positive bacterium growing in branched chains; they also stain with modified acid-fast protocols (Fite-Faraco stain).

- *Nocardia* are found in soil and cause opportunistic infections in immunocompromised hosts.
- *N. asteroides* causes indolent respiratory infections, often with CNS dissemination; *N. brasiliensis* infects the skin.
- *Nocardia* elicit suppurative responses, surrounded by granulation tissue and fibrosis.

Gram-Negative Bacterial Infections (p. 363)

Neisserial Infections (p. 363)

Neisserial infections are caused by aerobic, Gram-negative diplococci; they usually have stringent *in vitro* growth requirements e.g., sheep blood–enriched ("chocolate") agar.

- *N. meningitidis* is an important cause of bacterial meningitis, particularly in children younger than 2 years; there are 13 different serotypes.

  Bacteria colonize the oropharynx (10% of the population is colonized at any one time) and are spread by respiratory droplets.
  Meningitis occurs when people encounter serotypes to which they are not previously immune, e.g., in military barracks or college dormitories.

- *N. gonorrhoeae* is the second most common sexually transmitted bacterial infection in the United States (after *Chlamydia*).

  In men it causes symptomatic urethritis; in women it is often asymptomatic and can lead to pelvic inflammatory disease, infertility, and ectopic pregnancy.
  Disseminated adult infections cause septic arthritis and hemorrhagic rash.
  Neonatal infections cause blindness and, rarely, sepsis.

- Virulence factors include a capsule that inhibits opsonization, and antigenic variation to escape the immune response:

  Adhesive pili undergo genetic recombination.
  Outer membrane adhesive OPA proteins (so called because they make colonies opaque) undergo five-nucleotide frameshifts.
  Host defects in complement lead to more severe infections.

Whooping Cough (p. 364)

Whooping cough is caused by *Bordetella pertussis*, a Gram-negative coccobacillus; it is a highly communicable illness characterized by paroxysms of violent coughing.

- Coordinated expression of virulence factors is regulated by the *Bordetella* virulence gene locus *(bvg):*

  Hemagglutinin binds to respiratory epithelium carbohydrates and macrophage Mac-1 integrins.
  Pertussis toxin ADP ribosylates and inactivates guanine nucleotide-binding proteins; G proteins cannot transduce signals, and bronchial epithelium cilia are paralyzed.

- Infection causes laryngotracheobronchitis with mucosal erosion and mucopurulent exudates associated with striking peripheral lymphocytosis.

Pseudomonas Infection (p. 364)

Pseudomonas infection is due to *P. aeruginosa*, an opportunistic aerobic Gram-negative bacillus.

- This pathogen is frequently seen in patients with cystic fibrosis, burns, or neutropenia and is a common hospital-acquired infection. It also causes corneal keratitis in contact lens wearers and external otitis (i.e., swimmer's ear) in normal hosts.
- Virulence factors include:

  Pili and adherence proteins that bind to epithelial cells and lung mucin
  Endotoxin that cause Gram-negative sepsis and disseminated intravascular coagulation
  Exotoxin A that inhibits protein synthesis by the same mechanism as diphtheria toxin
  Phospholipase C that lyses red cells and degrades surfactant, and an elastase that degrades IgG and ECM
  Iron-containing compounds that are toxic to endothelium
  In patients with cystic fibrosis, the organism secretes an exopolysaccharide (alginate) that forms a slimy biofilm that protects bacteria from antibodies, complement, phagocytes, and antibiotics

- *Pseudomonas* pneumonia can cause extensive tissue necrosis by vascular invasion with subsequent thrombosis. Skin infections give rise to well-demarcated necrotic and hemorrhagic skin lesions, *ecthyma gangrenosum.*

Plague (p. 365)

Yersinia is a Gram-negative facultative intracellular bacterium with three clinically important species:

- *Yersinia pestis* causes plague; it is transmitted from rodents to humans by aerosols or flea bites.
- *Y. enterocolitica* and *Y. pseudotuberculosis* cause fecal-oral transmitted ileitis and mesenteric lymphadenitis.
- *Yersinia* proliferate in lymphoid tissues; virulence factors include:

  Yersinia toxins (called *Yops*) are injected into host phagocytes by a syringe-like mechanism; the toxins block phagocytosis and cytokine production.

  A biofilm that obstructs the flea gastrointestinal tract, forcing it to regurgitate prior to feeding and thus ensuring infection.

- Plague causes massive lymph node enlargement *(buboes)*, pneumonia, and sepsis, with extensive bacterial proliferation, tissue necrosis, and neutrophilic infiltrates.

Chancroid (Soft Chancre) (p. 366)

Chancroid (soft chancre) is an acute venereal, ulcerative genital infection caused by *Hemophilus ducreyi*, most common in Africa and Southeast Asia; the ulcerations probably serve as important co-factors in HIV transmission.

Granuloma Inguinale (p. 366)

Granuloma inguinale is a sexually transmitted disease caused by *Klebsiella granulomatis*, a minute, encapsulated coccobacillus.

- Infection begins as a papule on the genitalia or extragenital sites (oral mucosa or pharynx) that ulcerates and granulates to form a soft, painless mass with prominent epithelial hyperplasia at the borders.
- Left untreated, the lesion may scar and cause urethral, vulvar, or anal strictures; it is also associated with lymphatic scarring and lymphedema of the external genitalia.

Mycobacteria (p. 366)

Mycobacteria are aerobic bacilli that grow in chains and have a waxy cell wall composed of mycolic acid; the cell wall retains certain dyes after acid treatment (hence the name *acid-fast bacilli*).

Tuberculosis (p. 366)

Tuberculosis is caused by *M. tuberculosis*, the second leading infectious cause of death worldwide (after HIV); it affects 1.7 billion people worldwide and kills 1.6 million people annually. There are about 14,000 new cases of tuberculosis in the United States annually, most among immigrant, homeless, jailed, or HIV-infected individuals. It is transmitted person to person as an aerosol, and increasingly is multi-drug resistant.

- *Infection* represents only the presence of organisms and, in most cases, does not cause clinical *disease.*
- *M. tuberculosis* secretes no toxins, and its virulence is based on the properties of its cell wall.
- Outcomes of infection depend on host immunity; responses can both control infections and contribute to the pathologic manifestations of disease:

  Infection leads to the induction of a T_H1-mediated delayed hypersensitivity response (Chapter 6) that activates macrophages (via interferon-γ) to:

- Promote endocytosis and killing via nitric oxide
- Promote cidal activity though tumor necrosis factor production
- Surround microbes with granulomatous inflammation

Caseating granulomas are characteristic; central necrosis is surrounded by lymphocytes and activated macrophages.

T-cell immunity to mycobacteria can be detected by a tuberculin skin test (purified protein derivative [PPD]); the test signifies only prior T-cell sensitization to mycobacterial antigens and does not discriminate infection and disease.

- In most individuals (i.e., 95%), primary infection is asymptomatic.

Granulomas formed in response to infection typically involve the lung apex and draining lymph node; these are called a *Ghon complex.*

Eventual control of the infection leaves behind only a small residua—a tiny fibrocalcific nodule at the site where viable organisms may remain within granulomas, dormant for decades.

- Five percent of primary infections are symptomatic with lobar consolidation, hilar adenopathy, and pleural effusions.

Rarely, hematogenous spread leads to tuberculous meningitis and *miliary tuberculosis.*

Extrapulmonary involvement occurs in more than 50% of patients with severe immune deficiency.

- Secondary tuberculosis occurs in a previously exposed host.

If immunity wanes, the infection can reactivate to produce communicable disease with substantial morbidity and mortality.

Classically, because of prior T cell sensitization, there is more tissue damage with apical pulmonary cavitation and increased systemic manifestations with low-grade fever, night sweats, and weight loss.

- HIV is associated with an increased risk of tuberculosis, due to diminished T-cell immunity.
- Diagnosis of tuberculosis can be made by:

Identifying acid-fast bacilli in sputum or tissue
Culture from sputum or tissue (allows drug sensitivity testing)
Polymerase chain reaction (highly sensitive)

Mycobacterium Avium-Intracellulare Complex (p. 372)

These common environmental bacteria cause widely disseminated infections in immunocompromised hosts characterized by abundant acid-fast organisms within macrophages.

Leprosy (p. 372)

Leprosy, also known as *Hansen's disease,* is a slowly progressive infection caused by *M. leprae;* it affects skin and peripheral nerves with resultant deformities.

- Inhaled *M. leprae* are phagocytized by pulmonary macrophages and disseminated hematogenously; however, they replicate only in cooler tissues of the periphery.
- *M. leprae* secretes no toxins, and its virulence is based on the properties of its cell wall.
- Leprosy has two patterns of disease (depending on the host's immune response); *tuberculoid leprosy* is associated with a T_H1 response (IFN-γ), and *lepromatous leprosy* is associated with a relatively ineffective T_H2 response (Chapter 6).

Tuberculoid leprosy: Extensive granulomatous inflammation with few bacilli. Clinically, there are insidious, dry, scaly skin lesions lacking sensation, with asymmetric peripheral nerve involvement. Local anesthesia with skin and muscle atrophy increases the risk of trauma with chronic ulcers and autoamputation of digits.

Lepromatous (anergic) leprosy: Large collections of lipid-laden macrophages over-stuffed with bacilli. Clinically there are disfiguring cutaneous thickening and nodules, with nervous system damage due to mycobacterial invasion into perineural macrophages and Schwann cells. The testes are usually extensively involved, leading to sterility.

Spirochetes (p. 374)

Spirochetes are Gram-negative, corkscrew-shaped bacteria with flagella; an outer sheath membrane can mask bacterial antigens from host immune responses.

Syphilis (p. 374)

Syphilis is caused by *Treponema pallidum*, transmitted venereally or transplacentally (congenital syphilis). A T_H1 delayed type hypersensitivity response with macrophage activation appears important in reining in the infection, but it can also be the cause of disease manifestations (e.g., aortitis).

• *Primary syphilis* occurs about 3 weeks after contact:

A firm, non-tender, raised, red lesion *(chancre)* forms on the penis, cervix, vaginal wall, or anus; this will heal even without therapy.
Treponemes are plentiful (visualizable with silver or immunfluorescent stains) at the chancre surface; there is an exudate composed of plasma cells, macrophages, and lymphocytes, with a proliferative endarteritis.
Treponemes spread lymphohematogenously throughout the body even before the chancre appears.

• *Secondary syphilis* occurs 2 to 10 weeks later in 75% of untreated patients, with spread and proliferation of spirochetes in skin (including palms and soles) and mucocutaneous tissues (especially mouth)

Superficial lesions with erosions are painless and contain infectious spirochetes. Mucocutaneous lesions show plasma cell infiltrates and obliterative endarteritis.
Lymphadenopathy, mild fever, malaise, and weight loss are common.

• *Tertiary syphilis* occurs in one third of untreated patients, after a long latent period (more than 5 years).

Cardiovascular syphilis (more than 80% of tertiary syphilis) results in aortitis (due to endarteritis of the aortic vasa vasorum) with aortic root and arch aneurysms and aortic valve insufficiency.
Neurosyphilis can be symptomatic (meningovascular disease, *tabes dorsalis,* or diffuse brain parenchymal disease, so-called *general paresis*) or asymptomatic (cerebrospinal fluid [CSF] abnormalities only, with pleocytosis, increased protein, and decreased glucose).
"Benign" tertiary syphilis is associated with necrotic rubbery masses *(gummas* due to delayed type hypersensitivity to the organisms)*, which form in various sites (bone, skin, oral mucosa).

- *Congenital syphilis* usually occurs when the mother has primary or secondary syphilis.

  Intrauterine or perinatal death occurs in 50% of untreated cases.

  Early *(infantile)* congenital syphilis includes nasal discharge, a bullous rash with skin sloughing, hepatomegaly, and skeletal abnormalities (nose and lower legs are most distinctive). Diffuse lung or liver fibrosis can also occur.

  Late *(tardive)* manifestations include notched central incisors, deafness, and interstitial keratitis with blindness *(Hutchinson triad)*.

- Serologic tests for syphilis:

  Treponemal antibody tests measure antibodies reactive with *T. pallidum.*

  Nontreponemal tests (i.e., VDRL, RPR) measure antibody to cardiolipin, a phospholipid in treponemes and normal tissues.

  Both tests become positive about 6 weeks after infection and are positive during secondary syphilis; nontreponemal tests may become negative with time or treatment, but treponemal antibody tests remain positive.

Relapsing Fever (p. 377)

Relapsing fevers are insect-transmitted spirochetal diseases caused by *Borrelia* species; they are characterized by recurrent fevers, headache, and fatigue, followed by disseminated intravascular coagulation and multiorgan failure.

- *Epidemic relapsing fever* is caused by body louse–transmitted *Borrelia recurrentis,* often in conditions of poverty or overcrowding.
- *Endemic relapsing fever* is caused by several different *Borrelia* species, transmitted from small animals to humans by *Ornithodorus* (soft-bodied) ticks.
- Spirochetes are seen in blood smears during febrile periods; relapses are due to ongoing variation of the major surface protein, allowing the organism to repeatedly escape host antibody responses.

Lyme Disease (p. 377)

Lyme disease is caused by *B. burgdorferi* transmitted from rodents by *Ixodes* ticks; it is divided into three stages.

- Stage 1 (weeks): spirochetes multiply at the site of the tick bite, causing an expanding erythema, often with a pale center *(erythema chronicum migrans),* fever, and lymphadenopathy.
- Stage 2 (weeks to months): spirochetes spread hematogenously, causing secondary skin lesions, lymphadenopathy, migratory joint and muscle pain, cardiac arrhythmias, and meningitis.
- Stage 3 (years): encephalitis and polyneuropathy, and a chronic, occasionally destructive arthritis can arise.
- *B. burgdorferi* evades antibody-mediated immunity through antigenic variation.
- The bacterium does not make toxins; rather the pathology associated with infection is due to host immune responses. A distinctive feature of Lyme arthritis is an arteritis resembling that seen in lupus erythematosus.

Anaerobic Bacteria (p. 378)

These organisms normally reside in niches with low oxygen tension (intestine, vagina, oral recesses); they cause disease when they disproportionately expand (e.g., *C. difficile* colitis following antibiotic treatment) or when introduced into sterile sites. Environmental anaerobes also cause disease (e.g., tetanus, botulism).

Abscesses Caused by Anaerobes (p. 378)

Abscesses caused by anaerobes usually contain two or three different species of mixed bacteria flora; for each aerobic or facultative bacterial species present, there are one or two anaerobic species. The usual culprits are commensal bacteria from adjacent sites (e.g., oropharynx, intestines, or female genital tract), so that "normal flora" are typically cultured from abscesses.

- In head and neck abscesses, *Prevotella* and *Porphyromonas* are the usual anaerobes, while *S. aureus* and *S. pyogenes* are typical facultative aerobes.
- In abdominal abscesses, *Bacteroides fragilis* and *Peptostreptococcus* and *Clostridium* species are the common anaerobes, typically admixed with facultative *E. coli.*
- In genital tract abscesses in women, the anaerobes include *Prevotella* species, often mixed with facultative *E. coli* or *S. agalactiae.*
- Anaerobic abscesses are typically foul-smelling and poorly circumscribed but otherwise pathologically resemble other pyogenic infections.

Clostridial Infections (p. 378)

Clostridial infections are due to Gram-positive bacillus anaerobes that produce spores in the soil.

- *C. perfringens* and *Clostridium septicum* cause cellulitis and muscle necrosis in wounds (i.e., *gas gangrene),* food poisoning, and small bowel infection in ischemic or neutropenic patients.

  C. perfringens secretes 14 toxins, the most important being α-toxin; this has multiple activities including *phospholipase C,* which degrades erythrocyte, muscle, and platelet cell membranes, and sphingomyelinase, which causes nerve sheath damage.

  C. perfringens enterotoxin lyses gastrointestinal epithelial cells and disrupts tight junctions, causing diarrhea.

  Gas gangrene is reflected by marked edema and enzymatic necrosis of involved tissues; fermentation gas bubbles, hemolysis, and thrombosis with minimal inflammation are also characteristic.

- *Clostridium tetani* in wounds (or the umbilical stump of newborns) releases a neurotoxin (tetanospasmin) that causes *tetanus*—convulsive contractions of skeletal muscles—by blocking release of γ-aminobutyric acid, a neurotransmitter that inhibits motor neuron activity.

- *Clostridium botulinum* grows in canned foods; it releases a neurotoxin that causes flaccid paralysis of respiratory and skeletal muscles *(botulism)* by blocking acetylcholine release. Botulism toxin (Botox) is used in cosmetic surgery for its ability to paralyze strategically selected facial muscles.

- *C. difficile* overgrows other intestinal flora in antibiotic-treated patients and releases two glucosyl transferase toxins, causing *pseudomembranous colitis.*

  Toxin A stimulates chemokine production to recruit leukocytes. Toxin B (used for diagnosing *C. difficile* infections) causes cytopathic effects in cultured cells.

Obligate Intracellular Bacteria (p. 380)

Although some of these bacteria can survive in the extracellular environment, they can only proliferate within cells. They are well adapted to the intracellular environment with membrane transporters to capture amino acids and adenosine triphosphate (ATP).

Chlamydial Infections (p. 380)

Chlamydial infections are caused by small Gram-negative bacteria; *C. trachomatis* exists in two forms:

- A metabolically inactive but infectious spore-like *elementary body (EB)*. The EB is internalized by receptor-mediated endocytosis.
- Inside host cell endosomes, the EB differentiates into the metabolically active *reticulate body (RB)*; the RB replicates to form new EB for release.

    Specific *C. trachomatis* diseases are caused by particular serotypes:

- *Trachoma*, an ocular infection of children (serotypes A, B, and C).
- Urogenital infections and conjunctivitis are caused by serotypes D through K. Chlamydia is the most common bacterial sexually transmitted infection in the world. Although chlamydia is frequently asymptomatic, urogenital infections can cause epididymitis, prostatitis, pelvic inflammatory disease, pharyngitis, conjunctivitis, perihepatic inflammation, and proctitis.

    Infections exhibit a mucopurulent discharge containing neutrophils but no visible organisms by Gram stain.
    The CDC recommends treating both *C. trachomatis* and *N. gonorrhoeae* when either is diagnosed, due to frequent co-infections.

- Lymphogranuloma venereum (i.e., serotypes L1, L2, and L3) is a sporadic genital infection in the United States and western Europe; it is endemic in parts of Asia, Africa, the Caribbean, and South America.

    About 2 to 6 weeks after infection, organism growth and host immune response in draining lymph nodes leads to painful adenopathy.
    Lesions contain a mixed granulomatous and neutrophilic response with irregular foci of necrosis *(stellate abscesses)*; chlamydial inclusions can be seen in epithelial or inflammatory cells.

Rickettsial Infections (p. 380)

Rickettsial infections are caused by Gram-negative bacilli transmitted by arthropod vectors. They primarily infect endothelial cells, causing endothelial swelling, thrombosis, and vessel wall necrosis. Vascular thrombosis and increased permeability causing hypovolemic shock, pulmonary edema, and CNS manifestations. Natural killer cell and cytotoxic T-cell responses are necessary to contain and eradicate infections.

- Epidemic typhus *(Rickettsia prowazekii)* is transmitted by body lice.

    Lesions range from a rash with small hemorrhages to skin necrosis and gangrene with internal organ hemorrhages.
    CNS typhus nodules show microglial proliferations with T-cell and macrophage infiltration.

- Rocky Mountain spotted fever *(Rickettsia rickettsii)* is transmitted by dog ticks.

    A hemorrhagic rash extends over the entire body, including the palms of the hands and soles of the feet.

Vascular lesions in the CNS may involve larger vessels and produce microinfarcts.

Non-cardiogenic pulmonary edema is the major cause of death.

- *Ehrlichiosis* is transmitted by ticks.

  The bacteria predominantly infects neutrophils *(Anaplasma phagocytophila* and *Ehrlichia ewingii)* or macrophages *(Ehrlichia chaffeensis)* with characteristic intracytoplasmic inclusions *(morulae).*

  Infection is characterized by fever, headache, and malaise, progressing to respiratory insufficiency, renal failure, and shock.

Fungal Infections (p. 382)

Fungi are eukaryotes with cell walls; they grow as multicelluar filaments that grow and divide at their tips (molds), or as single cells or chains that typically propagate by budding (yeasts); dimorphic fungi assume a yeast form at body temperature and a mold form at room temperature.

Candidiasis (p. 382)

Candida species are part of the normal flora of the skin, mouth, and gastrointestinal tract; they occur as yeast and pseudohyphal forms. Candida can cause superficial infections in healthy individuals and disseminated visceral infections in neutropenic patients.

- *Candida* virulence factors include:

  Adhesins that mediate binding to host cells
  Enzymes that contribute to invasiveness
  Catalases that aid intracellular survival by resisting phagocyte oxidative killing
  Adenosine that blocks neutrophil degranulation and oxygen radical production
  Ability to grow as a biofilms on devices, thereby frustrating immune responses and anti-fungal agents

- Innate and T-cell responses are important for protection:

  Neutrophil and macrophage phagocytosis and oxidative killing are the first-line defense; these are induced by a T_H17 response.
  Yeast forms induce a protective T_H1 response; filamentous forms tend to induce a non-protective T_H2 response.

- *Candida* grows best on warm, moist surfaces; in healthy individuals, it can cause vaginitis and diaper rash.
- Superficial infections of the mouth and vagina are most common, producing superficial curdy white patches; these are easily detached to reveal a reddened, irritated mucosa.
- Chronic mucocutaneous candidiasis occurs in persons with AIDS, with defective T-cell immunity, or with polyendocrine deficiencies (e.g., hypoparathyroidism, hypoadrenalism, and hypothyroidism).
- Severe, invasive candidiasis occurs via blood-borne dissemination in neutropenic persons; typically, microabscesses (with fungi in the center) are surrounded by areas of tissue necrosis.

Cryptococcosis (p. 384)

Cryptococcus neoformans is an encapsulated yeast. In tissues, the capsule stains bright red with mucicarmine; in CSF, it is negatively stained with India ink.

- Virulence factors include:

  A capsular polysaccharide (glucuronoxylomannan) inhibits phago-cytosis, leukocyte migration, and inflammatory cell recruitment

  Regular alteration in the size and structure of the capsule poly-saccharide, which allows immune evasion

  Laccase, an enzyme that induces formation of a melanin-like pigment with antioxidant properties

  Enzymes that degrade fibronectin and basement membrane proteins and aid in tissue invasion

- In healthy individuals, *C. neoformans* can form solitary pulmo-nary granulomata (with reactivation if immunity wanes) and rarely causes meningoencephalitis.

- It occurs as an opportunistic infection in patients with AIDS, leukemia or lymphoid malignancies, lupus, sarcoidosis, or organ transplants or those receiving high-dose corticosteroids. In such patients, the major lesions involve the CNS, occurring as gray matter cysts ("soap bubble lesions"), occasionally with no inflammatory response.

Aspergillosis (p. 384)

Aspergillus (*A. fumigatus* is the most common species) is a ubiqui-tous mold transmitted by air-borne conidia; it grows as septated hyphae branching at acute angles occasionally with spore-produc-ing fruiting bodies. It causes allergy (allergic bronchopulmonary aspergillosis) in healthy individuals and severe sinusitis, pneumo-nia, and invasive disease in immunocompromised hosts.

- Neutrophils and macrophages are the major host defenses, kill-ing by phagocytosis and reactive oxygen species. Neutropenia is a major risk factor.

- Virulence factors include:

  Adhesion to albumin, surfactant, and a variety of ECM proteins.

  Antioxidant defenses including melanin pigment, mannitol, cata-lases, and superoxide dismutase.

  Phospholipases, proteases, and toxins including *aflatoxin* (synthe-sized by fungus growing on peanuts), a cause of liver cancer in Africa.

- Preexisting pulmonary lesions caused by tuberculosis, bronchi-ectasis, old infarcts, or abscesses can develop secondary *Aspergil-lus* colonization *(aspergillomas)* without tissue invasion.

- Invasive aspergillosis in immunosuppressed hosts usually presents as necrotizing pneumonia (forming "target lesions"), but often develops widespread hematogenous dissemination.

- Aspergillus tends to invade blood vessels with resulting throm-bosis; consequently, areas of hemorrhage and infarction are superimposed on necrotizing inflammation.

Zygomycosis (Mucormycosis) (p. 385)

Zygomycosis (mucormycosis) is an opportunistic infection in neu-tropenic patients and diabetics caused by *Zygomycetes* molds (*Mucor, Absidia, Rhizopus,* and *Cunninghamella*). Zygomycetes are non-septated with right-angle branching.

- The primary site of infection (nasal sinuses, lungs, or gastroin-testinal tract) depends on whether the spores are inhaled or ingested.

- In diabetics, fungus may spread from nasal sinuses to the orbit or brain.

- These fungi commonly invade arterial walls and cause necrosis.

Parasitic Infections (p. 386) (See Table 8-9 in *Robbins and Cotran Pathologic Basis of Disease,* ed 8, p. 386)

Protozoa (p. 386)

These are unicellular, eukaryotic organisms; parasitic protozoa are transmitted by insects or by the fecal-oral route. In humans, they mainly occupy the intestine or blood (extracellular or intracellular).

Malaria (p. 386)

Malaria is an intracellular parasite affecting 500 million people worldwide and killing 1 million annually. *Plasmodium falciparum* causes severe malaria; *vivax, ovale,* and *malariae* species cause less severe disease. All species are transmitted by female *Anopheles* mosquitoes.

- The *Plasmodium* life cycle is schematized in Figure 8-2:

  From the mosquito salivary gland, *sporozoites* in the bloodstream invade via the hepatocyte receptor for thrombospondin and properdin.

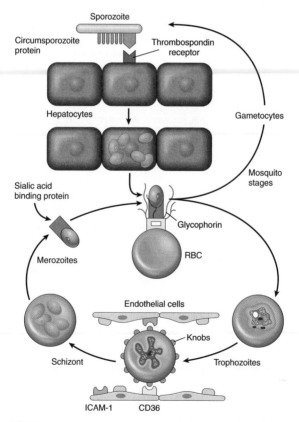

FIGURE 8-2 Life cycle of *Plasmodium falciparum. ICAM,* Intercellular adhesion molecule; *RBC,* red blood cell.

Parasites multiply rapidly, causing hepatocyte rupture and release of *merozoites* (asexual, haploid).

Merozoites bind to sialic acid residues on erythrocyte glycophorin and are internalized.

In erythrocytes, parasites hydrolyze red blood cell (RBC) hemoglobin to generate characteristic *hemozoin* pigment and undergo development.

Trophozoites (single chromatin mass) divide to form *schizonts* (multiple chromatin masses) that form new merozoites.

Merozoites released by red cell lysis cause another round of erythrocyte infection.

A small fraction of the parasites within RBCs develop into sexual forms *(gametocytes)* that infect mosquitoes when they feed.

- The greater pathogenicity of *P. falciparum* stems from its ability to:

  Infect erythrocytes of any age; other species infect only new or old cells.

  Cause infected erythrocytes to clump together or adhere to small vessel endothelium (via "knobs" on erythrocyte surfaces that bind to endothelial cells), causing vascular occlusion. Ischemia due to such occlusions causes the manifestations of cerebral malaria.

  Induce high levels of cytokines such as tumor necrosis factor (TNF) and interferon-γ (INF-γ) that suppress red cell production, cause fever, and stimulate nitric oxide (NO) production. This occurs through release of glycosyl phosphatidyl inositol–linked proteins (including merozoite surface antigens) from infected erythrocytes.

  Use antigenic variation to continuously modify surface proteins.

- Resistance to *Plasmodium* occurs through:

  Heritable erythrocyte traits:
  - Sickle cell trait (i.e., hemoglobin S [HbS]) and hemoglobin C (HbC) lessen malaria severity by reducing parasite proliferation.
  - Absence of Duffy blood group antigen prevents *P. vivax* from binding to erythrocytes.
  - Antibody and T-cell–mediated repertoires that develop after chronic infection.

Babesiosis *(p. 388)*

Babesiosis is caused by malaria-like protozoans transmitted from white-footed mice to humans by *Ixodes* ticks or rarely is contracted through blood transfusion.

- Babesiae cause fever and, through erythrocyte parasitization, hemolytic anemia.
- Babesiae resemble malaria schizonts but lack hemozoin pigment, are more pleomorphic, and form characteristic tetrads.

Leishmaniasis *(p. 388)*

Leishmaniasis is a chronic inflammatory disease of skin, mucous membranes, and viscera caused by *Leishmania* species, obligate intracellular parasites transmitted by sandfly bites. The life cycle involves two forms:

- Promastigotes develop and live extracellularly in the sandfly vector.
- Amastigotes multiply intracellularly in the macrophages of mammalian hosts.

  When sandflies bite infected hosts, infected macrophages are ingested; amastigotes differentiate into promastigotes in the insect digestive tract and migrate to the salivary gland.

Subsequent bite of a second host delivers the promastigotes; these are phagocytized by macrophages and undergo transformation in phagolysosomes into amastigotes that then proliferate.

- Disease manifestations vary with the species and host responses. Thus, whether a patient develops cutaneous disease, mucocutaneous disease, or visceral disease depends on which organism is in play; there are also different agents in the Old World *vs.* the New World.
- Virulence factors include the following:

  Lipophosphoglycan on promastigotes activates complement (leading to C3b deposition on the parasite surface and increasing phagocytosis) but also inhibits complement action (by preventing membrane attack complex assembly).

  gp63 on promastigotes binds fibronectin to promote promastigote adhesion to macrophages; it also cleaves complement and lysosomal antimicrobial enzymes to frustrate killing.

  A proton pump in amastigotes reduces macrophage phagolysosome acidity.

- Activation of macrophages by IFN-γ is necessary for adequate host defense; activated macrophages kill parasites through reactive oxygen species and NO.

African Trypanosomiasis *(p. 390)*

African trypanosomiasis is caused by extracellular parasites transmitted by tsetse flies.

- *Trypanosoma brucei rhodesiense* (East Africa) is an acute and virulent infection, whereas *Trypanosoma brucei gambiense* (West Africa) is chronic.
- Trypanosomiasis is a disease of intermittent fevers, lymphadenopathy, progressive brain dysfunction (sleeping sickness), cachexia, and death.

  In the fly, parasites multiply in the stomach and then in salivary glands before becoming non-dividing but infective trypomastigotes.

  A chancre forms at the insect bite site; large numbers of parasites are surrounded by a dense, largely mononuclear, inflammatory infiltrate.

  Lymph nodes and spleen enlarge as a result of hyperplasia and infiltration by lymphocytes, plasma cells, and parasite-laden macrophages.

  When parasites breach the blood-brain barrier, they induce a leptomeningitis and a demyelinating panencephalitis.

- Virulence factors include antigenic variation of a surface glycoprotein (VSG) specified by several different genes; as antibody responses clear one population of organisms expressing a particular VSG (causing a fever spike), a small number undergo genetic rearrangement and produce a new VSG.

Chagas Disease *(p. 391)*

Chagas disease is caused by *Trypanosoma cruzi,* an intracellular protozoan transmitted between animals (e.g., cats, dogs, rodents) and humans by "kissing bugs" (triatomids) that pass parasites in their feces as they bite.

- *T. cruzi* requires brief acid exposure in phagolysosomes to stimulate *amastigote* development; the organism then proliferates in the cytoplasm before developing flagella and rupturing the cell, traversing the blood to infect smooth, skeletal, and cardiac muscle.

- Acute Chagas disease:

  Is generally mild with cardiac damage secondary to direct invasion and associated inflammation

  Is rarely severe with high parasitemia, fever, and progressive cardiac dilation and failure

- Chronic Chagas disease occurs in 20% of patients, with late (i.e., 5 to 15 years):

  Myocardial inflammation, causing, cardiomyopathy and arrhythmias

  Damage to the myenteric plexus, causing colon and esophageal dilation

Metazoa (p. 391)

Metazoa are multicellular, eukaryotic organisms, typically contracted by eating undercooked meat, through insect bites, or by direct host invasion through the skin. Depending on the organism, they may ultimately dwell in the host intestine, skin, lung, liver, muscle, blood vessels, or lymphatics.

Strongyloidiasis (p. 391)

Strongyloides stercoralis larvae live in the soil.

- Larvae directly penetrate the skin of humans, traveling in the circulation to the lungs. From there they migrate up the trachea and are swallowed. Adult female worms produce eggs asexually in the mucosa of the small intestine; passed larvae contaminate soil to complete the cycle.
- In immunocompetent hosts, there may be diarrhea and malabsorption; larvae are present in the duodenal crypts with an underlying eosinophil-rich infiltrate.
- In immunocompromised hosts, larvae hatched in the gut can invade colonic mucosa and reinitiate infection. Such uncontrolled autoinfection results in massive larval burdens with widespread invasion—occasionally complicated by sepsis caused by bacteria carried into the bloodstream by parasites.

Tapeworms (Cestodes): Cysticercosis and Hydatid Disease (p. 392)

Disease is caused by larval development after the ingestion of eggs; *Taenia solium* causes *cysticercosis* and *Echinococcus granulosus* causes *hydatid disease.*

- Tapeworms have complex life cycles requiring two hosts—a definitive host where the worm reaches sexual maturity and an intermediate host.
- *T. solium* are transmitted to humans in two ways with distinct outcomes:

  Larval cysts (cysticerci) ingested in pork attach to the intestinal wall, where they mature and produce egg-laden proglottids (segments) that are passed in stool.

  If intermediate hosts (pigs or humans) ingest eggs in feces-contaminated food or water, hatching larvae penetrate the gut wall and disseminate to encyst in many organs, including the brain (causing severe neurologic manifestations).

- Humans are accidental hosts for *E. granulosus* and *E. multilocularis;* these are normally passed only between the definitive (dog or fox) and intermediate (sheep and rodents) hosts.

  Hydatid disease is caused by ingestion of echinoccal eggs in food contaminated with dog or fox feces.

Eggs hatch in the duodenum and invade the liver, lungs, or bones, where they form cysts.

- *T. saginata* (beef) and *Diphyllobothrium latum* (fish) are acquired by eating undercooked meat; in humans, these parasites live only in the gut and do not form cysticerci.

Trichinosis *(p. 393)*

Trichinella spiralis is typically acquired by ingestion of larvae in undercooked pork; pigs are infected by eating contaminated meat.

- In the gut, larvae develop into adults that mate and produce new larvae; these disseminate hematogenously and penetrate muscle cells, causing fever, myalgias, eosinophilia, and periorbital edema.
- Intracellular organisms increase dramatically in size and encapsulate; they may persist for years, subverting the cell to become a "nurse cell–parasite complex" surrounded by an eosinophil-rich infiltrate and a new host vascular plexus.
- *T. spiralis* stimulates T_H2 cells that activate eosinophils and mast cells (typical anti-nematodal inflammatory response; Chapter 6) and increase gut contractility to expel worms. Organisms usually die after a number of years, leaving behind characteristic calcified scars.

Schistosomiasis *(p. 393)*

Schistosomiasis is caused by *Schistosoma mansoni* (Latin America, Africa, and the Middle East), *S. haematobium* (Africa), and *S. japonicum* or *S. mekongi* (East Asia); these are transmitted from freshwater snails.

- Larvae penetrate human skin, migrate through the vasculature, and settle in the pelvic *(S. haematobium)* or portal (all others) venous systems.
- Females produce eggs that may disseminate and are shed in urine or stool. Proteases produced by eggs and the host inflammatory responses are necessary for eggs to penetrate mucosa (bladder or intestine) and be shed.
- The immune response is directed against eggs; early responses are T_H1-dominated, while in chronic infections, T_H2 responses predominate.
- Both T cell populations contribute to granuloma formation (often eosinophil-rich) and fibrosis; urinary schistosomiasis is also associated with urinary bladder squamous cell carcinoma.

Lymphatic Filariasis *(p. 395)*

Lymphatic filariasis is caused by two nematodes—*Wuchereria bancrofti* (i.e., 90% of cases) and *Brugia malay;* larvae are contracted from infected mosquitoes.

- Larvae develop into adults in lymphatic channels; those mate and release microfilariae that enter the bloodstream and can then infect secondary mosquitoes.
- Damage to lymphatics is mediated by T_H1-mediated inflammation, although T_H2 inflammation can also occur; differences in host immune responses likely accounts for the different manifestations of filariasis:

Asymptomatic microfilaremia
Recurrent lymphadenitis
Chronic lymphadenitis with swelling of the dependent limb or scrotum *(elephantiasis)*
Tropical pulmonary eosinophilia.

- Virulence factors:

    Antioxidant glycoproteins protect from oxygen radical injury.
    Homologues of cystatins (cysteine protease inhibitors) impair antigen presentation.
    Serpins (serine protease inhibitors) inhibit neutrophil proteases.
    Homologues of TGF-β bind to host TGF-β receptors and down-regulate inflammatory responses.
    Rickettsia-like *Wolbachia* bacteria infect filaria and are needed for nematode development and reproduction; these may also release LPS and stimulate inflammation.

Onchocerciasis (p. 395)

Onchocerca volvulus is a filarial nematode transmitted by black flies; it causes "river blindness," the second-most common cause of blindness in sub-Saharan Africa

- Nematodes mate in the host dermis, surrounded by host inflammatory cells that produce a subcutaneous nodule *(onchocercoma)*.
- Female worms release large numbers of microfilariae that accumulate in the skin and eye chambers, causing pruritic dermatitis and blindness.
- Treatment includes doxycycline to kill the symbiotic *Wolbachia* bacteria that live inside *O. volvulus* and are required for worm fertility.

9

Environmental and Nutritional Diseases

Environmental diseases refer to conditions caused by exposure to chemical or physical agents in the ambient, workplace, or personal environment (e.g., diet, drugs, alcohol, and tobacco), including diseases of nutritional origin (over- or undernutrition). Exposures may be acute or represent chronic contact with low-level contaminants. Worldwide, 2 million people die annually due to occupation-related injury or illness, and malnutrition is responsible for the death of another 2.7 million.

The Global Burden of Disease (p. 400)

Global health data is reported using a disability-adjusted life year (DALY) metric that combines years lost to premature mortality and years lived with illness and disability. By this measure, the burden of disease imposed by environmental causes (including infectious and nutritional diseases) shows several trends:

- Undernutrition is the single leading global cause of health loss; one third of the disease burden in developing countries is nutrition-related.
- Coronary and cerebrovascular diseases are the leading causes of death in developed countries; major risk factors include obesity, smoking, and high cholesterol.
- Infections constitute a significant global health burden; 5 of the top 10 causes of death in developing countries are infectious diseases, and the vast majority of mortality in children is infection-related.

  Malnutrition increases the risk of infection.

  Drug-resistant strains (due to clinical and agricultural antibiotic use) are the most important group of pathogens.

  Vector-borne diseases constitute almost a third of newly emerging infections, and in many cases can be linked to environmental changes, including global warming.

Health Effects of Climate Change (p. 401)

The dominant greenhouse gases (trapping energy from the earth that would otherwise radiate into space) are water vapor, carbon dioxide, methane, and ozone. Human activity has contributed materially to the last three and thereby contributed to global warming; depending on the model, global temperatures are predicted to rise 2° C to 5° C by 2100. While the outcome will depend on the tempo and extent of change, and the ability of humans to mitigate such changes, global warming will inevitably impact human disease:

- Cardiovascular and respiratory diseases will be amplified by heat waves and air pollution.
- Gastroenteritis and infection epidemics will be affected by water and food contamination following flooding and other environmental disruptions.
- Vector-borne infectious diseases are expected to increase as vector numbers and geographic distributions are altered.
- Malnutrition will increase as crop productivity wanes.

Toxicity of Chemical and Physical Agents (p. 402)

Toxicology studies the distribution, effects, and mechanisms of action of toxic agents. Xenobiotics are exogenous agents in the environment that may be inhaled, ingested, or directly absorbed. Four billion pounds of toxic chemicals, including 72 million pounds of known carcinogens, are released annually in the United States. Moreover, of the roughly 100,000 chemicals in commercial use in the United States, very few have been formally tested for adverse health effects.

- Toxicity depends on the structural properties of a compound, as well as the administered dose. Low doses of a given agent may be well tolerated *or even therapeutic*, whereas greater amounts are toxic.
- Toxic compounds may act locally at the site of entry into the body, or in other tissues after bloodstream transport.
- A lipophilic (fat-soluble) compound will have increased blood transport by associating with lipoproteins and will cross plasma membranes more readily.
- Compounds may be excreted in urine, feces, or expired air, or they may accumulate in bone, fat, brain, or other tissues.
- Some agents act directly and may be rendered less toxic (or more readily excreted) by metabolic activity; other compounds may become toxic only after being metabolized.
- Drug-metabolizing enzymes are divided into two general groups:

    Phase I:

    Enzyme activities include hydrolysis, oxidation, or reduction.
    The most important catalyst is the cytochrome P-450 (CYP) enzyme system.
    Cytochrome P-450 (CYP) are a large family of heme-containing endoplasmic reticulum enzymes.
    Enzymatic activity also releases oxygen-derived free radicals.
    Variation in CYP enzymatic activity may be due to genetic polymorphisms or to secondary compounds that augment or reduce CYP expression; tobacco and alcohol can enhance expression, whereas malnutrition may diminish it.

    Phase II:

    Enzyme activities include glucuronidation, sulfation, methylation, and conjugation.
    Generally increase water solubility and hence excretion.

Environmental Pollution (p. 403)

Air Pollution (p. 403)

Outdoor Air Pollution (p. 404)

The lung is the major organ affected, although other tissues can be affected by outdoor air pollutants (e.g., by carbon monoxide [CO] and lead). Decreased pulmonary function, lung inflammation, increased airway reactivity, diminished mucociliary clearance, and increased infections are all common effects.

- *Ozone* forms from the interaction of oxygen and ultraviolet (UV) radiation. Stratospheric ozone is critical in absorbing solar UV radiation; loss due to chlorofluorocarbon use increases skin cancer risk. However, ozone in the lower atmosphere is a major component of smog, which also contains nitrogen oxides and volatile organic compounds from industrial emissions and motor vehicle exhaust.

  Ozone toxicity is due to the production of free radicals; these injure alveolar epithelium and induce release of inflammatory mediators. The outcome is cough (upper airway hyperreactivity), chest discomfort, and pulmonary inflammation; the consequences are more severe in patients with asthma or emphysema.

- *Sulfur dioxide* is produced by the combustion of coal and oil, copper smelting, and paper manufacture. It is converted into sulfuric acid and sulfur trioxide, which cause burning, dyspnea, and airway hyperreactivity.
- *Particulate matter* (soot) is emitted by coal, oil, and diesel combustion; deposition and clearance of inhaled particulates depend on their size and shape with particles less than 10 microns being most deleterious (larger particles are usually trapped in nasal mucus or by the upper respiratory mucociliary clearance mechanisms). Toxic effects are attributed to macrophage and neutrophil uptake, with subsequent inflammatory mediator production.
- *CO* is a colorless, odorless, tasteless, non-irritating gas produced by incomplete oxidation of carbonaceous materials (internal combustion engines, wood burning, cigarette smoking, etc.). Ambient low-level exposure may contribute to impaired respiratory function, and chronic poisoning in confined spaces (e.g., tunnels, toll takers, underground garages) can cause serious injury. Acute lethality occurs through central nervous system (CNS) depression and systemic hypoxia (CO has 200-fold greater affinity for hemoglobin than oxygen). Acute poisoning is characterized by a cherry-red coloring of the victim due to high levels of carboxyhemoglobin.

Indoor Air Pollution (p. 405)

Levels of indoor air pollutants have increased owing to improved insulation and fewer air leaks in homes, coupled with increasing reliance on air conditioning rather than open window ventilation. Tobacco smoke, CO, nitrogen dioxide, and carcinogenic polycyclic aromatic hydrocarbons (from cooking) are all complicit. The following are some of the major indoor air pollutants:

- *Wood smoke* is a complex mixture of particulates and other toxic components (e.g., polycylic hydrocarbons); these are directly irritating, can increase the incidence of respiratory infections, and are potentially carcinogenic.
- *Bioaerosols* include the bacterial aerosols responsible for *Legionella* pneumonia and allergens from pet danders, dust mites, and molds.
- *Radon* is a radioactive gas formed as a decay product of uranium found naturally in the soil. Low-level radon in some homes may increase cancer risk in smokers.
- *Formaldehyde* is a soluble, volatile chemical used in the manufacture of many consumer products; it can cause acute irritation of the eyes and upper respiratory tract and is classified as a carcinogen.

Metals as Environmental Pollutants (p. 406)

Lead (p.406)

Lead is present in air where leaded gasoline is burned, soil and house dusts contaminated with leaded paint, and water supplies in the setting of lead plumbing. Inhalation is the most important route of occupational exposure, but it can also be ingested. Infants and children are particularly vulnerable due to greater gastrointestinal absorption and a more permeable blood-brain barrier. Lead competes with calcium ions, and 80% to 85% of absorbed lead accumulates in bones and teeth. Lead toxicity is due to the following:

- Neurotoxicity due to altered calcium homeostasis that disrupts neurotransmitter release. In children, this typically presents as psychomotor impairment; in adults, a peripheral demyelinating neuropathy is more common.
- Inhibition of enzymes involved in heme synthesis (δ-aminolevulinic acid dehydratase) and iron incorporation (ferrochelatase), leading to microcytic, hypochromic anemia (erythrocytes exhibit a characteristic punctate basophilic stippling).
- Altered cartilage remodeling in epiphyses (this leads to characteristic radiodense "lead lines") and inhibition of bone healing.
- Gastrointestinal changes include abdominal pain and anorexia (lead "colic").

Mercury (p. 407)

Mercury exposure is currently primarily through methyl mercury–contaminated fish (that concentrate environmental mercury over a million-fold), and mercury vapors released by metallic mercury in dental amalgams; mercury used in gold mining can contaminate water run-off. Lipid solubility of methyl mercury facilitates accumulation in the CNS where, toxicity is related to high binding affinity for cellular thiol groups; developing brains are particularly susceptible to neuronal toxicity.

Arsenic (p. 408)

Arsenic is found naturally in soil and water and is used in herbicides and as a wood preservative. The trivalent forms are most toxic (e.g., arsenic trioxide and sodium arsenite). Ingestion leads to gastrointestinal, cardiovascular, and neurologic sequelae by inhibiting mitochondrial oxidative phosphorylation. Chronic low-level exposure increases the risk of skin and lung cancer.

Cadmium (p. 408)

Cadmium is an environmental pollutant generated by mining, electroplating, and the production and improper disposal of nickel-cadmium batteries; ingestion of contaminated food is the most common route of human exposure. Toxicity is due to alveolar macrophage necrosis, causing obstructive lung disease, and to renal tubular damage; skeletal abnormalities may be related to calcium loss. An increased risk of lung cancer may be due to DNA damage induced by reactive oxygen species.

Occupational Health Risks: Industrial and Agricultural Exposures (p. 408)

More than 10 million injuries and 100,000 deaths annually in the United States are due to work-related illness or accident. Occupational exposures contribute to diseases that can range from mild irritation of the respiratory mucosa to lung cancer and leukemia; all organ systems can be affected (Table 9-1).

TABLE 9-1 Human Diseases Associated with Occupational Exposures

Organ	Effect	Toxicant
Cardiovascular system	Heart disease	Carbon monoxide, lead, solvents, cobalt, cadmium
Respiratory system	Nasal cancer	Isopropyl alcohol, wood dust
	Lung cancer	Radon, asbestos, silica, bis(chloromethyl)ether, nickel, arsenic, chromium, mustard gas
	Chronic obstructive lung disease	Grain dust, coal dust, cadmium
	Hypersensitivity	Beryllium, isocyanates
	Irritation	Ammonia, sulfur oxides, formaldehyde
	Fibrosis	Silica, asbestos, cobalt
Nervous system	Peripheral neuropathies	Solvents, acrylamide, methyl chloride, mercury, lead, arsenic, DDT
	Ataxic gait	Chlordane, toluene, acrylamide, mercury
	Central nervous system depression	Alcohols, ketones, aldehydes, solvents
	Cataracts	Ultraviolet radiation
Urinary system	Toxicity	Mercury, lead, glycol ethers, solvents
	Bladder cancer	Naphthylamines, 4-aminobiphenyl, benzidine, rubber products
Reproductive system	Male infertility	Lead, phthalate plasticizers
	Female infertility	Cadmium, lead
	Teratogenesis	Mercury, polychlorinated biphenyls
Hematopoietic system	Leukemia	Benzene, radon, uranium
Skin	Folliculitis and acneiform dermatosis	Polychlorinated biphenyls, dioxins, herbicides
	Cancer	Ultraviolet radiation
Gastrointestinal tract	Liver angiosarcoma	Vinyl chloride

Data from Leigh JP, et al: Occupational injury and illness in the United States. Estimates of costs, morbidity, and mortality, *Arch Intern Med* 157:1557, 1997; Mitchell FL: Hazardous waste. In Rom WN (ed): *Environmental and occupational medicine*, ed 2, Boston, 1992, Little, Brown, p 1275; Levi PE: Classes of toxic chemicals. In Hodgson E, Levi PE (eds): *A textbook of modern toxicology*, Stamford, Conn., 1997, Appleton & Lange, p 229.

- *Organic solvents* (e.g., chloroform and carbon tetrachloride) are widely used as industrial solvents and cleaning agents. These compounds are readily absorbed through the lungs, skin, and gastrointestinal tract. In addition to acute CNS depression, they can cause liver and kidney toxicity. *Aromatic hydrocarbons* (e.g., benzene) are metabolized by CYP2E1 to toxic metabolites that disrupt marrow hematopoiesis, leading to dose-dependent aplasia and an increased risk of acute myeloid leukemia.

- *Polycyclic hydrocarbons* are produced during fossil fuel combustion and by iron and steel foundries. These are potent carcinogens, and occupational exposure is associated with an increased risk of lung and bladder cancers.
- *Organochlorines* are synthetic lipophilic compounds that resist degradation; these include pesticides such as *dichlorodiphenyltrichloroethane (DDT)* and non-pesticides such as polychlorinated biphenyls (PCBs) and dioxin. Most are endocrine disrupters with anti-estrogenic and anti-androgenic effects. Dioxins and PCBs can also cause a folliculitis/dermatosis called chloracne, as well as hepatic and CNS abnormalities; they activate CYP and thus can alter drug metabolism.
- *Mineral dust inhalation* (e.g., coal, silica, asbestsos, beryllium) can cause chronic, non-neoplastic but diffusely fibrosing *pneumoconioses* (Chapter 15).
- *Vinyl chloride* monomers used to produce polyvinyl chloride resins are associated with angiosarcoma of the liver.
- *Phthalate* (found as a plasticizer in flexible plastic products) exposure leads to endocrine disruption and in laboratory animals causes a testicular dysgenesis syndrome.

Effects of Tobacco (p. 410)

Cigarette smoking is responsible for more than 400,000 deaths annually in the United States and 5 million deaths worldwide; lung cancer (one third of the total) and cardiovascular and chronic pulmonary disease account for the vast majority of the mortality. Indeed, tobacco use is the most common exogenous cause of human malignancy, responsible for 90% of lung cancers. Within 5 years of smoking cessation, overall mortality, and—more specifically—risk of death from cardiovascular disease is markedly reduced. Lung cancer risk decreases by 21% within 5 years, but the excess risk persists for 30 years.

- Cigarette smoke contains some 4000 constituents, of which 60 are known carcinogens.
- Nicotine is an addictive alkaloid found naturally in tobacco leaves; binding to CNS receptors releases catecholamines that increase heart rate, blood pressure, and cardiac contractility.

Smoking and Lung Cancer (p. 411)

Polycyclic hydrocarbons, benzopyrene, and nitrosamines in cigarette smoke are potent carcinogens, especially after CYP modification. Cancer risk is dose related (more cigarettes increases risk), and smoking synergizes with other carcinogenic influences in causing lung carcinoma (e.g., asbestos or radiation exposures). In addition to lung cancer, tobacco contributes to cancer development in the oral cavity, esophagus, pancreas, and bladder; smoke and smokeless tobacco both interact with alcohol in potentiating laryngeal cancer.

Smoking and Other Diseases (p. 411)

Formaldehyde, phenol, and nitrogen oxides in cigarette smoke are directly irritating, inducing tracheobronchial inflammation and increased mucus output *(bronchitis);* leukocyte recruitment leads to increased elastase production and subsequent *emphysema.*

- Cigarette smoking is strongly linked to development of atherosclerosis and myocardial infarction; increased platelet aggregation, endothelial dysfunction, and myocardial hypoxia are all implicated.

- Maternal smoking causes fetal hypoxia with intrauterine growth retardation, and it increases the risk of spontaneous abortions and preterm births.
- *Second-hand smoke (environmental smoke)* also increases the risk of lung cancer, ischemic heart disease, and acute myocardial infarction; relative risk of lung cancer in non-smokers exposed to second-hand smoke is 1.3 times greater than in individuals not exposed to environmental smoke.

Effects of Alcohol (p. 412)

- There are 10 million alcoholics in the United States. Roughly 100,000 deaths are attributable to alcohol abuse each year, with the majority due to drunken driving or alcohol-related homicides and suicides; 15% of alcohol-related deaths are due to cirrhosis.
- A blood alcohol concentration of 80 mg/dL is the legal definition for drunk driving in most states; drowsiness typically occurs at 200 mg/dL, stupor at 300 mg/dL, and coma (with possible respiratory arrest) at higher concentrations. Alcohol effects vary depending on age, gender, and body fat; for the *average individual,* 80 mg/dL occurs after 36 oz of beer, 15 oz of wine, or 4 to 5 oz of 80 proof distilled spirits. Chronic alcoholics can tolerate greater volumes due to hepatic CYP induction.
- After consumption, alcohol is absorbed unaltered in the stomach and small bowel; less than 10% is excreted unchanged in the urine, sweat, and breath. Ethanol is metabolized to acetaldehyde in hepatocytes mainly by cytosolic alcohol dehydrogenase (ADH); at high blood alcohol levels, the microsomal ethanol-oxidizing system (MEOS) also participates, while liver catalase metabolizes less than 5%. Hepatic acetaldehyde dehydrogenase (ALDH) then converts acetaldehyde to acetate that can be utilized by normal mitochondrial metabolic pathways.
- Induction of CYP (especially CYP2E1) by alcohol accelerates the metabolism of other drugs by the MEOS. However, when alcohol is present in high concentrations, it competes for the enzyme complex, and the metabolism of other compounds can be delayed.
- The metabolism of ethanol is directly responsible for most of its toxic and chronic effects:

  - Acetaldehyde is responsible for many of the acute toxicities of alcohol and the development of oral cancers. ADH and ALDH isoforms influence the relative rates of metabolite generation. Roughly half of Asians have low ALDH activity due to one copy of an inactive ALDH enzyme; homozygotes cannot oxidize acetaldehyde at all, and alcohol consumption is associated with nausea, flushing, tachycardia, and hyperventilation.
  - ADH oxidation of alcohol reduces nicotinamide adenine dinucleotide (NAD) to NADH; since NAD is required for fatty acid oxidation and for converting lactic acid to pyruvate, alcohol consumption leads to liver fat accumulation.
  - CYPE21 oxidation of alcohol leads to the formation of reactive oxygen species that may cause liver injury by membrane peroxidation; alcohol in the gastrointestinal tract also induces release of endotoxin from gut flora with subsequent inflammatory cytokine production.

  Adverse alcohol effects are due to:

- *Acute alcohol injury* including hepatic steatosis (fatty change), gastritis and ulceration, and the depression of CNS activity.

- *Chronic alcoholism* affecting virtually all organs, with substantial morbidity and mortality:

Liver: The liver is the main site of injury; besides fatty change, *alcoholic hepatitis* and *cirrhosis* can result (Chapter 18). Cirrhosis is associated with portal hypertension and increased risk of hepatocellular carcinoma.

Gastrointestinal tract: Massive bleeding may result from acute gastritis and ulceration or as a consequence of esophageal varices due to portal hypertension.

Nervous system: Thiamine deficiency (due to poor nutrition) is common in chronic alcoholics; it causes peripheral neuropathies and the *Wernicke-Korsakoff syndrome* (Chapter 28), as well as cerebral atrophy, cerebellar degeneration, and optic neuropathy.

Cardiovascular system: Chronic alcoholism can cause a dilated cardiomyopathy and is associated with an increased incidence of hypertension. Liver injury due to alcohol excess reduces HDL production and increase cardiovascular risk.

Pancreas: Alcohol use increases the risk of acute and chronic pancreatitis (Chapter 19).

Fetal alcohol syndrome: This is characterized by growth and developmental defects, including microcephaly, facial dysmorphology, and malformations of the brain, cardiovascular system, and genitourinary system. Consumption during the first trimester is most harmful, although the minimal amount that causes fetal alcohol syndrome is difficult to establish; frequent or binge drinking occurs in 6% of pregnant women, and fetal alcohol syndrome affects 0.1% to 0.5% of children born in the United States.

Ethanol and cancer: Alcohol use is associated with increased cancer rates in the oral cavity, pharynx, esophagus, liver, and possibly breast. The acetaldehyde metabolite may act as a tumor promoter.

Potential beneficial effects of alcohol:

Cardiovascular system: In moderation, alcohol can reduce cardiovascular disease risk by increasing HDL and reducing platelet aggregation. Red wine contains the polyphenolic compound *resveratrol* that at high doses far in excess of what is ingested with moderate wine consumption increases life span in a variety of animal models (by activating histone deacetylases of the *sirtuin* family) and protects mice against diet-induced obesity and insulin resistance.

Injury by Therapeutic Drugs and Drugs of Abuse (p. 414)

Injury by Therapeutic Drugs (Adverse Drug Reactions) (p. 414)

Adverse reactions refer to untoward effects of drugs given in conventional therapeutic settings (Table 9-2). Adverse drug reactions are common, affecting an estimated 10% of hospitalized patients, with fatal outcomes in 10% of that group. The following therapies are highlighted because they are commonly administered.

Hormonal Replacement Therapy (p. 414)

Although hormonal replacement therapy (HRT) alleviates menopausal symptoms (e.g., hot flashes) and reduces the incidence of fractures (presumably by reducing osteoporosis), prolonged therapy increases the risk of breast cancer and thromboembolism.

TABLE 9-2 Some Common Adverse Drug Reactions and Their Agents

Reaction	Major Offenders
Bone Marrow and Blood Cells*	
Granulocytopenia, aplastic anemia, pancytopenia	Antineoplastic agents, immunosuppressives, and chloramphenicol
Hemolytic anemia, thrombocytopenia	Penicillin, methyldopa, quinidine, heparin
Cutaneous	
Urticaria, macules, papules, vesicles, petechiae, exfoliative dermatitis, fixed drug eruptions, abnormal pigmentation	Antineoplastic agents, sulfonamides, hydantoins, some antibiotics, and many other agents
Cardiac	
Arrhythmias	Theophylline, hydantoins, digoxin
Cardiomyopathy	Doxorubicin, daunorubicin
Renal	
Glomerulonephritis	Penicillamine
Acute tubular necrosis	Aminoglycoside antibiotics, cyclosporin, amphotericin B
Tubulointerstitial disease with papillary necrosis	Phenacetin, salicylates
Pulmonary	
Asthma	Salicylates
Acute pneumonitis	Nitrofurantoin
Interstitial fibrosis	Busulfan, nitrofurantoin, bleomycin
Hepatic	
Fatty change	Tetracycline
Diffuse hepatocellular damage	Halothane, isoniazid, acetaminophen
Cholestasis	Chlorpromazine, estrogens, contraceptive agents
Systemic	
Anaphylaxis	Penicillin
Lupus erythematosus syndrome (drug-induced lupus)	Hydralazine, procainamide
Central Nervous System	
Tinnitus and dizziness	Salicylates
Acute dystonic reactions and parkinsonian syndrome	Phenothiazine antipsychotics
Respiratory depression	Sedatives

*Affected in almost half of all drug-related deaths.

In women younger than 60 years, HRT is protective against atherosclerosis and coronary disease (estrogen receptors regulate calcium homeostasis in vessels); in older women there is no cardiovascular risk benefit.

Oral Contraceptives (p. 415)

Oral contraceptives (OC) usually contain a synthetic estradiol and variable amounts of a progestin or can contain progestins alone; they work by preventing ovulation or implantation. Lower estrogen content is associated with fewer side effects, and current OC formulations reflect this understanding. Risks are therefore dependent on dosage and delivery modality:

- *Thromboembolism:* OC use results in a three-fold increased risk of venous thrombosis and pulmonary thromboembolism, likely due to increased hepatic synthesis of coagulation factors and decreased production of anti-coagulants (protein S and anti-thrombin III). Risk is further increased in carriers of mutations in factor V or prothrombin.
- *Cardiovascular disease:* OCs increase the risk of myocardial infarction in all smokers and in non-smoking women older than 35 years.
- *Cancer:* OCs increase the incidence of ovarian and endometrial cancers, but do not affect the lifetime risk of breast cancer.
- *Hepatic adenoma:* There is a well-defined association between OC and this benign tumor (Chapter 18).

Anabolic Steroids (p. 415)

Anabolic steroids are synthetic versions of testosterone; these are used at 10 to 100 times therapeutic doses to achieve enhanced athletic performance. In males, high doses feedback inhibit leutinizing hormone/follicle-stimulating hormone (FSH) production and lead to testicular atrophy; increased estrogens resulting from the catabolism of the anabolic steroids causes gynecomastia. In adolescents, use can lead to stunted growth; in women, use causes virilization and menstrual changes. Additional effects include psychiatric changes, premature myocardial infarctions, and hepatic cholestasis.

Acetaminophen (p. 416)

Acetaminophen is the most commonly used analgesic in the United States; it is also responsible for more than 50% of acute liver failure cases in the United States, with 30% mortality. At therapeutic doses, more than 95% is metabolized by phase II hepatic enzymes with urinary excretion as sulfate or glucuronate conjugates. The remainder is primarily metabolized by hepatic CYP2E to a highly reactive metabolite (*N*-acetyl-*p*-benzoquinoneimine; NAPQ1) that is conjugated by glutathione before it can cause any harm. In overdoses, glutathione stores are depleted, making the liver susceptible to reactive oxygen species–induced injury; moreover, excess NAPQ1 complexes with hepatocyte membrane proteins and mitochondria, causing their dysfunction or degradation. In overdoses, therapy is targeted to maintaining glutathione stores via the administration of *N*-acetylcysteine.

Aspirin (Acetylsalicylic Acid) (p. 417)

Initial consequences of an overdose are respiratory alkalosis, followed by metabolic acidosis that can prove fatal. *Chronic aspirin toxicity (salicylism)* can develop in persons taking 3 g or more daily; it is manifested by headache, dizziness, ringing in the ears (tinnitus), difficulty in hearing, mental confusion, drowsiness, nausea, vomiting, and diarrhea. Most common is acute erosive gastritis and ulcers; bleeding may be exacerbated by aspirin inhibition of platelet cyclooxygenase and the inability to make thromboxane A_2 to drive platelet aggregation. Long-term ingestion (years) of analgesic mixtures of aspirin and phenacetin is associated with renal papillary necrosis (*analgesic nephropathy;* Chapter 20).

Injury by Nontherapeutic Agents (Drug Abuse) (p. 417)

Common drugs of abuse and their molecular targets are listed in Table 9-3.

Cocaine (p. 417)

Cocaine is extracted from coca leaves and snorted or injected as the water-soluble cocaine hydrochloride; it is often diluted with powder look-alikes (e.g., talcum). Crack cocaine is the crystallized form of the pure alkaloid; its effects are the same, but its weight-for-weight potency is substantially greater. Cocaine induces euphoria and stimulation; there is no physical dependence, although psychologic withdrawal can be profound.

- *Cardiovascular effects* are due to excess dopaminergic and adrenergic stimulation (cocaine blocks neurotransmitter re-uptake and increases synaptic release of norepinephrine). The consequences are tachycardia, hypertension, and vascular spasm; in the coronary artery circulation, vasoconstriction can cause myocardial infarction. Cocaine causes arrhythmias through the enhanced sympathetic activity, as well as by disrupting normal myocardial K^+, Na^+, and Ca^{2+} channel transport.
- *CNS effects* include hyperpyrexia (due to disrupted dopaminergic signaling) and seizures.

TABLE 9-3 Common Drugs of Abuse

Class	Molecular Target	Example
Opioid narcotics	Mu opioid receptor (agonist)	Heroin, hydromorphone (Dilaudid) Oxycodone (Percodan, Percocet, Oxycontin) Methadone (Dolophine) Meperidine (Demerol)
Sedative-hypnotics	GABA$_A$ receptor (agonist)	Barbiturates Ethanol Methaqualone (Quaalude) Glutethimide (Doriden) Ethchlorvynol (Placidyl)
Psychomotor stimulants	Dopamine transporter (antagonist)	Cocaine
	Serotonin receptors (toxicity)	Amphetamines 3,4-methylenedioxymethamphetamine (MDMA, ecstasy)
Phencyclidine-like drugs	NMDA glutamate receptor channel (antagonist)	Phencyclidine (PCP, angel dust) Ketamine
Cannabinoids	CBI cannabinoid receptors (agonist)	Marijuana Hashish
Hallucinogens	Serotonin 5-HT$_2$ receptors (agonist)	Lysergic acid diethylamide (LSD) Mescaline Psilocybin

5-HT$_2$, 5-hydroxytryptamine; *GABA,* γ-aminobutyric acid; *NMDA, N*-methyl D-aspartate.
Data from Hyman SE: A 28-year-old man addicted to cocaine, *JAMA* 286:2586, 2001.

- In *pregnancy*, cocaine may reduce placental blood flow, leading to fetal hypoxia and neurologic deficits or spontaneous abortions.
- *Other effects* of chronic use include dilated cardiomyopathy and nasal septum perforation.

Heroin (p. 418)

Heroin is an alkaloid of the poppy plant, injected subcutaneously or intravenously along with any adulterants. It induces euphoria, hallucinations, somnolence, and sedation and is physically addictive. Adverse effects include:

- *Sudden death*, most commonly due to overdose leading to respiratory depression, pulmonary edema, and/or arrhythmia.
- *Pulmonary injury* with moderate to severe edema; foreign body granulomas to particulate matter are common.
- *Infection* due to contaminated needles or dirty skin at sites of injection. Tricuspid valve endocarditis is a frequent sequela, most often caused by normal skin flora. Sharing of needles is also a route for viral hepatitis and HIV transmission.
- *Skin pathology*, such as cellulitis, abscesses, and ulcerations, as well as thrombosed vessels.
- *Renal pathology*, such as amyloidosis (secondary to chronic skin infections) and focal segmental glomerulosclerosis; both result in proteinuria and nephrotic syndrome.

Amphetamines (p. 419)

Methamphetamine (also known as *speed*) is an addictive drug that induces CNS dopamine release and thereby slows glutamate release; administration induces euphoria. Long-term use can lead to violent behavior, confusion, paranoia, and hallucinations.

MDMA (3,4 methylenedioxymethamphetamine, also known as *ecstasy*) induces euphoria and hallucinogen-like feelings via enhanced CNS serotonin release.

Marijuana (p. 419)

Marijuana is isolated from the hemp plant *Cannabis sativa*; the major psychoactive substance is Δ^9-tetrahydrocannibinol (THC). THC binds to endogenous cannabinoid receptors (the normal ligands are *endocannabinoids*) that modulate the hypothalamic-pituitary-adrenal axis and regulate appetite, food intake, energy balance, fertility, and sexual behavior. Acute THC use distorts sensory perception and impairs motor coordination; it can also increase heart rate and blood pressure. Smoking marijuana is associated with the characteristic effects of inhaling gases from burning plant fibers (e.g., bronchitis, pharyngitis, and chronic obstructive pulmonary disease). Notably, the typical behaviors associated with marijuana smoking (deeper inhalation and breath holding) also lead to a three-fold increased deposition of tars and particulates compared to standard cigarette smoking. THC has therapeutic benefit in treating chemotherapy-induced nausea and chronic pain syndromes.

Injury by Physical Agents (p. 420)

Mechanical Trauma (p. 420)

Mechanical forces can injure soft tissues, bones, or head; outcomes depend on the shape of the colliding object, the force imparted, and the tissues that bear the brunt of impact:

- *Abrasion:* A superficial wound produced by rubbing or scraping; skin abrasions may only remove the epidermis.

- *Contusion:* A blunt force trauma that injures small blood vessels and causes interstitial bleeding, usually without disruption of the continuity of the tissue (bruise).
- *Incision:* Inflicted by a sharp instrument that cuts vessels and leaves relatively smooth edges.
- *Laceration:* A tear or disruptive stretching caused by blunt trauma; as opposed to an incision, lacerations typically have intact bridging blood vessels and jagged irregular edges.
- *Puncture:* Trauma caused by a long, narrow instrument or gunshot; it is *penetrating* when tissue is only pierced and *perforating* when the tissue is traverses to also create an exit wound.

Deep tissues and organs can sustain trauma from an external blow even without apparent superficial injury.

Thermal Injury (p. 421)

Thermal Burns (p. 421)

Burn injury and smoke inhalation cause roughly 4000 deaths annually in the United States; shock, sepsis, and respiratory insufficiency are the greatest threats to life. The clinical significance of burns depends on:

- Depth of the burn

  Superficial (confined to epidermis; formerly first-degree)
  Partial thickness (involving the dermis; formerly second-degree)
  Full-thickness (extending to subcutaneous tissue; formerly third- or fourth-degree)

- Percentage of body surface involved

  Burns involving more than 20% of surface area lead to rapid fluid mobilizations and potentially hypovolemic shock.
  Burns induce a hypermetabolic state; thus, injury involving 40% of surface area causes a doubling of metabolic demand.
  The greater the surface area involved, the greater the risk of infection; besides loss of barrier function and vast swaths of necrotic debris, burn injury causes depressed systemic innate and adaptive immune responses and compromises local blood flow that reduces local inflammatory cell recruitment. Opportunistic organisms such as *Pseudomonas* and antibiotic-resistant strains of hospital-acquired microbes such as *S. aureus* and *Candida* are common.

- Internal injuries from inhalation of hot and toxic fumes

  Airway and lung parenchymal injury typically develops within 1 to 2 days of exposure and can involve direct thermal injury or chemical toxicity
  Water-soluble gases (chlorine, sulfur oxides, and ammonia) react with water to form acids and alkalis that cause substantial upper airway edema and inflammation
  Lipid-soluble gases (nitrous oxide, burning plastic) reach deeper airways and cause pneumonitis

- Promptness and efficacy of postburn therapy

  Fluid and electrolyte management
  Prevention or control of wound infection

Hyperthermia (p. 422)

Prolonged exposure to elevated ambient temperatures can result in the following:

- *Heat cramps* (cramping of voluntary muscles) occur from loss of electrolytes through sweating; core body temperature is maintained.
- *Heat exhaustion* is the most common heat syndrome. It results from a failure of the cardiovascular system to compensate for

hypovolemia, secondary to water depletion. Its onset is sudden with prostration and collapse.
- *Heat stroke* is associated with high ambient temperatures, high humidity, and exertion. Thermoregulatory mechanisms fail, sweating ceases, and core body temperature markedly elevates (e.g., to 40° C). The body responds with generalized peripheral vasodilation with peripheral pooling of blood and a decreased effective circulating blood volume. Necrosis of muscles and myocardium can occur, associated with arrhythmias and disseminated intravascular coagulation.

Mutations in the ryanodine receptor type I—responsible for regulating skeletal muscle sarcoplasmic reticulum calcium release—can cause *malignant hyperthermia*, a rare situation where common anesthetics cause profound muscle contraction and elevated core body temperature.

Hypothermia *(p. 422)*

Hypothermia occurs with prolonged exposure to low ambient temperature. At a core temperature of 90° F, individuals lose consciousness; with further cooling, bradycardia and atrial fibrillation occur.

- Freezing of cells and tissues causes direct injury through the crystallization of intracellular and extracellular water.
- Indirect injury occurs due to circulatory changes. Slowly falling temperatures may induce vasoconstriction and increased vascular permeability, leading to edematous changes (e.g., *trench foot*). Persistent low temperatures may cause ischemic injury.

Electrical Injury *(p. 422)*

The passage of an electric current through the body may be without effect, may cause sudden death by disruption of neural regulatory impulses or cardiac conduction pathways, or may cause thermal injury. Variables include:

- Current strength, duration, and path; alternating current induces tetanic muscle spasm and prolongs the duration of exposure by causing involuntary clutching.
- Tissue resistance, which varies inversely with water content; dry skin is resistant, but wet skin has greatly decreased resistance. The greater the tissue resistance, the greater the heat generated.

Injury Produced by Ionizing Radiation *(p. 423)*

Radiation is energy traveling in the form of waves or high-speed particles; it has a wide range of energies spanning the electromagnetic spectrum:

- *Non-ionizing radiation* includes UV and infrared light, radiowaves, microwaves, and soundwaves; these sources are characterized by relatively longer wavelengths and lower frequencies and can produces vibration and rotation of atoms but have insufficient energy to displace bound electrons.
- *Ionizing radiation* includes x-rays and gamma rays, high-energy neutrons, alpha particles (composed of two neutrons and two protons), and beta particles (essentially electrons); these are typically of short wavelengths and high frequency and have sufficient energy to remove electrons from biologic molecules.

Radiation Units *(p. 423)*

Radiation doses are measured in three different ways—the amount of radiation emitted by a source, the radiation dose absorbed by a tissue, and the biologic effect of radiation:

- *Curie (Ci)* reflects the amount of radiation emitted from a source; it represents the disintegrations per second of a radioisotope such that 1 Ci $= 3.7 \times 10^{10}$ disintegrations per second.
- *Gray (Gy)* reflects the energy absorbed by a target tissue per unit mass; 1 Gy corresponds to 10^4 ergs/gm of tissue. This was previously expressed as "radiation absorbed dose" or "Rad" where 1 Rad $= 10^{-4}$ Gy.
- *Sievert (Sv)* reflects the biologic effect of a particular radiation dose (this was previously expressed by the term "rem"); some forms of radiation cause more injury than others, and some tissues are more susceptible. The *equivalent* dose—expressed in Sv—is the absorbed dose (expressed in Gy) multiplied by the relative biologic effectiveness of the type of radiation. For x-rays, 1 mSv = 1 mGy.

Main Determinants of the Biologic Effects of Ionizing Radiation (p. 423)

- *Rate of delivery:* A single dose can cause greater injury than divided or fractionated doses of the same cumulative amount. This is exploited in tumor therapy; normal tissues have intact repair pathways and divided doses allow time for cellular repair, whereas tumor cells putatively have poorer repair mechanisms and will not recover between doses.
- *Field size:* A single low dose of external radiation administered to the whole body is potentially more lethal than higher doses administered regionally with shielding.
- *Cell proliferation:* Since DNA is the main target of radiation injury, rapidly dividing cells are more susceptible than quiescent cells. Except at very high doses that impair DNA transcription, DNA damage is compatible with survival in non-dividing cells. Rapidly dividing normal cells (e.g., bone marrow, gonads, gastrointestinal epithelium) may be exquisitely sensitive to radiation injury because DNA damage can induce growth arrest and apoptosis.
- *Oxygen effects and hypoxia:* The generation of reactive oxygen species from water ionization is the major pathway by which DNA damage is initiated by radiation. Poorly vascularized tissues with relative hypoxia will therefore be less sensitive to radiation injury.
- *Vascular damage:* Endothelial cells are moderately sensitive to radiation injury; their damage leads to the production of pro-inflammatory cytokines and vascular wall healing with lumenal narrowing that will cause progressive tissue ischemia.

The acute effects of ionizing radiation range from overt necrosis at high doses (more than 10 Gy), killing of proliferating cells at intermediate doses (1 to 2 Gy), and no histopathologic effect at 0.5 Gy or less. If cells undergo extensive DNA damage or if they are unable to repair this damage, they may undergo apoptosis. Surviving cells may show delayed effects of radiation injury: mutations, chromosomal aberrations, and genetic instability. These genetically damaged cells may become malignant and cause cancers.

Total-Body Irradiation (p. 425)

Whole-body exposures of more than 1 Sv produce little or no effect. However, greater exposures cause *acute radiation syndromes*, which at progressively higher doses involve the hematopoietic, gastrointestinal, and central nervous system (Table 9-4).

Acute Effects on Hematopoietic and Lymphoid Systems (p. 425)

With high doses and large fields, peripheral lymphopenia with spleen and lymph node atrophy can develop within hours; at sub-lethal doses, repopulation occurs over weeks or months.

TABLE 9-4 Effects of Total-Body Ionizing Radiation				
	0-1 Sv	1-2 Sv	2-10 Sv	10-20 Sv	>50 Sv
Main site of injury	None	Lymphocytes	Bone marrow	Small bowel	Brain
Main signs and symptoms	None	Moderate granulocytopenia Lymphopenia	Leukopenia, hemorrhage, hair loss, vomiting	Diarrhea, fever, electrolyte imbalance, vomiting	Ataxia, coma, convulsions, vomiting
Time of development	—	1 day to 1 week	2-6 weeks	5-14 days	1-4 hours
Lethality	None	None	Variable (0% to 80%)	100%	100%

Hematopoietic precursors are similarly sensitive, resulting in a marrow aplasia; very high doses kill stem cells and will cause a permanent aplastic anemia. Reflecting their relative peripheral longevity, granulocyte numbers are first affected (roughly 12- to 24-hour lifespan), followed by platelets (10-day lifespan), and finally erythrocytes (120-day lifespan); full recovery may require months.

Fibrosis (p. 425)

Fibrosis can occur in the radiation field weeks to months after exposure. This occurs primarily as a consequence of replacing dead tissue with scar, but is also due to vascular injury (described previously), destruction of tissue stem cells, and the release of inflammatory cytokines that promote fiobroblast activation and matrix synthesis.

DNA Damage and Carcinogenesis (p. 425)

DNA damage from radiation includes single base damage, single- and double-strand breaks (DSB), and DNA-protein cross-links. In surviving cells, damage is repaired by a variety of mechanisms; DSB are most serious and repair requires either homologous recombination or non-homologous end-joining (Chapter 7). The latter is more common and also leads to mutations including deletions, duplications, inversions, or translocations. In the absence of cell cycle check-point controls, such mutations may initiate carcinogenesis.

Cancer Risks from Exposures to Low-Level Radiation (p. 426)

Although the level of radiation that increases cancer risk is difficult to unambiguously identify, any mutation has the potential to drive carcinogenesis. Doses more than 100 mSv clearly increase risk, but risk for doses in the range of 5 to 100 mSv is more difficult to quantify. To put this in context, a single chest x-ray delivers 0.01 mSv and chest computed tomography delivers 10 mSv.

Nutritional Diseases (p. 427)

Dietary Insufficiency (p. 427)

An appropriate diet provides adequate caloric intake to satisfy energy needs, amino acids and fats for protein and lipid synthesis, and necessary vitamins and minerals. In primary malnutrition, one or more components are missing; in secondary malnutrition, the nutrient supply is sufficient, but inadequate intake (e.g., due to anorexia), malabsorption, impaired utilization or storage, excess loss, or increased demand supervene. Poverty is a major determinant for primary malnutrition, although ignorance or failure of dietary supplement can contribute (e.g., iron-deficiency in infants exclusively receiving formula diets). Illness (e.g., cancers and infection) can dramatically increase metabolic demand, and alcoholism often leads to vitamin deficiencies due to diminished intake, abnormal utilization, or increased loss.

Protein-Energy Malnutrition (p. 428)

Protein-energy malnutrition (PEM) is characterized by inadequate dietary intake of protein and calories (or malabsorption) with resultant muscle, fat, and weight loss, lethargy, and generalized weakness. A body-mass index less than 16 kg/m^2 constitutes malnutrition; *body mass index (BMI)* is defined as weight (kg)/height^2 (m^2), where nl = 18.5-25 kg/m^2. More practically, a child whose weight falls to less than 80% of normal is considered to be malnourished. Other helpful measures are fat stores, muscle mass, and circulating levels of serum proteins (e.g., albumin and transferrin). In elderly nursing home patients, more than 5% weight loss associated with PEM increases mortality risk 5-fold.

Marasmus and Kwashiorkor (p. 428)

Marasmus and kwashiorkor are two ends of the PEM spectrum but also have substantial overlap:

- Marasmus:

  Weight loss of 60% or more compared to normal for sex and age
  Growth retardation and loss of muscle mass
  Protein and fat are mobilized from the *somatic compartment* of the body (largely skeletal muscle and subcutaneous fat); this provides energy from amino acids and triglycerides
  Serum protein levels are largely maintained
  Diminished leptin synthesis may drive increased pituitary-adrenal axis production of glucocorticoids that induce lipolysis
  Anemia and immune deficiency are common, with recurrent infections

- Kwashiokor:

  Occurs when protein deprivation is relatively greater than overall calorie reduction
  Associated with protein loss from the *visceral compartment* of the body (largely liver); there is relative sparing of muscle and adipose tissue
  Resulting hypoalbuminemia causes generalized edema that may mask weight loss
  An enlarged fatty liver is due to inadequate lipoprotein synthesis and thus hepatic accumulation of peripherally mobilized triglycerides
  Apathy, listlessness, and anorexia occur
  Small bowel mucosal atrophy (reversible) can lead to malabosrption
  Immune deficiency is common, with secondary infections

Cachexia (p. 429)

Cachexia is a term used to describe PEM that occurs in chronically ill patients (e.g., with cancer or AIDS). Cachexia occurs in roughly 50% of cancer patients and is the cause of death in a third (often due to atrophy of muscles of respiration). Tumors cause cachexia via proteolysis-inducing factor (PIF) and lipid-mobilizing factor, the latter likely by driving the production of pro-inflammatory cytokines such as tumor necrosis factor and interleukin-6. PIF and the inflammatory cytokines cause skeletal muscle catabolism through NF-κB–induced activation of ubiquitin-proteasome pathways.

Anorexia Nervosa and Bulimia (p. 430)

These disorders occur as a result of obsession with body image; altered serotonin metabolism is implicated.

- Anorexia nervosa is self-induced starvation

  Highest death rate of any psychiatric disorder
  Clinical findings are similar to those in severe PEM
  Amenorrhea is common due to suppression of the hypothalamus-pituitary axis
  Decreased thyroid hormone production causes cold intolerance, bradycardia, constipation, dry scaly skin, and hair thinning
  Decreased bone density is associated with low estrogen levels
  Sudden death due to arrhythmias in the setting of hypokalemia

- Bulimia is characterized by food binging followed by self-induced vomiting; diuretic or laxative abuse may also occur

  More common than anorexia, afflicting 1% to 2% of women and 0.1% of men

  Better overall prognosis

  Amenorrhea is less common due to relatively normal weights and hormonal levels

  Medical complications are related to persistent vomiting and include electrolyte abnormalities (hypokalemia) that can cause arrhythmias, aspiration of gastric contents, and esophageal or gastric laceration

Vitamin Deficiencies (p. 430)

Thirteen vitamins are necessary for health. Nine are water-soluble and are primarily renally excreted. Four—vitamins A, D, E, and K—are fat soluble, and thus readily stored but also may be poorly taken up in malabsorption syndromes. Vitamins D and K, biotin, and niacin can be synthesized endogenously, but dietary intake is also generally necessary. Table 9-5 is a summary of the essential vitamins and their deficiency syndromes. Table 9-6 is the equivalent table for selected trace elements.

Vitamin deficiency may be primary (dietary in origin) or secondary to abnormalities of absorption, transport, storage, loss, or metabolic conversion. Isolated single-vitamin deficiencies are relatively uncommon.

Vitamin A (p. 430)

Vitamin A is a group of related compounds with similar activities. *Retinol* is the transport and storage form of vitamin A, *retinal* is the aldehyde, and *retinoic acid* is the acid form. Dietary intake includes pre-formed vitamin A (found in meat, eggs, milk) and carotenoids (primarily β-carotene, found in yellow and leafy green vegetables); carotenoids are efficiently metabolized to active vitamin A and constitute roughly a third of dietary intake. Ninety percent of vitamin A is stored in the perisinusoidal stellate (Ito) cells in the liver and in healthy adults constitutes a 6-month reserve. Retinol is transported bound to retinol-binding protein, synthesized in the liver.

Function (p. 431)

- Vision: Rhodopsin (rods) and iodopsins (cones) are synthesized from retinal and membrane protein opsins. Photons convert bound 11-*cis* retinal to all-*trans*-retinal, triggering opsin conformational changes that are ultimately converted into nerve impulses that enable vision. Most all-*trans*-retinal is reduced to retinol and is lost to the retina, thus requiring constant replenishing.
- Differentiation of mucus-secreting epithelial cells: Interaction of retinoic acid with intracellular receptors (RARs) releases repressor molecules and permits heterodimer formation with retinoic X receptors (RXR); these then activate a variety of genes by binding to specific promoter elements. Vitamin A deficiency leads to squamous metaplasia of epithelium.
- Metabolic effects: Interaction of retinoic acid with RXR leads to heterodimer formation with other nuclear receptors involved in regulating metabolism and vitamin D activity. Peroxisome proliferators–activated receptors (PPARs) interact with RXR and are key regulators of lipid metabolism and adipogenesis.
- Enhancing immunity to infections, in part by maintaining epithelial integrity.

TABLE 9-5   Vitamins: Major Functions and Deficiency Syndromes

Vitamin	Functions	Deficiency Syndrome
Fat-Soluble		
Vitamin A	A component of visual pigment Maintenance of specialized epithelia Maintenance of resistance to infection	Night blindness, xerophthalmia, blindness Squamous metaplasia Vulnerability to infection, particularly measles
Vitamin D	Facilitates intestinal absorption of calcium and phosphorus and mineralization of bone	Rickets in children Osteomalacia in adults
Vitamin E	Major antioxidant; scavenges free radicals	Spinocerebellar degeneration
Vitamin K	Cofactor in hepatic carboxylation of procoagulants—factors II (prothrombin), VII, IX, and X; and protein C and protein S	Bleeding d'athesis
Water-Soluble		
Vitamin B1 (thiamine)	As pyrophosphate, is coenzyme in decarboxylation reactions	Dry and wet beriberi, Wernicke syndrome, Korsakoff syndrome
Vitamin B2 (riboflavin)	Converted to coenzymes flavin mononucleotide and flavin adenine dinucleotide, cofactors for many enzymes in intermediary metabolism	Ariboflavincsis, cheilosis, stomatitis, glossitis, dermatitis, corneal vascularization
Niacin	Incorporated into nicotinamide adenine dinucleotide (NAD) and NAD phosphate, involved in a variety of redox reactions	Pellagra—three "Ds": dementia, dermatitis, diarrhea

Continued

TABLE 9-5   Vitamins: Major Functions and Deficiency Syndromes—cont'd

Vitamin	Functions	Deficiency Syndrome
Vitamin B6 (pyridoxine)	Derivatives serve as coenzymes in many intermediary reactions	Cheilosis, glossitis, dermatitis, peripheral neuropathy
Vitamin B12	Required for normal folate metabolism and DNA synthesis Maintenance of myelinization of spinal cord tracts	Combined system disease (megaloblastic pernicious anemia and degeneration of posterolateral spinal cord tracts)
Vitamin C	Serves in many oxidation-reduction (redox) reactions and hydroxylation of collagen	Scurvy
Folate	Essential for transfer and use of 1-carbon units in DNA synthesis	Megaloblastic anemia, neural tube defects
Pantothenic acid	Incorporated in coenzyme A	No nonexperimental syndrome recognized
Biotin	Cofactor in carboxylation reactions	No clearly defined clinical syndrome

TABLE 9-6 Functions of Trace Metals and Deficiency Syndromes

Nutrient	Functions	Deficiency Syndromes
Iron	Essential component of hemoglobin as well as a number of iron-containing metalloenzymes	Hypochromic microcytic anemia
Zinc	Component of enzymes, principally oxidases	Acrodermatitis enteropathica, growth retardation, infertility
Iodine	Component of thyroid hormone	Goiter and hypothyroidism
Selenium	Component of glutathione peroxidase	Myopathy, rarely cardiomyopathy
Copper	Component of cytochrome *c* oxidase, dopamine β-hydroxylase, tyrosinase, lysyl oxidase, and unknown enzymes involved in cross-linking keratin	Muscle weakness, neurologic defects, hypopigmentation, abnormal collagen cross-linking
Manganese	Component of metalloenzymes, including oxidoreductases, hydrolases, and lipases	No well-defined deficiency syndrome
Fluoride	Mechanism unknown	Dental caries

Vitamin A Deficiency (p. 432)

Vitamin A deficiency affects vision (especially in reduced light [night blindness]), immunity, and the normal differentiation of various epithelia.

- *Xerophthalmia* (dry eye) occurs when conjunctival and lacrimal epithelium become keratinized; this causes conjunctival dryness (xerosis), formation of small opaque spots on the cornea due to keratin debris (Bitot spots), and eventual destruction of the cornea (keratomalacia) with blindness.
- Keratinizing metaplasia of epithelial surfaces results in respiratory tract infections due to airway squamous metaplasia, and causes renal and urinary bladder calculi due to desquamation of keratinized epithelium.

Vitamin A Toxicity (p. 433)

- Acute manifestations include headache, vomiting, stupor, and papilledema.
- Chronic toxicity is associated with weight loss, nausea and vomiting, lip dryness, and bone and joint pain. Retinoic acid activates osteoclasts, leading to increased bone resorption and risk of fracture.
- Synthetic retinoids can be teratogenic and should be avoided in pregnancy.

Vitamin D (p. 433)

Vitamin D is critical for maintenance of normal plasma levels of calcium and phosphorus and is therefore involved in maintaining normal bone mineralization and neuromuscular transmission.

Metabolism of Vitamin D (p. 433)

Metabolism of vitamin D is outlined in Figure 9-1, *A:*

- Vitamin D_3 (cholecalciferol, hereinafter vitamin D) is absorbed in the gut (10% of requirement) or synthesized by UV-induced conversion from a 7-dehydrocholesterol precursor in the skin; limited sun exposure or melanin in dark skin may result in less conversion.
- Vitamin D is transported to liver bound to a plasma α_1-globulin (D-binding protein), where it is converted to 25-hydroxyvitamin D (25[OH]D) by a 25-hydroxylase CYP.
- In the kidney, α_1-hydroxylase converts 25(OH)D to 1,25(OH)$_2$D, the most biologically-active form; the enzyme activity is regulated in the following way:

  1,25(OH)$_2$D feed-back inhibits α_1-hydroxylase activity
  Parathyroid hormone (induced by low calcium) activates α_1-hydroxylase
  Hypophosphatemia activates $\alpha_1$hydroxylase

Mechanisms of Action (p. 433)

Vitamin D is essentially a steroid hormone that binds to high-affinity intracellular receptors and induces their association with RXR. The heterodimer binds to promoters of vitamin D target genes in small bowel, bone, and kidney to regulate plasma calcium and phosphorous (see later); it also has immunomodulatory and anti-proliferative effects. Vitamin D can also bind to membrane receptors that directly activate protein kinase C and open calcium channels.

Effects of Vitamin D on Calcium and Phosphorous Homeostasis (p. 433)

- *Intestinal calcium absorption* is augmented by vitamin D–induced increases in TRPV6, a calcium transport channel.
- *Renal tubular epithelial resorption of calcium* is augmented by vitamin D–induced increases of TRPV5, another calcium transport channel.
- *Osteoclast maturation and activity* is induced by vitamin D–driven increases of RANKL expression on osteoblasts (Chapter 26).
- *Bone mineralization* is increased by vitamin D–induced stimulation of osteoblasts to synthesize osteocalcin, a protein involved in calcium deposition

Deficiency States (p. 435)

Deficiency states are schematized in Figure 9-1, *B:*

- Vitamin D deficiency primarily results from inadequate intake, inadequate sun exposure, or altered vitamin D absorption or metabolism (e.g., renal disease).
- Deficiency causes deficient absorption of calcium and phosphorus from the gut with consequent depressed serum levels of both.
- Hypocalcemia activates the parathyroid glands, causing PTH-induced mobilization of calcium and phosphorus from bone; PTH also induces calcium retention in the urine with phosphate wasting. Although serum levels of calcium may thereby be maintained, phosphate level is low, impairing bone mineralization.
- Vitamin D deficiency causes *rickets* in growing children and *osteomalacia* in adults; both forms of skeletal disease arise from an excess of unmineralized matrix.
- In *rickets,* inadequate provisional calcification of epiphyseal cartilage deranges endochondral bone growth, resulting in skeletal deformation, including frontal bossing, deformation of the chest plate, lumbar lordosis, and bowing legs.
- In osteomalacia, weakening of the bone increases fracture susceptibility.

NORMAL VITAMIN D METABOLISM

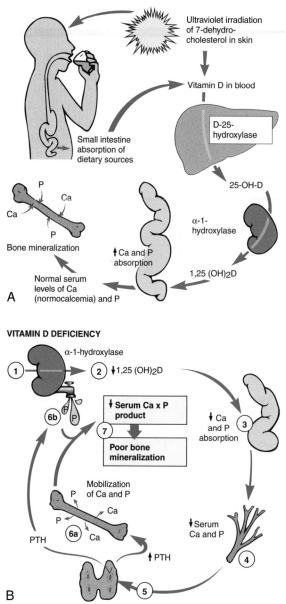

FIGURE 9-1 A, Vitamin D metabolism. **B,** Vitamin D deficiency. Inadequate substrate for the renal hydroxylase *(1)* results in 1,25(OH)$_2$D deficiency *(2)* and insufficient GI calcium and phosphorus absorption *(3),* with consequent depressed serum levels of both *(4).* Hypocalcemia activates the parathyroid glands *(5),* with parathyroid hormone *(PTH)* release causing mobilization of calcium and phosphorus from bone *(6a).* PTH also induces renal calcium retention and phosphate wasting; this maintains serum calcium near normal levels, but with low serum phosphate, mineralization is impaired *(7).*

Non-Skeletal Effects of Vitamin D (p. 436)

1,25$(OH)_2$D can be synthesized by macrophages and a variety of epithelia; vitamin D receptors are also present in numerous tissues that do not regulate calcium and phosphorus homeostasis. Vitamin D activity in these cells may be related to innate immunity; moreover, of the more than 200 genes whose expression is regulated by vitamin D, several influence cell proliferation, differentiation, apoptosis, and angiogenesis. Chronic vitamin D insufficiency is associated with 30% to 50% increased incidence of colon, prostate, and breast cancers.

Vitamin D Toxicity (p. 436)

Vitamin D toxicity due to over-ingestion can cause hypercalcemia, and can cause metastatic calcification in soft tissues.

Vitamin C (Ascorbic Acid) (p. 437)

Vitamin C (ascorbic acid) is present in many foods and is abundant in fruits and vegetables, so that all but the most restricted diets provide adequate amounts.

Function (p. 437)

- Activating prolyl and lysyl hydroxylases, providing for hydroxylation of procollagen and thereby facilitating collagen cross-linking.
- Scavenging free radicals and regenerating the antioxidant form of vitamin E.

Deficiency States (p. 437)

Insufficient vitamin C leads to *scurvy,* characterized in children by inadequate osteoid (and therefore inadequate bone formation), and by hemorrhage and poor healing in all ages.

Obesity (p. 438)

Obesity is a massive problem (pun not intended). Individuals with a BMI of 30 kg/m^2 or more are considered obese; those with BMI between 25 and 30 kg/m^2 are overweight. By these standards, 66% of adults in the United States are overweight or obese, and 16% of children are overweight. Excess adiposity is associated with increased incidence of type 2 diabetes, dyslipidemias, cardiovascular disease, hypertension, and cancer.

Obesity is a simple consequence of caloric imbalance with intake greater than expenditure; however, the regulation of the neural and humoral mechanisms controlling appetite, satiety, and energy balance is complex (Fig. 9-2):

- Peripheral sites generate signals to indicate adequacy of metabolites or stores; *leptin* and *adiponectin* in fat cells, *ghrelin* in the stomach, *peptide YY (PYY)* from ileum and colon, and *insulin* from the pancreas.
- The arcuate nucleus in the hypothalamus integrates the peripheral input and outputs efferent signals through pro-opiomelanocortin (POMC) and cocaine- and amphetamine-regulated transcript (CART) neurons, as well as neurons containing neuropeptide Y (NPY) and agouti-related peptide (agRP).
- The efferent output to second-order hypothalamic neurons controls food intake and energy expenditure.

  POMC/CART neurons enhance energy expenditure and weight loss by production of anorexigenic α-melanocyte stimulating hormone that binds to melanocortin receptors

  NPY/AgRP neurons promote food intake and weight gain

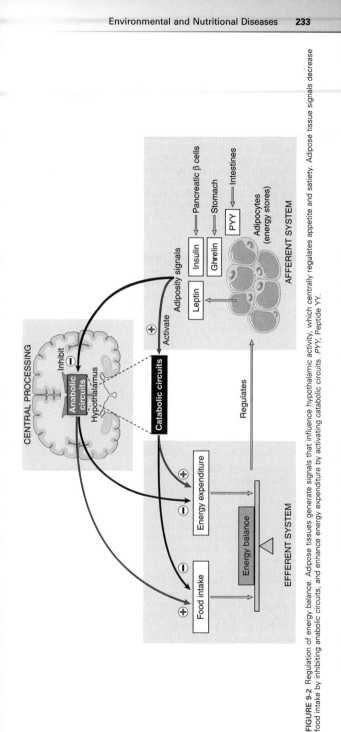

FIGURE 9-2 Regulation of energy balance. Adipose tissues generate signals that influence hypothalamic activity, which centrally regulates appetite and satiety. Adipose tissue signals decrease food intake by inhibiting anabolic circuits, and enhance energy expenditure by activating catabolic circuits. *PYY,* Peptide YY.

Leptin (p. 439)

Leptin is a peptide hormone secreted by adipose tissue when fat stores are abundant. Leptin stimulates hypothalamic POMC/CART neurons and inhibits NPY/AgRP neurons; food intake is accordingly diminished. If adipose stores are low, leptin secretion is diminished and food intake is increased. Through other circuits, an abundance of leptin also stimulates physical activity, heat production, and energy expenditure. Loss of function in the leptin signaling pathway is a rare cause of massive obesity; melanocortin receptor mutations account for perhaps 5% of severe obesity.

Adiponectin (p. 441) is a polypeptide hormone produced by adipocytes; it diminishes liver influx of triglycerides and stimulates skeletal muscle fatty oxidation. It also decreases hepatic gluconeogenesis and increases insulin sensitivity.

Adipose tissue (p. 441) is also a source of pro-inflammatory cytokines such as TNF, IL-6, and Il-1. These lead to chronic subclinical inflammatory states that influence hepatic acute phase reactant levels.

Absolute adipocyte number is established during childhood and adolescence and does not significantly vary after that time. Thus, weight loss is due to reduced volume of adipocytes but not change in their quantity.

Gut Hormones (p. 441)

Gut hormones include ghrelin, PYY, and insulin; these act as short-term meal initiators and terminators. Ghrelin is the only known gut hormone that increases food intake, likely acting through NPT/AgRP neurons; in obese individuals post-prandial ghrelin suppression is attenuated. PYY administration reduces food intake; PYY levels are low during fasting and increase after meals, and PYY levels are increased after gastric bypass surgery. PYY levels are generally low in patients with Prader-Willi syndrome and may contribute to their obesity.

General Consequences of Obesity (p. 442)

Obesity increases the risk for a number of conditions, including:

- *Metabolic syndrome*, characterized by visceral adiposity, insulin resistance, hypertension, and dyslipidemia.
- *Type 2 diabetes*, with insulin resistance and hyperinsulinemia (Chapter 24).
- Hypertension, hypertriglyceridemia, and low HDL cholesterol, which all increase the risk of *coronary artery disease.*
- *Nonalcoholic steatohepatitis* is marked by fatty change with inflammation and focal liver cell injury, and can progress to cirrhosis (Chapter 18).
- *Cholelithiasis* (gallstones), which is six times more common in obese than in lean individuals.
- *Hypoventilation syndrome,* a group of respiratory abnormalities in obese individuals associated with hypersomnolence, polycythemia, and right-sided heart failure.
- *Osteoarthritis*, which is attributable to the cumulative effects of added wear and tear on the joints.

Obesity and Cancer (p. 443)

Approximately 5% of cancers are associated with obesity. In men, a BMI more than 25 kg/m^2 strongly correlates with esophageal adenocarcinoma, and cancers of thyroid, colon, and kidney; in women with BMI more than 25 kg/m^2, there is an increased incidence of esophageal adenocarcinoma, and cancers of endometrium, gallbladder, and kidney.

Increased risk is attributed to peripheral insulin resistance and the associated hyperinsulinemia. High insulin levels activate a variety of kinases (e.g., phosphatidylinositol-3-kinase and Ras) that influence proliferation; hyperinsulinemia also induces insulin-like growth factor-1 production, a peptide that is mitogenic and anti-apoptotic. Finally, obesity influences the production of steroid hormones that regulate growth and differentiation of breast, uterus, and other tissues; greater adiposity increases adrenal and ovarian synthesis of androgens, and fat cell aromatases increase estrogen production from androgen precursors.

Diets, Cancer, and Atherosclerosis (p. 443)

Diet and Cancer (p. 443)

Epidemiologic studies demonstrate impressive geographic and population variation in cancer incidence, some of which can be associated with diet. Issues include:

- *Exogenous carcinogens:* Examples include aflatoxin in the development of hepatocellular carcinoma and the possible carcinogenicity of selected food additives, artificial sweeteners, and pesticide contaminants.
- *Endogenous synthesis of carcinogens from dietary components:* Examples include nitrosamines and nitrosamides derived from amides in digested proteins, derived from nitrites in food preservatives, or produced by gut flora reduction of vegetable nitrates.

Increased fat intake also increases bile acid production that modifies gastrointestinal flora; subsequent bile acid catabolism produces carcinogenic metabolites. Conversely, increased dietary fiber can bind and remove potential carcinogens while also decreasing bowel transit time, thus effectively lessening mucosal exposure to noxious metabolites. Although these are attractive hypotheses, the data are conflicting.

- *Lack of protective factors:* Selenium, β-carotene, and vitamins C and E are presumed to be anti-carcinogenic by virtue of their antioxidant properties; the data again are incomplete.

Diet and Atherosclerosis (p. 444)

Reduced consumption of cholesterol and saturated animal fats and increased levels of unsaturated fatty acids can lower serum cholesterol levels and may lessen atherosclerotic complications. Consumption of omega-3 fatty acids (e.g., from fish) is also protective against cardiovascular complications—potentially attributable to the different spectrum of eicosanoids that these fats engender. Caloric restriction, related to effects on sirtuin activation and insulin lowering, lowers the risk of atherosclerosis and also extends life span.

10

Diseases of Infancy and Childhood

The major causes of death in infancy and childhood are listed in Table 10-1; the greatest mortality occurs in the first year and declines progressively until accidents and suicide supervene beginning in middle adolescence. The relative incidences of the various causes of mortality also depend on age, with congenital anomalies, prematurity, and sudden infant death syndrome (SIDS) topping the list in the first year of life; overall, congenital anomalies and malignancies are the most important causes across all ages.

Congenital Anomalies (p. 448)

Congenital anomalies are morphologic defects present at birth; occasionally, these become apparent only later in life. About 3% of newborns in the United States have a congenital anomaly; clearly such abnormalities are still compatible with life. It is estimated, however, that more than 20% of all fertilized ova are so anomalous that they never develop into a viable conceptus.

DEFINITIONS

Organ-Specific Terms:
Agenesis: Complete absence of an organ and its associated primordium
Aplasia: Absence of an organ due to failure of the developmental anlage
Atresia: Absence of an opening, usually of a hollow visceral organ (e.g., intestine)
Dysplasia: In the context of malformations; refers to abnormal cellular organization
Hyperplasia: Enlargement of an organ associated with increased numbers of cells
Hypoplasia: Underdevelopment of an organ with decreased numbers of cells
Hypertrophy: Increased organ size due to increased cell size
Hypotrophy: Decreased organ size due to decreased cell size

General Terms:
Malformations: These are intrinsic disturbances in morphogenesis; these are typically multifactorial and not caused by a single genetic defect.
Disruptions: These are extrinsic disturbances in morphogenesis causing a secondary destruction of a previously developmentally normal tissue; disruptions are not heritable. The classic example is an amniotic band, resulting from an amniotic rupture that causes fibrous stranding that encircles, compresses, or attaches to a developing body part.

Deformations: These are common, affecting 2% of neonates; like disruptions, deformations result from an external disturbance in morphogenesis. Deformations are caused by localized or generalized compression by abnormal mechanical forces, and they manifest as abnormalities in shape, form, or position (e.g., clubfeet). Most have a low risk of recurrence. The most common underlying factor is uterine constraint:

- Maternal factors include first pregnancies, a small uterus, or leiomyomas
- Fetal and placental factors include oligohydramnios, multiple fetuses, or abnormal fetal presentations

Sequence: This is a constellation of anomalies resulting from one initiating aberration that leads to multiple secondary effects. A classic example is the oligohydramnios (Potter) sequence. Thus, oligohydramnios (i.e., decreased amniotic fluid) can occur through a variety of mechanisms: renal agenesis (fetal urine is a major component of amniotic fluid), placental insufficiency due to maternal hypertension, or an amniotic leak. Regardless of the cause, oligohydramnios leads in sequence to fetal compression with characteristic findings including facial flattening, hand and foot malpositioning, hip dislocation, and chest compression with lung hypoplasia.

Syndrome: This is a combination of anomalies that cannot be explained on the basis of one initiating aberration and a subsequent cascade. Most syndromes are caused by a single pathology that simultaneously affects several tissues (e.g., viral infection or chromosomal abnormality).

Causes of Anomalies (p. 450)

The causes of congenital anomalies are known in only 25% to 50% of cases; these are grouped into three major categories (Table 10-2):

Genetic Causes (p. 450)

- *Chromosomal abnormalities* are present in 10% to 15% of live-born infants with congenital anomalies, although it is important to note that 80% to 90% of fetuses with chromosomal abnormalities die *in utero*. Most cytogenetic aberrations arise as defects in gameto-genesis and are therefore not familial. The most common chromosomal abnormalities in live-born infants are (in order):

  Trisomy 21 (Down syndrome)
  Klinefelter syndrome (47,XXY)
  Turner syndrome (45,XO)
  Trisomies 13 (Patau) and 18 (Edwards) (Chapter 5)

- *Single-gene mutations* are relatively uncommon but follow men-delian patterns of inheritance; many involve loss of function in genes that drive organogenesis or development (e.g., Hedgehog signaling pathway and holoprosencephalic developmental defects of the forebrain and midface)

Environmental Causes (p. 451)

- *Viruses* (p. 451): The effect is related to gestational age at time of infection.

  Cytomegalovirus is the most common fetal viral infection; the highest at-risk period is the second trimester. Although organo-genesis is largely complete and congenital malformations are therefore less common, central nervous system (CNS) infection results in mental retardation, microcephaly, and deafness.

TABLE 10-1 Cause of Death Related to Age	
Causes*	**Rate†**
Younger Than 1 Year	685.2
Congenital malformations, deformations, and chromosomal anomalies	
Disorders related to short gestation and low birth weight	
Sudden infant death syndrome (SIDS)	
Newborn affected by maternal complications of pregnancy	
Newborn affected by complications of placenta, cord, and membranes	
Respiratory distress of newborn	
Accidents (unintentional injuries)	
Bacterial sepsis of newborn	
Intrauterine hypoxia and birth asphyxia	
Diseases of the circulatory system	
1 to 4 years	29.9
Accidents and adverse effects	
Congenital malformations, deformations, and chromosomal abnormalities	
Malignant neoplasms	
Homicide	
Diseases of the heart‡	
Influenza and pneumonia	
5 to 14 years	16.8
Accidents and adverse effects	
Malignant neoplasms	
Homicide	
Congenital malformations, deformations, and chromosomal abnormalities	
Suicide	
Diseases of the heart	
15 to 24 years	80.1
Homicide	
Suicide	
Malignant neoplasms	
Diseases of the heart	

*Causes are listed in decreasing order of frequency. All causes and rates are final 2004 statistics.
†Rates are expressed per 100,000 people from all causes within each age group.
‡Excludes congenital heart disease.
Data from Minino AM, et al: Deaths: final data for 2004, *National Vital Statistics Rep* 55:19, 2007.

Rubella infection occurring before 16 weeks of gestation can result in a tetrad of defects (congenital rubella syndrome): cataracts, heart defects, deafness, and mental retardation.

- *Drugs and other chemicals* (p. 452): These cause less than 1% of congenital anomalies. Teratogens include thalidomide, folate antagonists, androgenic hormones, anticonvulsants, and 13-*cis*-retinoic acid.
- *Alcohol:* Alcohol is the most widely used teratogen; it is responsible for several structural anomalies, as well as cognitive and behavioral deficits, collectively termed *fetal alcohol spectrum disorders.* The most severely affected infants have a classic teratogenic phenotype called *fetal alcohol syndrome* (e.g., growth retardation, microcephaly, atrial septal defects, short palpebral fissures, and maxillary hypoplasia).
- *Radiation* (p. 452): High doses during organogenesis can result in microcephaly, blindness, skull defects, and spina bifida.

TABLE 10-2 Causes of Congenital Anomalies in Humans	
Cause	Frequency (%)
Genetic	
Chromosomal aberrations	10-15
Mendelian inheritance	2-10
Environmental	
Maternal/placental infections	2-3
Rubella	
Toxoplasmosis	
Syphilis	
Cytomegalovirus	
Human immunodeficiency virus (HIV)	
Maternal disease states	6-8
Diabetes	
Phenylketonuria	
Endocrinopathies	
Drugs and chemicals	1
Alcohol	
Folic acid antagonists	
Androgens	
Phenytoin	
Thalidomide	
Warfarin	
13-*cis*-retinoic acid	
Others	
Irradiations	1
Multifactorial (Multiple Genes and Environmental Influences)	20-25
Unknown	40-60

Data from Stevenson RE, et al (eds): *Human malformations and related anomalies,* New York, 1993, Oxford University Press, p 115.

- *Maternal diabetes* (p. 452): The incidence of major malformations in diabetic mothers is 6% to 10%. Maternal hyperglycemia-induced fetal hyperinsulinemia causes increased body fat, muscle mass and organomegaly *(fetal macrosomia)*, cardiac anomalies, neural tube defects, and other CNS malformations.

Multifactorial Causes (p. 452)

Anomalies may involve the interaction of environmental factors with mutated genes; independently, these may have no or minimal effect. Examples are congenital hip dislocation (requiring a shallow acetabular socket *and* a breech delivery) and neural tube defects (requiring a genetic predisposition *and* low maternal folate).

Pathogenesis of Congenital Anomalies (p. 452)

- The timing of any teratogenic insult influences the nature and incidence of the anomaly produced—a given agent can have significantly different outcomes depending on when it is encountered (Fig. 10-1).

  In the early *embryonic period* (first 3 weeks after fertilization), injury either kills so many cells that death and spontaneous abortion results or such limited numbers of cells are affected that the fetus can recover without much consequence.

  Between the third and ninth week of the *embryonic period*, organs are developing from germ layers and the embryo is exquisitely sensitive to teratogenesis.

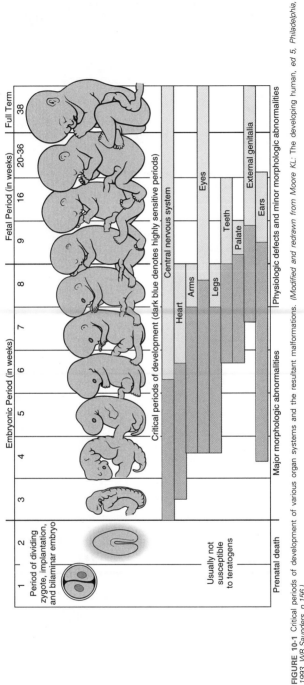

FIGURE 10-1 Critical periods of development of various organ systems and the resultant malformations. *(Modified and redrawn from Moore KL: The developing human, ed 5, Philadelphia, 1993, WB Saunders, p 156.)*

The *fetal period* following organogenesis is marked chiefly by further maturation and growth, with greatly reduced sensitivity to teratogenic agents. The fetus is susceptible, however, to growth retardation.

- Teratogens and genetic defects can act on the same developmental pathways, as well as result in similar anomalies. Thus, valproic acid (an anti-seizure medication) is teratogenic through disruption of the expression of several *homeobox (HOX)* transcription factors; moreover, *HOX* gene mutations give rise to congenital anomalies that mimic the valproate embryopathy.

Disorders of Prematurity (p. 453)

Morbidity and mortality rates are greater for infants born before the normal gestation period is completed; prematurity is the second most common cause of neonatal mortality after congenital anomalies. Babies born before 37 weeks of gestation are considered *preterm* (12% of births in the United States); those born after 42 weeks of gestation are denoted *post-term*. Infants who fail to grow normally during gestation are also at increased risk, but a small full-term neonate generally has fewer adverse consequences than a premature infant of the same weight. To take into account both developmental age *and* weight, infants are classified as:

- Appropriate for gestational age (i.e., between the 10th and 90th percentiles)
- Small for gestational age (i.e., below the 10th percentile)
- Large for gestational age (i.e., above the 90th percentile)

Causes of Prematurity and Fetal Growth Restriction (p. 454)

Major risk factors for prematurity are:

- *Preterm* (i.e., before 37 weeks of gestation) *premature rupture of placental membranes (PPROM):* PPROM complicates 3% of pregnancies and is the most common cause of prematurity (33%). PPROM is associated with maternal smoking or malnutrition, preterm labor, and gestational vaginal bleeding. The pathophysiology involves placental inflammation and matrix metalloproteinase activation.
- *Intrauterine infection* (25% of preterm births): This occurs with inflammation of the placental membrane (chorioamnionitis) and/or umbilical cord (funisitis). Organisms include *Ureaplasma urealyticum, Mycoplasma hominis, Gardnerella vaginalis, Trichomonas, Gonorrhoea,* and *Chlamydia*. Toll-like receptor (TLR) activation may deregulate prostaglandin production, leading to uterine smooth muscle contraction.
- *Uterine, cervical, and placental structural abnormalities* (e.g., uterine fibroids or "cervical incompetence")
- *Multiple gestation* (i.e., twin pregnancy)

Infants with *fetal growth restriction (FGR; also called intrauterine growth retardation)* are small for gestational age. Three main factors contribute:

- *Fetal* (p. 455): Despite adequate maternal nutritional supply, there is compromised fetal growth potential; typically, there is symmetric growth restriction—all organ systems are proportionately affected. Causes include:

  Chromosomal abnormalities (e.g., triploidy and trisomy 18, 13, and 21)
  Congenital anomalies
  Congenital infections, most commonly the TORCH group (*to*xoplasmosis, *r*ubella, *c*ytomegalovirus, *h*erpesvirus)

- *Placenta* (p. 455): Vigorous fetal growth in the third trimester demands adequate placental growth and development; defects in placental supply typically cause asymmetric (or *disproportionate*) growth retardation, with relative sparing of the brain. Causes include:

  Umbilical-placental vascular anomalies (e.g., single umbilical artery, abnormal insertion)
  Placental abruption
  Placenta previa (i.e., low-lying placenta)
  Placental thrombosis and infarctions
  Placental infections
  Multiple gestations
  Placental mosaicism (15% of pregnancies with FGR): Viable genetic mutations arising after zygote formation (Trisomy 7 is most common.) lead to two genetic populations of cells within the placenta (90% of the time) and/or fetus; the phenotypic outcome is dependent on the specific mutation and which cells and what percentage are involved.

- *Maternal causes* (p. 455) of FGR are the most common; essentially, these all result in decreased placental blood supply. These impose significant risks for CNS dysfunction, learning disability, and hearing or visual impairment. Causes include:

  Preeclampsia
  Hypertension
  Inherited thrombophilias (e.g., factor V Leiden mutations [Chapter 4])
  Malnutrition
  Narcotic or alcohol intake
  Cigarette smoking
  Certain drugs (e.g., teratogens)

  Risks associated with prematurity include:

- Hyaline membrane disease (neonatal respiratory distress syndrome)
- Necrotizing enterocolitis
- Sepsis
- Intraventricular hemorrhage
- Long-term complications, including developmental delay

Neonatal Respiratory Distress Syndrome (p. 456)

Among many causes of neonatal respiratory distress (e.g., maternal sedation, blood or amniotic fluid aspiration, fetal head injury, or umbilical cord around the neck), the most common is *respiratory distress syndrome (RDS)*, also known as *hyaline membrane disease.*

Etiology and Pathogenesis (p. 456) (Fig. 10-2)

Lung immaturity is the most important substrate; the incidence of RDS is 60% in infants born before 28 weeks of gestation and less than 5% in infants born after 37 weeks of gestation. Inadequate pulmonary surfactant is the key feature; surfactant synthesis by type II pneumocytes (Chapter 15) is accelerated beginning at 35 weeks of gestation, with production of phospholipids and glycoproteins that impact innate immunity and alveolar surface tension:

- Decreased surfactant results in increased alveolar surface tension, progressive alveolar atelectasis, and increasing inspiratory pressures required to expand alveoli.
- Hypoxemia results in acidosis, pulmonary vasoconstriction, pulmonary hypoperfusion, capillary endothelial and alveolar epithelial damage, and plasma leakage into alveoli.

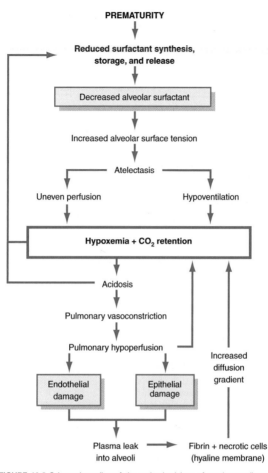

PREMATURITY

↓

Reduced surfactant synthesis, storage, and release

↓

Decreased alveolar surfactant

↓

Increased alveolar surface tension

↓

Atelectasis

Uneven perfusion · Hypoventilation

↓

Hypoxemia + CO$_2$ retention

↓

Acidosis

↓

Pulmonary vasoconstriction

↓

Pulmonary hypoperfusion

↓

Endothelial damage · Epithelial damage

Increased diffusion gradient

↓

Plasma leak into alveoli → Fibrin + necrotic cells (hyaline membrane)

FIGURE 10-2 Schematic outline of the pathophysiology of respiratory distress syndrome.

- Plasma proteins combine with fibrin and necrotic alveolar pneumocytes to form *hyaline membranes* that further impede gas exchange.
- *Corticosteroids* reduce RDS by inducing surfactant lipid and apoprotein production. Increased fetal insulin levels, due to maternal diabetes, suppress surfactant production.

Morphology (p. 456)

- *Grossly:* Lungs are solid, airless, and reddish purple.
- *Microscopically:* Alveoli are poorly developed and frequently collapsed; proteinaceous "membranes" line respiratory bronchioles, alveolar ducts, and random alveoli.

Clinical Course (p. 457)

The typical infant with RDS is preterm but appropriate for gestational age. Lung maturity (reflecting surfactant synthesis) is assessed by measuring the amniotic fluid lecithin/sphingomyelin ratio. Antenatal corticosteroid therapy can induce surfactant production. If delivery cannot be delayed until there is adequate surfactant synthesis, therapy involves surfactant replacement and oxygen therapy. In uncomplicated cases, recovery begins in 3 to 4 days; however, because of high-concentration oxygen therapy, infants are at risk for developing *retinopathy of prematurity* (Chapter 29) and *bronchopulmonary dysplasia (BPD)*.

- Retinopathy occurs when hyperoxic therapy reduces VEGF expression and causes endothelial cell apoptosis; subsequent return to the relative hypoxia of room air causes the characteristic retinal vessel proliferation.
- BPD is attributed to impaired alveolar septation in the setting of hyperoxia, hyperventilation, and inflammatory cytokines; BPD is manifested by decreased alveolar number *(alveolar hypoplasia)* and a dysmorphic capillary configuration.

Infants recovering from RDS may also have other complications of prematurity, including patent ductus arteriosus, intraventricular hemorrhage, and necrotizing enterocolitis (NEC).

Necrotizing Enterocolitis (p. 458)

NEC occurs most commonly in premature infants; the incidence is inversely proportional to gestational age (10% of very low birth weight infants; i.e., weighing 1500 g or less). Predisposing conditions include bacterial colonization of the gut and enteral feeding that induce inflammatory mediators; in particular, platelet activating factor production is implicated in promoting enterocyte apoptosis and increased intercellular permeability. This augments transmural bacterial migration with a vicious cycle of associated inflammation and mucosal necrosis.

Clinical Consequences

NEC typically involves the terminal ileum, cecum, and right colon. Affected infants present with bloody stools, abdominal distention, and progressive circulatory collapse; gas within the intestinal wall *(pneumatosis intestinalis)* can occur. Microscopically, there is mucosal to transmural coagulative necrosis, ulceration, bacterial colonization, and submucosal gas bubbles. Early NEC can often be managed conservatively, although 20% to 60% require resection of necrotic bowel segments, and perinatal mortality is high; survivors may have post-NEC bowel strictures due to healing-associated fibrosis.

Perinatal Infections (p. 458)

Infections are typically acquired either transcervically (i.e., ascending) or transplacentally (i.e., hematologic); occasionally, ascending microbes infect the endometrium and then the fetus via the chorionic villi.

Transcervical (Ascending) Infections (p. 458)

Most bacterial and a few viral infections occur via the cervicovaginal route. Infection may be acquired *in utero* by inhaling infected amniotic fluid into the lungs or at parturition by passing through an infected birth canal. Chorioamnionitis and funisitis are usually present, and preterm birth is a common outcome. In the fetus, pneumonia, sepsis, and meningitis are the most common sequelae.

Transplacental (Hematologic) Infections (p. 459)

Most parasitic (e.g., toxoplasma, malaria) and viral infections, as well as a few bacterial infections (e.g., *Listeria*, syphilis) enter the fetal bloodstream via chorionic villi. Infection may occur at any time during gestation or, occasionally at parturition (e.g., hepatitis B virus [HBV] and human immunodeficiency virus [HIV]). Sequelae are highly variable, depending on the gestational timing and microorganism; adverse outcomes include spontaneous abortion, stillbirth, hydrops fetalis (see later discussion), and congenital anemia (e.g., parvovirus B19).

TORCH infections all have similar manifestations, including fever, encephalitis, chorioretinitis, hepatosplenomegaly, pneumonitis, myocarditis, hemolytic anemia, and vesicular or hemorrhagic skin lesions; long-term sequelae include growth and mental retardation, cataracts, congenital cardiac anomalies, and bone defects.

Sepsis (p. 459)

Early-onset (i.e., during the first 7 days of life) sepsis is most commonly due to group B streptococcus, acquired at or shortly before birth; besides sepsis, infants present with pneumonia and occasionally meningitis. Late-onset (i.e., up to 3 months) sepsis is often due to *Listeria* or *Candida*.

Fetal Hydrops (p. 459)

Fetal hydrops refers to fetal edema fluid collection during intrauterine growth; Table 10-3 lists the possible causes. Accumulation can be variable, ranging from severe and generalized (*hydrops*

TABLE 10-3   Selected Causes of Non-Immune Fetal Hydrops
Cardiovascular
Malformations
Tachyarrhythmia
High-output failure
Chromosomal
Turner syndrome
Trisomy 21, trisomy 18
Thoracic causes
Cystic adenomatoid malformation
Diaphragmatic hernia
Fetal Anemia
Homozygous α-thalassemia
Parvovirus B19
Immune hydrops (Rh and ABO)
Twin Gestation
Twin-to-twin transfusion
Infection (Excluding Parvovirus)
Cytomegalovirus
Syphilis
Toxoplasmosis
Genitourinary Tract Malformations
Tumors
Genetic/Metabolic Disorders

Note: The cause of fetal hydrops may be undetermined ("idiopathic") in up to 20% of cases. Data from Machin GA: Hydrops, cystic hygroma, hydrothorax, pericardial effusions, and fetal ascites. In Gilbert-Barness E, et al (eds): *Potter's pathology of the fetus, infant, and child*, St Louis, 2007, Mosby, p 33.

fetalis, usually lethal), to more localized, non-lethal forms, for example, isolated pleural and peritoneal effusions, or postnuchal fluid accumulations (cystic hygroma).

Immune Hydrops (p. 460)

Immune hydrops is a hemolytic disorder caused by blood group incompatibility between mother and fetus. If fetal erythrocytes express paternal antigens that are foreign to the mother, those will elicit antibody responses that can cause red cell hemolysis. The most important molecules are the Rh D antigen and ABO blood group antigens.

Etiology and Pathogenesis (p. 460)

The underlying basis of disease is the immunization of the mother by antigens present on fetal erythrocytes, followed by free passage of maternal antibodies across the placenta and into the fetus. These antibodies bind to erythrocytes and mediate complement-dependent lysis and/or phagocytosis by Fc receptor–bearing cells.

- Fetal erythrocytes can reach the maternal circulation during childbirth or during the last trimester of pregnancy (due to loss of the cytotrophoblast barrier).
- The first exposure to the antigenic stimulus elicits immunoglobulin M (IgM) antibodies that do not cross the placenta; however, subsequent pregnancies can elicit brisk maternal immunoglobulin G (IgG) responses that do cross the placenta.
- Concurrent ABO incompatibility tends to reduce Rh immunization, since any leaked red blood cells (RBCs) are promptly coated by maternal antibodies to A/B and cleared.
- Although ABO incompatibility is more common than Rh incompatibility, hemolytic disease is rare in such mismatches because:

  Most ABO antibodies are IgM and do not cross the placenta.
  Neonatal erythrocytes express A and B antigens poorly.
  Many cells in addition to RBCs express A/B antigens and therefore absorb the majority of any antibody that enters the fetal bloodstream.

Clinical Consequences (p. 461)

- *Anemia* is a major sequela. If it is mild, fetal extramedullary hematopoiesis can keep pace. If it is severe, there is progressive heart and liver ischemia; liver injury leads to diminished protein synthesis while cardiac hypoxia causes decompensation and failure. The combination of reduced oncotic pressure and increased venous hydrostatic pressure (i.e., heart failure) results in generalized edema.
- *Jaundice* develops because hemolysis produces unconjugated bilirubin; this passes across the poorly developed fetal blood-brain barrier and causes CNS injury *(kernicterus).*
- Phototherapy can oxidize toxic unconjugated bilirubin to harmless water-soluble dipyrroles. In severe cases, exchange transfusion may be necessary.
- In Rh-negative mothers, prophylaxis with anti-D immunoglobulin at the time of initial delivery usually prevents sensitization and subsequent hemolytic disease.

Nonimmune Hydrops (p. 461)

Major causes include the following:

- *Cardiovascular defects* occur; congenital defects or arrhythmias can lead to congestive failure.
- *Chromosomal anomalies* (Turner syndrome, trisomies 21 and 18) occur, which are often due to cardiac structural abnormalities.

In Turner syndrome, aberrant lymphatic drainage in the neck can lead to local fluid accumulations *(cystic hygromas).*

- *Fetal anemia unrelated to immune hemolysis* occurs, for example, homozygous α thalassemia, or parvovirus B19; in the latter, virus replicates within erythroid precursors (normoblasts), leading to apoptosis and aplastic anemia.
- Monozygous twin pregnancies and twin-twin transfusions occur via anastomoses between the two circulations (10% of nonimmune hydrops).

Morphology of Hydrops Fetalis (p. 461)

Anatomic findings vary with hydrops severity and the underlying cause. With fetal anemia, both the fetus and placenta are pale; there is hepatosplenomegaly from cardiac failure and congestion. Except in parvovirus infections, the bone marrow exhibits compensatory erythroid hyperplasia and multiple organs exhibit extramedullary hematopoiesis; increased hematopoiesis deposits large numbers of immature RBCs in the peripheral blood (hence the name *erythroblastosis fetalis*).

Inborn Errors of Metabolism and Other Genetic Disorders (p. 462)

Phenylketonuria (p. 463)

Phenylketonuria (PKU) is an autosomal recessive disease, most commonly associated with bi-allelic mutations of the gene encoding *phenylalanine hydroxylase (PAH),* an enzyme that irreversibly converts phenylalanine to tyrosine.

There are more than 500 disease-associated alleles; disease severity correlates with the loss of enzyme activity and the associated increase in phenylalanine levels. Some PAH mutations result in only modestly elevated phenylalanine levels without neurologic sequelae, called *benign hyperphenylalaninemia.* About 2% of PKU cases are caused by defects in regenerating tetrahydrobiopterin (BH_4), a necessary co-factor for PAH activity.

Although normal at birth, affected infants exhibit rising plasma phenylalanine within the first few weeks of life, followed by impaired brain development and mental retardation. Screening for elevated phenylalanine metabolite in the urine allows early diagnosis; subsequent phenylalanine dietary restriction prevents most clinical sequelae. Phenylalanine and its metabolites are teratogenic—infants born to PKU mothers with high phenylalanine levels are microcephalic and mentally retarded.

Galactosemia (p. 464)

Intestinal mucosal lactase converts lactose into glucose and galactose; galactose is then metabolized to glucose by three additional enzymes. Enzymatic defects lead to accumulation of toxic metabolites *(galactosemia).* The most common and clinically significant form is an autosomal recessive mutation in *galactose-1-phosphate uridyl transferase (GALT);* affected patients accumulate galactose-1-phosphate and elevated levels of galactitol and galactonate.

The clinical picture is variable, depending on the GALT mutations. Classically, infants present with vomiting and diarrhea after milk ingestion, with failure to thrive. Liver, eyes, and brain are most severely affected; changes include hepatomegaly due to hepatic fat accumulation, cirrhosis, cataracts, and nonspecific CNS alterations (including mental retardation).

Urinary screening reveals the presence of an abnormal reducing sugar. Removal of dietary galactose for at least the first 2 years of life prevents most of the sequelae. Nevertheless, older patients may exhibit speech disorders, ataxia, and gonadal failure.

Cystic Fibrosis (Mucoviscidosis) (p. 465)

Cystic fibrosis (CF) is an autosomal recessive disorder that affects epithelial cell ion transport and causes abnormal fluid secretion in exocrine glands, as well as in respiratory, gastrointestinal, and reproductive mucosa. It occurs in 1 of 2500 live births in the United States (i.e., 1 in 20 carrier frequency among Caucasians, but lower in other groups), and it is the most common lethal genetic disease affecting Caucasian populations. Heterozygote carriers also have a higher incidence of respiratory and pancreatic pathology relative to the general population.

The Cystic Fibrosis–Associated Gene: Normal Structure and Function (p. 465)

- The gene mutated in CF encodes the *cystic fibrosis transmembrane conductance regulator (CFTR)* protein—a chloride channel; activation of the channel occurs via agonist-induced increases in intracellular cyclic AMP, followed by protein kinase A activation and CFTR phosphorylation.
- *CFTR regulates other ion channels and cellular processes.* Although CF mutations specifically affect the CFTR, disease manifestations are related to the interactions of CFTR with other ion channels and cellular processes. These include potassium, sodium, and gap junction channels, as well as ATP transport and mucus secretion.
- *CFTR association with the epithelial sodium channel (ENaC)* has the most pathophysiologic relevance to CF. ENaC is an apical membrane protein in exocrine epithelium that is responsible for sodium transport.
- *CFTR functions are tissue-specific* (Fig. 10-3).

  In *eccrine sweat duct epithelium,* normal CFTR *augments* ENaC activity. In CF, ENaC activity is lost, resulting in hypertonic sweat (hence the sweat chloride test used for clinical diagnosis).

  In *respiratory and intestinal epithelium,* normal CFTR *inhibits* ENaC activity. In CF, augmented ENaC activity increases sodium movement into cells; coupled with reduced luminal chloride, there is increased osmotic water resorption from the lumen, leading to dehydration of mucus secretions. Defective mucociliary action and the accumulation of hyperconcentrated, viscous secretions ultimately obstruct ductal outflow from the organs (hence the alternative name for the disease—*mucoviscidosis*).

- *CFTR mediates bicarbonate transport.* CFTR is co-expressed with a family of anion exchangers called *SLC26.* Alkaline fluids (containing bicarbonate) are secreted in normal tissues, whereas in the setting of some CFTR mutations, acidic fluids are secreted, leading to an acidic environment that causes mucin precipitation and duct obstruction.

The Cystic Fibrosis Gene: Mutational Spectra and Genotype-Phenotype Correlation (p. 466)

At least 1300 disease-causing mutations of *CFTR* have been identified; these affect different regions of CFTR, resulting in distinct functional consequences and differing severity of clinical sequelae. The most common (70% world-wide) is a three-nucleotide deletion

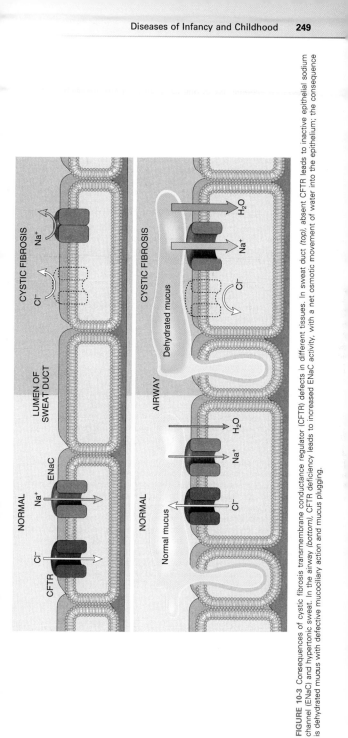

FIGURE 10-3 Consequences of cystic fibrosis transmembrane conductance regulator (CFTR) defects in different tissues. In sweat duct *(top)*, absent CFTR leads to inactive epithelial sodium channel (ENaC) and hypertonic sweat. In the airway *(bottom)*, CFTR deficiency leads to increased ENaC activity, with a net osmotic movement of water into the epithelium; the consequence is dehydrated mucus with defective mucociliary action and mucus plugging.

coding for phenylalanine at position 508 (i.e., ΔF508); this results in defective intracellular CFTR processing with degradation before it reaches the cell surface. Other mutations affect primary protein synthesis, ATP binding (preventing activation), chloride conductance, or associated ion channels.

Patients homozygous for the ΔF508 mutation (or a combination of any two "severe" mutations) have virtual absence of CFTR function; they present with severe clinical disease (*classic* CF), including early pancreatic insufficiency and various degrees of pulmonary damage. Patients with other combinations may present with features of *atypical* or *variant CF,* including isolated chronic pancreatitis, late-onset chronic pulmonary disease, or infertility only (caused by bilateral absence of the vas deferens).

Genetic and Environmental Modifiers (p. 468)

Genetic and environmental modifiers impact CF severity. Thus, reduced expression of mannose-binding lectin 2 (involved in microbial opsonization) confers a three-fold increased risk of end-stage lung disease; polymorphisms that influence transforming growth factor-β expression (a direct inhibitor of CFTR function) also exacerbate the pulmonary phenotype.

The nature of secondary pulmonary infections (e.g., *Pseudomonas*), with more or less mucoid polysaccharide biofilm production, also impact subsequent inflammation and lung destruction.

Morphology (p. 468)

Features are variable depending on the affected epithelium and the severity of involvement:

- *Pancreas:* Abnormalities occur in 85% to 90% of patients, ranging from mucus accumulation in small ducts with mild dilation to total atrophy of the exocrine pancreas. Absence of pancreatic exocrine secretions impairs fat absorption, and the resulting avitaminosis A partly explains ductal squamous metaplasia.
- *Intestine:* Thick viscous plugs of mucus (*meconium ileus*) can cause small bowel obstruction (5% to 10% of affected infants).
- *Liver:* Bile canalicular plugging by mucinous material (5% of patients) results in diffuse hepatic cirrhosis.
- *Salivary glands:* Like pancreas, these commonly show progressive duct dilation, ductal squamous metaplasia, and glandular atrophy.
- *Lungs:* Lungs are involved in most cases and are the most serious complication of CF. Mucus cell hyperplasia and viscous secretions block and dilate bronchioles. Superimposed infections and pulmonary abscesses are common. *Staphylococcus aureus, Haemophilus influenzae,* and *Pseudomonas aeruginosa* are most common; *Burkholderia cepacia* is associated with fulminant illness.
- *Male genital tract:* Azoospermia and infertility occur in 95% of male patients surviving to adulthood, frequently with congenital absence of the vas deferens.

Clinical Features (p. 469)

The different molecular variants and the presence of secondary modifiers result in highly variable clinical manifestations. In classic CF, pancreatic exocrine insufficiency is universal, associated with malabsorption that manifests as large, foul-smelling stools, abdominal distention, and poor weight gain. Poor fat absorption results in fat-soluble vitamin deficiencies (i.e., A, D, and K). Cardiorespiratory complications (e.g., chronic cough, persistent lung infections, obstructive pulmonary disease, and *cor pulmonale*) are the most common causes of death (~80%). Median life expectancy is now approximately 36 years.

Sudden Infant Death Syndrome (p. 471)

SIDS is officially defined by the National Institute of Clinical Health and Human Development as: *"sudden death of an infant less than 1 year of age, that remains unexplained after a thorough case investigation, including performance of a complete autopsy, examination of the death scene, and review of the clinical history."* Thus, by definition, SIDS is a diagnosis of exclusion and a disease of unknown cause; sudden death in infancy with an anatomical or biochemical basis uncovered at autopsy should not be labeled SIDS. Table 10-4 lists post-mortem abnormalities detected in cases of sudden unexpected death.

An aspect not emphasized in the definition of SIDS is that infants usually die while asleep, mostly in the prone or side position. Most SIDS deaths occur between 2 and 4 months of life, and 90% of SIDS deaths occur within 6 months of birth; in the United States, it is the leading cause of death in children between 1 month and 1 year of age and the third leading cause of infant death overall.

Morphology (p. 472)

Autopsy findings are usually subtle and of uncertain significance. Multiple petechiae (e.g., thymus, visceral and parietal pleura, epicardium) and histologic evidence of recent infection in the upper respiratory tract are common. The CNS demonstrates astrogliosis of the brain stem and cerebellum; arcuate nucleus hypoplasia may be present.

Pathogenesis (p. 472)

The pathogenesis of SIDS is poorly understood; SIDS is most likely a heterogeneous, multifactorial disorder. The most compelling hypothesis is that SIDS reflects developmental immaturity of critical brain stem regions (e.g., arcuate nucleus) involved in arousal and cardiorespiratory control and that environmental influences (e.g., infection) further fatally impair these regulatory mechanisms.

TABLE 10-4 Postmortem Abnormalities Detected in Cases of Sudden Unexpected Infant Death*

Infections
- Viral myocarditis
- Bronchopneumonia

Unsuspected congenital anomaly
- Congenital aortic stenosis
- Anomalous origin of the left coronary artery from the pulmonary artery

Traumatic child abuse
- Intentional suffocation (filicide)

Genetic and metabolic defects
- Long QT syndrome (*SCN5A* and *KCNQ1* mutations)
- Fatty acid oxidation disorders (*MCAD, LCHAD, SCHAD* mutations)
- Histiocytoid cardiomyopathy (*MTCYB* mutations)
- Abnormal inflammatory responsiveness (partial deletions in *C4a* and *C4b*)

---

*SIDS is not the only cause of sudden unexpected death in infancy but rather is a *diagnosis of exclusion.* Therefore, an autopsy may often reveal findings that would explain the cause of sudden unexpected death. These cases should *not*, strictly speaking, be labeled "SIDS."

C4, Complement component 4; *KCNQ1,* potassium voltage-gated channel, KQT-like subfamily, member 1; *LCHAD,* long-chain 3-hydroxyacyl coenzyme A dehydrogenase; *MCAD,* medium-chain acyl coenzyme A dehydrogenase; *MTCYB,* mitochondrial cytochrome *b*; *SCHAD,* short-chain 3-hydroxyacyl coenzyme A dehydrogenase; *SCN5A,* sodium channel, voltage-gated, type V, alpha polypeptide.

Parental risk factors include young maternal age, short inter-gestational interval, inadequate prenatal care, low socioeconomic status, and maternal smoking or drug abuse.

Infant risk factors include prematurity or low birth weight, SIDS in a prior sibling (suggesting a genetic component such as polymorphisms in autonomic nervous system genes), and male gender; most SIDS babies have an immediate prior history of a mild respiratory tract infection, but no single causative organism has been isolated.

Environmental risk factors include sleeping prone, hyperthermia, and sleeping on a soft surface.

Tumors and Tumor-Like Lesions of Infancy and Childhood (p. 473)

Benign tumors are much more common than malignant tumors; however, 2% of all cancers occur in infancy and childhood, and these are the leading cause of death (after accidents) in United States children between ages 4 and 14 years.

Benign Tumors and Tumor-Like Lesions (p. 473)

Because displaced tissue masses can be present from birth, distinguishing true tumors from "tumor-like" lesions can be difficult; the latter are frequently histologically normal and grow at approximately the same rate as the infant.

- *Heterotopia* (also called *choristomas*) represents microscopically normal cells or tissues present in abnormal locations (e.g., a rest of pancreatic tissue in the wall of the stomach); these cells are usually of little significance but can be the origin of true neoplasms (e.g., adrenal carcinoma in an ovary).
- *Hamartomas* are excessive (but focal) overgrowth of mature cells or tissues native to the organ or site in which they occur, that do not recapitulate normal architecture (e.g., a hamartoma of cartilaginous tissue in the lung parenchyma). These are histologically benign but can be clinically significant.

Hemangiomas (p. 473) are the most common tumors of infancy; most are cutaneous, with a predilection for face and scalp. They may enlarge along with the growth of the child but commonly spontaneously regress; they rarely become malignant. Hemangiomas may represent one facet of hereditary disorders such as *von Hippel-Lindau disease* (Chapter 28).

Lymphatic tumors (p. 473) may occur on the skin but also within deeper regions of the neck, axilla, mediastinum, and retroperitoneal tissue. They tend to increase in size and, depending on location, become clinically significant if they encroach on vital structures. Histologically, lymphangiomas are composed of cystic and cavernous lymphatic spaces, with variable numbers of associated lymphocytes.

Fibrous tumors (p. 474) range from sparsely cellular proliferations (*fibromatosis*) to richly cellular lesions indistinguishable from adult fibrosarcomas. The histology does not predict the biology of the infantile tumors. Thus, as compared to their malignant adult counterparts, congenital infantile fibrosarcomas have an excellent prognosis; in these tumors, a characteristic chromosomal translocation produces an *ETV6-NTRK3* fusion gene that codes for a constitutively active tyrosine kinase.

Teratoma (p. 474) incidence has two peaks—at age 2 years and in late adolescence. Those occurring in infancy and childhood are congenital lesions with 40% arising in the sacrococcygeal region.

- Approximately 10% of sacrococcygeal teratomas are associated with congenital anomalies, primarily defects of the hindgut and cloacal region, and other midline defects.
- Approximately 75% are benign mature teratomas, while 12% are unequivocally malignant and lethal; the remaining lesions, designated immature teratomas, contain mature and immature tissue, with malignant potential correlating with the percentage of immature tissues.

Malignant Tumors (p. 474)

Childhood malignancies differ biologically and histologically from their adult counterparts by:

- Incidence and type of tumor
- A close relationship between abnormal development (i.e., teratogenesis) and tumor induction (i.e., oncogenesis)
- A greater prevalence of underlying familial or genetic germline aberrations
- A tendency to spontaneously regress or cytodifferentiate
- Better survival and cure rates, with attention being increasingly focused on preventing subsequent therapy-induced malignancies

Incidence and Types (p. 475)

The most frequent childhood cancers involve:

- Hematopoietic system (e.g., leukemia, some lymphomas)
- CNS (e.g., astrocytoma, medulloblastoma, ependymoma)
- Adrenal medulla (e.g., neuroblastoma)
- Retina (e.g., retinoblastoma)
- Soft tissue (e.g., rhabdomyosarcoma)
- Bone (e.g., Ewing sarcoma, osteogenic sarcoma)
- Kidney (e.g., Wilms tumor)

Leukemia accounts for more deaths in children younger than 15 years of age than all other tumors combined.

Many pediatric cancers tend to have a more primitive, *embryonal* rather than a frankly anaplastic histology, with features of organogenesis consistent with the site of origin (hence the suffix "-blastoma"). Such tumors are often collectively labeled "small, round blue cell tumors"; included in this designation are lymphoma, Wilms tumor, rhabdomyosarcoma, Ewing sarcoma/peripheral neuroectodermal tumor (PNET), neuroblastoma, medulloblastoma, and retinoblastoma.

The Neuroblastic Tumors (p. 475)

Neuroblastic tumors arise in the adrenal medulla or sympathetic ganglia. Characteristic features include spontaneous regression, spontaneous or therapy-induced differentiation into mature elements, and a wide range of biologic behaviors; neuroblastoma is the most important entity in this group. Most neuroblastic tumors occur sporadically, but 1% to 2% of neuroblastic tumors are familial, associated with *anaplastic lymphoma kinase (ALK)* mutations. In high-risk subsets of neuroblastic tumors, the 5-year survival is only 40%.

Morphology (p. 476)

Neuroblastoma is the most common histologic subtype; 40% occur in the adrenal. These tumors are characterized by sheets of small, round blue neuroblasts within a neurofibrillary background (neuropil) and characteristic *Homer-Wright pseudorosettes*. Some tumors display variable differentiation toward ganglion cells, accompanied by the appearance of a so-called *schwannian stroma* (organized fascicles of neuritic processes, Schwann cells, and fibroblasts). Depending on the degree of differentiation, these latter tumors are called *ganglioneuroblastomas* or *ganglioneuromas*.

Clinical Course and Prognostic Features (p. 478)

Prognosis is based on staging (size and spread), patient's age (i.e., younger than 18 months is favorable), histologic features (schwannian stroma is favorable), and specific genetic changes (near-normal ploidy and *N-MYC* amplification are unfavorable). In addition to local infiltration and lymph node spread, hematogenous spread commonly involves the liver, lungs, bones, and marrow. About 90% of neuroblastomas produce catecholamines; elevated levels of blood or urine catecholamine metabolites can aid in diagnosis. Newer therapeutic approaches involve retinoids to direct differentiation of neuroblastomas into mature tissues, and tyrosine kinase inhibitors.

Wilms Tumor (p. 479)

Wilms tumor of the kidney is usually diagnosed between ages 2 and 5 years; although the tumor is malignant, the overall survival rate is more than 90%. Most tumors (90%) are sporadic; bilateral tumors occur in 5% to 10% of patients, and are presumed related to germline mutations; the tumors in this group are associated with malformation syndromes, all involving chromosome 11p:

- *WAGR syndrome* (*W*ilms tumor, *a*niridia, *g*enital anomalies, mental *r*etardation) is associated with a deletion on chromosome 11p band 13; patients have a 33% chance of developing Wilms tumor. The deleted chromosomal segment contains the *Wilms tumor 1 (WT1)* and aniridia *(PAX6)* genes. *WT1* encodes a DNA binding transcription factor critical for normal renal and gonadal development; patients heterozygous for the deletion ("first hit") can develop a Wilms tumor when the second *WT1* allele acquires a frameshift or nonsense mutation ("second hit").
- *Denys-Drash syndrome* patients have gonadal dysgenesis and nephropathy (diffuse mesangial sclerosis) leading to renal failure; 90% develop Wilms tumors. The genetic abnormality is a dominant negative mutation in the *WT1* gene that affects DNA binding; Wilms tumors arise when the wild-type *WT1* allele is also inactivated. Denys-Drash patients are also at increased risk for gonadoblastomas.
- *Beckwith-Wiedemann syndrome* patients have enlarged body organs, hemihypertrophy, adrenal cytomegaly, and a predisposition to developing Wilms and other primitive tumors; the genetic abnormality is localized to chromosome 11p band 15.5 distal to the *WT1* locus. Several candidate genes map to this locus, including *insulin-like growth factor-2 (IGF-2); IGF-2* is normally imprinted (transcribed from only one parental allele) but demonstrates loss of imprinting (biallelic expression) in many of the tumors.
- Less than 10% of sporadic Wilms tumors are associated with *WT1* mutations, indicating that there are other tumorigenic pathways. In 10% of sporadic tumors, gain-of-function mutations in β-catenin are implicated.

Morphology (p. 480)

Wilms tumors are soft, large, well-circumscribed renal masses characterized by triphasic histologic features: (1) blastema, (2) immature stroma, and (3) tubules—an attempt to recapitulate nephrogenesis. Histologic anaplasia (i.e., approximately 5% of tumors) is associated with a worse prognosis. *Nephrogenic rests* are putative precursor lesions of Wilms tumors and are seen in renal parenchyma adjacent to 40% of unilateral tumors. This frequency rises to nearly 100% in bilateral Wilms tumors, so that identifying rests on a unilateral Wilms tumor resection mandates watchful waiting for a malignancy on the cotralateral side.

Clinical Features (p. 481)

Patients typically present with large abdomenal masses; hematuria, pain, hypertension, or bowel obstruction is common. Resection and some combination of radio- and chemotherapy will be curative in 85% of patients, although second malignancies related to earlier treatment can occur.

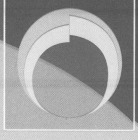

Systemic Pathology: Diseases of Organ Systems

11

Blood Vessels

Congenital Anomalies (p. 489)

- *Variants of the usual anatomic pattern* of vascular supply are important during surgery and vascular interventions.
- *Berry aneurysms* are outpouchings in cerebral vessels due to congenital wall weakness; rupture can cause fatal intracerebral hemorrhage (Chapter 28).
- *Arteriovenous fistulas* are abnormal communications between arteries and veins. They can be congenital or secondary to trauma, surgery, inflammation, or a healed ruptured aneurysm. Fistula rupture can cause extensive hemorrhage, and large fistulas can create significant left-to-right vascular shunting, with increased venous return that leads to high-output heart failure.
- *Fibromuscular dysplasia* is focal irregular thickening and attenuation of the arterial wall due to intimal and medial hyperplasia and fibrosis. In the renal artery, the associated luminal stenosis causes renovascular hypertension (see later discussion); areas of medial thinning can also lead to aneurysm formation with possible vascular rupture.

Vascular Wall Cells and their Response to Injury (p. 490)

Endothelial Cells (p. 490)

Normal endothelial function maintains vessel wall homeostasis and circulatory function through:

- Maintenance of a permeability barrier
- Elaboration of prothrombotic, antithrombotic, and fibrinolytic mediators
- Extracellular matrix production
- Modulation of blood flow and vasomotor tone
- Regulation of inflammation
- Regulation of cell growth

Endothelial dysfunction is defined as an altered phenotype that affects vasoreactivity, induces a thrombogenic surface, or is abnormally adhesive for inflamatory cells.

Vascular Smooth Muscle Cells (p. 491)

Vascular smooth muscle cells are the dominant cell type of the vessel media and can:

- Migrate and proliferate in response to various mediators (e.g., platelet-derived growth factor, endothelin, thrombin, and fibroblast growth factor)

- Elaborate cytokines and growth factors
- Synthesize and remodel extracellular matrix (ECM)
- Cause vasoconstriction or dilation in response to physiologic or pharmacologic stimuli

Intimal Thickening—A Stereotypical Response to Vascular Injury (p. 491)

Regardless of the nature of injury (e.g., traumatic, inflammatory, toxic, infectious), injured endothelium and underlying vessel wall heals by stimulating smooth muscle cell (SMC) ingrowth and ECM production leading to intimal thickening, called *neointima*. The neointimal cells have a proliferative and synthetic phenotype distinct from the underlying media, and the cells may derive from vessel wall or circulating precursors. In small to medium-sized vessels (e.g., coronary artery) such intimal thickening can cause lumenal stenosis and downstream tissue ischemia.

Hypertensive Vascular Disease (p. 492)

Blood pressure needs to be maintained within certain parameters to prevent untoward consequences. *Hypotension* (low pressure) leads to inadequate organ perfusion, causing dysfunction or tissue death, while *hypertension* (high pressure) can cause significant vessel and end-organ damage. Indeed, hypertension is a major risk factor for coronary heart disease, cerebrovascular accidents, heart failure, renal failure, and aortic dissection.

Blood pressure is a continuously distributed variable and detrimental effects increase continuously as the pressure rises; thus, no rigidly defined level distinguishes safety from risk, and other concomitant risk factors (e.g., diabetes) can lower the threshold for what is deleterious. Nevertheless, clinically significant hypertension is defined as sustained diastolic pressures more than 89 mm Hg or systolic pressures more than 139 mm Hg; by these criteria, 25% of the United States population is hypertensive.

Some 5% of hypertensive patients have a rapidly rising blood pressure that can cause death within 1 to 2 years if untreated. Such *malignant hypertension* is characterized by systolic blood pressure more than 200 mm Hg, diastolic pressure more than 120 mm Hg, renal failure, and retinal hemorrhages.

Regulation of Normal Blood Pressure (p. 492). Blood pressure is a function of cardiac output and peripheral vascular resistance, which are, in turn, influenced by genetic and environmental factors (Fig. 11-1).

- Cardiac output is determined by myocardial contractility, heart rate, and blood volume. Blood volume is affected by:

  Sodium load
  Mineralocorticoids (aldosterone)
  Natriuretic factors that induce sodium excretion

- Vascular resistance is determined primarily at the level of the arterioles

  Vasoconstrictors: angiotensin II, catecholamines, thromboxane, leukotrienes, and endothelin
  Vasodilators: kinins, prostaglandins, nitric oxide, and adenosine

- Regional autoregulation occurs when increased blood flow leads to local vasoconstriction; local hypoxia or acidosis can also cause vasodilation

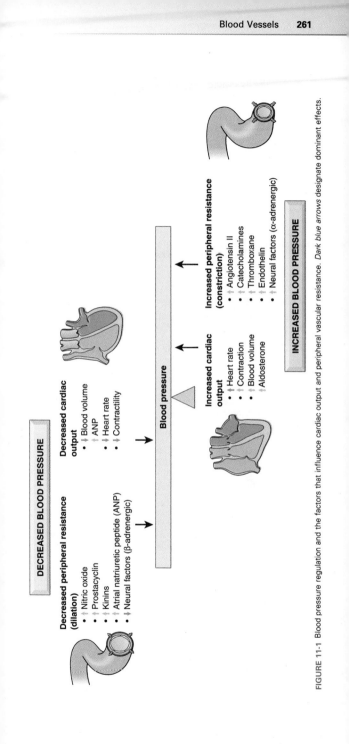

FIGURE 11-1 Blood pressure regulation and the factors that influence cardiac output and peripheral vascular resistance. *Dark blue arrows* designate dominant effects.

- Kidneys have a major influence on blood pressure by producing renin in the setting of hypotension:

  Renin converts angiotensinogen to angiotensin I, which is subsequently converted to angiotensin II
  Angiotensin II causes vasoconstriction
  Angiotensin II also increases blood volume by inducing aldosterone production, which increases renal sodium resorption

Mechanisms of Essential Hypertension (p. 493). In 90% to 95% of cases, hypertension is idiopathic *(essential hypertension)*. This does not mean that there is no cause, but rather that cumulative effects of non-genetic environmental factors (e.g., stress, salt intake) and multiple (individually minor) genetic polymorphisms in vasomotor tone or blood volume regulation conspire to cause high blood pressure.

Sodium homeostasis is a key element of blood volume control, and it is primarily regulated at the level of renal sodium resorption in the distal tubule; this, in turn, is largely influenced by the renin-angiotensin system, which regulates aldosterone production. Although *single gene disorders* in these pathways (see later discussion) are rare causes of hypertension, it is apparent that subtle variations in their activity might influence blood pressure in the broader population:

- Mutations in enzymes that influence aldosterone synthesis (11β-hydroxylase, 17α-hydroxylase) lead to increased aldosterone production
- Mutations in the renal epithelial Na^+ channel protein lead to increased sodium resorption *(Liddle syndrome)*

In the remainder of cases *(secondary hypertension)*, causes include intrinsic renal disease, renal artery stenosis (renovascular hypertension), endocrine abnormalities, vascular malformations, or neurologic disorders (Table 11-1).

Vascular Pathology in Hypertension (p. 495)

Hypertension accelerates the development of atherosclerosis and also causes arteriolar structural changes that potentiate both aortic dissection and cerebrovascular hemorrhage. Hypertension is also associated with two forms of small arteriolar disease:

- *Hyaline arteriolosclerosis* is due to endothelial cell (EC) injury, with subsequent plasma leakage into arteriolar walls and increased SMC matrix synthesis. The same lesions occur in diabetic angiopathy due to EC hyperglycemic injury. Microscopically, there is diffuse pink hyaline arteriolar wall thickening, with associated lumenal stenosis.
- *Hyperplastic arteriolosclerosis* occurs in malignant hypertension; there is concentric laminated *(onion-skin)* arteriolar thickening with reduplicated basement membrane and SMC proliferation, frequently associated with fibrin deposition and wall necrosis, called *necrotizing arteriolitis*.

Arteriosclerosis (p. 496)

Arteriosclerosis is a term denoting arterial wall thickening and loss of elasticity; three patterns are recognized:

- *Arteriolosclerosis* primarily affects small and medium-sized arteries and arterioles, and associated with downstream ischemia (see preceding discussion).
- *Mönckeberg medial sclerosis* is characterized by medial calcification in muscular arteries typically occurring after age 50 years.

TABLE 11-1   Types and Causes of Hypertension

Essential Hypertension

Secondary Hypertension
Renal
    Acute glomerulonephritis
    Chronic renal disease
    Polycystic disease
    Renal artery stenosis
    Renal artery fibromuscular dysplasia
    Renal vasculitis
    Renin-producing tumors
Endocrine
    Adrenocortical hyperfunction (Cushing syndrome, primary
      aldosteronism, congenital adrenal hyperplasia, licorice ingestion)
    Exogenous hormones (glucocorticoids, estrogen [including
      pregnancy induced and oral contraceptives], sympathomimetics,
      tyramine-containing foods, and monoamine oxidase inhibitors
    Pheochromocytoma
    Acromegaly
    Hypothyroidism (myxedema)
    Hyperthyroidism (thyrotoxicosis)
    Pregnancy induced
Cardiovascular
    Coarctation of aorta
    Polyarteritis nodosa (or other vasculitides)
    Increased intravascular volume
    Increased cardiac output
    Rigidity of the aorta
Neurologic
    Psychogenic
    Increased intracranial pressure
    Sleep apnea
    Acute stress, including surgery

The calcific deposits are non-obstructive and not usually clinically significant.

- *Atherosclerosis* is the most frequent and clinically important (see later discussion).

Atherosclerosis (p. 496)

Atherosclerosis is a slowly progressive disease of large- to medium-sized muscular and elastic arteries. The lesions are characterized by elevated intimal-based plaques composed of lipids, proliferating SMC, inflammatory cells, and increased ECM. They cause pathology by:

- Mechanically obstructing flow, especially in smaller-bore vessels
- Plaque rupture leading to vessel thrombosis
- Weakening the underlying vessel wall and leading to aneurysm formation

Epidemiology (p. 496)

The prevalence and severity of atherosclerosis and its complications are related to a number of risk factors, some constitutional and some modifiable. The major classic risk factors emerging from the Framingham Heart Study are family history, hypercholesterolemia, hypertension, smoking, and diabetes.

Constitutional Risk Factors in Ischemic Heart Disease (p. 496)

- *Age:* Atherosclerotic burden progressively increases with age, typically reaching a critical mass with clinical manifestations beginning between ages 40 and 60 years.
- *Gender:* Relative to age-matched men, premenopausal women are relatively protected against atherosclerosis and its complications. In postmenopausal women, the risk rapidly increases and can exceed that for men. Besides affecting the progression to atherosclerosis, female gender also influences hemostasis, infarct healing, and myocardial remodeling.
- *Genetics:* Family history is the most significant independent risk factor for atherosclerosis. Monogenic disorders such as familial hypercholesterolemia account for only a minor percentage, and numerous genetic polymorphisms (including predilection for hypertension and diabetes) are contributory.

Modifiable Risk Factors in Ischemic Heart Disease (p. 497)

- *Hypercholesterolemia:* Increased risk is associated with increased low-density lipoprotein (LDL) and decreased high-density lipoprotein (HDL; clears cholesterol from vessel wall lesions). Levels can be favorably modified by diet, exercise, moderate alcohol intake, and statins (inhibitors of hydroxymethylglutaryl-coA reductase, the rate-limiting enzyme in cholesterol biosynthesis).
- *Hypertension:* Both diastolic and systolic hypertension are important and independent of other risk factors; high blood pressure increases the risk of atherosclerotic ischemic heart disease by 60%.
- *Smoking:* Smoking of one pack of cigarettes daily over many years doubles the death rate from ischemic heart disease.
- *Diabetes mellitus:* Directly and indirectly (by inducing hypercholesterolemia), diabetes accelerates atherosclerosis and doubles the risk of myocardial infarction and markedly increases the risk of stroke or extremity gangrene.

Additional Risk Factors (p. 498)

Up to 20% of all cardiovascular events occur in the absence of the major identified risk factors, suggesting other contributions:

- *Inflammation:* Present at all stages of atherosclerosis, inflammation plays a significant causal role. A number of circulating markers of inflammation correlate with risk of ischemic heart disease; C-reactive protein (CRP; a liver-synthesized acute phase reactant involved in bacterial recognition and complement activation) has emerged as one of the simplest and most sensitive to measure. It strongly and independently predicts risk of cardiovascular events, even in healthy individuals.
- *Hyperhomocystinemia:* Elevated levels of homocysteine are associated with increased atherosclerotic vascular disease. Levels can be increased in the setting of low folate or vitamin B12 or with hereditary homocystinuria.
- *Metabolic syndrome:* A constellation of findings including central obesity, hypertension, glucose intolerance, dyslipidemia, and a systemic pro-inflammatory state. Adipose tissue cytokines have been implicated.
- *Lipoprotein(a):* This is an altered form of the lipoprotein constituent in LDL; elevated levels confer increased risk independent of LDL or total cholesterol levels.
- *Hemostatic factors:* Systemic markers of hemostasis or fibrinolysis are predictors of risk for atherosclerotic events.

Pathogenesis of Atherosclerosis (p. 498)

Atherosclerosis is a chronic inflammatory and healing response of the arterial wall to EC injury. In turn, EC injury causes increased endothelial permeability, white blood cell (WBC) and platelet adhesion, and coagulation activation. These events induce chemical mediator (e.g., growth factors and inflammatory mediators) release and activation, followed by recruitment and subsequent proliferation of SMC in the intima to produce the characteristic intimal lesion (Fig. 11-2).

Endothelial Injury (p. 499)

Even without causing EC loss, endothelial injury leads to *endothelial cell dysfunction* with increased adhesivity and procoagulant activity; injury mechanisms include hypercholesteromia, hemodynamic disturbances (e.g., disturbed flow), smoking, hypertension, toxins, and infectious agents. Regardless of the inciting stimulus, the vessel responds with a fairly stereotyped intimal thickening; in the presence of circulating lipids, typical atheromas ensue.

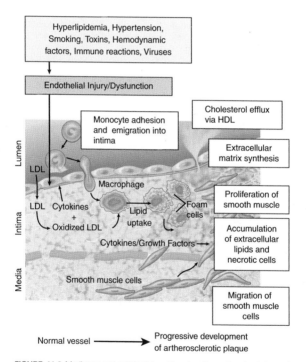

FIGURE 11-2 Mediators and cellular interactions in atherosclerosis. A host of noxious insults (e.g., hyperlipidemia, hypertension, smoking) cause endothelial injury or dysfunction. This results in monocyte (and platelet) adhesion and growth factor release, leading to smooth muscle cell recruitment, and proliferation in the intima; matrix synthesis is also increased. Foam cells result when macrophages and smooth muscle cells accumulate cholesterol through the uptake of low-density lipoprotein (LDL; e.g., in the form of oxidized LDL). These lipids derive from insudation from the vessel lumen, particularly in the presence of hypercholesterolemia, and also from degenerating foam cells. Circulating high-density lipoprotein (HDL) can help remove cholesterol from these accumulations.

Hemodynamic Disturbances (p. 500)

Despite presumably uniformly distributed injurious agents (e.g., hypercholesterolemia, cigarette toxins, hyperglycemia), atherosclerotic plaques are not randomly distributed and, in fact, characteristically develop at vascular branch points and other areas of disturbed flow. Indeed, non-turbulent laminar flow activates EC genes whose products are *protective* against atherosclerosis.

Lipids (p. 500)

Defects in lipid uptake, metabolism, or binding to circulating apoproteins can lead to elevated lipids. Increased circulating levels accumulate in the vessel wall and cause EC dysfunction by increasing local oxygen free radical formation. Accumulated lipoproteins also become oxidized; oxidized LDL in particular are directly toxic to EC and SMC, causing dysfunction. Moreover, oxidized LDLs are ingested by macrophages through scavenger receptors, causing the formation of *foam cells* and leading to pro-inflammatory macrophage activation.

Inflammation (p. 500)

Dysfunctional EC express increased levels of adhesion molecules (e.g., vascular cell adhesion molecule-1 [VCAM-1]) promoting increased inflammatory cell recruitment. Subsequent T cell and macrophage accumulation and activation leads to local increased cytokine production that drives SMC proliferation and matrix synthesis.

Infection (p. 500)

Herpesvirus, cytomegalovirus, and *Chlamydia pneumoniae* have all been detected in atherosclerotic plaques. It is not clear whether this is coincidence (these are common organisms) or causal (e.g., by driving inflammatory responses).

Smooth Muscle Proliferation (p. 501)

SMC precursors recruited from the circulation or the vessel wall are induced to proliferate and sythesize ECM through the activities of platelet-derived growth factor (released by adherent platelets and inflammatory cells), fibroblast growth factor, and transforming growth factor-α (TGF-α). Activated inflammatory cells can also cause medial SMC apoptosis and increase ECM dgradation, leading to unstable plaques (see later discussion).

Morphology (p. 502)

- *Fatty streaks* are early lesions composed of intimal collections of foamy macrophages and SMC that gently protrude into the vascular lumen. These can occur at virtually any age and even in infants. A causal relationship between fatty streaks and atheromatous plaques is suspected but remains unproved.
- The characteristic atheromatous plaque *(atheroma or fibrofatty plaque)* is a raised white-yellow intimal-based lesion. Plaques are composed of superficial fibrous caps containing SMC, inflammatory cells, and dense ECM overlying necrotic cores, containing dead cells, lipid, cholesterol (manifesting as empty "clefts" on most routine histologic processing), foam cells, and plasma proteins; small blood vessels proliferate at the intimal-medial interface
- Plaques are denoted as *complicated* when they exhibit calcification, hemorrhage, fissuring, or ulceration; such changes are often also associated with local thrombosis, medial thinning, cholesterol microemboli, and aneurysmal dilation.

Consequences of Atherosclerotic Disease (p. 504)

Atherosclerosis is a dynamic process with periods of growth and remodeling beginning in childhood. Most plaques are typically asymptomatic for decades until manifesting via one of the following mechanisms. The resulting restricted flow can cause tissue atrophy or infarction, depending on the severity of the narrowing and the rate at which it develops.

Atherosclerotic Stenosis (p. 504)

Artherosclotic stenosis restricts blood flow to downstream tissues; effects depend on the degree of stenosis and the metabolic demands of the affected tissues.

- Slow insidious narrowing of vascular lumens occurs by gradual accumulation of plaque matrix
- At early stages of stenosis, outward remodeling of the vessel media (leading to overall vessel dilation) can preserve the luminal diameter
- At approximately 70% stenosis *(critical stenosis)*, the vascular supply typically becomes inadequate to meet demand, and ischemia supervenes

Acute Plaque Change (p. 504)

Acute plaque change means that there is plaque erosion, frank rupture, or hemorrhage into the plaque, which expands the plaque volume and can increase luminal stenosis. When plaques are disrupted, the blood can be exposed to highly thrombogenic plaque contents or subendothelial basement membrane, leading to partial or complete vascular thrombosis.

- In most cases of myocardial infarction, plaque disruption and associated precipitous thrombosis occurs at areas of sub-critical stenoses (i.e., less than 70%).
- Intrinsic factors that influence disruption include plaque structure and composition (Fig. 11-3).

    Vulnerable plaques have large deformable atheromatous cores, thin fibrous caps, and/or increased inflammatory cell content (leading to the elaboration of matrix metalloproteinases [MMPs] that degrade ECM).
    Stable plaques have minimal atheromatous cores and thicker, well-collagenized fibrous caps, with relatively less inflammation.

- Extrinsic factors that influence plaque disruption include systemic hypertension and focal vasoconstriction.
- Not all plaque ruptures result in completely occlusive thromboses with catastrophic consequences. Indeed, plaque disruption with partial thrombosis is probably a common, clinically silent complication; organization of such sub-total thromboses is an important mechanim in the growth of atherosclerotic lesions.

Thrombosis (p. 506)

Thrombus that forms over a disrupted plaque or contents of a friable atherosclerotic plaque can embolize and obstruct downstream vessels.

Vasoconstriction (p. 506)

Vasoconstriction can occur at sites of plaque formation due to endothelial dysfunction (with loss of nitric oxide production that normally promotes vasorelaxation) or to products elaborated by aggregated platelets or inflammatory cells.

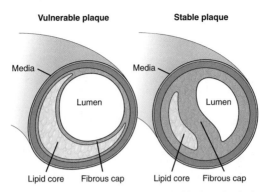

Vulnerable plaque   **Stable plaque**

Media — Lumen — Lipid core — Fibrous cap

FIGURE 11-3 Schematic comparing vulnerable and stable atherosclerotic plaque. Stable plaques have thick, densely fibrotic caps with minimal atheromatous cores and inflammation; vulnerable plaques are prone to rupture due to thin fibrous caps, large deformable lipid cores, and increased inflammation.

Vessel Wall Weakening

Vessel wall weakening can be followed by aneurysm formation and possible rupture (see later discussion).

Aneurysms and Dissections (p. 506)

Aneurysms are abnormal vascular dilations. A *true aneurysm* is bounded by all three vessel wall layers (i.e., intima, media, and adventitia), although the layers can be individually attenuated. In contrast, a *false aneurysm (pseudoaneurysm)* is an extravascular hematoma that communicates with the intravascular space; part of the vessel wall has been lost. A *dissection* occurs when blood enters the arterial wall itself, as a hematoma dissecting between the layers. Morbidity and death due to aneurysms and dissections are secondary to:

- Rupture
- Impingement on adjacent structures
- Occlusion of proximal vessels by extrinsic pressure or superimposed thrombosis
- Embolism from a mural thrombus

Pathogenesis of Aneurysms (p. 506)

Arteries are dynamically remodeling, and the various constituents are constantly turning over. Aneurysms can occur due to:

- *Poor intrinsic quality of the vessel matrix*: In *Marfan syndrome*, inadequate fibrillin synthesis leads to aberrant transforming growth factor-β (TGF-β) activation and progressive loss of elastic tissue matrix; in *Loeys-Dietz syndrome*, TGF-β receptor mutations likewise cause elastic tissue loss. In both cases, aneurysms result from progressive remodeling of an inelastic media. Defective collagen III synthesis in *Ehlers-Danlos syndrome*, or defective collagen cross-linking in vitamin C deficiency *(scurvy)* also lead to aneurysm formation.
- *Imbalance of matrix synthesis matrix and degradation*: Increased MMP activity by inflammatory cells (e.g., in atherosclerotic plaque or in vasculitis) can cause a net loss of medial ECM.
- *Loss of medial SMC or change in SMC matrix synthesis*: Ischemia of the innermost aspect of the aortic media occurs when thick atherosclerotic plaque impedes adequate oxygen and nutritional

diffusion from the lumen. Similarly, mid-medial ischemia of the aorta can occur when vessels of the vasa vasorum are stenosed due to inflammation or hypertension. Such ischemia is reflected in SMC loss and/or "degenerative changes," with loss of normal ECM synthesis and increased production of amorphous ground substance (glycosaminoglycan). These changes are collectively denoted as *cystic medial degeneration* and can be seen in a variety of settings including Marfan syndrome or scurvy.

The most common causes of aortic aneurysms include *atherosclerosis* (particularly in the abdominal aorta) and *hypertension* (particularly in the ascending thoracic aorta). Other causes include syphilis, trauma, vasculitis, and congenital defects (e.g., berry aneurysms). Aneurysms due to infections *(mycotic aneurysms)* can originate from septic embolization (e.g., from bacterial endocarditis), from an adjacent suppurative process, or from systemic bacteremia. The intense, acute inflammation in mycotic aneurysms accelerates vascular wall destruction and potentiates rapid aneurysmal dilation.

Abdominal Aortic Aneurysm (p. 507)

Abdominal aortic aneurysms (AAAs) are true aneurysms; they classically occur in male smokers older than 50 years and are positioned below the renal arteries and above the iliac bifurcation. Pathogenesis involves medial SMC loss and increased matrix degradation by MMP; histology reveals severe complex atherosclerosis with markedly attenuated media. Due to the aneurysmal dilation and abnormal vascular flow, the lumen typically contains a laminated, poorly organized mural thrombus.

Complications include occlusion of a branch vessel, atheroembolism, compression of adjacent structures, or rupture. Risk of rupture increases with the maximal diameter of the AAA: it is low if smaller than 5 cm but 11% annually when 5 to 6 cm and 25% per year when more than 6 cm. Operative mortality rate for AAA repair is 5% for unruptured aneurysms but more than 50% after rupture. Because aortic atherosclerosis is usually accompanied by severe coronary atherosclerosis, patients with AAA also have a high incidence of ischemic heart disease.

Inflammatory AAA is a variant of AAA characterized by dense periaortic fibrosis and an exuberant transmural lymphoplasmacytic infiltrate.

Thoracic Aortic Aneurysms (p. 508)

The most common etiology is hypertension, although Marfan and Loeys-Dietz syndromes are increasingly recognized; syphilis is a rare cause in the United States. Signs and symptoms are referrable to aortic root dilation (aortic valve insufficiency), rupture, or encroachment on mediastinal structures, including airways (dyspnea), esophagus (dysphagia), recurrent laryngeal nerves (cough), or vertebral bodies (bone pain).

Aortic Dissection (p. 508)

Dissection of blood within the aortic media often leads to rupture, causing sudden death through massive hemorrhage or cardiac tamponade. Aortic dissection is not usually associated with marked preexisting aortic dilation. Aortic dissection occurs principally in two groups:

- Hypertensive men between the ages of 40 and 60 years; the aortas typically exhibit variable degrees of cystic medial degeneration
- Younger individuals with connective tissue defects that affect the aorta (e.g., Marfan syndrome)

Other causes of aortic dissection include trauma, complications from therapeutic or diagnostic arterial cannulation, and hormonal and physiologic changes associated with pregnancy. Dissection is uncommon in atherosclerosis or in other conditions with medial scarring, presumably because the fibrosis limits dissection propagation.

Pathogenesis (p. 509)

Medial degeneration (described previously) is the important underlying substrate; the trigger for the intimal tear that begins the dissection is often unknown. Nevertheless, once the tear is initiated, blood flow under systemic pressures advances the dissection plane. In some cases, rupture of the penetrating vessels of the vasa vasorum can give rise to an intramural hematoma without an intimal tear.

Morphology (p. 509)

The most common pre-existing histologic change is cystic medial degeneration, most often without accompanying inflammation. The vast majority of dissections begin as a tear within the first 10 cm above the aortic valve annulus. The dissection plane can extend retrograde to the heart, which causes coronary compression or hemopericardium with tamponade, and/or anterograde, which extends into the great arteries or other major branches. Rupture through the wall of the aorta causes massive hemorrhage; occasionally, re-entry into the lumen gives rise to a double-barreled aorta (i.e., *chronic dissection*).

Clinical Features (p. 509)

The complications following dissection depend strongly on the portion of the aorta affected; dissections are classified into:

- The more common (and dangerous) *proximal* lesions, involving the ascending aorta (called *type A*)
- *Distal lesions not involving the ascending part* and usually beginning distal to the subclavian artery *(type B)*

The classic clinical presentation involves sudden onset of excruciating pain, usually beginning in the anterior chest, radiating to the back, and moving downward as the dissection progresses. Death is usually the result of rupture into the pericardium, thorax, or abdomen; early recognition, institution of anti-hypertensive therapy, and surgical plication allows 65% to 75% survival.

Vasculitis (p. 510)

Vasculitis is vessel wall inflammation; symptoms are typically referable to the ischemia that occurs in the downstream tissues (due to vessel injury and thrombosis), as well as constitutional manifestations (e.g., fever, myalgias, arthralgias, and malaise). Any vessel can be involved, but many of the vasculitides have a predilection for specific vascular sizes or beds. Vasculitides are classified according to vessel size and site, lesion histology, clinical manifestations, and pathogenesis (Fig. 11-4). The two most common pathogenic mechanisms are immune-mediated inflammation and infections; physical and chemical injury (e.g., irradiation, trauma, toxins) can also be causal.

Noninfectious Vasculitis (p. 510)

Immune Complex–Associated Vasculitis (p. 510)

Immune complex–associated vasculitis is caused by vascular deposition of circulating antigen-antibody complexes (e.g., DNA/anti-DNA complexes in systemic lupus erythematosus). Vascular injury arises from complement activation or the recruitment of

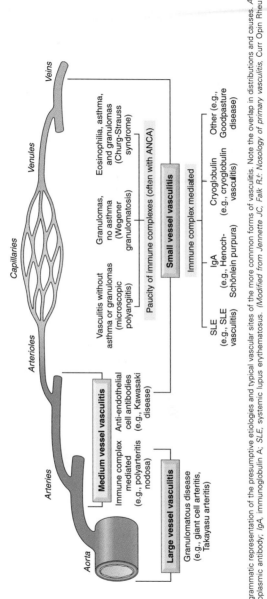

FIGURE 11-4 Diagrammatic representation of the presumptive etiologies and typical vascular sites of the more common forms of vasculitis. Note the overlap in distributions and causes. *ANCA,* Antineutrophil cytoplasmic antibody; *IgA,* immunoglobulin A; *SLE,* systemic lupus erythematosus. *(Modified from Jennette JC, Falk RJ: Nosology of primary vasculitis,* Curr Opin Rheumatol *19:10, 2007.)*

Fc-receptor-bearing cells (Chapter 6). Although the nature of the initiating antigen is not always known, immune complex deposition typically underlies the vasculitis associated with drug hypersensitivities (antibodies against the agent itself or directed against modified self-proteins); in vasculitis secondary to viral infections, antibodies are directed against viral proteins (e.g., hepatitis B surface antigen in 30% of patients with polyarteritis nodosa).

Antineutrophil Cytoplasmic Antibodies (p. 511)

Antineutrophil cytoplasmic antibodies (ANCAs) are a heterogeneous group of autoantibodies directed against the constituents of neutrophil primary granules, monocyte lysosomes, or EC:

- *Anti-myeloperoxidase (MPO-ANCA)* is directed against the lysosomal constituent involved in generating oxygen free radicals; it is also called *perinuclear-ANCA (p-ANCA)*. This antibody is characteristically seen in *microscopic polyangiitis* and *Churg-Strauss syndrome.*
- *Anti-proteinase 3 (PR3-ANCA)* is directed against a neutrophil azurophiic granule constituent, also called *cytoplasmic ANCA (c-ANCA)*. This is characteristically associated with *Wegener granulomatosis.*

ANCAs are useful diagnostic markers for ANCA-associated vasculitides, and titers often mirror inflammation levels, suggesting a pathogenic association. These autoantibodies may be induced via cross-reactive microbial antigens; once formed, they can directly activate neutrophils and thereby cause release of proteolytic enzymes and reactive oxygen species that damage endothelium.

Anti-Endothelial Cell Antibodies (p. 512)

Anti-endothelial cell antibodies may underlie certain vasculitides such as *Kawasaki disease* (see later discussion).

Giant Cell (Temporal) Arteritis (p. 512)

This is the most common form of vasculitis in the United States elderly population; it is characterized by focal granulomatous inflammation of medium-sized and small arteries, chiefly cranial vessels (most commonly the temporal arteries). It can also involve the aorta *(giant cell aortitis)*. The primary etiology is likely a T cell–mediated immune response to vessel wall antigen(s).

Morphology (p. 512)

- Granulomatous vasculitis with elastic tissue fragmentation; multinucleated giant cells are seen in up to 75% of cases.
- Intimal fibrosis with medial scarring and luminal narrowing
- Biopsy may be negative in one third of patients, presumably owing to lesion focality.

Clinical Features (p. 513)

Temporal arteritis typically manifests with headache and facial pain; most patients also have systemic symptoms, including a flu-like syndrome with fever, fatigue, and weight loss. Ophthalmic artery involvement with ocular symptoms appears abruptly in about 50% of patients and can cause permanent blindness. The disease responds well to steroids.

Takayasu Arteritis (p. 513)

This is a granulomatous vasculitis of medium to large arteries characterized by transmural fibrous thickening of the aortic arch and virtual obliteration of the great vessel branches. An immune etiology is likely causal.

Morphology (p. 513)

- *Grossly:* There is irregular aortic thickening with intimal hyperplasia.
- *Microscopically:* Early stages show adventitial perivascular (vasa vasorum) mononuclear cell infiltrates, followed in later stages by medial fibrosis, with granulomas and acellular intimal thickening; the changes are indistinguishable from giant cell arteritis.

Clinical Features (p. 514)

Initial symptoms are usually non-specific (e.g., fatigue, fever, weight loss). Ocular and neurologic disturbances and marked weakening of upper extremity perfusion pressures (hence the name *pulseless disease*) are common. The pulmonary artery is involved in half of cases, and coronary and renal arteries can also be affected; hypertension occurs secondary to the renal artery disease. Takayasu arteritis is diagnosed when the affected patient is younger than 50 years; the same gross and histologic features in older individuals are designated giant cell aortitis.

Polyarteritis Nodosa (p. 514)

Polyarteritis nodosa (PAN) is a systemic disease characterized by necrotizing vasculitis involving small to medium arteries; kidney, heart, liver, and gastrointestinal tract are involved in descending order, and the pulmonary circulation is spared. Immune complex deposition is causal in the third of cases associated with chronic hepatitis, but the etiology of the classic idiopathic and cutaneous forms of PAN is unknown. ANCAs are not involved.

Morphology (p. 514)

PAN lesions are sharply demarcated and often induce thrombosis, causing distal ischemic injury. Lesions at different histologic stages may be present concurrently.

- *Acute* lesions are characterized by sharply circumscribed arterial *fibrinoid necrosis* (hyaline proteinaceous depositions in a degenerating vessel wall) with associated neutrophilic infiltrates that may extend into the adventitia.
- *Healed* lesions show only marked fibrotic thickening of the artery with associated elastic lamina fragmentation and occasionally aneurysmal dilation.

Clinical Features (p. 515)

PAN is largely a disease of young adults with nonspecific systemic symptoms (e.g., fever, malaise, weight loss) and clinical presentations related to the tissues involved (e.g., hematuria, albuminuria, and hypertension [kidneys]). Untreated, the disease is generally fatal, but a 90% remission rate is achieved with immunosuppressive therapy.

Kawasaki Disease (p. 515)

This is an acute febrile, usually self-limited illness of infants and children; it is associated with a medium-large vessel arteritis. The etiology is a T-cell hypersensitivity to yet-unidentified antigens.

Morphology (p. 515)

Lesions resemble those of PAN.

Clinical Features (p. 515)

Also known as mucocutaneous lymph node syndrome, the disease is typically heralded by fever, lymphadenopathy, skin rash, and oral/conjunctival erythema. Its clinical significance stems largely from its propensity to cause coronary arteritis (20% of untreated patients), forming aneurysms that rupture or thrombose, and leading to myocardial infarction. Aspirin and intravenous (IV) gamma globulin reduce the coronary arteritis incidence roughly five-fold.

Microscopic Polyangiitis (p. 515)

This is a necrotizing vasculitis of vessels (i.e., arterioles, capillaries, and venules) smaller than those involved in PAN, with lesions typically all at the same histologic stage. In some cases, an antibody response to drugs, microbes, or tumor proteins (e.g., in lymphoproliferative disorders) has been implicated with immune complex deposition; however, most lesions are pauci-immune, and MPO-ANCAs are increasingly implicated.

Morphology (p. 515)

There is typically fibrinoid necrosis although affected vessels may show only fragmented neutrophilic nuclei within and around vessel walls *(leukocytoclastic vasculitis)*. Necrotizing glomerulonephritis (90% of patients) and pulmonary capillaritis are particularly common. Little or no immunoglobulin deposition is seen in most lesions.

Clinical Features (p. 515)

The clinical consequences depend on the vascular bed involved and can include hemoptysis (lungs), hematuria and proteinuria (kidneys), purpura (skin), or bowel pain and bleeding. Cyclosporine and steroids induce remission and improve long-term survival.

Churg-Strauss Syndrome (p. 516)

Also called *allergic granulomatosis and angiitis,* this is a small-vessel necrotizing vasculitis associated with asthma, allergic rhinitis, peripheral eosinophilia, and extravascular necrotizing granulomas. ANCAs are identified in less than 50% of cases. Vascular lesions resemble PAN but are also characteristically accompanied by eosinophils and granulomas. Eosinophilic infiltrates are causally implicated in the cardiomyopathy that develops in 60% of patients; the cardiac involvement is the cause of mortality in roughly half the patients.

Wegener Granulomatosis (p. 516)

This is a necrotizing vasculitis associated with the triad:

- Necrotizing or granulomatous vasculitis of small to medium vessels mostly in the lung and upper airway
- Necrotizing granulomas of the upper and lower respiratory tract
- Glomerulonephritis

A T-cell hypersensitivity to an inhaled agent or microbe is likely causal, although PR3-ANCAs are present in 95% of cases.

Morphology (p. 516)

- Granulomas occur with geographic necrosis and accompanying vasculitis
- Granulomas may coalesce to produce nodules that cavitate.
- Renal lesions vary from focal and segmental necrosis and scarring to proliferative (crescentic) glomerulonephritis.

Clinical Features (p. 517)

Men older than 40 years are the most commonly affected group. Without treatment, there is 80% 1-year mortality; treatment with cyclophosphamide, steroids, and tumor necrosis factor (TNF) antagonists is largely effective.

Thromboangiitis Obliterans (Buerger Disease) (p. 517)

Typically encountered in heavy cigarette smokers younger than 35 years, this is a segmental, thrombosing, acute, and chronic inflammation of intermediate and small arteries and veins in the extremities. A T-cell hypersensitivity response to smoke-modified self antigens is implicated.

Morphology (p. 517)

- Acute lesions include neutrophilic infiltrates with mural thrombi containing microabscesses, often with giant cell formation and secondary involvement of the adjacent vein and nerve
- Late lesions show organization and recanalization

Clinical Features (p. 517)

Clinical consequences include nodular phlebitis, Raynaud-like cold sensitivity (see later discussion), and leg claudication. The vascular insufficiency can lead to excruciating pain (even at rest, suggesting neural involvement), skin ulcers, and ultimately gangrene.

Vasculitis Associated with Other Disorders (p 517)

Vasculitis that clinically and histologically resembles PAN or hypersensitivity angiitis may be attributable to other disorders such as rheumatoid arthritis, malignancy, or antiphospholipid antibody syndrome. Identifying the underlying etiology has important therapeutic implications (e.g., immunosuppression versus anti-coagulation).

Infectious Vasculitis (p. 517)

Arteritis can be caused by direct invasion from an adjacent source (especially *Aspergillus* and *Mucor*) or can originate from septic embolization (e.g., from bacterial endocarditis). Vascular infections can result in mycotic aneurysms or cause thrombosis and downstream infarction.

Raynaud Phenomenon (p. 518)

Raynaud phenomenon results from exaggerated vasoconstriction of digital (and sometimes facial) arteries and arterioles, producing pain, pallor, and even cyanosis; prolonged vasospasm can result in tissue necrosis.

- *Primary Raynaud phenomenon* occurs in 3% to 5% of the general population and most commonly affects young women; it reflects exaggerated vasomotor responses to cold or emotion. The clinical course is usually benign.
- *Secondary Raynaud phenomenon* is vascular insufficiency due to arterial narrowing induced by other conditions (e.g., atherosclerosis, systemic lupus erythematosus, systemic sclerosis [scleroderma], or Buerger disease).

Veins and Lymphatics (p. 518)

Vein disorders are extremely common; 90% involve *varicose veins* or *thrombophlebitis/phlebothrombosis*.

Varicose Veins (p. 518)

These are typically superficial lower extremity veins that are dilated and tortuous due to chronically elevated intraluminal pressure. They occur in 10% to 20% of men, and 25% to 33% of women; the increased frequency in women is due to the venous stasis occurring in pregnancy. Other causes include hereditary venous defects, obesity, prolonged dependent leg position, proximal thrombosis, and compressive tumor masses.

Vein dilation renders the valves incompetent, with stasis, persistent edema, and trophic skin changes, ultimately resulting in stasis dermatitis; affected tissues may have impaired circulation and poor healing with *varicose ulcers*. Although thrombosis is common, superficial varicosities are rarely sources of clinically significant emboli.

Varicosities in two other sites merit mention:

• *Esophageal varices* are typically due to portal vein hypertension (secondary to cirrhosis, or hepatic or portal vein thrombosis); portal hypertension opens porto-systemic shunts, which increase flow into veins at the gastro-esophageal junction (esophageal varices), rectum (hemorrhoids), and periumbilical veins *(caput medusa)*. Esophageal varices are most important since their rupture can lead to exsanguination.

• *Hemorrhoids* can also result from primary dilation of the anorectal venous plexus (e.g., secondary to pregnancy or chronic constipation). They can ulcerate and bleed or thrombose and become painfully inflamed.

Thrombophlebitis and Phlebothrombosis (p. 519)

These are largely interchangeable terms for venous thrombosis and inflammation. Predisposing factors for *deep vein thrombosis (DVT)* include congestive heart failure, prolonged immobilization, local infection, or systemic hypercoagulability (e.g., neoplasia, pregnancy, or the postoperative state). Although 90% of thromboses occur in deep leg veins, the periprostatic plexus in men and ovarian and pelvic veins in women are other important sites. *In contrast to superficial vein thromboses, DVT are common sources of pulmonary emboli.*

Migratory thrombophlebitis (Trousseau syndrome) is a malignancy-associated hypercoagulability due to procoagulant elaboration (Chapter 7); it is characterized by sporadic thrombosis at various sites.

Superior and Inferior Vena Caval Syndromes (p. 519)

• Superior vena cava (SVC) syndrome is usually caused by neoplasms compressing or invading the SVC (e.g., primary bronchogenic carcinoma). The resulting vascular obstruction produces a distinctive dusky cyanosis and marked dilation of head, neck, and arm veins.

• Inferior vena cava (IVC) syndrome is caused by extrinsic IVC compression or occlusion. In addition, certain neoplasms, particularly hepatocellular and renal cell carcinomas, tend to grow within veins and ultimately obstruct the IVC. IVC obstruction induces marked leg edema, distention of the lower abdominal superficial collateral veins, and—when renal veins are involved—massive proteinuria.

Lymphangitis and Lymphedema (p. 519)

Lymphangitis denotes the inflammation occurring when infections spread into lymphatics; β-hemolytic streptococci are a common cause. Lymphangitis presents as painful subcutaneous red streaks, often with tender regional lymphadenopathy *(lymphadenitis)*. Dilated lymphatics are filled with neutrophils and macrophages; inflammation can extend into adjacent tissues with cellulitis or abscess formation.

Lymphedema is due to lymphatic obstruction and dilation, with associated increases in interstitial fluid. Primary hereditary causes include *Milroy disease* (primary lymphatic agenesis). Common secondary causes of lymphedema are:

* Malignancy
* Surgical resection of regional lymph nodes
* Post-radiation fibrosis
* Filariasis
* Postinflammatory thrombosis with lymphatic scarring

Prolonged lymphedema causes interstitial fibrosis, and in cutaneous tissues it causes a *peau d'orange* (orange peel) appearance, with associated ulcers and *brawny induration*. Rupture of obstructed lymphatics in a body cavity leads to milky *chylous* accumulations.

Tumors (p. 520)

Primary tumors of blood vessels and lymphatics run the gamut from common (i.e., benign *hemangiomas*) to intermediate frequency, locally aggressive lesions, to rare (i.e., highly malignant *angiosarcomas*). Congenital or developmental malformations and non-neoplastic reactive vascular proliferations (e.g., *bacillary angiomatosis*) can also present as tumor-like lesions.

Vascular neoplasms can be EC-derived or can arise from cells that support or surround blood vessels. In general, benign vascular neoplasms are composed of well-formed vascular channels lined by EC; at the other end of the spectrum, malignant tumors show few or poorly developed vascular channels with solid, cellular, anaplastic endothelial proliferation.

Benign Tumors and Tumor-Like Conditions (p. 520)

Hemangiomas (p. 520)

Hemangiomas are very common lesions, accounting for 7% of all benign pediatric tumors.

* *Capillary hemangiomas* (p. 520) are the most common type of vascular tumor, occurring primarily in skin or mucous membranes. These are unencapsulated lesions 1 mm to several centimeters in size, composed of closely packed aggregates of capillary-sized, thin-walled vessels. They may be partially or completely thrombosed. The *juvenile (strawberry) hemangioma* variant is present at birth in 1 of 200 children, grows rapidly for a few months, and begins regressing at 1 to 3 years; most disappear by age 7 years.
* *Cavernous hemangiomas* (p. 521) are unencapsulated lesions usually 1 to 2 cm in diameter (with rare giant forms), exhibiting large thin-walled vascular spaces. In addition to the skin, the liver is a common site, and lesions can also occur in the central nervous system (CNS) or other viscera. These can be locally destructive and generally do not regress; thrombosis and dystrophic calcification are common. Cavernous hemangiomas in the cerebellum, brain stem, or eye grounds are associated with angiomatous or cystic neoplasms in pancreas and liver in *von Hippel-Lindau disease* (Chapter 28).
* *Pyogenic granulomas* (p. 521) are an ulcerated polypoid variant of capillary hemangiomas, often following trauma. Composed of proliferating capillaries with interspersed edema and inflammatory infiltrates, they resemble exuberant granulation tissue. Pregnancy tumor *(granuloma gravidarum)* is essentially the same lesion, occurring in the gingiva of 1% of pregnant women; they regress postpartum.

Lymphangiomas *(p. 522)*

Lymphangiomas are the benign lymphatic analog of hemangiomas.

- *Simple (capillary) lymphangiomas* (p. 522) are 1 to 2 cm exudate-filled blister-like blebs composed of small lymphatic channels lined by EC; they have a predilection for head, neck, and axillary subcutaneous tissue.
- *Cavernous lymphangiomas* (*cystic hygromas*) (p. 522) are the analog to cavernous hemangioma, occurring in children in the neck or axilla (and rarely retroperitoneally). They can occasionally be large (up to 15 cm) and produce gross deformities; they are not well encapsulated, and complete surgical resection can be difficult.

Glomus Tumor (Glomangioma) *(p. 522)*

Glomus tumor (glomangioma) is a benign, exquisitely painful tumor of modified smooth muscle cells arising from the glomus body, a specialized arteriovenous structure involved in thermoregulation. Tumors occur most commonly in the distal phalanges, especially beneath nail beds. Excision is curative.

Morphology *(p. 522)*

Tumors are less than 1 cm and may be pinpoint; they consist of aggregates, nests, and masses of specialized glomus cells associated with branching vascular channels.

Vascular Ectasias *(p. 522)*

Vascular ectasias are common lesions characterized by local dilations of pre-existing vessels; they are *not* true neoplasms.

- *Nevus flammeus* (p. 522) is the classic "birthmark." It is a macular cutaneous lesion that histologically shows only dermal vessel dilation; most eventually regress. *Port-wine stains* are an important variant that tend to persist and grow along with the child, thickening the involved skin. Such lesions associated with leptomeningeal angiomatous masses, mental retardation, seizures, hemiplegia, and skull radiopacities compose the *Sturge-Weber syndrome*.
- *Spider telangiectasias* (p. 522) are minute subcutaneous arterioles, often pulsatile, arranged in radial fashion around a central core. They typically occur above the waist and are associated with hyperestrogenic states (e.g., pregnancy or cirrhosis).
- *Hereditary hemorrhagic telangiectasia (Osler-Weber-Rendu disease)* (p. 522) is a rare autosomal dominant disorder characterized by multiple small (less than 5 mm) aneurysmal telangiectasias on skin and mucous membranes. Patients present with epistaxis, hemoptysis, or gastrointestinal or genitourinary bleeding.

Bacillary Angiomatosis *(p. 522)*

Bacillary angiomatosis is a vascular proliferation resulting from opportunistic infection in an immunocompromised host; lesions can involve skin, bone, brain, and other organs. It is caused by a Gram-negative bacillus of the *Bartonella* family.

Morphology *(p. 522)*

Skin lesions have one or more red papules or nodular subcutaneous masses; microscopically, these are capillary proliferations composed of atypical EC admixed with neutrophils, nuclear dust, and the causal bacteria. The vascular proliferation results from hypoxia-inducible transcription factor-1α (HIF-1α) induction, which in turn drives vascular endothelial growth factor (VEGF) production. Treatment with erythromycin is curative.

Intermediate-Grade (Borderline) Tumors (p. 523)

Kaposi Sarcoma (p. 523)

Epidemiologically, Kaposi sarcoma (KS) is categorized into four varieties; all share the same underlying viral pathogenesis:

- *Chronic/classic/European KS* occurs typically in elderly men of Eastern European (especially Ashkenazi Jewish) or Mediterranean descent; it is not associated with HIV. Lesions are red-purple cutaneous plaques and nodules on the lower extremities, rarely with visceral involvement.
- *Lymphadenopathic/African/endemic KS* has the same general geographic distribution as Burkitt lymphoma; it is not associated with HIV. Cutaneous lesions are sparse, and the KS occurs largely in lymph node but with occasional visceral involvement that can be quite aggressive.
- *Transplant-associated KS* occurs in patients receiving chronic immunosuppression. Nodal, mucosal, and visceral involvement can be aggressive (and fatal); lesions may regress when immunosuppression is discontinued.
- *Acquired immunodeficiency syndrome (AIDS)-associated (epidemic) KS* may occur anywhere in the skin and mucous membranes, lymph nodes, gastrointestinal tract, or viscera. Wide visceral dissemination occurs early. With antiretroviral therapy, the incidence in the United States AIDS population is now less than 1%; most patients die of opportunistic infections and not KS. In combination with the endemic form of the disease (see preceding), KS constitutes the most common tumor in central Africa.

Pathogenesis (p. 523)

More than 95% of KS lesions are infected with *human herpesvirus-8 (HHV-8)*, also known as *KS-associated herpesvirus (KSHV)*; this agent is both necessary and sufficient for KS development, although a local proliferative milieu (potentially related to inflammatory cell cytokine production) is an important cofactor in disease pathogenesis and clinical expression.

Morphology (p. 524)

Three stages of lesions are recognized:

- *Patches* are pink-purple macules usually confined to the distal lower extremities. Microscopically, these contain dilated, irregular EC-lined spaces, with interspersed lymphocytes, plasma cells, and macrophages (sometimes containing hemosiderin).
- *Raised plaques* have dilated, jagged vascular channels lined by plump spindle cells accompanied by perivascular aggregates of similar spindled cells.
- *Nodular lesions* are more distinctly neoplastic and often herald lymph node and visceral involvement, particularly in the African and AIDS-associated diseases. Microscopically, lesions consist of sheets of plump, spindle-shaped cells creating slit-like vascular spaces filled with erythrocytes; there are intermingled small vessels, with marked hemorrhage and mononuclear inflammatory cell infiltration.

Clinical Features (p. 524)

The course varies widely, depending on the clinical setting; most primary KSHV infections are asymptomatic. Classic KS is generally restricted to the skin, and surgical resection is usually adequate for an excellent prognosis. Radiation and/or chemotherapy is generally effective for the lymphadenopathic form, and withdrawal of immunosuppression can ameliorate the transplantation-associated form. For AIDS-associated KS, antiretroviral therapy is helpful; interferon-α, angiogenesis inhibitors, and blockade of intracellular kinase pathways are also used.

Hemangioendothelioma (p. 524)

Hemangioendotheliomas are neoplasms with clinical behavior straddling benign and malignant. *Epithelioid hemangioepithelioma* is an example; most lesions are cured by excision, although 40% recur, 20% eventually metastasize, and 15% of patients die from their tumor.

Malignant Tumors (p. 524)

Angiosarcoma (p. 524)

Angiosarcomas are malignant endothelial neoplasms on a spectrum from well-differentiated *(hemangiosarcoma)* to anaplastic; they can occur anywhere, but they tend to arise in skin, soft tissue, breast, and liver. Angiosarcomas are aggressive tumors and metastasize readily; 5-year survival rates are roughly 30%.

Hepatic angiosarcomas are associated with exposure to arsenic (some pesticides), polyvinylchloride (some plastics), and Thorotrast (a radio-contrast agent no longer used).

Angiosarcomas can also develop in long-term chronic lymphedema—classically in the ipsilateral arm years after radical mastectomy for breast cancer; the tumor putatively arises from dilated lymphatic vessels *(lymphangiosarcoma)*. Angiosarcomas may also be induced by radiation and are rarely associated with foreign bodies.

Morphology (p. 525)

Cutaneous lesions begin as small, well-demarcated red nodules evolving into large, fleshy, gray-white soft-tissue masses. *Microscopically,* all degrees of differentiation are found, from plump anaplastic EC to undifferentiated lesions with marked cellular atypia (including giant cells), lacking vascular lumens.

Hemangiopericytoma (p. 525)

Hemangiopericytomas are pericyte tumors, commonly arising on the lower extremities or in the retroperitoneum; 50% metastasize. Presenting as slowly enlarging, painless masses, they consist of branching capillary channels encased by nests and masses of spindle-shaped to round cells extrinsic to the EC basement membrane.

Pathology of Vascular Interventions (p. 525)

In the same way that various forms of vascular wall injury result in healing that leads to intimal hyperplasia (e.g., in atherosclerosis), the trauma consequent to vascular intervention tends to induce a concentric intimal thickening composed of recruited SMC and associated ECM.

Angioplasty and Endovascular Stents (p. 526)

Angioplasty dilates arterial stenoses (typically coronary arteries) using a balloon catheter. Balloon dilation of an atherosclerotic vessel causes plaque fracture and medial dissection; complications include abrupt re-closure (uncommon) and proliferative restenosis in 30% to 50% of patients within the post-procedural 4 to 6 months. Angioplasty is rarely now performed without concurrent stent placement.

Vascular stents are expandable tubes of metallic mesh that pre-serve luminal patency at angioplasty sites. Stents can ameliorate the untoward effects of angioplasty by providing a larger and more regular lumen, acting as a scaffold to support the intimal flaps and dissections that occur during angioplasty, limiting elastic recoil and preventing vascular spasm, and increasing blood flow. Neverthe-less, both early thrombosis and late intimal thickening can occur and lead to vascular occlusion. Use of anticoagulation and incorporation of anti-proliferative drugs in the stents (*drug-eluting stents*) are current therapeutic approaches to these issues.

Vascular Replacement (p. 526)

Large-diameter (i.e., more than 10 cm) synthetic grafts in high-flow locations such as the aorta perform well. In contrast, small-diameter vascular conduits (i.e., less than 6 to 8 mm)—autologous saphenous vein or expanded polytetrafluoroethylene—perform less durably. Graft failure is related to thrombotic occlusion (i.e., early) or intimal fibrous hyperplasia (i.e., months to years), either generalized (i.e., vein grafts) or at anastomoses only (i.e., synthetic grafts).

The patency of saphenous veins used as coronary artery bypass grafts is 50% at 10 years. In comparison, internal mam-mary arteries used as coronary bypass grafts have more than 90% patency at 10 years.

12

The Heart

Effects of Aging on the Heart (p. 531)

- Reduced ventricular cavity size (base-to-apex) leading to bulging of the basal ventricular septum and partial functional outflow obstruction *(sigmoid septum)*
- Valve sclerosis and calcification leading to stenosis (aortic valve)
- Valve degenerative changes leading to insufficiency (mitral valve)
- Reduced myocyte number and increased interstitial fibrosis causing reduced contractility and compliance

Heart Disease: Overview of Pathophysiology (p. 532)

Heart disease is the leading cause of morbidity and death worldwide; it accounts for 40% of deaths in the United States. Cardiac disease occurs as a consequence of one (or more) of the following general mechanisms:

- *Failure of the pump,* due to either poor contractile function or inability to relax to allow filling
- *Blood flow obstruction* (e.g., due to atherosclerosis, thrombosis, hypertension, or valvular stenosis)
- *Regurgitant flow* (e.g., due to valvular insufficiency); output from each contraction is directed backward, causing volume overload and diminished forward flow
- *Shunts* that allow abnormal blood flow either right-to-left (bypassing the lungs) or left-to-right (causing volume overload)
- *Abnormal cardiac conduction* leading to uncoordinated myocardial contractions
- *Rupture of the heart or major vessels*

Heart Failure (p. 533)

Congestive heart failure (CHF) is the common end point of many forms of heart disease and affects 2% of the United States population; it is the cause of death in roughly 300,000 patients annually. CHF occurs when impaired function renders the heart unable to maintain output sufficient for the metabolic requirements of the body or when it can only do so at elevated filling pressures. CHF is characterized by diminished cardiac output (forward failure), accumulation of blood in the venous system (backward failure), or both.

When cardiac function is impaired or the workload increases, compensatory mechanisms attempt to maintain arterial pressure and organ perfusion:

- *Frank-Starling mechanism*: Increased filling pressures dilate the heart, thereby increasing functional cross-bridge formation within sarcomeres and enhancing contractility
- *Myocardial hypertrophy* with increased expression of contractile apparatus proteins
- *Activation of neurohumoral systems*

  Autonomic nervous system adrenergic stimulation, which increases heart rate, contractility, and vascular reistance
  Modulating blood volume and pressures by activation of renin-angiotensin-aldosterone system and release of atrial natriuretic peptide

  While initially adaptive, these compensatory changes impose further demands on cardiac function. Moreover, when superimposed on further pathologic insults (e.g., myocyte apoptosis, cytoskeletal changes, and increased extracellular matrix), CHF may supervene.

- Most frequently heart failure occurs due to progressive deterioration of myocardial contractile function *(systolic dysfunction)*; causes include ischemia, pressure or volume overload due to valvular disease, or primary myocardial failure.
- Occasionally, CHF results from the inability of the heart chamber to relax and fill during diastole *(diastolic dysfunction)*; causes include hypertrophy (most common), fibrosis, amyloid deposition, or constrictive pericarditis. Diastolic failure occurs predominantly in patients over the age of 65, and more often in women than men.
- With the exception of frank myocyte death, the *mechanisms* of myocardial decompensation in CHF are not well understood.

Cardiac Hypertrophy: Pathophysiology and Progression to Failure (p. 533)

- Because adult myocytes cannot classically proliferate, the heart responds to pressure or volume overload by increasing myocyte size *(myocyte hypertrophy)*; similar hypertrophy is stimulated by chronic trophic signals (i.e., driven by β-adrenergic receptor activation). The result is an enlarged heart. Notably, similar compensatory changes can occur in residual viable myocardium after myocardial infarction irreversibly damages part of the heart.
- Although the mechanism(s) that translate exogenous stressors into cellular changes is uncertain, individual myocytes exhibit increased DNA ploidy, increased numbers of mitochondria, and increased numbers of sarcomeres. The genetic expression pattern also shifts to a more embryonic phenotype, including fetal isoforms of β-myosin heavy chain, natriuretic peptides, and collagen.
- While hypertrophy is initially adaptive, it can make myocytes vulnerable to injury. The capillary density does not increase in proportion to the cell size increase or metabolic demands. Hypertrophy is also accompanied by interstitial matrix deposition that can diminish cardiac compliance.
- Heart failure may eventually result from a combination of aberrant myocyte metabolism, alterations in intracellular calcium flux, apoptosis, and genetic reprogramming. Increased heart mass is also an independent risk factor for sudden (presumably arrhythmic) cardiac death.
- *Physiologic hypertrophy* (with aerobic exercise) is a volume-load hypertrophy that tends also to induce beneficial effects including increased capillary density, decreased resting heart rate, and decreased blood pressure.

Left-Sided Heart Failure (p. 535)

Major causes include ischemic heart disease, hypertension, aortic and mitral valve disease, and intrinsic myocardial disease. Left-sided failure is manifested by:

- *Pulmonary congestion and edema* due to regurgitant flow or impaired pulmonary outflow
- *Left atrial dilation with atrial fibrillation*
- *Reduced renal perfusion:*

  Salt and water retention
  Ischemic acute tubular necrosis (ATN)
  Impaired waste excretion, causing prerenal azotemia

- *Hypoxic encephalopathy* due to reduced central nervous system perfusion

Right-Sided Heart Failure (p. 536)

Right-sided heart failure is most commonly caused by left-sided failure; thus, in most cases, patients present with biventricular CHF. Isolated right-sided heart failure is caused by tricuspid or pulmonic valvular disease or by intrinsic pulmonary or pulmonary vascular disease causing functional right ventricular outflow obstruction (e.g., cor pulmonale). Right-sided failure is manifested by:

- Right atrial and ventricular dilation and hypertrophy
- Edema, typically in dependent peripheral locations (e.g., feet, ankles, sacrum) with serous effusions in pericardial, pleural, or peritoneal spaces
- Hepatomegaly with centrilobular congestion and atrophy, producing a nutmeg appearance (chronic passive congestion). With severe hypoxia, there is centrilobular necrosis, and elevated right-sided pressures cause central hemorrhage. Subsequent central fibrosis creates "cardiac cirrhosis."
- Congestive splenomegaly with sinusoidal dilation, focal hemorrhages, hemosiderin deposits, and fibrosis
- Renal congestion, hypoxic injury, and ATN (more marked in right- versus left-sided CHF)

Congenital Heart Disease (p. 537)

Congenital heart disease (CHD) refers to cardiac or great vessel abnormalities present at birth; most are attributable to faulty embryogenesis during weeks 3 to 8 of gestation, when major cardiovascular structures develop. Severe anomalies are incompatible with intrauterine survival; thus, defects that permit development to birth generally involve only specific chambers or regions, with the remainder of the heart being normal. Congenital disorders constitute the most common cardiac disease among children, with an incidence of 1% of live births; the incidence is higher in premature infants and stillborns. The most frequent disorders (constituting 85% of cases) are listed in Table 12-1.

Pathogenesis (p. 538)

- The main known causes of CHD are sporadic genetic abnormalities, either single-gene mutations or chromosomal deletions or additions.

  Single-gene mutations typically involve signaling pathways or transcription factors that regulate cardiac development; some of the transcription factors (e.g., GATA-4) are mutated in rare forms of adult-onset cardiomyopathy, suggesting an additional role in maintaining normal post-natal cardiac function.

TABLE 12-1   Frequencies of Congenital Cardiac Malformations*

Malformation	Incidence per Million Live Births	%
Ventricular septal defect	4482	42
Atrial septal defect	1043	10
Pulmonary stenosis	836	8
Patent ductus arteriosus	781	7
Tetralogy of Fallot	577	5
Coarctation of aorta	492	5
Atrioventricular septal defect	396	4
Aortic stenosis	388	4
Transposition of great arteries	388	4
Truncus arteriosus	136	1
Total anomalous pulmonary venous connection	120	1
Tricuspid atresia	118	1
Total	9757	

*Presented as upper quartile of 44 published studies. Percentages do not add to 100% owing to rounding.
From Hoffman JIE, Kaplan S: The incidence of congenital heart disease, *J Am Coll Cardiol* 39:1890, 2002.

Deletion of chromosome 22q11.2 in DiGeorge syndrome affects the development of the third and fourth pharyngeal pouches with thymic, parathyroid, and cardiac defects.

The *most common genetic cause of CHD is trisomy 21* (i.e., Down syndrome); 40% of patients have one or more cardiac defects.

- Beyond known associations, genetics likely also contribute to many lesions; first-degree relatives of affected patients are at increased risk of CHD relative to the general population.
- Environmental (e.g., congenital rubella infection or teratogens) and maternal factors (e.g., gestational diabetes) also contribute to the incidence of CHD.

Clinical Features (p. 539)

Children with CHD have direct hemodynamic sequelae, as well as retarded development and failure to thrive. They are at increased risk for chronic illness and infective endocarditis due to abnormal valves or endocardial injury from jet lesions.

- CHD are either *obstructions* or *shunts*.

Obstructions include abnormal narrowing of chambers, valves, or vessels; a complete obstruction is called an *atresia*.
Shunts denote abnormal communications between heart chambers, between vessels, or between chambers and vessels. Depending on pressure relationships, blood is shunted from right to left, or from left to right (more common).

- *Right-to-left shunts* bypass the lungs, leading to hypoxia and tissue *cyanosis*. Right-to-left shunts also allow venous emboli to enter the systemic circulation *(paradoxical emboli)*. Secondary findings in long-standing cyanotic heart disease include finger and toe *clubbing* (also called *hypertrophic osteoarthropathy*) as well as polycythemia.

- *Left-to-right shunts* cause pulmonary volume overload. If the shunt is prolonged, the vasculature responds with medial hypertrophy and increased vascular resistance to maintain normal pulmonary capillary and venous pressures. As pulmonary resistance approaches systemic levels, a right-to-left shunt occurs *(Eisenmenger syndrome)*. Once there is significant pulmonary hypertension, the underlying structural defects are no longer candidates for surgical correction.

Altered hemodynamics usually cause chamber dilation and/or hypertrophy; however, defects occasionally lead to diminished chamber volume and muscle mass. This is called *hypoplasia* if it occurs during development or *atrophy* if it occurs postnatally.

Left-to-Right Shunts (p. 540)

The major congenital left-to-right shunts are (Fig. 12-1):

- Atrial septal defect (ASD)
- Ventricular septal defect (VSD)
- Patent ductus arteriosus (PDA)

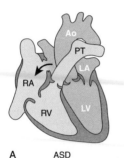
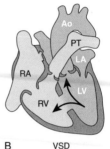
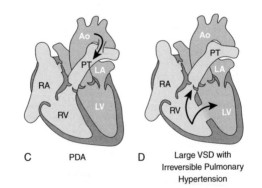

FIGURE 12-1 Schematic of the most important congenital left-to-right shunts. *Arrows* indicate the direction of blood flow. **A,** Atrial septal defect (ASD). **B,** Ventricular septal defect (VSD). In VSD, the shunt is left to right with equilibration of pressures in both ventricles. Pressure hypertrophy of the right ventricle, and volume hypertrophy of the left ventricle are usually present. **C,** Patent ductus arteriosus (PDA). **D,** Large VSD with irreversible pulmonary hypertension. Long-standing pressure overload in the pulmonary circulation has led to increased resistance, and eventually sufficient right ventricular hypertrophy to generate pressures in excess of the left ventricle; at this point, flow reversal occurs with a right-to-left shunt. *Ao,* Aorta; *LA,* left atrium; *LV,* left ventricle; *PT,* pulmonary trunk; *RA,* right atrium; *RV,* right ventricle.

Atrial Septal Defect (p. 541) (see Fig. 12-1, A)

Atrial spetal defects *are the most common congenital cardiac anomalies seen in adults.* Even large ASDs are usually asymptomatic until adulthood, when either right-sided heart failure can occur or right-sided hypertrophy and pulmonary hypertension can induce right-to-left shunting with cyanosis.

*   *Primum type:* 5% of ASD; these occur adjacent to mitral and tricuspid valves.
*   *Secundum type:* 90% of ASD; results from deficient or fenestrated fossa ovalis in the central atrial septum, and is usually not associated with other anomalies.
*   *Sinus venosus type:* 5% of ASD; occurs near the superior vena cava entrance and can be associated with anomalous right pulmonary vein drainage.

Patent Foramen Ovale (p. 541)

Patent foramen ovale is a small hole resulting from defective postnatal closure of the fossa ovalis flap; these occur in 20% of individuals and can be a conduit for paradoxical emboli in the setting of elevated right-sided pressures.

Ventricular Septal Defect (p. 541) (Fig. 12-1, B)

Ventricular septal defects *are the most common congenital cardiac anomaly overall.* Depending on VSD size, the clinical outcome ranges from fulminant CHF to late cyanosis to spontaneous closure (50% of those that are less than 0.5 cm diameter). Surgical correction is desirable before right-sided overload and pulmonary hypertension develop.

*   VSD are frequently associated with other anomalies, particularly *tetralogy of Fallot (TOF),* but 20% to 30% are isolated.
*   90% involve the membranous septum *(membranous VSD)* near the aortic valve, while the remainder are muscular.

Patent Ductus Arteriosus (p. 541) (Fig. 12-1, C)

The ductus arteriosus (just distal to the left subclavian artery) allows blood flow between the aorta and pulmonary artery during fetal development, thus bypassing the lungs. The ductus normally closes within 1 to 2 days of life; depending on its caliber, persistent patency can cause left-to-right shunting that eventually induces Eisenmenger physiology.

*   90% of PDAs are isolated defects; the remainder are associated with VSD, aortic coarctation, or valvular stenosis.
*   Most are initially asymptomatic but produce a harsh continuous *machinery-like* heart murmur. Large PDAs cause right-sided volume and pressure overload.
*   Early closure—surgically or with prostaglandin synthesis inhibitors—is advocated, unless other concurrent CHD (e.g., aortic valve atresia) is present; in the later case, the PDA may be the only means to provide systemic perfusion.

Right-to-Left Shunts (p. 542) (Fig. 12-2)

The major congenital right-to-left shunts (Fig. 12-2) are:

*   Tetralogy of Fallot
*   Transposition of the great arteries (TGA)

Tetralogy of Fallot (p. 542) (Fig. 12-2, A)

The cardinal findings are:

*   VSD
*   Pulmonary stenosis with right ventricle outflow obstruction

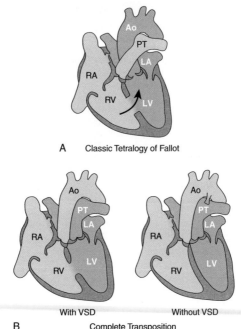

A   Classic Tetralogy of Fallot

With VSD   Without VSD

B   Complete Transposition

FIGURE 12-2 Schematic of the most important congenital right-to-left (cyanotic) shunts. **A,** Tetralogy of Fallot (TOF). The degree of shunting across the VSD depends on the degree of subpulmonic stenosis; if the pulmonary stenosis is severe, a right-to-left shunt occurs *(arrow)*. **B,** Transposition of the great arteries with and without VSD. *Ao,* Aorta; *LA,* left atrium; *LV,* left ventricle; *PT,* pulmonary trunk; *RA,* right atrium; *RV,* right ventricle.

- Overriding aorta
- Right ventricular hypertrophy

Symptom severity is directly related to the extent of right ventricle outflow obstruction. With a large VSD and mild pulmonary stenosis, there is minimal left-to-right shunt and no cyanosis. More severe pulmonary stenosis produces a cyanotic right-to-left shunt.

With complete pulmonary obstruction, survival can occur only by flow through a PDA or dilated bronchial arteries. Surgical correction can be delayed provided that the child can tolerate the level of oxygenation. Pulmonary outflow stenosis protects the lung from volume and pressure overload, and right ventricular failure is rare.

Transposition of the Great Arteries (p. 543) (Fig. 12-2, B)

Systemic and pulmonary venous return—to the right and left atria, respectively—are normal; however, the aorta arises from the right ventricle and the pulmonary artery from the left, so that the pulmonary and systemic circulations are functionally separated.

- Normal fetal development occurs because venous and systemic blood mixes through the ductus arteriosus and a patent foramen ovale.
- Postnatal life critically depends on ongoing blood mixing (e.g., a PDA, VSD, ASD, or patent foramen ovale).

- Prognosis depends on the severity of tissue hypoxia and the ability of the right ventricle to maintain systemic aortic pressures. Untreated, most infants die within months.

Obstructive Congenital Anomalies (p. 544)

Although these will cause ventricular hypertrophy, none cause cyanosis unless there is an additional shunt present.

Coarctation of the Aorta (p. 544)

Coarctation of the aorta is a constriction of the aorta; 50% occur as isolated defects; the remainder occur with other anomalies, most commonly a bicuspid aortic valve. Males are affected twice as often as females, although coarctations are common in Turner syndrome. Besides left ventricular hypertrophy, additional clinical manifestations depend on the location and severity of the constriction and on ductus arteriosus patency.

- *Preductal* coarctation manifests early in life ("infantile form") and can be rapidly fatal. Survival depends on the ability of a PDA to provide adequate systemic blood flow.
- *Postductal* coarctation ("adult form") can be asymptomatic unless severe; effects are also dependent on ductus arteriosus patency:

  An associated PDA leads to right-to-left shunting with lower body cyanosis; survival requires surgical intervention.

  A closed ductus may be asymptomatic but can lead to upper extremity hypertension and lower extremity hypotension with arterial insufficiency (claudication, cold sensitivity). Flow around the coarctation generally develops via internal mammary and axillary artery collaterals; such vascular dilation causes intercostal rib notching notable on x-ray films.

  Surgical resection and end-to-end anastomoses or conduit insertion yields an excellent outcome.

Pulmonary Stenosis and Atresia (p. 544)

Pulmonary stenosis and atresia can be isolated or occur with other anomalies (e.g., transposition or TOF).

- *Valvar stenoses* are associated with right ventricular hypertrophy and post-stenotic pulmonary artery dilation.
- In *subvalvar stenoses*, the right ventricular pressures are not transmitted to the pulmonary circulation; the pulmonary trunk is not dilated, and it may be hypoplastic.
- In *complete pulmonary atresia*, blood flow to the lungs occurs via an ASD and PDA, and the right ventricle is hypoplastic.

Aortic Stenosis and Atresia (p. 544)

- *Valvar aortic stenosis* can be caused by a small hypoplastic valve, thickened dysplastic cusps, or abnormal numbers of cusps (i.e., bicuspid or unicuspid)
- Infants with severe aortic stenosis or atresia can only survive via PDA flow to the aorta and coronaries; there is left ventricular under-development (i.e., *hypoplastic left heart syndrome*).
- *Subaortic stenosis* due to a discrete ring or diffuse collar of endocardial fibrosis is associated with infective endocarditis, left ventricle hypertrophy, post-stenotic aortic dilation, and sudden death.
- *Supravalvar stenosis* is a heritable form of aortic dysplasia with a thickened wall; it may be due to elastin gene mutations, or it may be part of a multi-organ developmental disorder due to partial chromosome 7 deletion (Williams-Beuren syndrome).

Ischemic Heart Disease (p. 545)

Ischemic heart disease (IHD) comprises multiple pathophysiologically related syndromes related to myocardial ischemia, that is, mismatch between cardiac demand and vascular supply of oxygenated blood. The consequences are oxygen insufficiency *(hypoxia, anoxia)*, inadequate nutrient supply, and diminished metabolite removal. In the United States, IHD is annually responsible for 500,000 deaths.

Ischemia results from three possible causes:

- *Reduced coronary blood flow* is commonly due to coronary atherosclerosis (more than 90% of cases), vasospasm, and/or thrombosis. Atherosclerosis causes chronic progressive narrowing of the coronary lumens, a process that can be punctuated by acute plaque disruption and thrombosis (Chapter 11). Uncommon causes of compromised flow include arteritis, emboli, and hypotension (e.g., shock).
- *Increased myocardial demand* (e.g., tachycardia, hypertrophy).
- *Hypoxia due to diminished oxygen transport* (nutrient supply and metabolite removal are not affected); causes include anemia, lung disease, cyanotic CHD, carbon monoxide (CO) poisoning, or cigarette smoking.

There are four overlapping ischemic syndromes, differing in severity and tempo:

- Angina pectoris
- Myocardial infarction
- Chronic IHD
- Sudden cardiac death

Angina Pectoris (p. 546)

This is paroxysmal substernal pain; ischemia duration and severity are not sufficient to cause infarction. Three patterns are recognized based on etiology:

- *Stable angina* reliably occurs with the same level of exertion and diminishes with rest; this is typically associated with 70% or greater chronic stable stenosis (i.e., a fixed supply that becomes limiting with increased demand).
- *Prinzmetal angina* is due to vasospasm; symptoms are unrelated to exertion and respond promptly to vasodilators.
- *Unstable (crescendo) angina* is a pattern of pain occurring with successively lesser amounts of exertion or even at rest; it occurs when atherosclerotic plaque is disrupted—often with associated thrombosis or vasospasm. Myocardial death does not occur, because thrombi either fragment spontaneously or undergo fibrinolysis; alternatively, vasospasm can subside. Although the duration and extent of luminal obstruction in unstable angina is insufficient to cause cell death, it is a harbinger of myocardial infarction.

Myocardial Infarction (p. 547)

Myocardial infarction (MI) is myocyte cell death caused by vascular occlusion. In the United States, 1.5 million MIs occur annually with risk increasing progressively with age; 10% occur in individuals who are 40 years old or younger; 45% occur in people who are 65 years of age or younger.

Pathogenesis (p. 547)

MIs are most commonly due to intraplaque hemorrhage, plaque erosion, or plaque rupture with superimposed thrombosis. In 10% of cases, vascular occlusion is a consequence of vasospasm or embolization in the coronary circulation or due to smaller vessel obstruction (e.g., vasculitis, amyloidosis, sickle cell disease, etc.).

- Coronary occlusion causes myocardial ischemia, dysfunction, and, potentially, myocyte death; the outcome depends on the severity and duration of flow deprivation (Fig. 12-3).

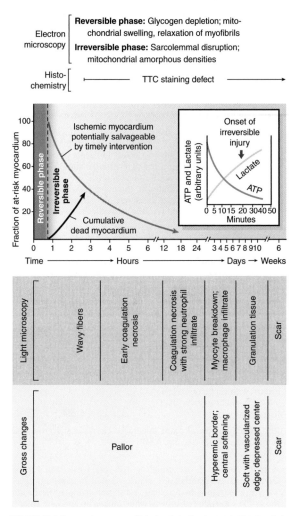

FIGURE 12-3 Temporal sequence of biochemical, ultrastructural, histochemical, and histologic findings after onset of severe myocardial ischemia. For approximately half an hour after onset of ischemia, myocardial injury is potentially reversible. Thereafter, progressive loss of viability occurs and is complete by 6 to 12 hours. The benefits of reperfusion are greatest when it is achieved early with progressively smaller benefit occurring as reperfusion is delayed. *ATP,* Adenosine triphosphate; *TTC,* triphenyl tetrazolium chloride. *(Data from Schoen FJ: Pathologic considerations of the surgery of adult heart disease. In Edmunds LH (ed): Cardiac surgery in the adult, New York, 1997, McGraw-Hill, p. 85.)*

Severe ischemia leads to ATP depletion and loss of contractile function (but not cell death) within 60 seconds; this may precipitate myocardial failure long before there is cell death.

Complete deprivation of blood flow for 20 to 30 minutes leads to irreversible myocardial injury.

Severe compromise of flow for prolonged periods (i.e., 2 to 4 hours) can also cause irreversible injury; this delay before cell death provides impetus for "late" therapeutic interventions to salvage myocardium during an MI.

Necrosis is usually complete within 6 hours of severe ischemia; however, with extensive coronary collateral circulation, necrosis can follow a more protracted course (i.e., more than 12 hours).

- The distribution of myocardial necrosis depends on the vessel involved (e.g., left anterior descending versus right coronary artery) and collateral perfusion, as well as the location of the occlusion within the vessel and the cause of diminished perfusion.

  Most MIs occur within the distribution of a single coronary artery and are *transmural* (the full thickness of the ventricular wall); these are due to atherosclerosis and acute plaque change with thrombosis. These characteristically show electrocardiographic ST elevations ("ST elevation MI")

  Subendocardial MIs are limited to the inner 30% to 50% of the ventricle and may involve more territory than is perfused by a single coronary. These result in *non-ST elevation MI*. Causes include:

  - Lysis of a thrombotic occlusion before full-thickness infarction
  - Chronic atherosclerotic disease in the setting of increased myocardial demand (e.g., tachycardia) or systemically diminished supply (e.g., hypotension, anemia, lung disease)

- Reflow to (i.e., *reperfusion* of) precariously injured cells (e.g., by intervention with thrombolytics) may restore viability but leave the cells poorly contractile *(stunned)* for 1 to 2 days (p. 553). Reperfused myocardium is usually somewhat hemorrhagic due to ischemic vascular injury; irreversibly injured myocytes that are reperfused also show *contraction band necrosis* due to calcium overload and hyper-tetanic contraction. Finally, reperfusion can potentially cause additional injury by heightened recruitment of inflammatory cells and perfusion-induced microvascular injury with capillary occlusion.

Morphology (p. 550)

After infarction, myocardium undergoes characteristic gross and microscopic changes (see Fig. 12-3):

  Gross changes:

- *6 to 12 hours:* MIs are usually grossly inapparent but can be highlighted by histochemical stains; triphenyltetrazolium chloride is a lactate dehydrogenase substrate; viable myocardium turns the substrate red-brown, while nonviable areas are pale.
- *18 to 24 hours:* Infarcted tissue becomes apparent as pale to cyanotic areas.
- *1 week:* Lesions become progressively more defined, yellow, and softened.
- *7 to 10 days:* Hyperemic granulation tissue appears at the infarct edges; with time, granulation tissue progressively fills in the infarct.
- *1 to 2 months:* White fibrous scar is usually well established.

Microscopic changes:

- *Less than 1 hour:* Intercellular edema, and wavy myocytes at the infarct margin; coagulative necrosis is not yet evident.
- *12 to 72 hours:* Dead myocytes become hypereosinophilic with loss of nuclei *(coagulative necrosis);* neutrophils also progressively infiltrate necrotic tissue.
- *3 to 7 days:* Dead myocytes are digested by invading macrophages.
- *7 to 10 days:* Granulation tissue progressively replaces necrotic tissue.
- *More than 2 weeks:* Granulation tissue is progressively replaced by fibrous scar.

Clinical Features (p. 553)

MI diagnosis is based on symptoms (e.g., chest pain, nausea, diaphoresis, dyspnea), electrocardiographic changes, and serum elevation of cardiomyocyte-specific proteins released from dead cells (e.g., creatine kinase MB [CK-MB] isoform or various troponins). In 10% to 15% of patients (especially diabetic or geriatric), symptoms are absent (silent MI).

- Nearly all transmural MIs affect the left ventricle; 15% also involve the right ventricle, particularly in posterior-inferior left ventricle infarcts. Isolated right ventricle infarction occurs in 1% to 3% of cases.
- Half of MI-associated deaths occur within the first hour; most patients die before reaching a hospital. Overall, mortality is 30% in the first year after an MI, with 3% to 4% mortality per annum thereafter.
- Therapies in the acute setting include anticoagulation, oxygen, nitrates, β-adrenergic blockade, angiotensin-converting enzyme inhibitors, and fibrinolytics; coronary angioplasty, stenting, or surgical bypass can also be performed.

Complications of an MI depend on the size and location of injury, as well as functional myocardial reserves.

- Contractile dysfunction occurs roughly in proportion to the extent of infarction; effects include systemic hypotension and pulmonary edema (e.g., CHF). Severe pump failure (cardiogenic shock) occurs in 10% to 15% of patients, typically with loss of 40% or more left ventricular mass. Cardiogenic shock has a 70% mortality rate.
- Arrhythmias.
- Ventricular rupture (1% to 2% of transmural MIs) can occur typically within the first 10 days (median, 4 to 5 days). Rupture of the free wall causes pericardial tamponade; septal rupture causes a left-to-right shunt with right-sided volume overload; papillary muscle infarction (with or without ventricular rupture) causes mitral regurgitation.
- Fibrinous pericarditis (Dressler syndrome) is common 2 to 3 days after MI.
- Mural thrombosis adjacent to a noncontractile area can be a source of peripheral embolization.
- Stretching of a large area of transmural infarction *(expansion)* may heal into a *ventricular aneurysm;* both are prone to mural thrombosis.
- Infarction adjacent to existing MI *(extension)* can occur.

After MI, non-infarcted myocardium undergoes hypertrophy and dilation *(ventricular remodeling).* While initially hemodynamically beneficial, such changes can become substrate for aneurysms or for areas of secondary ischemia and arrhythmia.

Chronic Ischemic Heart Disease (p. 558)

The term designates progressive heart failure due to ischemic myocardial damage; it may result from postinfarction cardiac decompensation or slow ischemic myocyte degeneration.

- Invariably, there is some degree of obstructive coronary atherosclerosis, often with evidence of prior healed infarcts. *Microscopically,* there is myocyte hypertrophy, diffuse subendocardial myocyte vacuolization, and interstitial and replacement fibrosis.
- Patients need not have a prior diagnosed MI; diagnosis depends on excluding other causes of CHF.

Sudden Cardiac Death (p. 558)

Sudden cardiac death (SCD) is defined as *unexpected cardiac death within 1 hour of symptom onset.* More than 300,000 cases occur annually in the United States, and the vast majority of cases are due to lethal arrhythmia. IHD is the dominant cause, with 80% to 90% of victims having significant atherosclerotic stenoses, often with acute plaque disruption. In patients who survive SCD (by cardiac resuscitation), only 25% actually develop an MI, indicating that a fatal arrhythmia (e.g., asystole or ventricular fibrillation) is the most common cause of death. Arrhythmias are presumably triggered by conduction system scarring, acute ischemic injury, or electrical instability resulting from an ischemic focus. SCD is infrequently a consequence of myocardial hypertrophy (e.g., due to aortic valvular stenosis or hypertrophic cardiomyopathy), hereditary or acquired conduction system abnormalities, electrolyte derangements, mitral valve prolapse, myocardial depositions, or myocarditis.

Some SCD is attributable to heritable conditions with recognizable structural abnormalities (e.g., mitral valve prolapse or hypertrophic cardiomyopathy). Others are primarily electrical disorders related to defects either in conduction pathways (e.g., *Wolff-Parkinson-White syndrome*) or mutations in ion channels. The latter, called *channelopathies,* are typically autosomal dominant disorders involving ion channel proteins (for Na^+, K^+, or Ca^{2+} transport) or accessory molecules that conduct the electrical currents that control myocardial contraction. *Long QT syndrome* is prototypical; mutations in one of at least seven different genes result in diminished K^+ currents that, in turn, prolong the QT repolarization interval and increase the susceptibility to malignant arrhythmias.

Hypertensive Heart Disease (p. 559)

Systemic (Left-Sided) Hypertensive Heart Disease (p. 559)

Hypertrophy of the heart is an adaptive response to chronically elevated pressures; with continued overload, the result can be dysfunction, dilation, CHF, or SCD. The minimal criteria for diagnosing systemic hypertensive heart disease is a history or pathologic evidence of hypertension plus left ventricular hypertrophy (typically concentric) in the absence of other lesions that induce cardiac hypertrophy (e.g., aortic valve stenosis, aortic coarctation).

- Myocyte hypertrophy increases the content of contractile proteins. However, thickened myocardium reduces left ventricle compliance, impairing diastolic filling while increasing oxygen demand. Hypertrophy is also usually accompanied by interstitial fibrosis that also reduces compliance.
- Depending on the severity and duration of underlying hypertension (and adequacy of therapy) patients can have normal

longevity, develop IHD as a consequence of the potentiating effects of hypertension and atherosclerosis, suffer the renal or cerebrovascular complications of hypertension, or experience progressive CHF or even SCD.

Pulmonary (Right-Sided) Heart Disease (Cor Pulmonale) (p. 559)

Cor pulmonale is the right-sided counterpart to systemic hypertensive heart disease; disorders that affect lung structure or function (e.g., emphysema or primary pulmonary hypertension) can cause pulmonary vascular hypertension, resulting in right ventricular hypertrophy, dilation, and/or failure. Recall that the most common cause of pulmonary venous hypertension is left-sided heart disease.

- *Acute cor pulmonale* with right ventricular dilation occurs after massive pulmonary embolization
- *Chronic cor pulmonale* results from chronic right ventricular pressure overload (e.g., CHD or primary lung disease)

Valvular Heart Disease (p. 560)

Causes of *acquired* valvular heart disease (CHD constitutes a third of total valvular disease):

- Degeneration (e.g., calcific aortic stenosis, mitral annular calcification, mitral valve prolapse)
- Inflammatory processes (e.g., rheumatic heart disease)
- Infection (e.g., infective endocarditis)
- Changes secondary to myocardial disease (e.g., IHD causing *ischemic mitral regurgitation*)

The clinical consequences depend on the valve involved, the degree of impairment, whether the lesion is stenotic (pressure overload) or regurgitant (volume overload), the tempo of onset, compensatory changes, and any co-morbid disease.

Calcific Aortic Stenosis (p. 561)

Calcific aortic stenosis is a common (i.e., occurs in 2% of the population) degenerative age-related lesion that typically becomes clinically significant in individuals older than 70 years. Earlier onset (i.e., patients between the ages of 50 and 60 years) occurs most commonly in congenitally bicuspid valves (about 1% of the population); bicuspid valves are responsible for roughly half of adult aortic stenosis. Although "wear and tear" has been cited as an etiology for calcific aortic stenosis, newer data implicate chronic injury due to hypertension, hyperlipidemia, and inflammation.

Morphology (p. 562)

- *Sclerosis* (valve fibrosis) is an early, hemodynamically inconsequential stage.
- Nodular, rigid calcific subendothelial masses on the valve outflow surface impede mobility and aortic outflow.
- There is no commissural fusion, and the thickening spares the cuspal free edges.
- Concentric left ventricular hypertrophy is common due to chronic pressure overload.

Clinical Features (p. 562)

The failure of compensatory hypertrophy mechanisms is heralded by angina (reduced perfusion in hypertrophied myocardium), syncope (with increased risk of SCD), or CHF; if untreated, there is a 50% mortality within 2 to 5 years. Surgical valve replacement improves survival.

Mitral Annular Calcification (p. 563)

Mitral annular calcificiation is due to degenerative, non-inflammatory calcific deposits, most commonly in women older than 60 years or in individuals with mitral valve prolapse (see later discussion). While usually inconsequential, annular calcification can cause:

- Regurgitation due to poor systolic contraction of the mitral valve ring
- Stenosis due to poor leaflet excursion over bulky deposits
- Impingement on conduction pathways, causing arrhythmias
- Rarely, a focus for infective endocarditis.

Mitral Valve Prolapse (p. 563)

One or both mitral valve leaflets are enlarged, redundant, myxomatous, and floppy; they balloon back (prolapse) into the left atrium during systole. Mitral valve prolapse affects 3% of the United States population, most commonly young women. The etiology is uncertain; a high frequency in Marfan syndrome suggests abnormal extracellular matrix synthesis potentially related to dysregulated TGF-β signaling.

Morphology (p. 563)

- *Grossly:* Redundancy and ballooning is seen with elongated, attenuated, or occasionally ruptured chordae tendineae.
- *Microscopically:* The *fibrosa* layer (on which the strength of the leaflet depends) shows thinning and degeneration with myxomatous expansion of the *spongiosa*.
- Secondary changes include: fibrous thickening of valve leaflets at points of contact; thickened ventricular endocardium at sites of contact with prolapsing leaflets; atrial thrombosis behind the ballooning cusps.

Clinical Features (p. 563)

Some patients also have aortic, tricuspid, or pulmonary valve myxomatous degeneration. *Mitral valve prolapse is generally asymptomatic* and discovered only as a mid-systolic click on auscultation; more severe cases may also have mitral regurgitation. Importantly, 3% of patients develop complications secondary to:

- Infective endocarditis
- Mitral insufficiency resulting in CHF
- Arrhythmias and/or SCD
- Embolization of atrial or leaflet thrombi

Rheumatic Fever and Rheumatic Heart Disease (p. 565)

Rheumatic fever (RF) is an acute inflammatory disease classically occurring in children after group A streptococcal infection (usually pharyngitis). It is attributed to host anti-streptococcal antibodies and/or T cells that cross-react with cardiac antigens. The cell and antibody responses in turn cause progressive valve damage with fibrosis (rheumatic heart disease [RHD]). Solitary mitral involvement occurs in 65% to 70% of cases with combined aortic and mitral involvement in 20% to 25%; tricuspid and pulmonary valves are less frequently affected. RHD is virtually the only cause of acquired mitral valve stenosis.

Morphology (p. 565)

Acute phase:

- *Aschoff bodies* are pathognomonic for RF; these are myocardial, pericardial, or endocardial foci of fibrinoid necrosis surrounded by mononuclear inflammatory cells. Activated macrophages in these lesions, called *Anitschkow cells,* have characteristic wavy chromatin aggegation, giving rise to the designation *caterpillar cells.*

- Inflammatory valvulitis is characterized by beady fibrinous vegetations *(verrucae)* along the lines of valve closure.
- With time, these inflammatory foci are replaced by scar.

Chronic (or healed) phase:

- Diffuse fibrous thickening of valve leaflets, with fibrous commissural fusion generating "fishmouth" or "buttonhole" stenoses
- Thickened, fused, and shortened chordae
- Subendocardial collections of Aschoff nodules, usually in the left atrium, forming thickened *MacCallum plaques*

Clinical Features (p. 566)

Diagnosis of RF is based on clinical history and a constellation of findings, called *Jones criteria,* that include: *erythema marginatum* (a skin rash), *Sydenham chorea* (a neurologic disorder with rapid, involuntary, purposeless movements), *carditis* (involving myocardium, endocardium, or pericardium), *subcutaneous nodules,* and/or *migratory large joint polyarthritis.* Death (most frequently secondary to *myocarditis*) occurs rarely in acute rheumatic fever. Typically, myocarditis and arthritis are transient and resolve without complications; however, valvular involvement can deform and scar the valve, causing permanent dysfunction (RHD) and subsequent CHF. RHD is most likely when the first attack is in early childhood, when it is particularly severe, or if there are recurrent attacks. Changes secondary to mitral stenosis include:

- Left atrial hypertrophy and enlargement, occasionally with mural thrombi
- Atrial fibrillation secondary to atrial dilation
- CHF with chronic pulmonary congestive changes
- Increased risk of infective endocarditis

Infective Endocarditis (p. 566)

Infective endocarditis (IE) reflects microbial colonization or invasion of valves, leading to friable, infected vegetations, often with valve damage. Traditionally, these are classified as *acute* or *subacute* forms:

- *Acute IE* is caused by highly virulent organisms (e.g., *Staphylococcus aureus*), typically seeding a previously normal valve to produce necrotizing, ulcerative, and invasive infections. Clinically, there is rapid onset of fever with rigors, malaise, and weakness. Larger vegetations can cause embolic complications; splenomegaly is common.
- *Subacute IE* is typically caused by moderate to low-virulence organisms (e.g., *Streptococcus viridans*) seeding an abnormal or previously injured valve; there is less valvular destruction than in acute infective endocarditis. This pattern occurs insidiously with nonspecific malaise, low-grade fever, weight loss, and a flulike syndrome. Vegetations tend to be small so that embolic complications occur less frequently. The disease tends to have a protracted course even without treatment and has a lower mortality rate than acute IE.

Pathogenesis (p. 567)

IE is caused by blood-borne organisms, usually bacteria that derive from infections elsewhere in the body, intravenous (IV) drug abuse, dental or surgical procedures, or otherwise trivial injury to gut, urinary tract, oropharynx, or skin. Contributory conditions include neutropenia and immunosuppression.

- Although endocarditis can occur on normal valves, infection is more likely to occur in the setting of previous valve pathology (e.g., CHD [particularly tight shunts or stenoses with jet streams], RHD, MVP, degenerative calcific stenoses, bicuspid aortic valves, or prosthetic valves).
- IE in IV drug abusers is most commonly caused by *S. aureus* infecting a normal valve; right-sided valves are involved more commonly than left.
- Besides *S. viridans* (50% to 60% of cases), low virulence organisms include enterococci and the so-called *HACEK group of oral commensals* (i.e., *Haemophilus, Actinobacillus, Cardiobacterium, Eikenella,* and *Kingella*).
- IE on prosthetic valves is caused most commonly by *S. epidermidis*; sewing ring abscesses are a common feature.
- In 10% to 15% of IE, no organisms are identified (culture-negative).

Morphology (p. 567)

- Acute IE is typically associated with bulky (i.e., 1 to 2 cm) vegetations causing valve destruction; invasion into adjacent myocardium or aorta can cause abscesses. Distal embolization with septic infarcts or mycotic aneurysms can occur.
- Subacute IE has smaller vegetations that rarely penetrate the leaflets.

Clinical Features (p. 568)

- Valvular and myocardial damage as described earlier
- Embolic complications as described earlier
- Renal injury, including embolic infarction or infection and antigen-antibody complex–mediated glomerulonephritis (with nephrotic syndrome, renal failure, or both).
- Diagnosis is confirmed by the Duke criteria; blood cultures are critically important for directing therapy.

Nonbacterial Thrombotic Endocarditis (p. 568)

Nonbacterial thrombotic endocarditis (NBTE), also called *marantic endocarditis,* characteristically occurs in settings of cancer (particularly adenocarcinomas) or prolonged debilitating illness (e.g., renal failure, chronic sepsis) with disseminated intravascular coagulation or other hypercoagulable states.

- Small (i.e., 1 to 5 mm) sterile, bland fibrin and platelet thrombi are loosely adherent to valve leaflets along closure lines, without significant inflammation or valve damage.
- Vegetations can embolize systemically.

Endocarditis of Systemic Lupus Erythematosus (Libman-Sacks Disease) (p. 569)

Endocarditis of systemic lupus erythematosus (Libman-Sacks disease) occurs in systemic lupus erythematosus and in anti-phospholipid syndrome, presumably due to immune complex deposition. Findings include small fibrinous, sterile vegetations on *either* side of valve leaflets, with associated fibrinoid necrosis and inflammation. Valve scarring and deformation can result; these resembles RHD and may require surgery.

Carcinoid Heart Disease (p. 569)

Carcinoid tumors (Chapter 17) elaborate bioactive products (e.g., serotonin, kallikrein, bradykinins, histamine, prostaglandins, and tachykinins P and K) that can cause cardiac lesions. The precise agent responsible is uncertain, although it is presumably rapidly metabolized in lung and liver, because cardiac lesions do not occur unless there is extensive hepatic metastatic spread. Right-sided heart lesions (valvular and endocardial) predominate.

Morphology (p. 569)

- Lesions are characterized by plaque-like intimal thickening (composed of smooth muscle cells and associated ECM) of the tricuspid and pulmonary valves and right ventricular outflow tract; left-sided lesions are uncommon except in primary pulmonary carcinoids.
- Tricuspid insufficiency and pulmonic stenosis are the typical valvular consequences.
- Similar lesions occur in the setting of drugs that have serotoninergic effects (e.g., methylsergide, ergotamine, some antiparkinsonian medications, and fenfluramine [part of the fen-phen appetite suppressant combination with phentermine]).

Complications of Artificial Valves (p. 570)

Prosthetic valves are of two basic types: mechanical (rigid, synthetic) and bioprosthetic (chemically fixed animal tissues). Roughly 60% of valve recipients develop a significant valve-related complication within 10 years of surgical implantation:

- *Thromboembolic complications*, either local obstruction by thrombus or distal embolization, are the major complications of mechanical valves; this complication necessitates long-term anticoagulation in such valve recipients, with the attendant risks of hemorrhagic stroke or other bleeding complication.
- *Infective endocarditis*, infection at the valve sewing ring, often leads to ring abscesses and paravalvular regurgitation.
- *Structural deterioration* is uncommon with mechanical valves, but valvular calcification or degenerative tears often cause bioprosthetic valve failure.
- *Occlusion* occurs due to tissue overgrowth.
- Intravascular *hemolysis* occurs due to high shear forces or *paravalvular leak* due to poor healing.

Cardiomyopathies (p. 571)

Although myocardial dysfunction can occur secondary to ischemic, valvular, hypertensive, or other heart diseases, the term *cardiomyopathy* implies a *principal* cardiac dysfunction. Causes of such myocardial disease can be *primary* (i.e., predominantly affecting heart) or *secondary* (i.e., part of a larger systemic disorder):

- Infections (e.g., viral, bacterial, fungal, protozoal)
- Toxic exposures (e.g., alcohol, cobalt, chemotherapeutic agents)
- Metabolic disorders (e.g., hyperthyroidism, nutritional deficiency)
- Genetic abnormalities in cardiomyocytes (e.g., storage disorders, muscular dystrophies)
- Infiltrative lesions (e.g., sarcoid, carcinoma, radiation-induced fibrosis)
- Immunologic disorders (e.g., autoimmune myocarditis, rejection)

Cardiomyopathy is divided into three main functional and pathologic patterns: *dilated, hypertrophic,* and *restrictive* (Fig. 12-4 and Table 12-2).

Dilated Cardiomyopathy (p. 572)

Dilated cardiomyopathy (DCM) is characterized by gradual four-chamber hypertrophy and dilation; there is systolic dysfunction

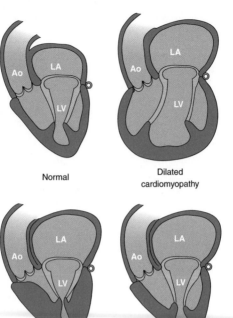

Normal

Dilated
cardiomyopathy

Hypertrophic
cardiomyopathy

Restrictive
cardiomyopathy

FIGURE 12-4 Schematics of the three distinctive forms of cardiomyopathy; each form can have a variety of causes. *Ao,* Aorta; *LA,* left atrium; *LV,* left ventricle.

with hypocontraction. It typically presents as indolent, progressive CHF. Only 25% of patients survive more than 5 years after symptom onset. Although the cause is frequently unknown *(idiopathic DCM),* certain pathologic mechanisms can contribute (Fig. 12-5):

- *Genetic influences:* 20% to 50% of DCM is familial; autosomal dominant inheritance is most common. Known genetic abnormalities commonly involve cytoskeletal proteins (e.g., dystrophin in X-linked cardiomyopathy [Duchenne and Becker muscular dystrophies]). Others involve mutations of enzymes involved in fatty acid β-oxidation or mitochondrial gene deletions causing abnormal oxidative phosphorylation.
- *Alcohol toxicity:* DCM is attributed to direct toxicity of alcohol or a metabolite (especially acetaldehyde) on the myocardium. No morphologic features distinguish alcohol-induced cardiac damage from other forms of idiopathic DCM or chronic thiamine deficiency.
- *Peripartum cardiomyopathy:* DCM is discovered within several months before or after delivery. Although the mechanism is uncertain, the association with pregnancy suggests possible etiologies of chronic hypertension, volume overload, nutritional deficiency, metabolic derangement, or immunologic response.
- *Myocarditis* (see later discussion): even after resolution of the infection, injury related to myocarditis can progress to DCM.

TABLE 12-2   Cardiomyopathy and Indirect Myocardial Dysfunction: Functional Patterns and Causes

Functional Pattern	Left Ventricular Ejection Fraction*	Mechanisms of Heart Failure	Causes	Indirect Myocardial Dysfunction (Not Cardiomyopathy)
Dilated	<40%	Impairment of contractility (systolic dysfunction)	Idiopathic; alcohol; peripartum; genetic; myocarditis; hemochromatosis; chronic anemia; doxorubicin (Adriamycin); sarcoidosis	Ischemic heart disease; valvular heart disease; hypertensive heart disease; congenital heart disease
Hypertrophic	50% to 80%	Impairment of compliance (diastolic dysfunction)	Genetic; Friedreich ataxia; storage diseases; infants of diabetic mothers	Hypertensive heart disease; aortic stenosis
Restrictive	45% to 90%	Impairment of compliance (diastolic dysfunction)	Idiopathic; amyloidosis; radiation-induced fibrosis	Pericardial constriction

*Normal, approximately 50% to 65%.

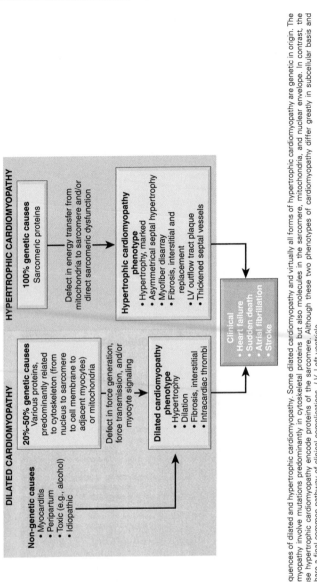

FIGURE 12-5 Causes and consequences of dilated and hypertrophic cardiomyopathy. Some dilated cardiomyopathy and virtually all forms of hypertrophic cardiomyopathy are genetic in origin. The genetic causes of dilated cardiomyopathy involve mutations predominantly in cytoskeletal proteins but also molecules in the sarcomere, mitochondria, and nuclear envelope. In contrast, the several mutated genes that cause hypertrophic cardiomyopathy encode proteins of the sarcomere. Although these two phenotypes of cardiomyopathy differ greatly in subcellular basis and morphologic phenotypes, they share a final common pathway of clinical complications. *LV*, Left ventricle.

Morphology (p. 572)

- *Grossly*, the heart is flabby with cardiomegaly (i.e., up to 900 g); wall thickness may not reflect the degree of hypertrophy due to chamber dilation.
- Poor contractile function and stasis predispose to mural thrombi.
- Valves and coronary arteries are generally normal.
- *Microscopic changes* in DCM are often subtle and entirely non-specific; most commonly there is diffuse myocyte hypertrophy and variable interstitial fibrosis.

Arrhythmogenic Right Ventricular Cardiomyopathy (p. 575)

Arrhythmogenic right ventricular cardiomyopathy is a recently recognized cardiomyopathy with distinct presentation and morphology. It is an autosomal dominant disorder (with variable penetrance) characterized by predominantly right-sided failure and arrhythmia. The defect is most commonly caused by defective adhesive molecules in desmosomes. Morphologically, the right ventricular wall is severely thinned with myocyte loss and profound fatty infiltration. Death occurs secondary to progressive CHF or fatal arrhythmias.

Hypertrophic Cardiomyopathy (p. 575)

Hypertrophic cardiomyopathy (HCM) is characterized by heavy, muscular, *hypercontractile*, poorly compliant hearts with poor diastolic relaxation; in a third of cases there is also ventricular outflow obstruction.

Morphology (p. 575)

- Classically, there is disproportionate thickening of the interventricular septum (asymmetric septal hypertrophy), although 10% have concentric hypertrophy.
- The left ventricular cavity is compressed into a *banana-like configuration* by the asymmetric bulging of the septum.
- Septal thickening at the level of the mitral valve compromises left ventricular systolic outflow by contact of the anterior mitral leaflet with the septum *(systolic anterior motion)*; this causes *hypertrophic obstructive cardiomyopathy*, reflected by a fibrous plaque on the septum.
- *Microscopically*, there is marked myofiber hypertrophy, classically with helter-skelter *myocyte disarray*, accompanied by myofilament disorganization within muscle cells, most prominent in the interventricular septum. There is also patchy interstitial and replacement fibrosis.

Pathogenesis (p. 576)

- HCM is predominantly caused by mutations of sarcomeric proteins (β-myosin heavy chain mutations being most common); most are autosomal dominant mutations with variable penetrance.
- Prognosis varies widely depending on the specific mutations.
- The pathogenic sequence leading from specific mutations to disease manifestations is not understood (see Fig. 12-5). Different mutations in the same gene can even give rise to DCM or HCM.

Clinical Features (p. 577)

The major feature is reduced stroke volume due to a combination of impaired diastolic filling and left ventricular outflow tract obstruction.

- Focal myocardial ischemia is common due to increased ventricular pressures, massive myocyte hypertrophy, diminished stroke volume, and frequently abnormal intramyocardial arterioles.
- HCM can be entirely asymptomatic. Symptomatic disease usually presents in young adults with dyspnea, angina, and/or syncope.
- The clinical course can be highly variable; major complications include atrial fibrillation with mural thrombus and embolization, IE, CHF, and SCD. Indeed, HCM is one of the most common causes of sudden death in young athletes.

Restrictive Cardiomyopathy (p. 577)

Relatively rare and with multiple etiologies, this entity is marked by a restriction of ventricular filling leading to reduced cardiac output. Contractile function is usually normal. Ventricle size is normal, although there is typically biatrial dilation. Non-specific interstitial myocardial fibrosis is usually present; biopsy frequently reveals a specific etiology. Causes include:

- *Endomyocardial fibrosis* is a disease mainly of African children and young adults; the cause is unknown. It is characterized by dense ventricular subendocardial fibrosis extending from the apex upward, often with superimposed organizing mural thrombus.
- *Loeffler endocarditis* is morphologically similar to endomyocardial fibrosis but is classically associated with peripheral eosinophilia and eosinophilic infiltration of multiple organs (especially the heart). The cardiac changes are probably due to toxic products of eosinophils, and the course can be rapidly fatal. A subset of these patients has a myeloproliferative disorder with eosinophilia and associated chromosomal rearrangements of PDGF receptor genes; kinase inhibitors are effective in inducing hematologic remission.
- *Endocardial fibroelastosis* is an uncommon disorder of obscure etiology (and possibly the end point of different injuries), characterized by focal to diffuse, *fibroelastic* thickening of the endocardium, and left ventricle greater than right. It occurs at all ages but is most common in patients less than 2 years old. CHD is present in a third of cases.

Myocarditis (p. 578)

Infectious etiologies or primary autoimmune responses underlie myocarditis.

- The clinical spectrum is broad, from entirely asymptomatic to abrupt onset of arrhythmia, CHF, or SCD; most patients recover quickly and without sequelae, although DCM can occur (see earlier discussion).
- Most cases in the United States are viral in origin (e.g., Coxsackievirus A and B, echovirus). Cardiac involvement occurs days to weeks after a primary viral infection; cardiac involvement can be due to a direct infection or secondary to immunologic cross-reactivity between pathogen and myocardium.
- *Trypanosoma cruzi* (causal organism in *Chagas disease*) causes myocarditis in the majority of infected individuals with 10% dying acutely and others progressing to cardiac failure over 10 to 20 years.
- Toxin released by *Corynebacterium diptheriae* is responsible for the myocardial injury in diptheria.
- Myocarditis occurs in 5% of patients with Lyme disease (*Borrelia burgdorferi*). Lyme myocarditis is usually mild and reversible but occasionally requires a temporary pacemaker for atrioventricular block.

- Myocarditis in acquired immunodeficiency syndrome (AIDS) patients results from inflammation and damage without a clear etiologic agent or directly from human immunodeficiency virus (HIV) or some other opportunistic pathogen.
- Noninfectious myocarditis may be immune mediated (e.g., associated with rheumatic fever, systemic lupus erythematosus, or drug allergies).
- In some cases, the cause is unknown (e.g., sarcoidosis, giant cell myocarditis) or the microbe is unidentifiable.

Morphology (p. 578)

Gross manifestations include a flabby heart, often with four-chamber dilation and patchy hemorrhagic mottling.

- Mural thrombi can form in dilated chambers.
- Endocardium and valves are typically unaffected.
- Long-term remodeling can lead to dilation or hypertrophy.

Microscopically, there is a myocardial inflammatory infiltrate with associated myocyte necrosis or degeneration. Lesions are often focal (and may be missed by routine endomyocardial biopsy). Inflammatory lesions typically resolve over days to weeks, leaving either no residua or variable interstitial and replacement fibrosis.

- In *Chagas disease,* trypanosomes parasitize myocytes and produce acute and chronic inflammation, including eosinophils.
- *Hypersensitivity myocarditis* is characterized by perivascular mononuclear and eosinophilic infiltrates; this variant is often induced by therapeutic drugs.
- In *giant cell myocarditis,* there is focal to occasionally extensive myocyte necrosis associated with multinucleated giant cells. This variant of myocarditis has a poor prognosis.

Other Causes of Myocardial Disease (p. 579)

- *Cardiotoxic agents* commonly cause myofiber swelling, fatty change, and individual cell lysis. Anthracycline chemotherapeutic agents doxorubicin and daunorubicin induce dose-dependent cardiotoxicity, attributed primarily to lipid peroxidation in myofiber membranes. Tyrosine kinase inhibitors and certain forms of immunotherapy are increasingly recognized as cardiotoxic. Both the physiologic and the morphologic patterns of cardiotoxic agents may be indistinguishable from those of idiopathic DCM.
- *Catecholamines,* either administered exogenously (e.g., epinephrine) or produced endogenously (e.g., by pheochromocytomas), induce tachycardia and vasomotor constriction (with superimposed platelet aggregation); this can result in diffuse but patchy ischemic necrosis. *Cocaine* can have a similar effect by blocking catecholamine reuptake at adrenergic nerve terminals. Sudden emotional or physical stress—presumably by release of adrenergic mediators—can also induce left ventricular dysfunction, called *Takotsubo cardiomyopathy.*
- *Amyloidosis* occurs as patchy nodular and perivascular/interstitial hyaline protein deposits; the amyloid nature of the protein is confirmed by Congo red staining, yielding a characteristic apple-green birefringence under polarized light. Cardiac amyloid can be secondary to systemic amyloidosis (Chapter 6) or may be isolated, for example, *senile cardiac amyloidosis* due to transthyretin deposition (transthyretin is a normal serum protein involved in *trans*porting *thy*roxine and *retin*ol). Mutant forms of transthyretin (more common in African Americans) can accelerate cardiac and systemic amyloidosis. Isolated atrial

amyloid (or uncertain clinical significance) is due to atrial natri-uretic peptide deposition. Amyloid accumulation typically causes a restrictive physiology, although DCM, arrhythmias, or CHF symptoms mimicking IHD can occur.

- *Iron overload* with myocyte hemosiderin deposits occurs in hereditary hemochromatosis and hemosiderosis from multiple blood transfusions. Injury is thought to occur through iron-induced free radical generation, or by interfering with metal-dependent enzyme systems. Patients present most commonly with DCM.
- *Hyper- and hypothyroidism* commonly affect the heart; indeed, cardiac manifestations are among the most consistent features of thyroid disease. Hyperthyroidism causes supraventricular tachyarrhythmias and cardiomegaly, although CHF is uncom-mon; hypothyroidism causes reduced heart rate and stroke vol-ume, and in conjunction with increased peripheral resistance leads to decreased tissue perfusion.

Pericardial Disease (p. 581)

Pericardial disease is typically secondary to diseases of adjacent structures or part of a systemic disorder; isolated disease is less common.

Pericardial Effusion and Hemopericardium (p. 581)

The normal pericardial sac contains 30 to 50 mL of serous *nonin-flammatory* fluid. Slow fluid accumulation can be well tolerated, resulting in chronic collections greater than 500 mL; rapidly accumulating fluids can cause fatal *tamponade* with as little as 200 mL.

Pericarditis (p. 581)

Pericarditis is usually secondary to disorders involving the heart or mediastinal structures (e.g., after MI, surgery, trauma, radiation, tumors, infections); it can also be due to systemic abnormalities (e.g., uremia, autoimmune diseases). Acute primary pericarditis is chiefly viral in origin. Chronic pericarditis also occurs (e.g., with tuberculosis and fungal infections).

Acute Pericarditis (p. 581)

- *Serous pericarditis:* Although the etiology is frequently unknown, it is characteristically non-bacterial; causes include: rheumatic fever, systemic lupus erythematosus, tumors, uremia, and primary viral infections. Microscopically, there is scant pericardial acute and chronic inflammatory infiltration (mostly lymphocytes).
- *Fibrinous and serofibrinous pericarditis:* These are the most com-mon forms of pericarditis, occurring as serous fluid mixed with a fibrinous exudate; patients classically present with a loud friction rub, pain, and fever. Causes include acute MI, post-infarction *(Dressler)* syndrome, cardiac surgery, uremia, irradia-tion, RF, SLE, and trauma. Exudates can be completely resolved or can organize, leaving fibrous adhesions.
- *Purulent (suppurative) pericarditis* usually signifies bacterial, fun-gal, or parasitic infection reaching the pericardium by direct extension, by hematogenous or lymphatic spread, or during cardiotomy. Purulent pericarditis is typically composed of 400 to 500 mL of a thin-to-creamy pus with marked inflammation and erythematous, granular serosal surfaces. It presents with high fevers, rigors, and a friction rub and can organize to

produce *mediastinopericarditis* or *constrictive pericarditis* (see following discussion).

- *Hemorrhagic pericarditis* denotes an exudate of blood admixed with fibrinous-to-suppurative effusion. Most commonly, it follows cardiac surgery or is associated with tuberculosis or malignancy.
- *Caseous pericarditis* is due to tuberculosis (typically by direct extension from neighboring lymph nodes) or, less commonly, mycotic infection. This pattern is the most frequent antecedent to fibrocalcific constrictive pericarditis.

Chronic or Healed Pericarditis (p. 582)

Healing of acute lesions can lead to resolution or to pericardial fibrosis ranging from a thick, pearly, nonadherent epicardial plaque (i.e., "soldier's plaque") to thin, delicate adhesions to massive fibrosis.

- *Adhesive mediastinopericarditis* obliterates the pericardial sac, and the parietal layer is tethered to mediastinal tissue. The heart thus contracts against all the surrounding attached structures, with subsequent hypertrophy and dilation.
- *Constrictive pericarditis* is marked by thick (i.e., up to 1 cm), dense, fibrous obliteration, often with calcification of the pericardial sac encasing the heart, limiting diastolic expansion and restricting cardiac output.

Heart Disease Associated with Rheumatologic Disorders (p. 583)

Rheumatoid arthritis involves the heart in 20% to 40% of severe chronic cases. Most common is fibrinous pericarditis; this can organize to form dense, fibrous, and potentially restrictive adhesions. Less frequently, granulomatous rheumatoid nodules involve the myocardium, endocardium, aortic root, or valves, where they are particularly damaging. Rheumatoid valvulitis can produce changes similar to those seen in RHD.

Tumors of the Heart (p. 583)

Cardiac metastases occur *much* more frequently than primary heart tumors; metastases can involve the pericardium (with or without effusions) or penetrate into the myocardium.

Primary cardiac tumors:

- *Myxomas are the most common primary cardiac tumor in adults.* Usually isolated, 90% arise in the left atrium in the region of the fossa ovale. Roughly 10% of patients with myxomas have an autosomal dominant *Carney syndrome*, with cardiac and extra-cardiac myxomas, pigmented skin lesions, and endocrine hyperactivity.

  Grossly: Myxomas range from 1 cm to more than 10 cm and are sessile-to-pedunculated masses varying from globular and hard to papillary and myxoid. They may cause symptoms by physical obstruction, by trauma to the atrioventricular valves, or by peripheral embolization.

  Microscopically: They are composed of stellate multipotential mesenchymal myxoma cells, embedded in an acid mucopolysaccharide matrix, with vessel-like and occasionally gland-like structures.

- *Lipomas* are well-circumscribed benign accumulations of adipose tissue, more commonly in the left ventricle, right atrium, or septum. Symptoms depend on location and on encroachment on valve function or conduction pathways.

- *Papillary fibroelastomas* are sea-anemone–like lesions with centimeter-long filaments radiating out from a central core; they are characteristically found on valves and can cause emboli but are usually incidental findings at autopsy. Microscopically, the filaments have a core of myxoid connective tissue with concentric elastic fibers, all covered by endothelium.
- *Rhabdomyomas* are the most common primary heart tumor in children; they can cause valvular or outflow tract obstruction. Most are probably hamartomas and can be associated with tuberous sclerosis, caused by defects in the *TSC1* and *TSC2* tumor-suppressor genes. Microscopically, they are composed of large rounded-to-polygonal cells rich in glycogen and containing myofibrils. Fixation and histologic processing leaves characteristic artifactual cytoplasmic stranding radiating from the central nucleus to plasma membrane, forming so-called *spider cells*.
- *Angiosarcomas and rhabdomyosarcomas* are malignant neoplasms resembling their counterparts in other locations.

Cardiac Effects of Noncardiac Neoplasms (p. 584)

The heart can also be *indirectly* affected by tumors at other sites:

- Metastases or direct extension; 5% of patients dying from malignancy have heart involvement
- Hypercoagulable states leading to nonbacterial thrombotic endocarditis (NBTE)
- Carcinoid heart disease
- Myeloma-associated amyloidosis
- Pheochromocytoma-associated (catecholamine) heart disease
- Effects of tumor therapy (e.g., radiation or cardiotoxic agents)

Cardiac Transplantation (p. 585)

Cardiac transplantation (about 3000 cases annually worldwide) is performed most commonly for DCM and ischemic heart disease. The 1-year survival is 70% to 80%, with 5-year survival rates of 60% or more.

Acute allograft rejection is characterized by interstitial lymphocytic inflammation with associated myocyte damage; severe rejection is accompanied by inflammatory vascular injury and extensive myocyte necrosis. Other complications in immunosuppressed transplant recipients include opportunistic infections and malignancies, particularly B-cell lymphomas (due to Epstein-Barr virus). The major current long-term limitation to cardiac transplantation is progressive diffuse intimal proliferation of the coronary arteries *(graft arteriosclerosis)* causing downstream myocardial ischemia.

13

Diseases of White Blood Cells, Lymph Nodes, Spleen, and Thymus

Development and maintenance of hematopoietic tissues (p. 590)

- The formed blood elements—erythrocytes, granulocytes, monocytes, platelets, and lymphocytes—have a common origin from hematopoietic stem cells (HSCs); the characteristic features of HSC are their *pluripotency* (ability for one cell to produce all lineages) and *capacity for self-renewal.*
- The self-renewing divisions of HSC occur in specialized marrow niches where stromal cells and secreted factors maintain the appropriate milieu. Under stress conditions, other tissues (e.g., liver and spleen) can provide the requisite niche environment, leading to *extramedullary hematopoiesis.*
- Marrow responses to physiologic needs are regulated by lineage-specific hematopoietic growth factors acting on committed progenitor cells. Some growth factors (e.g., stem cell factor) may act on very early committed multipotent progenitors, whereas others (e.g., erythropoietin, granulocyte-macrophage colony-stimulating factor [GM-CSF], etc.) act on committed progenitors with more restricted potential. Feedback loops mediated through growth factor production maintain the numbers of formed blood elements within appropriate ranges (Table 13-1).
- Tumors of hematopoietic origin are typically associated with mutations that either block progenitor cell maturation or abrogate their dependence on growth factors.

Disorders of white blood cells (WBCs) are broadly classified as either deficiencies *(leukopenias)* or proliferations *(leukocytosis);* the latter can be reactive or neoplastic.

Leukopenia (p. 592)

Leukopenia can reflect decreased numbers of any of the specific leukocyte types; this most commonly involves neutrophils (*neutropenia,* granulocytopenia). *Lymphopenia* is less common; besides congenital immunodeficiency diseases, it can occur with human immunodeficiency virus (HIV) or other viral infections, glucocorticoid or cytotoxic drug therapy, autoimmune disorders, or malnutrition.

TABLE 13-1 Adult Reference Ranges for Blood Cells*	
Cell Type	
White cells ($\times 10^3/\mu L$)	4.8-10.8
Granulocytes (%)	40-70
Neutrophils ($\times 10^3/\mu L$)	1.4-6.5
Lymphocytes ($\times 10^3/\mu L$)	1.2-3.4
Monocytes ($\times 10^3/\mu L$)	0.1-0.6
Eosinophils ($\times 10^3/\mu L$)	0-0.5
Basophils ($\times 10^3/\mu L$)	0-0.2
Red cells ($\times 10^6/\mu L$)	4.3-5, men; 3.5-5.0, women
Platelets ($\times 10^3/\mu L$)	150-450

*Reference ranges vary among laboratories. The reference ranges for the laboratory providing the result should always be used.

Neutropenia, Agranulocytosis (p. 592)

Pathogenesis (p. 593)

- Inadequate or ineffective granulopoiesis

  HSC suppression, as in aplastic anemia (Chapter 14)
  Infiltrative marrow disorders (e.g., tumors, granulomatous disease)
  Suppression of committed granulocytic precursors (e.g., after drug exposure)
  Disease states characterized by ineffective granulopoiesis (e.g., megaloblastic anemias [vitamin B_{12} deficiency] and myelodysplastic syndromes)
  Rare inherited conditions (e.g., Kostmann syndrome, impairing differentiation)

- Accelerated removal or destruction of neutrophils

  Neutrophil injury caused by immunologic disorders (e.g., systemic lupus erythematosus) or drug exposures
  Splenic sequestration
  Increased peripheral utilization in overwhelming infections

Drug toxicity is the most common cause of agranulocytosis. Some agents act in a predictable dose-dependent fashion, and can cause general marrow suppression; this includes many chemotherapeutic cancer drugs (e.g., alkylating agents and antimetabolites). Others act in an *idiosyncratic and unpredictable* way related to metabolic polymorphisms or the development of autoantibodies (e.g., chloramphenicol, sulfonamides, chlorpromazine, thiouracil, and phenylbutazone).

Morphology (p. 593)

Marrow *hypocellularity* occurs with agents that suppress granulocyte progenitor cell growth and survival; these may be granulocyte-specific, or they can potentially affect erythroid and megakaryocytic progenitors, leading to pancytopenia and aplastic anemia (empty marrow). Marrow *hypercellularity* can occur in conditions with ineffective granulopoiesis (myelodysplastic syndromes) or when there is increased peripheral destruction of neutrophils.

Clinical Features (p. 593)

Symptoms and signs relate to intercurrent infections and include malaise, chills, and fever, often with marked weakness and fatigability. Serious infections are most likely when the neutrophil count is 500 cells/mm^3 or less. Ulcerating necrotizing lesions of the gingiva, buccal mucosa, or pharynx are characteristic. Severe life-threatening invasive bacterial or fungal infections can occur in the lungs, kidney, or urinary tract; neutropenic patients are at high risk for deep *Candida* or *Aspergillus* infections.

Infections are often fulminant; neutropenic patients are therefore treated with broad-spectrum antibiotics at the first sign of infection. Granulocyte colony-stimulating factor therapy decreases the duration and severity of the neutrophil nadir caused by chemotherapeutic drugs.

Reactive (Inflammatory) Proliferations of White Cells and Lymph Nodes (p. 593)

Leukocytosis (p. 593)

Leukocytosis occurs commonly in a variety of inflammatory states. The peripheral leukocyte count is a function of the size of precursor pools in the marrow, circulation, and peripheral tissues; rate of precursor release; the proportion of cells adherent to the cell wall; and the rate of extravasation into tissues. Infection is the major driving force for leukocytosis; inflammatory cytokines not only increase marrow egress but also increase proliferation and differentiation of committed precursors. Growth factors can preferentially stimulate select lineages, or more broadly promote proliferation of several different leukocyte lines:

- *Polymorphonuclear leukocytosis* accompanies acute inflammation associated with infection or tissue necrosis. Sepsis or severe inflammatory disorders yield neutrophils with *toxic granulations* (coarse, dark cytoplasmic granules) and/or *Döhle bodies* (sky-blue, dilated endoplasmic reticulum).
- *Eosinophilic leukocytosis* (eosinophilia) can occur with allergic disorders, parasitic infestations, drug reactions, lymphomas, and some vasculitides.
- *Basophilic leukocytosis* (basophilia) is rare; it suggests an underlying myeloproliferative disease (e.g., chronic myelogenous leukemia).
- *Monocytosis* occurs with chronic infections (e.g., tuberculosis, bacterial endocarditis, and malaria), collagen vascular diseases (e.g., systemic lupus erythematosus), and inflammatory bowel diseases (e.g., ulcerative colitis).
- *Lymphocytosis* accompanies monocytosis in many disorders associated with chronic immunologic stimulation (e.g., tuberculosis, brucellosis), viral infections (e.g., hepatitis A, cytomegalovirus, Epstein-Barr virus), and *Bordetella pertussis* infections.

In childhood acute viral infections, atypical lymphocytes can appear in blood or bone marrow and simulate a lymphoid neoplasm. At other times, particularly with severe infections, copious immature granulocytes can appear in the blood and simulate myelogenous leukemia, called a *leukemoid reaction*.

Lymphadenitis (p. 595)

Activation of resident immune cells in lymph nodes and spleen leads to morphologic changes in the lymphoid architecture. Following antigenic stimulation, the primary follicles enlarge and are transformed into *germinal centers*, highly dynamic structures in which B cells develop the capacity for making high-affinity antibodies; paracortical T cells may also be hyperplastic.

Acute Nonspecific Lymphadenitis (p. 595)

Acute nonspecific lymphadenitis can be localized or systemic.

- The *localized* form is commonly caused by direct microbiologic drainage, most frequently in the cervical area associated with dental or tonsillar infections.
- The *systemic* form is associated with bacteremia and viral infections, particularly in children.

Affected nodes are enlarged, tender, and fluctuant with extensive abscess formation. Histologically, there are large germinal centers with numerous mitotic figures. With pyogenic organisms, a neutrophilic infiltrate occurs and the follicular centers can undergo necrosis. Overlying skin is frequently red; penetration of the infection to the skin surface produces draining sinuses. With control of the infection, lymph nodes can revert to their normal appearance, but scarring is common after suppurative reactions.

Chronic Nonspecific Lymphadenitis (p. 595)

Chronic nonspecific lymphadenitis is common in axillary and inguinal nodes, and is characteristically non-tender (due to slow enlargement).

Morphology (p. 595)

Follicular hyperplasia is caused by inflammatory processes that activate B cells; these include rheumatoid arthritis, toxoplasmosis, and early stages of HIV infection. Follicular hyperplasia is distinguished by prominent large germinal centers (secondary follicles) surrounded by a rim of resting naive B cells (the *mantle zone*):

- Dark zones in the germinal centers contain proliferating blast-like B cells *(centroblasts)*
- Light zones in the germinal center are composed of B cells with irregular or cleaved nuclear contours *(centrocytes)*
- Interspersed are dendritic cells, and *tingible-body macrophages* containing the nuclear debris of apoptotic B cells that failed to generate sufficiently high antibody affinities

Although follicular hyperplasia can be confused morphologically with follicular lymphomas, features favoring a reactive process include:

- Preservation of the lymph node architecture
- Marked variation in follicular shape and size
- Frequent mitotic figures, phagocytic macrophages, and recognizable light and dark zones

Paracortical hyperplasia is caused by stimuli that trigger T cell-mediated responses, such as acute viral infections (e.g., infectious mononucleosis). Paracortical hyperplasia is characterized by reactive changes within the T-cell regions of the lymph node:

- Activated parafollicular T-cell immunoblasts (3 to 4 times larger than resting lymphocytes) proliferate and partially efface B-cell follicles

Sinus histiocytosis (reticular hyperplasia) is nonspecific, but it is often observed in lymph nodes draining tissues involved by epithelial cancers. Sinus histiocytosis is characterized by prominent, distended lymphatic sinusoids caused by marked hypertrophy of lining endothelial cells and infiltration with macrophages (histiocytes).

Neoplastic Proliferations of White Cells (p. 596)

White cell malignancies fall into three broad categories:

- *Lymphoid neoplasms*, encompassing tumors of B-cell, T-cell, or natural killer (NK) cell origin
- *Myeloid neoplasms*, originating from early hematopoietic progenitors

  Acute myeloid leukemias: Immature progenitor accumulation in the marrow
  Myelodysplastic syndromes: Ineffective hematopiesis
  Chronic myeloproliferative disorders: Increased production of one or more terminally differentiated myeloid elements

- *Histiocytoses*, representing proliferative lesions of macrophages ("histiocytes") and dendritic cells

Etiologic and Pathogenetic Factors in White Cell Neoplasia: Overview (p. 596)

Chromosomal Translocations and Other Acquired Mutations (p. 596)

Nonrandom karyotypic abnormalities, most commonly *translocations*, are present in most WBC neoplasms. They can cause inappropriate expression of normal proteins or synthesis of novel fusion oncoproteins.

- Altered genes often play crucial roles in the development, growth, or survival of the normal counterpart of the malignant cell; the altered genes may result in dominant negative loss-of-function mutations or increased activity gain-of-function changes.
- Oncoproteins generated by genomic aberrations often block normal maturation.
- Proto-oncogenes are often activated in lymphoid cells by errors that occur during antigen receptor rearrangement and diversification. Among lymphoid cells, oncogenic mutations occur most frequently in germinal center B cells during attempted antibody diversification. Thus, after antigen stimulation, germinal center B cells up-regulate activation-induced deaminase (AID), a DNA-modifying enzyme that allows immunoglobulin (Ig) class switching (e.g., IgM to IgG), and somatic hypermutation to increase antibody affinities. Remarkably the same AID enzyme can also induce *c-MYC/Ig* translocations that can put *c-MYC* oncogene expression under control of an immunoglobulin promoter and can also activate other proto-oncogenes such as *BCL6*. Genomic instability can also be generated by the activities of the V(D)J recombinase responsible for antigen receptor variation.

Inherited Genetic Factors (p. 597)

Genetic diseases that promote genomic instability (e.g., Bloom syndrome, Fanconi anemia, and ataxia-telangiectasia) increase the risk of leukemia. Down syndrome (i.e., trisomy 21) and neurofibromatosis type I are also associated with an increased incidence.

Viruses (p. 597)

Three viruses—human T-cell leukemia virus type 1 (HTLV-1), Epstein-Barr virus (EBV), and human herpesvirus-8 (HHV-8)—are implicated (see Chapter 7 for mechanisms). EBV is found in a subset of Burkitt lymphoma, 30% to 40% of Hodgkin lymphoma, many B-cell lymphomas occurring in the setting of T-cell immunodeficiency, and NK cell lymphomas. HTLV-1 is associated with adult T-cell leukemia, and HHV-8 is found in unusual large B-cell lymphomas presenting as lymphomatous effusions.

Chronic Immune Stimulation (p. 598)

Environmental agents that cause chronic immune stimulation can predispose to lymphoid neoplasia. The most clear-cut associations are *H. pylori* infection with gastric B-cell lymphoma and gluten-sensitive enteropathy with intestinal T-cell lymphoma. HIV-induced T cell dysregulation also leads to germinal center B-cell hyperplasia that can progress to B-cell lymphoma, arising in virtually any organ.

Iatrogenic Factors and Smoking (p. 598)

Radiotherapy and many cancer chemotherapies increase the risk of myeloid and lymphoid neoplasms, stemming from the mutagenic effects of such treatments on progenitor cells. The incidence of acute myeloid leukemia is increased 1.3- to 2-fold in smokers, presumably due to inhaled carcinogens (e.g., benzene in tobacco smoke).

Lymphoid Neoplasms (p. 598)

DEFINITIONS AND CLASSIFICATIONS (P. 598)

Leukemia: Neoplasms with widespread involvement of bone marrow and often (but not always) the peripheral blood.

Lymphoma: Proliferations that arise as discrete tissue masses (e.g., within lymph nodes, spleen, or extranodal tissues). Among the *lymphomas*, two broad categories are recognized:

Hodgkin lymphoma (HL), with important clinical and histologic features

Non-Hodgkin lymphoma (NHL), comprising all forms besides HL

Plasma cell neoplasms are another important group of lymphoid tumors; these typically arise in marrow (infrequently involving lymph nodes) and are composed of terminally differentiated B cells.

Whether a particular neoplasm is designated a "leukemia" or "lymphoma" is based on the *usual* tissue distribution. Thus, entities formally classified as "lymphomas" can have leukemic presentations or may evolve to leukemias; similarly, tumors categorized as leukemias can occasionally arise as soft-tissue masses without marrow involvement.

As a corollary to this classification, lymphomas characteristically present as enlarged, non-tender lymph nodes, whereas the leukemias come to attention because of signs and symptoms related to the suppression of normal hematopoiesis (e.g., infection, bleeding, and/or anemia). The most common plasma cell neoplasm *(multiple myeloma)* causes bone destruction and often presents with pain and/or pathologic fractures.

The *World Health Organization (WHO)* classification scheme sorts the various lymphoid neoplasms into five broad categories based on clinical features, morphology, immunophenotype, and genotype:

- Precursor B-cell neoplasms (immature B cells)
- Peripheral B-cell neoplasms (mature B cells)
- Precursor T-cell neoplasms (immature T cells)
- Peripheral T-cell and NK-cell neoplasms (mature T cells and NK cells)
- Hodgkin lymphoma (neoplasms of Reed-Sternberg cells)

Important principles regarding lymphoid neoplasms:

- Diagnosis requires histologic examination of lymph nodes or other involved tissues.

- In most lymphoid neoplasms, antigen receptor gene rearrangement precedes transformation; hence, all daughter cells share the same antigen receptor sequence and synthesize identical proteins (either immunoglobulins or T-cell receptors). In contrast, normal immune responses are polyclonal. Thus, clonality analyses of lymphoid populations can distinguish neoplastic versus reactive proliferations. Moreover, a unique antigen receptor rearrangement can be used as a highly specific clonal marker to detect small numbers of malignant cells.
- Most lymphoid neoplasms (85% to 90%) are of B-cell origin, with most of the remainder being T-cell tumors; only rare tumors are of NK cell or histiocytic origin. Most lymphoid neoplasms resemble some recognizable stage of B- or T-cell development, a feature used in their classification (Fig. 13-1).
- Lymphoid neoplasms tend to disrupt normal immune regulatory mechanisms, leading frequently to immunologic dysfunction.
- Neoplastic B and T cells circulate widely but tend to home to and grow in areas where their normal counterparts reside.
- While NHL spread widely and somewhat unpredictably early in their course, HL spreads in an orderly fashion; hence, staging in HL is of substantial utility in guiding therapy.

The salient features of the major types of lymphoid leukemias, NHL, and plasma cell tumors are summarized in Table 13-2.

Precursor B- and T-Cell Neoplasms (p. 600)

ACUTE LYMPHOBLASTIC LEUKEMIA/LYMPHOMA (p. 600)

Acute lymphoblastic leukemia/lymphoma (ALL) are neoplasms of immature precursor B (pre-B) or precursor T (pre-T) lymphocytes (lymphoblasts). These constitute the most common childhood cancers.

- Most (about 85%) are pre-B tumors manifesting as childhood acute leukemias with extensive marrow and peripheral blood involvement.
- Pre-T ALL tend to occur in adolescent boys as thymic lymphomas (50% to 70% of cases).

Morphology (p. 602)

In leukemic presentations, the marrow is hypercellular and packed with lymphoblasts showing a high mitotic activity; tumor cells have scant basophilic cytoplasm with nuclei slightly larger than small lymphocytes exhibiting finely stippled chromatin and inconspicuous nucleoli; the nuclear membrane typically exhibits a convoluted appearance. Pre-B and pre-T lymphoblasts are morphologically identical.

Immunophenotype (p. 602)

Terminal deoxytransferase (TdT), a DNA polymerase expressed only by pre-B and pre-T lymphoblasts, is present in more than 95% of cases.

- Pre-B ALL cells are arrested at stages preceding surface immunoglobulin expression; most lymphoblasts express the pan B-cell antigen CD19, the transcription factor PAX5, and CD10.
- Pre-T ALL cells are arrested at early intrathymic stages of maturation; the lymphoblasts often express CD1, CD2, CD5, and CD7.

Molecular Pathogenesis (p. 602)

Approximately 90% of ALL have chromosomal changes. Many of the chromosomal aberrations dysregulate the expression or function of transcription factors that control normal B- and T-cell

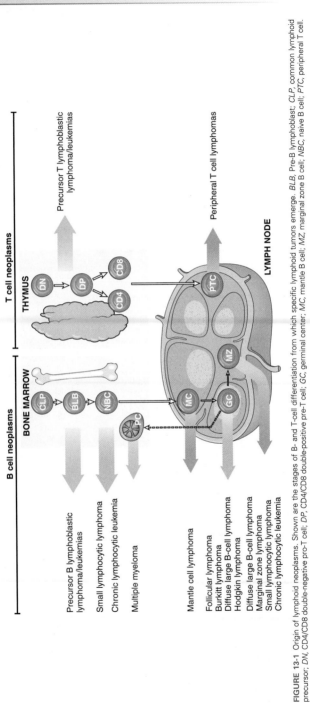

FIGURE 13-1 Origin of lymphoid neoplasms. Shown are the stages of B- and T-cell differentiation from which specific lymphoid tumors emerge. *BLB*, Pre-B lymphoblast; *CLP*, common lymphoid precursor; *DN*, CD4/CD8 double-negative pro-T cell; *DP*, CD4/CD8 double-positive pre-T cell; *GC*, germinal center; *MC*, mantle B cell; *MZ*, marginal zone B cell; *NBC*, naive B cell; *PTC*, peripheral T cell.

TABLE 13-2 Summary of Major Types of Lymphoid Leukemias and Non-Hodgkin Lymphomas

Diagnosis	Cell of Origin	Genotype	Salient Clinical Features
Neoplasms of Immature B and T cells			
B-cell acute lymphoblastic leukemia/lymphoma	Bone marrow precursor B cell	Diverse chromosomal translocations; t(12;21) involving *CBFα* and *ETV6* present in 25%	Predominantly children; symptoms relating to marrow replacement and pancytopenia; aggressive
T-cell acute lymphoblastic leukemia/lymphoma	Precursor T cell (often of thymic origin)	Diverse chromosomal translocations, *NOTCH1* mutations (50% to 70%)	Predominantly adolescent boys; thymic masses and variable bone marrow involvement; aggressive
Neoplasms of Mature B Cells			
Burkitt lymphoma	Germinal-center B cell	Translocations involving c-*MYC* and Ig loci, usually t(8;14); subset EBV-associated	Adolescents or young adults with extranodal masses; uncommonly presents as "leukemia"; aggressive
Diffuse large B-cell lymphoma	Germinal-center or post-germinal-center B cell	Diverse chromosomal rearrangements, most often of *BCL6* (30%), *BCL2* (10%), or c-*MYC* (5%)	All ages, but most common in adults; often appears as a rapidly growing mass; 30% extranodal; aggressive
Extranodal marginal zone lymphoma	Memory B cell	t(11;18), t(1;14), and t(14;18) creating *MALT1-IAP2*, *BCL10-IgH*, and *MALT1-IgH* fusion genes, respectively	Arises at extranodal sites in adults with chronic inflammatory diseases; may remain localized; indolent
Follicular lymphoma	Germinal-center B cell	t(14;18) creating *BCL2-IgH* fusion gene	Older adults with generalized lymphadenopathy and marrow involvement; indolent
Hairy cell leukemia	Memory B cell	No specific chromosomal abnormality	Older men with pancytopenia and splenomegaly; indolent
Mantle cell lymphoma	Naive B cell	t(11;14) creating *CyclinD1-IgH* fusion gene	Older men with disseminated disease; moderately aggressive
Multiple myeloma/solitary plasmacytoma	Post-germinal-center bone marrow homing plasma cell	Diverse rearrangements involving *IgH*; 13q deletions	Myeloma: older adults with lytic bone lesions, pathologic fractures, hypercalcemia, and renal failure; moderately aggressive Plasmacytoma: isolated plasma cell masses in bone or soft tissue; indolent

Continued

TABLE 13-2 Summary of Major Types of Lymphoid Leukemias and Non-Hodgkin Lymphomas—cont'd

Diagnosis	Cell of Origin	Genotype	Salient Clinical Features
Small lymphocytic lymphoma/chronic lymphocytic leukemia	Naïve B cell or memory B cell	Trisomy 12, deletions of 11q, 13q, and 17p	Older adults with bone marrow, lymph node, spleen, and liver disease; autoimmune hemolysis and thrombocytopenia in a minority; indolent
Neoplasms of Mature T Cells or NK Cells			
Adult T-cell leukemia/ lymphoma	Helper T cell	HTLV-1 provirus present in tumor cells	Adults with cutaneous lesions, marrow involvement, and hypercalcemia; occurs mainly in Japan, West Africa, and the Caribbean; aggressive
Peripheral T-cell lymphoma, unspecified	Helper or cytotoxic T cell	No specific chromosomal abnormality	Mainly older adults; usually presents with lymphadenopathy; aggressive
Anaplastic large-cell lymphoma	Cytotoxic T cell	Rearrangements of ALK	Children and young adults, usually with lymph node and soft-tissue disease; aggressive
Extranodal NK/T-cell lymphoma	NK-cell (common) or cytotoxic T cell (rare)	EBV-associated; no specific chromosomal abnormality	Adults with destructive extranodal masses, most commonly sinonasal; aggressive
Mycosis fungoides/Sézary syndrome	Helper T cell	No specific chromosomal abnormality	Adult patients with cutaneous patches, plaques, nodules, or generalized erythema; indolent
Large granular lymphocytic leukemia	Two types: cytotoxic T cell and NK cell	No specific chromosomal abnormality	Adult patients with splenomegaly, neutropenia, and anemia, sometimes accompanied by autoimmune disease

EBV, Epstein-Barr virus; *HIV,* human immunodeficiency virus; *Ig,* immunoglobulin; *NK,* natural killer.

development and lead to maturation arrest. Pre-B and pre-T ALL have different genetic aberrations, indicating that different molecular mechanisms underlie their pathogenesis. Characteristic changes include:

- *Hyperdiploidy* (i.e., more than 50 chromosomes) is most common, although hypodiploidy and balanced translocations also occur. Hyper- and hypodiploidy only occur in B-ALL.
- Seventy percent of T-ALL have gain-of function mutations in *NOTCH1*, a gene essential for T-cell development.
- Many B-ALL have loss-of function mutations in *PAX5, E2A,* or *EBF*—genes involved in B-cell development; they may also have balanced t(12;21) translocations involving genes important in early hematopoiesis.

Importantly, *single mutations are not sufficient to cause ALL;* rather, additional, complementary, mutations, which typically increase proliferation or survival, are necessary to convert a preleukemic clone into full-blown malignancy.

Clinical Features (p. 603)

Approximately 2500 new cases of ALL are diagnosed each year in the United States. The peak incidence for B-ALL is 3 years, and the peak for T-ALL is adolescence; both B- and T-ALL occur less frequently in adults. The clinical features of ALL stem from accumulation of neoplastic blast cells in the marrow:

- *Abrupt, stormy onset* within days to weeks of symptom onset
- *Symptoms related to depressed marrow function* fatigue due to anemia; fever due to infections in the setting of neutropenia; and bleeding due to thrombocytopenia
- *Bone pain and tenderness,* due to marrow expansion and infiltration of the subperiosteum by blasts
- *Generalized lymphadenopathy, splenomegaly, hepatomegaly* and *testicular enlargement* due to neoplastic infiltration; pre-T cell ALL with thymic involvement can cause compression of mediastinal vessels and airways
- *Central nervous system (CNS) manifestations* (e.g., headache, vomiting, and nerve palsies) due to meningeal spread

Prognosis (p. 603)

With aggressive chemotherapy 95% of children with ALL achieve complete remission, and 75% to 85% are cured; however ALL is the leading cause of cancer deaths in children. Roughly 35% to 40% of adults are cured.

Features with worse prognosis:

- Age younger than 2 years (largely due to translocations involving the *MLL* gene)
- Age older than 10 years
- Peripheral blast counts more than 100,000/μL
- Presence of t(9;22) (Philadelphia chromosome; see later discussion)

Features with better prognosis include hyperploidy, trisomy of chromosomes 4, 7, and 10, and a t(12;21) translocation.

Peripheral B-Cell Neoplasms (p. 603)

CHRONIC LYMPHOCYTIC LEUKEMIA/SMALL LYMPHOCYTIC LYMPHOMA (p. 603)

Chronic lymphocytic leukemia (CLL)/small lymphocytic lymphoma (SLL) are morphologically, phenotypically, and genotypically indistinguishable, differing only in the degree of peripheral blood lymphocytosis.

Morphology (p. 603)

Lymph node architecture is diffusely effaced by small lymphocytes with round to slightly irregular nuclei; these are admixed with variable numbers of larger dividing cells *(prolymphocytes)*. The mitotically active cells often cluster in loose aggregates *(proliferation centers)* that are pathognomonic for CLL/SLL. In CLL, peripheral smears contain increased numbers of small lymphocytes, some of which are disrupted, producing so-called *smudge cells*. Involvement of marrow, spleen, and liver is common.

Immunophenotype (p. 604)

CLL/SLL cells express pan-B cell markers (CD19 and CD20) as well as CD5, found on a small subset of normal B cells. Low-level surface immunoglobulin expression (usually IgM) is typical.

Molecular Pathogenesis (p. 604)

Chromosomal translocations are rare in CLL/SLL. The most common findings are trisomy 12q as well as deletions of 13q12-14 (related to the loss of two microRNAs), 11q, or 17p. Tumor growth is largely confined to the proliferation centers where tumor cells receive critical cues from the surrounding microenvironment; factors that induce NF-κB transcription factor production promote neoplastic cell growth and survival.

Clinical Features (p. 605)

CLL, defined as an absolute lymphocyte count more than 4000 cells/μL, is the most common adult leukemia in the Western world; 15,000 new cases arise each year in the United States with a median age of 60 years and a 2:1 male predominance. A minority of cases do not have lymphocytosis and are classified as SLL (constituting 4% of NHL). Characteristic features include:

- Nonspecific symptoms (e.g., easy fatigability, weight loss, and anorexia)
- Generalized lymphadenopathy and hepatosplenomegaly (50% to 60% of patients)
- Lymphocytosis in CLL (up to 200,000/μL)
- Immune abnormalities, including hypogammaglobulinemia (common, leading to increased susceptibility to bacterial infections) and autoantibodies against erythrocytes or platelets (10% to 15% of patients)

The prognosis is extremely variable, depending primarily on the clinical stage. Median survival is 4 to 6 years, but patients with minimal tumor burden often survive more than 10 years. Worse outcomes are associated with:

- Deletions of 11q or 17p
- Lack of somatic hypermutation
- Expression of ZAP-70, a protein that augments Ig receptor signaling activity

Transformation of CLL/SLL to a more-aggressive histologic type is a common, ominous event; most patients survive less than 1 year. Two forms are seen:

- *Prolymphocytic transformation* (15% to 30% of patients) is heralded by worsening cytopenias, increasing splenomegaly, and large numbers of *prolymphocytes* in the circulation.
- *Transformation to diffuse large B-cell lymphoma (Richter syndrome)* occurs in 5% to 10% of patients, and presents as a rapidly enlarging mass within a lymph node or the spleen.

FOLLICULAR LYMPHOMA (p. 605)

Follicular lymphoma is the most common form of NHL in the United States (15,000 to 20,000 cases per year). It arises from germinal center cells and is stringly associated with translocations involving *BCL2*.

Morphology (p. 605)

In lymph nodes, follicular (nodular) and diffuse proliferations are composed of two principal cell types: (1) *centrocytes*, small cells with cleaved nuclear contours and scant cytoplasm and (2) *centroblasts*, larger cells with open nuclear chromatin, several nucleoli, and modest amounts of cytoplasm. Centrocytes predominate in most tumors. Involvement of spleen, liver, and marrow is common; peripheral blood involvement occurs in 10% of patients.

Immunophenotype (p. 606)

Neoplastic cells resemble normal follicular center B cells and express CD19, CD20, CD10, BCL6, and surface Ig. More than 90% of tumor cells also express BCL2 protein (normal follicular center B cells are BCL2 negative).

Molecular Pathogenesis (p. 606)

A characteristic (14;18) translocation juxtaposes the *IgH* locus on chromosome 14 and the *BCL2* locus on chromosome 18, leading to BCL2 protein overexpression; BCL2 prevents apoptosis and promotes tumor cell survival.

Clinical Features (p. 606)

Follicular lymphoma characteristically presents as painless, generalized lymphadenopathy in middle-aged adults. It is not curable but typically follows an indolent waxing-waning course with a median survival of 7 to 9 years. Histologic transformation to diffuse large B-cell lymphoma occurs in 30% to 50% of cases; after transformation, median survival is less than 1 year.

DIFFUSE LARGE B-CELL LYMPHOMA (p. 606)

Diffuse large B-cell lymphoma (DLBCL) is the most common form of NHL, with 25,000 new cases annually in the United States.

Morphology (p. 606)

Common features are a relatively large cell size (4 to 5 times the diameter of small lymphocytes) and a diffuse growth pattern obliterating the underlying architecture. The nuclear shape is variable and vesicular in appearance, with 2 to 3 nucleoli; the cytoplasm is moderately abundant and can be pale or basophilic.

Immunophenotype (p. 606)

These mature B-cell tumors express pan-B cell markers CD19 and CD20, with variable expression of germinal center B-cell markers (e.g., CD10 and BCL6); most have surface Ig.

Molecular Pathogenesis (p. 607)

DLBCL is a heterogeneous group of lymphomas. Nevertheless, two chromosomal rearrangements are relatively common:

• Thirty percent have *translocations involving the BCL6 locus*. *BLC6* encodes a zinc-finger transcription factor that regulates the development and growth of germinal center B cells; over-expression holds cells in a relatively undifferentiated and proliferative state. BCL6 can also silence the expression of p53. Somatic mutations in the *BCL6* promoter can also lead to aberrant BCL6 expression.

- Between 1% and 20% have *t(14;18)* leading to over-expression of the anti-apoptotic *BCL2* gene and may arise from transformation of previously unrecognized follicular lymphomas. Tumors with *BCL2* rearrangements also typically lack *BCL6* rearrangements, suggesting that these constitute distinct molecular classes of DLBCL.

Special Subtypes of DLBCL Associated with Oncogenic Herpesviruses (p. 607)

- *Immunodeficiency-associated large B-cell lymphomas* occur in the setting of severe T-cell immunodeficiency (e.g., HIV and bone marrow transplantation). The neoplastic cells are often latently infected with EBV, which plays a critical pathogenic role. Restoration of T-cell immunity can lead to regression of the proliferations.
- *Primary effusion lymphomas* arise as malignant pleural or ascitic effusions, mostly in advanced HIV infection or the elderly. Tumor cells are anaplastic and lack T- or B-cell markers but have clonal Ig heavy chain gene rearrangements. Tumor cells are infected with human Kaposi sarcoma herpesvirus (KSHV)/ HHV8, which plays a causal role.

Clinical Features (p. 607)

DLBCL occur most frequently in older adults (median age of 60 years) as a rapidly enlarging, symptomatic mass at a single nodal or extranodal site (e.g., gastrointestinal tract, skin, bone, or brain). Involvement of liver, spleen, and marrow can occur but usually later in the course.

DLBCL are aggressive, rapidly fatal tumors if left untreated. With intensive chemotherapy, complete remission is achieved in 60% to 80%, and 40% to 50% are cured; anti-CD20 immunotherapy improves initial responses and overall outcomes. Patients with limited disease fare better than patients with widespread disease or a large bulky tumor mass.

BURKITT LYMPHOMA (p. 607)

Burkitt lymphoma (BL) occurs in three different settings; although they are histologically identical, they have distinct clinical, genotypic, and virologic features:

- African (endemic) BL
- Sporadic (nonendemic) BL
- A subset of aggressive lymphomas occurring in patients infected with HIV

Morphology (p. 608)

Involved tissues are diffusely effaced by intermediate-sized tumor cells with round-oval nuclei, coarse chromatin, several nucleoli, and moderate cytoplasm. A high mitotic index and numerous apoptotic cells are typical; apoptotic cells ingested by scattered macrophages with abundant clear cytoplasm produce a characteristic "starry sky" appearance.

Immunophenotype (p. 608)

Tumors comprise relatively mature B cells expressing surface IgM, CD19, CD20, CD10, and BCL6, consistent with a germinal center B-cell origin; BCL2 is rarely expressed.

Molecular Pathogenesis (p. 608)

BL are associated with *c-MYC* gene (chromosome 8) translocations; the partner is usually the IgH locus (t[8;14]) but can be the Ig κ (t[2;8]) or λ (t[8;22]) light chain loci. The outcome is *c-MYC* positioned adjacent to strong Ig enhancer and promoter elements that increase *c-MYC* expression. Inactivating p53 mutations are also common.

Virtually all African (endemic) tumors are latently infected with EBV; EBV is also present in 25% of HIV-associated tumors and 15% to 20% of sporadic cases. Molecular analysis shows that the viral DNA configuration is identical in all tumor cells within a given case, indicating that infection precedes cellular transformation.

Clinical Features (p. 608)

Both endemic and sporadic BL occur largely in children or young adults; in the United States, BL accounts for 30% of childhood NHL. Most tumors arise at extranodal sites as rapidly growing masses; endemic BL often presents in the mandible (with a secondary predilection for kidneys, ovaries, and adrenals), whereas sporadic BL most often occurs as an ileocecal or peritoneal mass. Marrow and peripheral blood involvement are uncommon.

BL is aggressive but responds well to intensive chemotherapy; most children and young adults can be cured, whereas the outcome in older adults is more guarded.

PLASMA CELL NEOPLASMS AND RELATED DISORDERS (p. 609)

Plasma cell neoplasms and related disorders are neoplasms of terminally differentiated B cells. They represent the expansion of a single clone of Ig-secreting plasma cells, with resulting serum elevations in a single homogeneous immunoglobulin or its fragments. These tumors cause 15% of deaths due to lymphoid neoplasms; 15,000 cases of multiple myeloma (the most common and lethal form) occur annually in the United States.

A monoclonal Ig identified in the blood is called an *M component* or M protein. In many cases, neoplastic cells secrete excess free light (L) or heavy (H) chains; occasionally, only L or H chains are produced. Because of their small size, free L chains are excreted in the urine, called *Bence Jones proteins*. Terms to describe abnormal Ig include *monoclonal gammopathy, dysproteinemia,* and *paraproteinemia.*

There are several different clinicopathologic entities associated with monoclonal gammopathies:

Multiple Myeloma (p. 609)

Multiple myeloma is a plasma cell neoplasm with a peak incidence between 65 and 70 years; it is characterized by multifocal destructive bony lesions.

Molecular Pathogenesis (p. 609)

- Ig genes show somatic hypermutation, indicating that the cell of origin is a post-germinal center B cell that has migrated to the marrow and differentiated into a plasma cell.
- Proliferation and survival are dependent on tumor cell and stromal cell cytokines, particularly IL-6.
- Factors produced by the tumor cells, for example, MIP1α, which that drives stromal cell production of RANKL (receptor activator of NF-κB ligand), lead to osteoclast activation and osteoblast inactivation; the net result is bone resorption with hypercalcemia and pathologic fractures.
- Translocations of the Ig heavy chain gene is common; translocation partners include *FGFR3* receptor gene, and cell cycle regulatory genes cyclin D1 and cyclin D3.

Morphology (p. 609)

- Bone involvement by destructive plasma cell tumors (plasmacytomas) is most common in the vertebral column, ribs, skull, pelvis, and femur. Skull lesions have a sharply defined, punched-out radiologic appearance; generalized osteoporosis can also be seen.

- Away from overt masses, bone marrow shows increased numbers of plasma cells (more than 30% of total cells), often with abnormal features. The cells can diffusely infiltrate or occur as sheet-like masses that completely replace normal elements.
- High levels of M proteins cause erythrocytes in peripheral smears to stick together in linear arrays, called *rouleaux formation.*
- Bence Jones proteinuria leads to *myeloma kidney* (Chapter 20).

Clinical Features (p. 610)

The clinical features of multiple myeloma stem from organ infiltration (particularly bones) by neoplastic plasma cells, excess immunoglobulin production (often having abnormal physicochemical properties), and suppression of normal humoral immunity.

- *Bone infiltration, bone pain, and pathologic fractures are due to bone resorption.* Secondary hypercalcemia contributes to renal disease and polyuria and can cause neurologic manifestations including confusion, weakness, lethargy, and constipation.
- *Recurrent bacterial infections* result from decreased production of normal immunoglobulins.
- *Hyperviscosity syndrome* has multiple manifestations (see later discussion).
- *Renal insufficiency* (up to 50% of patients) is multifactorial; notably, light chains are toxic to tubular epithelial cells.
- Certain light chains are prone to causing *amyloidosis* of the AL type (Chapter 6).

In 99% of patients, electrophoresis reveals increased blood monoclonal Ig (M protein) and/or Bence Jones proteinuria. IgG (55%) and IgA (25%) are the most common M proteins. In 20% of patients, Bence Jones proteinuria is an isolated finding, and 1% of myelomas are non-secretory.

Prognosis is variable but generally poor with median survivals of 4 to 6 years. If untreated, patients with multiple bony lesions survive only 6 to 12 months. Cyclin D1 translocations are associated with better outcomes; 13q or 17q deletions or t(4;14) portend a more aggressive course. Chemotherapy induces remission in 50% to 70%, and proteasome inhibitors are showing efficacy against myeloma cells; thalidomide has efficacy by blocking tumor-stromal interactions and by inhibiting angiogenesis. Infection and renal failure are the two most common causes of death.

Solitary Myelomas (Plasmacytomas) (p. 611)

Solitary myelomas (plasmacytomas) represent 3% to 5% of plasma cell neoplasms. Modest elevations of serum or urinary M proteins occur in a minority. Solitary bony lesions almost inevitably progress to multiple myeloma but can take 10 to 20 years to do so. Extraosseous lesions often localize to lung, nasal sinuses, or oronasopharynx; these rarely disseminate and can be cured by local resection.

Monoclonal Gammopathy of Uncertain Significance (p. 611)

Monoclonal gammopathy of uncertain significance (MGUS) is the most common plasma cell dyscrasia. By definition, patients are asymptomatic; nevertheless, serum M proteins (less than 3 g/dL) are detected in 3% of people older than 50 years and 5% of people older than 70 years. Most patients follow a completely benign clinical course; however, 1% annually progress to a symptomatic monoclonal gammopathy, typically multiple myeloma.

Lymphoplasmacytic Lymphoma *(p. 612)*

Lymphoplasmacytic lymphoma is a B-cell neoplasm of older adults (typical onset between 60 and 70 years of age) that characteristically secretes monoclonal IgM, often in amounts sufficient to cause a *hyperviscosity syndrome* known as *Waldenström macroglobulinemia.* Unlike multiple myeloma, H- and L-chain synthesis is balanced so that complications of excess light chains (e.g., amyloidosis or renal failure) are rare. Bone destruction is also not observed.

Morphology (p. 612)

Diffuse marrow infiltrates of neoplastic lymphocytes, plasma cells, and plasmacytoid lymphocytes, mixed with reactive mast cells, are seen. With disseminated disease, similar polymorphous infiltrates can occur in lymph nodes, spleen, or liver.

Clinical Features (p. 612)

Patients present with weakness, fatigue, and weight loss; half have lymphadenopathy, hepatomegaly, and splenomegaly.

- Marrow infiltration causes anemia; this can be exacerbated by autoimmune hemolysis due to cold agglutinins of the IgM type (10% of patients).
- IgM secretion frequently results in a *hyperviscosity syndrome:*

  Visual impairment is due to venous congestion; there is striking *tortuosity* and distention of retinal veins, often with hemorrhages and exudates.

  Neurologic problems including headaches, dizziness, deafness, and stupor are attributable to sluggish blood flow and sludging.

  Bleeding is related to the formation of complexes containing macroglobulins and clotting factors, as well as interference with platelet function.

  Cryoglobulinemia reflects precipitation of macroglobulins at low temperatures; symptoms include Raynaud phenomenon and cold urticaria.

Lymphoplasmacytic lymphoma is an incurable progressive disease with a median survival time of 4 years. Symptoms related to increased levels of IgM (e.g., hyperviscosity and hemolysis) can be treated with plasmapheresis.

MANTLE CELL LYMPHOMA (p. 612)

Mantle cell lymphoma accounts for about 2.5% of NHL in the United States and 7% to 9% of NHL in Europe.

Morphology (p. 612)

Tumor cells closely resemble the normal mantle zone B cells that surround germinal centers; they are small lymphocytes with irregular/clefted nuclei, condensed nuclear chromatin, inconspicuous nucleoli, and scant cytoplasm. Expansion of these cells in nodes can produce a nodular appearance or efface the normal architecture.

Immunophenotype (p. 613)

Tumor cells characteristically *overexpress cyclin D1*; most also express CD19, CD20, CD5, and moderate surface Ig. The IgH genes lack somatic hypermutation, consistent with a naive B cell origin.

Molecular Pathogenesis (p. 613)

A distinctive t(11;14) translocation, detected in more than 70% of cases, results in the juxtaposition of the cyclin D1 and IgH loci.

Clinical Features (p. 613)

Men are affected more than women, and typical onset is between ages 50 and 60 years. Patients have generalized lymphadenopathy, and peripheral blood involvement occurs in 20% to 40% of patients. Extranodal disease is relatively common; marrow and splenic involvement (i.e., 50% of patients) are not unusual, and there is frequently multifocal mucosal involvement of the small bowel and colon *(lymphomatoid polyposis)*. The prognosis is poor with median survivals of 3 to 4 years; patients succumb to complications of organ dysfunction due to tumor infiltration.

MARGINAL ZONE LYMPHOMAS (p. 613)

Marginal zone lymphomas are a heterogeneous group of B-cell tumors arising in lymph nodes, spleen, or extranodal tissues. Because mucosa is a typical extranodal site, these are also called *mucosa-associated lymphoid tumors, or MALTomas*. Although cells have different stages of B lymphoid differentiation, *the predominant population resembles a normal marginal zone B cell*; there is evidence of Ig somatic hypermutation, suggesting an origin from memory B cells.

Notable characteristics of the extranodal marginal zone lymphomas:

- Tendency to occur at sites of *chronic immune or inflammatory reactions* (e.g., salivary glands in Sjögren disease, thyroid in Hashimoto thyroiditis, stomach in *H. pylori* infection).
- Lymphomas remain localized at sites of origin for long periods, spreading systemically only late in their course.
- Tumors can regress if the inciting stimulus (e.g., *Helicobacter*) is eradicated.

These features suggest that marginal zone lymphomas lie on a continuum between reactive hyperplasia and full-blown lymphoma. Following a reactive, polyclonal immune response, a monoclonal B-cell neoplasm emerges, probably due to acquired genetic changes; cell growth is still dependent, however, on local factors (e.g., factors produced by reactive T-helper cells). With additional genetic aberrations, the neoplasm becomes factor independent; (11;18), (1;14) or (11;14) translocations are relatively specific and lead to up-regulation of BCL10 or MALT1—proteins that activate the NF-κB pathway and promote B cell growth and survival. With further clonal evolution, distant spread and transformation to DLBCL can occur.

HAIRY CELL LEUKEMIA (p. 614)

Hairy cell leukemia constitutes about 2% of all leukemias; it predominantly affects middle-aged Caucasian men (male to female ratio of 5:1).

Morphology (p. 614)

The name derives from fine hairlike projections on the tumor cells; routine blood smears reveal variably shaped nuclei and modest amounts of pale-blue cytoplasm with thread- or bleb-like extensions. Because tumor cells are trapped in ECM, they frequently cannot be recovered from aspirates (resulting in a so-called *dry tap*) and can only be visualized on marrow biopsies. Splenic red pulp is usually heavily infiltrated, leading to white pulp obliteration and a beefy red gross appearance.

Immunophenotype and Molecular Pathogenesis (p. 614)

Cells typically express pan B-cell markers (CD19 and 20), surface Ig, CD11c, CD25, and CD103. Most tumors have hypermutated Ig genes, suggesting an origin from post-germinal center memory B cells.

Clinical Features (p. 614)

Clinical consequences result from marrow, liver, or splenic infiltration. *Splenomegaly,* often massive, is the most common and sometimes only abnormal physical finding. *Hepatomegaly* is less common and not as marked; lymphadenopathy is rare. *Pancytopenia,* resulting from marrow infiltration and splenic sequestration, occurs in more than 50%. *Infections* are the presenting feature in one third of cases. Monocytopenia may contribute to the high incidence of atypical mycobacterial infections. This is an indolent disorder with good prognosis. It is exquisitely sensitive to certain chemotherapies, typically producing long-lasting remissions.

Peripheral T-Cell and Natural Killer Cell Neoplasms (p. 614)

Peripheral T-cell and NK cell neoplasms are a heterogeneous group united by phenotypes that resemble normal mature T or NK cells. Peripheral T-cell tumors account for 5% to 10% of NHL in the United States and Europe, while NK cell tumors are rare. Both types are more common in Asia.

PERIPHERAL T-CELL LYMPHOMAS, UNSPECIFIED (p. 614)

These lymphoma cells are largely a "wastebasket" category for tumors that do not fit any other WHO criteria. No morphologic feature is pathognomonic, but certain findings are characteristic:

- Tumor cells diffusely efface lymph nodes and are commonly composed of a pleomorphic mixture of variably sized malignant T cells.
- Infiltrates of reactive cells (e.g., eosinophils and macrophages) are common, as is brisk angiogenesis.
- By definition, these all have a mature T-cell phenotype; they express pan T-cell markers (e.g., CD2, CD3, CD5) and have clonal T-cell receptor rearrangements.

Most patients have generalized lymphadenopathy, sometimes with eosinophilia, pruritus, fever, and weight loss. Although cures are reported, the prognosis is worse than for comparably aggressive mature B-cell neoplasms (e.g., DLBCL).

ANAPLASTIC LARGE-CELL LYMPHOMA (p. 615)

Anaplastic large-cell lymphoma is an entity defined by chromosomal rearrangements involving the *anaplastic lymphoma kinase (ALK)* gene on chromosome 2p23. These rearrangements create *ALK* fusion genes that encode constitutively active forms of ALK—a tyrosine kinase upstream of Janus kinase/signal transducers and activation of transcription (JAK/STAT) signaling pathways.

Tumor cells are large with reniform, embryoid, or horseshoe-shaped nuclei and voluminous cytoplasm.

These tumors occur most commonly in children and young adults, frequently involve soft tissues, and carry a very good prognosis; cure rates approach 80%. Morphologically similar tumors lacking *ALK* rearragemnts usually arise in older adults and have a poor prognosis, similar to peripheral T-cell lymphoma, unspecified.

ADULT T-CELL LEUKEMIA/LYMPHOMA (p. 615)

Adult T-cell leukemia/lymphoma occurs in patients infected by *HTLV-1*; it is most common where HTLV-1 is endemic (southern Japan, West Africa, and Caribbean basin). Tumor cells contain clonal HTLV-1 provirus, suggesting a pathogenic role; notably, HTLV-1 encodes a Tax protein that activates NF-κB and thereby enhances lymphocyte growth and survival. Tumor cells with multilobular (cloverleaf) nuclei are characteristic. Clinical findings include skin involvement, generalized lymphadenopathy and hepatosplenomegaly, peripheral blood lymphocytosis, and hypercalcemia. This is a rapidly fatal lesion, often with mortality within a year despite aggressive chemotherapy.

MYCOSIS FUNGOIDES/SÉZARY SYNDROME (p. 616)

Mycosis fungiodes/Sézary syndrome are different manifestations of a tumor of CD4+ helper T cells that home to the skin. Tumor cells characteristically express the CLA adhesion molecule, as well as CC4 and CCR10 chemokine receptors; all these surface molecules contribute to the cutaneous localization of tumor cells.

*   *Mycosis fungoides* progresses from an inflammatory *premycotic phase* through a *plaque phase* to a *tumor phase*. Histologically, the epidermis and upper dermis are infiltrated by neoplastic T cells with *cerebriform* nuclei (marked infolding of the nuclear membrane). Disease progression involves extracutaneous spread, most commonly to lymph nodes and marrow.
*   *Sézary syndrome* is a variant where skin involvement is manifested as a generalized exfoliative erythroderma with an associated leukemia of *Sézary* cells (also with cerebriform nuclei).

These tumors are usually indolent with median survivals of 8 to 9 years; transformation to aggressive T-cell lymphoma can be a terminal event

LARGE GRANULAR LYMPHOCYTIC LEUKEMIA (p. 616)

This form of leukemia is a rare neoplasm occurring mainly in adults.

*   Tumor cells are large lymphocytes with abundant blue cytoplasm containing scattered coarse azurophilic granules. Marrow involvement is usually sparse; hepatic and splenic infiltrates are usually present.
*   Two variants are recognized: CD3+ T-cell tumors and CD56+ NK cell tumors.
*   Despite the paucity of marrow involvement, *neutropenia* (with maturation arrest of myeloid elements in the marrow) and *anemia* dominate the clinical picture; *pure red blood cell aplasia* can rarely occur.
*   There is also an increased incidence of *rheumatologic disorders;* some patients present with Felty syndrome, characterized by a triad of rheumatoid arthritis, splenomegaly, and neutropenia.
*   The course is variable, being largely dependent on the severity of the cytopenias.

EXTRANODAL NATURAL KILLER/T-CELL LYMPHOMA (p. 616)

Extranodal NK/T-cell lymphoma is rare in the United States and Europe but constitutes 3% of Asian NHL.

*   It presents most commonly as a destructive nasopharyngeal mass; less common sites include skin or testis. Tumor cells infiltrate small vessels, leading to extensive ischemic necrosis.
*   Histologic appearance is variable; tumor cells can contain large *azurophilic granules* resembling those in normal NK cells.
*   This lymphoma is highly associated with EBV; tumor cells in any given patient contain identical EBV episomes, indicating an origin from a single EBV-infected cell. Most tumors express NK cell markers and lack T-cell receptor rearrangements, supporting an NK cell origin.
*   These are highly aggressive neoplasms that respond well to radiotherapy but are resistant to chemotherapy.

Hodgkin Lymphoma (p. 616)

HL accounts for 0.7% of all new cancers in the United States; the average age at diagnosis is 32 years. *As opposed to* NHL—that often occurs in extranodal sites and spreads in an unpredictable fashion:

- HL arises in a single node or chain and spreads in a predictable way to anatomically contiguous lymphoid tissue.
- HL is characterized by the presence of distinctive neoplastic giant cells called *Reed-Sternberg (RS)* cells, derived primarily from germinal center or post-germinal center B cells. These cells release factors that induce the accumulation of the reactive lymphocytes, macrophages, and granulocytes that constitute more than 90% of tumor cellularity.

Morphology (p. 617)

RS cells and their variants are the neoplastic element; their identification is essential for histologic diagnosis:

- *Classic, diagnostic RS cells* are large (45 μm or more) with either a multi-lobed nucleus or multiple nuclei, each with a large, inclusion-like nucleolus roughly the size of a small lymphocyte (5 to 7 μm diameter); cytoplasm is abundant.
- *Mononuclear variants* contain only a single round or oblong nucleus with a large inclusion-like nucleolus.
- *Lacunar cells* have more delicate folded or multilobate nuclei surrounded by abundant pale cytoplasm that retracts during tissue processing, leaving the nucleus in an empty hole (i.e., the lacune).
- *Lymphohistiocytic variants (L&H cells)* have polypoid nuclei resembling popcorn kernels, inconspicuous nucleoli, and moderately abundant cytoplasm.

"Classic" RS cells express PAX5 (a B-cell transcription factor), and CD15 and CD30, but are negative for other B- and T-cell markers and CD45. L&H variants express B-cell markers typical of germinal-center B cells (e.g., CD20 and BCL6) and are negative for CD15 and CD30.

Cells similar or identical in appearance to RS cells occur in other conditions (e.g., infectious mononucleosis, solid tissue cancers, and NHL). Thus, RS cells must be present in an appropriate background of reactive, non-neoplastic inflammation to make the diagnosis.

There are five subtypes of HL in the standard classification scheme, each with somewhat unique diagnostic and/or clinical features (Table 13-3).

- *Nodular sclerosis type* is the most common form of HL, constituting 65% to 75% of cases; it tends to involve the lower cervical, supraclavicular, and mediastinal lymph nodes. This type is characterized by the presence of *lacunar variant* RS cells and *collagen bands* that divide the lymphoid tissue into circumscribed nodules. It is uncommonly associated with EBV. The prognosis is excellent.
- *Mixed cellularity type* constitutes 20% to 25% of cases. It is more likely to be associated with older age, so-called *B symptoms* (i.e., fever and weight loss), and advanced tumor stage. Classic RS cells and mononuclear variants are usually plentiful and are infected by EBV in 70% of cases. The overall prognosis is good.
- *Lymphocyte-rich type* is an uncommon variant. Reactive lymphocytes make up the vast majority of the non-neoplastic portion of the infiltrate, while mononuclear variants and diagnostic RS cells with a classical immunophenotype are reasonably common. This form is associated with EBV in about 40% of cases. Prognosis is very good to excellent.

TABLE 13-3 Subtypes of Hodgkin Lymphoma		
Subtype	**Morphology and Immunophenotype**	**Typical Clinical Features**
Nodular sclerosis	Frequent lacunar cells and occasional diagnostic RS cells; background infiltrate composed of T lymphocytes, eosinophils, macrophages, and plasma cells; fibrous bands dividing cellular areas into nodules. RS cells CD15+, CD30+; usually EBV−	Most common subtype; usually stage I or II disease; frequent mediastinal involvement; equal occurrence in males and females, most patients young adults
Mixed cellularity	Frequent mononuclear and diagnostic RS cells; background infiltrate rich in T lymphocytes, eosinophils, macrophages, plasma cells; RS cells CD15+, CD30+; 70% EBV+	More than 50% present with stage III or IV disease; M greater than F; biphasic incidence, peaking in young adults and again in adults older than 55 years
Lymphocyte rich	Frequent mononuclear and diagnostic RS cells; background infiltrate rich in T lymphocytes; RS cells CD15+, CD30+; 40% EBV+	Uncommon; M greater than F; tends to be seen in older adults
Lymphocyte depletion	Reticular variant: Frequent diagnostic RS cells and variants and a paucity of background reactive cells; RS cells CD15+, CD30+; most EBV+	Uncommon; more common in older men and HIV-infected individuals and in developing countries; often present with advanced disease
Lymphocyte predominance	Frequent L&H (popcorn cell) variants in a background of follicular dendritic cells and reactive B cells; RS cells CD20+, CD15−, C30−; EBV−	Uncommon; young males with cervical or axillary lymphadenopathy; mediastinal

L&H, Lymphohistiocytic; *RS,* Reed-Sternberg.

- *Lymphocyte-depletion type* is the least common form of HL (5% or less) and has a somewhat worse prognosis than other subtypes. RS cells and variants are frequent and reactive cells are relatively sparse; RS cells are infected with EBV in more than 90% of cases. Advanced stage and systemic symptoms are common, and the overall prognosis is somewhat worse than the other varieties.

- *Lymphocyte predominance type* accounts for approximately 5% of all cases, and typically presents with axillary or cervical lymphadenopathy. It is characterized by nodal effacement due to nodular infiltrates of small lymphocytes admixed with variable numbers of benign macrophages and *L&H RS cell variants* (classic RS cells are extremely difficult to find). There is no EBV association. The overall prognosis is excellent.

Molecular Pathogenesis (p. 620)

- In the vast majority of cases, the Ig genes of RS cells have undergone both V(D)J recombination and somatic hypermutation, establishing an origin from germinal center or post-germinal center cells. Nevertheless, for unclear reasons, RS cells of classic HL fail to express most B cell–specific genes (including Ig).
- NF-κB transcription factor activation is a common event in classic HL, either through EBV infection or other mechanisms. This promotes lymphocyte survival and proliferation.
- The different kinds of tissue reaction observed in various HL subtypes are partly due to cytokines and chemokines secreted by the RS cells and reactive background cells. In turn, cytokines produced by the reactive cells may support the growth and survival of tumor cells.
- RS cells are aneuploid with diverse clonal chropmosomal aberrations. Copy number gains in the *c-REL* proto-oncogene on chromosome 2p are common and may contribute to increased NF-κB activity.

Clinical Features (p. 620)

HL typically presents with painless lymphadenopathy. Younger patients with more favorable histologic types tend to present in clinical stage I or II without systemic manifestations. Patients with disseminated disease (stages III and IV) and mixed cellularity or lymphocyte depletion types are more likely to present with B symptoms. Cutaneous anergy due to depressed cell-mediated immunity (attributed to factors released from RS cells that suppress T_H1 responses) is common.

Since HL spreads predictably from its site of origin to contiguous lymphoid groups and then on to spleen, liver, and marrow, staging not only is prognostically important but also guides therapy; patients with limited disease can be cured with local radiotherapy. Staging involves careful physical examination and several investigative procedures, including computed tomography (CT) of the abdomen and pelvis, chest radiography, and marrow biopsy.

Tumor burden (i.e., stage) rather than histologic type is the most important prognostic variable. The 5-year survival rate for stage I or IIA disease approaches 90%, and many are likely cured. Even with advanced disease (stage IVA or IVB), a 60% to 70% 5-year disease-free survival rate is common.

Long-term HL survivors treated with alkylating chemotherapy and radiotherapy have an increased risk of developing second hematologic cancers (myelodysplastic syndromes, acute myelogenous leukemia, NHL) or solid cancers of the lung, breast, stomach, skin, or soft tissues. Non-neoplastic complications of radiotherapy include pulmonary fibrosis and accelerated atherosclerosis.

Myeloid Neoplasms (p. 620)

The common feature of these neoplasms is an origin from hematopoietic progenitor cells. Myeloid neoplasms primarily involve the marrow with lesser involvement of the secondary hematopoietic organs (spleen, liver, and lymph nodes); clinical presentations are related to altered normal hematopoiesis. There are three broad categories:

- *Acute myeloid leukemias* are characterized by marrow accumulation of immature myeloid cells (blasts) that suppress normal hematopoiesis.
- *Myelodysplastic syndromes* exhibit ineffective hematopoiesis that leads to cytopenias.
- *Myeloproliferative disorders* are characterized by increased production of one or more blood cell types.

Acute Myeloid Leukemia (p. 621)

Acute myeloid leukemia (AML) is a tumor of hematopoietic progenitors caused by acquired oncogenic mutations that impede differentiation, leading to the accumulation of immature myeloid blasts.

Classification (p. 622)

AML is quite heterogeneous, reflecting the complexities of myeloid cell differentiation. A new WHO system takes into account the molecular lesions that cause AML and is gaining favor largely because it predicts clinical outcome more reliably. In this classification (Table 13-4), AML is divided into four categories based on the presence or absence of characteristic cytogenetic abnormalities, the presence of dysplasia, prior exposure to drugs known to induce AML, and the type and degree of differentiation.

TABLE 13-4	Major Subtypes of AML in the WHO Classification	
Class	**Prognosis**	**FAB Subtype**
I. AML with Genetic Aberrations		
AML with t(8;21)(q22;q22); *CBFα/ETO* fusion gene	Favorable	M2
AML with inv(16)(p13;q22); *CBFβ/MYH11* fusion gene	Favorable	M4eo
AML with t(15;17)(q22;11-12); *RARα/PML* fusion gene	Intermediate	M3, M3v
AML with t(11q23;v); diverse *MLL* fusion genes	Poor	M4, M5
AML with normal cytogenetics and mutated *NPM*	Favorable	Variable
II. AML with MDS-like Features		
With prior MDS	Poor	Variable
AML with multilineage dysplasia	Poor	Variable
AML with MDS-like cytogenetic aberrations	Poor	Variable
III. AML, Therapy-Related	Very poor	Variable
IV. AML, Not Otherwise Specified		
AML, minimally differentiated	Intermediate	M0
AML without maturation	Intermediate	M1
AML with myelocytic maturation	Intermediate	M2
AML with myelomonocytic maturation	Intermediate	M4
AML with monocytic maturation	Intermediate	M5a, M5b
AML with erythroid maturation	Intermediate	M6a, M6b
AML with megakaryocytic maturation	Intermediate	M7

AML, Acute myeloid leukemia; *FAB*, French-American-British; *MDS*, myelodysplasia; *NPM*, nucleophosmin.

Morphology (p. 622)

The number of leukemic cells in the circulation is highly variable: more than 100,000 cells/μL in some but less than 10,000 cells/μL in 50% of patients. Occasionally, the peripheral smear does not contain any blasts *(aleukemic leukemia)*, and marrow biopsy is required for diagnosis. Myeloid versus lymphoid blasts are distinguished by immunohistochemistry specific for unique surface markers.

AML diagnosis is based on more than 20% myeloid blasts in the marrow; these have different morphologic features depending on the AML type.

- *Myeloblasts* have delicate nuclear chromatin, two to four nucleoli, and voluminous cytoplasm containing fine, azurophilic, peroxidase-positive granules or distinctive red-staining, peroxidase-positive, needle-like structures called *Auer rods*.
- *Monoblasts* have folded or lobulated nuclei, lack Auer rods, and usually do not express peroxidase but can be identified by staining for non-specific esterase.

Cytogenetics (p. 623)

A combination of standard cytogenetic techniques and high-resolution banding modalities reveal chromosomal abnormalities in 90% of cases. Several associations have emerged:

- AML arising *de novo* in patients with no risk factors is often associated with balanced chromosomal translocations (e.g., t[8;21], inv[16], and t[15;17]).
- AMLs that follow a myelodysplastic syndrome or occur after exposure to DNA-damaging agents (e.g., chemotherapy or radiation therapy) usually lack chromosomal translocations; instead, they are commonly associated with deletions or monosomies involving chromosomes 5 and 7.
- AMLs occurring after treatment with drugs that inhibit the enzyme topoisomerase II are often associated with translocations involving the *MLL* gene on chromosome 11 at band q23.

Molecular Pathogenesis (p. 624)

Most genetic aberrations in AML interfere with transcription factor activities required for normal myeloid cell differentiation. For example, in acute promyelocytic leukemia (APML), a t(15;17) translocation results in the fusion of the *retinoic acid receptor-α gene (RARα)* on chromosome 17 to the *promyelocytic leukemia (PML)* gene on chromosome 15. The fusion product encodes an abnormal retinoic acid receptor that interacts with transcriptional repressors and thus blocks myeloid cell differentiation.

Mutations in genes that promote proliferation and survival (e.g., in tyrosine kinases) also likely synergize with transcription factor mutations to cause full-blown AML. Thus, AML with the t(15;17) translocation frequently also have activating mutations in FLT3, a receptor tyrosine kinase that promotes cell growth and inhibits apoptosis.

The t(15;17) translocation not only has pathogenic significance but also guides therapy. Thus, tumors with this translocation respond to high doses of all-*trans*-retinoic acid (ATRA); ATRA binds to the PML-RARα fusion protein and antagonizes its inhibitory effects on gene transcription.

Clinical Features (p. 624)

Although AML constitutes 20% of childhood leukemias, it primarily affects adults, with incidence rising throughout life and peaking after the age of 60 years.

- Most patients present with findings related to *anemia, neutropenia,* and *thrombocytopenia,* most notably fatigue, fever, and spontaneous mucosal and cutaneous bleeding.
- The *bleeding diathesis* caused by thrombocytopenia is often the most striking clinical feature; patients exhibit cutaneous petechiae and ecchymoses, as well as hemorrhages into serosal linings, gingiva, and gastrointestinal and urinary tracts.
- *Procoagulants* released by leukemic cells, especially in APML, can produce *disseminated intravascular coagulation.*
- *Neutropenia leads to infections (frequently opportunistic, e.g., fungi),* particularly in the oral cavity, skin, lungs, kidneys, urinary bladder, and colon.
- In AML with monocytic differentiation and gingival and skin infiltration *(leukemia cutis)* can occur.
- CNS spread is less common than in ALL.
- Rarely, patients present with localized masses composed of myeloblasts (called *myeloblastomas* or *chloromas*). Without systemic treatment, these typically progress to typical AML.

Prognosis is variable, depending on the underlying molecular pathogenesis. Overall, 60% achieve complete remission with chemotherapy, but only 15% to 30% remain disease-free for 5 years. The prognosis is especially dismal for patients with AML arising out of a myelodysplastic syndrome (see the following section) or after previous chemotherapy, since *normal* hematopoietic stem cells in such patients have likely been damaged.

Myelodysplastic Syndromes (p. 624)

Myleodysplastic syndromes (MDS) are a group of clonal stem cell disorders characterized by maturation defects associated with ineffective hematopoiesis and a high risk of transformation to AML. The marrow is partly or wholly replaced by the clonal progeny of a mutant multipotent stem cell that retains the capacity to differentiate but in a manner that is both ineffective and disordered. The marrow is usually hypercellular or normocellular, but the peripheral blood shows pancytopenia; myeloblasts are less than 10% of peripheral leukocytes.

MDS can be *idiopathic or primary*—developing insidiously in patients older than 50 years—or can be secondary to previous myelosuppressive chemotherapy or radiotherapy (usually appearing 2 to 8 years after treatment). All forms of MDS can transform to AML; transformation occurs most rapidly and with highest frequency in patients with therapy-related MDS.

Molecular Pathogenesis (p. 625)

Although the pathogenesis is largely unknown, MDS typically arises in a background of stem cell damage. Progenitors undergo apoptosis at increased rates, a hallmark of ineffective hematopoiesis. Cytogenetic analysis can help confirm an MDS diagnosis since certain chromosomal aberrations are characteristic. Thus, both primary and therapy-related MDS are associated with monosomy 5 and monosomy 7, deletions of 5q and 7q, trisomy 8, and deletions of 20q.

Morphology (p. 625)

The most characteristic finding is disordered (dysplastic) differentiation affecting all three lineages (i.e., erythroid, myeloid, and megakaryocytic).

- *Erythroid lineage effects:*

  Ringed sideroblasts, that is erythroblasts with iron-laden mitochondria visible as perinuclear granules on Prussian blue stain

Megaloblastoid maturation, resembling that seen in vitamin B_{12} or folate deficiency

Nuclear budding abnormalities, producing misshapen nuclei, often with polypoid outlines

- *Granulocytic lineage effects:*

  Neutrophils with decreased numbers of secondary granules, toxic granulations, or Döhle bodies

  Pseudo-Pelger-Huet cells (neutrophils with only two nuclear lobes)

  Myeloblasts may be increased but account for less than 20% of overall marrow cellularity

- *Megakaryocytic lineage effects:* Megakaryocytes with single nuclear lobes or multiple separate nuclei ("pawn ball" megakaryocytes)

Clinical Course (p. 626)

Mean age of onset is 70 years; half of patients are asymptomatic and MDS is discovered only incidentally on routine blood testing. Symptoms that arise stem from pancytopenia. Median survival varies from 9 to 29 months (4 to 8 months for therapy-related MDS), but individuals in good prognostic groups can live 5 years or longer. Death is related to infections and bleeding complications. Progression to AML occurs in 10% to 40% of individuals, accompanied by the appearance of additional clonal cytogenetic changes. In older patients, therapy is largely supportive (antibiotics and transfusions); in younger patients, bone marrow transplantation offers the best hope of long-term survival.

Myeloproliferative Disorders (p. 626)

The common pathogenic feature of myeloproliferative disorders (MPD) is the presence of mutated, constitutively active tyrosine kinases. These tyrosine kinases circumvent normal proliferative control pathways that regulate hematopoiesis and lead to growth factor–independent proliferation and survival of marrow progenitors. These disorders are classified based on clinical, laboratory, and molecular criteria. Common clinical features include:

- Increased proliferative drive in the marrow
- Homing of hematopoietic stem cells to non-marrow sites, causing extramedullary hematopoiesis
- Variable transformation to a spent phase characterized by marrow fibrosis and peripheral cytopenia
- Variable transformation to acute leukemia

CHRONIC MYELOID LEUKEMIA (p. 627)

Chronic myeloid leukemia (CML) is a neoplasm of pluripotent hematopoietic stem cells leading to preferential proliferation of granulocytic progenitors. It is distinguished from other MPD by the presence of a *chimeric, constitutively active* BCR-ABL *tyrosine kinase.*

Molecular Pathogenesis (p. 627)

In more than 90% of CML, the *BCR-ABL* fusion gene is generated by the reciprocal t(9;22) translocation designated the Philadelphia chromosome. In the remaining cases, the fusion gene is created by cytogenetically complex rearrangements.

- t(9;22) leads to fusion of portions of the *BCR* gene (chromosome 22) and the *ABL* gene (chromosome 9).
- The resultant *BCR-ABL* fusion gene directs the synthesis of a 210-kD fusion protein with constitutive tyrosine kinase activity.

The BCR portion provides a dimerization domain leading to the activation the ABL kinase; ABL phosphorylates downstream targets to drive proliferation and survival.

Morphology (p. 627)

CML marrow specimens are markedly hypercellular, with most of the increased cellularity comprising maturing granulocytic precursors. Peripheral blood shows leukocytosis, often more than 100,000 cells/μL. A mixture of neutrophils, metamyelocytes, and myelocytes, with less than 10% myeloblasts, is typical. Peripheral blood eosinophilia, basophilia, and thrombocytosis are also common. Extramedullary hematopoiesis within the splenic red pulp produces marked splenomegaly, often complicated by focal infarction.

Clinical Features (p. 627)

CML primarily occurs in adults with a peak incidence from 50 to 60 years of age. Onset is insidious; initial symptoms (e.g., fatigability, weakness, weight loss, and anorexia) are due to anemia and hypermetabolism owing to increased cell turnover. Other presentations are related to splenomegaly or splenic infarction.

• After a variable *stable phase* period averaging 3 years, 50% of patients enter an *accelerated phase* marked by worsening anemia and thrombocytopenia, increased basophilia, and refractoriness to treatment. Additional clonal cytogenetic abnormalities (e.g., trisomy 8, isochromosome 17q, or duplication of the Philadelphia chromosome) may appear.
• Within 6 to 12 months, the accelerated phase terminates in acute leukemia *(blast crisis)*.
• In the remaining 50%, blast crises occur abruptly without an intermediate accelerated phase.
• In 70% of patients, blasts have the morphologic and cytochemical features of myeloblasts; in about 30%, blasts are of pre-B cell origin (lymphoid blast crisis).

CML is curable in 75% of patients by allogeneic bone marrow transplantation during the stable phase. Imatinib, a BCR-ABL kinase inhibitor, markedly decreases (but does not eliminate) the number of BCR-ABL-positive cells and yields sustained hematologic remissions in 90% of patients. It also substantially decreases the risk of transformation to the accelerated phase and blast crisis; once in accelerated phase or blast crisis, CML becomes rapidly resistant to kinase inhibitor therapy.

POLYCYTHEMIA VERA (p. 628)

Polycythemia vera (PCV) is characterized by increased marrow production of erythrocytes, granulocytes, and platelets. However, *the absolute increase in red blood cell (RBC) mass is responsible for most of the clinical symptoms. PCV is strongly associated with activating point mutations in the JAK2 tyrosine kinase* that participates in JAK/STAT signaling pathways.

Molecular Pathogenesis (p. 628)

Due to constitutive JAK2 signaling, progenitor cells in PCV have diminished requirements for erythropoietin and other hematopoietic growth factors leading to substantial ongoing proliferation.

Morphology (p. 628)

There is hypercellular marrow involving all three lineages; 10% of patients have increased marrow reticulin fibers. Peripheral blood exhibits basophilia and abnormally large platelets. Late in the disease, 15% to 20% of PCV patients progress to a spent phase with substantial marrow fibrosis that displaces hematopoietic cells. This, in turn, leads to *extramedullary hematopoiesis* in the spleen and liver, producing prominent organomegaly. Transformation to AML occurs in just 1% of patients.

Clinical Features (p. 629)

PCV appears insidiously, usually in late middle age:

- *Erythrocytosis* causes patients to be plethoric and cyanotic due to vascular stagnation and deoxygenation. Headache, dizziness, and hypertension are common findings.
- *Basophilia* with histamine release may underlie gastrointestinal symptoms, increased tendency to peptic ulceration, and intense pruritus.
- *High cell turnover* causes hyperuricemia and symptomatic gout in 5% to 10% of cases.
- *Platelet dysfunction* coupled with abnormal blood flow leads to increased risk of both major bleeding and thrombotic events. About 25% of patients first come to clinical attention with thrombosis; life-threatening hemorrhages occur in 5% to 10% of cases.

With no treatment, death from bleeding or thrombosis occurs within months. Simple phlebotomy to normalize the hematocrit results in median survival of roughly 10 years. JAK2 inhibitors are in clinical trials.

ESSENTIAL THROMBOCYTOSIS (p. 629)

Essential thrombocytosis (ET) is an MPD arising in multipotent stem cells, but the increased proliferation and production is largely confined to the megakaryocytic elements. *ET is associated with activating point mutations in JAK2 (i.e., 50% of cases) or MPL (i.e., 5% to 10% of cases), a tyrosine kinase that is normally activated by thrombopoietin.* These mutations render megakaryocytic lineage progenitors thrombopoietin-independent and lead to hyperproliferation. The reason some patients with JAK2 mutations develop PCV and others ET is not understood.

Marrow cellularity is usually only mildly increased, but megakaryocytes are often markedly increased and include abnormally large forms. Peripheral smears reveal thrombocytosis and abnormally large platelets, accompanied by mild leukocytosis. Neoplastic extramedullary hematopoiesis can produce mild organomegaly (i.e., 50% of cases). Uncommonly, ET can evolve to a spent phase of marrow fibrosis or transform to AML.

Qualitative and quantitative abnormalities in platelets underlie the major clinical manifestations of thrombosis and hemorrhage. *Erythromelalgia,* the throbbing and burning of hands and feet caused by occlusion of small arterioles by platelet aggregates, is a characteristic symptom.

Essential thrombocytosis has an indolent course; long asymptomatic periods are punctuated by thrombotic or hemorrhagic crises. Median survival time is 12 to 15 years.

PRIMARY MYELOFIBROSIS (p. 630)

Primary myelofibrosis is characterized by the development of obliterative marrow fibrosis, which—in turn—leads to diminished hematopoiesis, cytopenias, and extensive extramedullary hematopoiesis (spleens can be more than 4000 g).

Molecular Pathogenesis (p. 630)

Activating JAK2 mutations are present in 50% to 60% of cases and activating MPL mutations in 1% to 5%. The resulting marrow fibrosis and obliteration may be secondary to release of fibrogenic factors from neoplastic megakaryocytes; platelet-derived growth factor and transforming growth factor-β (TGF-β) are both implicated. With displacement of hematopoietic elements to extramedullary sites (e.g., spleen, liver, and sometimes lymph nodes), the resulting blood cell production is often disordered.

Morphology (p. 630)

* Early, the marrow is often hypercellular and contains large, dysplastic, and abnormally clustered megakaryocytes. With progression, diffuse fibrosis displaces hematopoietic elements. Late in the course, the fibrotic marrow space can be largely converted to bone (osteosclerosis).
* Nucleated erythroid progenitors and early granulocytes are inappropriately released from the fibrotic marrow and sites of extramedullary hematopoiesis; their appearance in the circulation is termed *leukoerythroblastosis*. Other frequent peripheral blood findings include tear-drop erythrocytes, increased basophils, and abnormally large platelets.
* Moderate to severe normochromic, normocytic anemia is common. The WBC count is usually normal or reduced but can be markedly elevated (i.e., 80,000 to 100,000 cells/μL) during the early cellular marrow phase. Thrombocytopenia, often severe, appears with disease progression.

Clinical Features (p. 631)

Primary myelofibrosis typically occurs in patients older than 60 years; it is less common than PCV or ET. It often presents with anemia or marked splenic enlargement. Nonspecific symptoms (e.g., fatigue, weight loss, and night sweats) result from increased metabolism associated with the expanded mass of hematopoietic cells. Owing to high cell turnover, hyperuricemia and secondary gout can complicate the picture. Prognosis is variable, with median survival periods of 3 to 5 years. Causes of death include infections, thrombotic episodes or bleeding related to platelet abnormalities, and transformation to AML (5% to 20% of cases).

Langerhans Cell Histiocytosis (p. 631)

There are three types of *histiocytoses* (an archaic term for proliferations of dendritic cells and macrophages):

* True histiocytic lymphomas (rare)
* Benign, reactive histiocytoses
* Langerhans cell histiocytoses; these represent monoclonal proliferations of an immature dendritic cell population.

In the last group, the proliferating Langerhans cells have abundant, often vacuolated cytoplasm, with vesicular oval to indented nuclei; expression of HLA-DR, S100, and CD1a is characteristic. Electron microscopy also reveals cytoplasmic structures called *Birbeck granules*; these are pentalaminar tubules resembling tennis racquets and containing the protein *langerin*. Homing of the neoplastic Langerhans cells is dependent on their expression of CCR6 and CCR7.

Langerhans histiocytoses present as several different clinicopathologic entities:

* *Multifocal multisystem Langerhans cell histiocytosis (Letterer-Siwe disease)* is an aggressive systemic disorder in which Langerhans

cells infiltrate and proliferate within skin (there resembling a seb-orrheic eruption), spleen, liver, lung, and bone marrow; anemia and destructive bony lesions are also seen. Usually occurring before age 2 years, Letterer-Siwe disease is rapidly fatal if untreated. Intensive chemotherapy yields 5-year survival rates of about 50%.

- *Unifocal and multifocal unisystem Langerhans cell histiocytosis (eosinophilic granuloma)* usually affects the skeleton as an erosive, expanding accumulation of Langerhans cells (commonly admixed with lymphocytes, plasma cells, neutrophils, and especially eosinophils) within calvarium, ribs, or femur; it can also occur in skin, lungs, or stomach. Lesions can be asymptomatic or painful; pathologic fractures may occur, and lesions can sometimes expand into adjacent soft tissues. Involvement of the posterior hypothalamus causes diabetes insipidus in 50% of patients; the triad of calvarial bone defects, diabetes insipidus, and exophthalmos is called *Hand-Schuller-Christian syndrome.* Lesions can remit spontaneously or may be cured by local excision or irradiation.

- *Pulmonary Langerhans cell histiocytosis* typically occurs in adult smokers and may represent a reactive hyperplasia rather than a true neoplasm; it can spontaneously regress with smoking cessation.

Splenomegaly (p. 633)

Splenomegaly is a common feature of hematolymphoid disorders, but spleens can be enlarged in a wide variety of non-neoplastic conditions (Table 13-5). *Hypersplenism* is a syndrome that can occur with splenic enlargement; it is characterized by reduction of one or more cellular elements of the blood (due to increased splenic macrophage sequestration and destruction). The cytopenias typically resolve after splenectomy.

Nonspecific Acute Splenitis (p. 633)

Splenic enlargement can occur with any blood-borne infection, largely due to the microbes themselves, as well as cytokine-induced proliferation. Grossly, the spleen is red and extremely soft. Microscopically, there is red pulp congestion with lymphoid follicle effacement, occasionally with white pulp follicular necrosis.

Congestive Splenomegaly (p. 634)

Passive chronic venous congestion and enlargement can result from:

- Systemic congestion, encountered in right-sided cardiac failure
- Intrahepatic derangement of portal venous drainage (e.g., due to cirrhosis)
- Extrahepatic portal vein obstruction (e.g., spontaneous portal vein thrombosis); inflammatory involvement of the portal vein *(pylephlebitis)*, with intraperitoneal infections; and thrombosis of the splenic vein

There is moderate to marked splenic enlargement (i.e., 1000 to 5000 g), with a thickened, fibrous capsule. Microscopically, the red pulp is acutely congested but becomes increasingly fibrous and cellular with time, leading to the vascular stasis and increased macrophage clearance.

Splenic Infarcts (p. 634)

Embolic infarcts occur in the setting of endocarditis or severe atherosclerosis. Infarction due to enlargement and compromise of intrasplenic blood flow can occur in virtually any condition that causes significant splenomegaly (see Table 13-5). Grossly, infarcts are

TABLE 13-5 Disorders Associated with Splenomegaly

I. Infections

Nonspecific splenitis of various blood-borne infections (particularly infective endocarditis)
Infectious mononucleosis
Tuberculosis
Typhoid fever
Brucellosis
Cytomegalovirus
Syphilis
Malaria
Histoplasmosis
Toxoplasmosis
Kala-azar
Trypanosomiasis
Schistosomiasis
Leishmaniasis
Echinococcosis

II. Congestive States Related to Portal Hypertension

Cirrhosis of the liver
Portal or splenic vein thrombosis
Cardiac failure

III. Lymphohematogenous Disorders

Hodgkin lymphoma
Non-Hodgkin lymphomas and lymphocytic leukemias
Multiple myeloma
Myeloproliferative disorders
Hemolytic anemias
Thrombocytopenic purpura

IV. Immunologic-Inflammatory Conditions

Rheumatoid arthritis
Systemic lupus erythematosus

V. Storage Diseases

Gaucher disease
Niemann-Pick disease
Mucopolysaccharidoses

VI. Miscellaneous

Amyloidosis
Primary neoplasms and cysts
Secondary neoplasms

wedge-shaped and subcapsular. Fresh infarcts are hemorrhagic and red; older infarcts are yellow-gray and fibotic.

Neoplasms (p. 634)

Neoplastic involvement of the spleen is rare except in cases of myeloid and lymphoid tumors. Benign splenic tumors include fibromas, osteomas, chondromas, lymphangiomas, and hemangiomas.

Congenital Anomalies (p. 634)

Complete absence of the spleen is rare and is usually associated with other congenital anomalies such as *situs inversus*; hypoplasia is considerably more common. *Accessory spleens* are fairly common (up to a third of individuals) and can be found anywhere in the abdominal cavity.

Rupture (p. 635)

Splenic rupture is typically a sequela of blunt force trauma; so-called "spontaneous ruptures" without antecedent injury usually result from some minor physical insult to a spleen already rendered fragile due to an underlying disorder (e.g., infectious mononucleosis), other infections, or splenic neoplasms. Rupture leads to significant intraperitoneal hemorrhag and must be treated with prompt splenectomy to prevent exsanguination. Interestingly, chronically enlarged spleens often have reactive capsular fibrosis that resists rupture.

Thymic Developmental Disorders (p. 635)

- *Thymic hypoplasia or aplasia* is accompanied by parathyroid aplasia and variable defects involving the heart and great vessels; these changes occur in *DiGeorge syndrome* (Chapter 5).
- *Thymic cysts* are uncommon lesions lined by stratified or columnar epithelium; they are mostly developmental in origin and of little clinical significance. Occasionally, thymic cysts herald an adjacent thymic neoplasm, especially lymphoma or thymoma.

Thymic Hyperplasia (p. 635)

Thymic hyperplasia refers to the appearance of reactive B-cell lymphoid follicles within the thymus. It is seen in chronic inflammatory and immunologic states, particularly myasthenia gravis (65% to 75% of cases).

Thymomas (p. 636)

Thymomas are neoplasms derived from *thymic epithelial cells.* These may be cytologically benign and non-invasive, cytologically benign but invasive or metastatic, or cytologically malignant *(thymic carcinoma).*

Morphology (p. 636)

- *Grossly:* Thymomas are usually lobulated, firm, gray-white masses up to 15 to 20 cm; they can exhibit focal cystic necrosis and calcification. Most are encapsulated but in 20% to 25% adjacent structures are invaded; benign tumors are typically well encapsulated.
- *Microscopically:*

  Noninvasive thymomas are composed of medullary (spindled) and/or cortical (plump with rounded vesicular nuclei) epithelial cells, often with a sparse thymocyte infiltrate.

  Invasive thymomas more commonly exhibit cortical-type epithelial cells and more numerous thymocytes. Occasionally, neoplastic cells exhibit atypia, presaging a more aggressive phenotype. Invasive thymomas—by definition—penetrate through the capsule into surrounding structures.

  Thymic carcinoma represents 5% of thymomas; they are fleshy, invasive masses that are most commonly *squamous cell carcinomas.* The second most common variant is *lymphoepithelioma-like carcinoma,* microscopically resembling nasopharyngeal carcinomas, and in 50% of cases containing monoclonal EBV genomes.

Clinical Features (p. 637)

These are tumors primarily of adults older than 40 years; about 40% present with symptoms referable to compression of mediastinal structures, and an additional 30% to 45% present with *myasthenia gravis.* Thymomas are associated with other paraneoplastic syndromes (e.g., acquired hypogammaglobulinemia, pure RBC aplasia, Graves disease, pernicious anemia, dermatomyositis-polymyositis, and Cushing syndrome). For minimally invasive lesions, complete excision results in more than 90% 5-year survivals; more extensive invasion is associated with 5-year survivals less than 50%.

14

Red Blood Cells and Bleeding Disorders

Anemias (p. 639)

Anemia is a reduction in the total circulating red blood cell (RBC) mass below normal limits; the consequences are reduced oxygen-carrying capacity and tissue hypoxia. Patients are pale, weak, and easily fatigued. Anemia is formally diagnosed based on a reduction in the hematocrit and/or hemoglobin concentration (Table 14-1). The classification of anemias is usually based on the underlying mechanism (see the following sections); the specifics of RBC morphology (size, shape, and hemoglobinization) can often provide etiologic clues. Thus, microcytic, hypochromic anemias suggest disorders of hemoglobin synthesis (most often iron deficiency), while macrocytic anemias suggest abnormalities in bone marrow erythroid precursor maturation; normochromic, normocytic anemias have diverse etiologies.

Anemias of Blood Loss (p. 641)

Clinical features depend on the rate of hemorrhage and whether it is external or internal; interstitial bleeding allows recapture of red cell iron, but bleeding into the gut or externally can lead to iron deficiency and hamper restoration of normal RBC counts.

- *Acute blood loss*: Any clinical effects are due mainly to the loss of intravascular volume; shock and/or death can result. If the patient survives, fluid shifts from the interstitium rapidly restore the blood volume; however, there will be hemodilution and lowering of the hematocrit. The resulting reduction in oxygen-carrying capacity triggers renal erythropoietin production, with increased proliferation of committed erythroid progenitors. Release of new RBCs begins at day 5; it is heralded by increased numbers of reticulocytes (large, immature RBCs) peaking at 10% to 15% of the peripheral RBC count by day 7. Significant bleeding (with hypotension) also triggers an adrenergic response that mobilizes granulocytes from the intravascular marginated pool (causing leukocytosis); thrombocytosis also occurs due to increased platelet production.
- *Chronic blood loss*: Anemia will occur only if the rate of loss exceeds the marrow regenerative capacity, or when iron reserves are depleted.

Hemolytic Anemias (p. 641)

Hemolytic anemias feature premature RBC destruction (i.e., less than the normal 120-day lifespan), elevated erythropoietin with increased erythropoiesis, and increased hemoglobin catabolites

TABLE 14-1	Adult Reference Ranges for Red Blood Cells*	
Measurement (units)	**Men**	**Women**
Hemoglobin (g/dL)	13.6-17.2	12.0-15.0
Hematocrit (%)	39-49	33-43
RBC count ($10^6/\mu L$)	4.3-5.9	3.5-5.0
Reticulocyte count (%)	0.5-1.5	
Mean cell volume (fL)	82-96	
Mean corpuscular hemoglobin (pg)	27-33	
Mean corpuscular hemoglobin concentration (g/dL)	33-37	
RBC distribution width (expressing the degree of anisocytosis)	11.5-14.5	

*Reference ranges vary among laboratories. The reference ranges for the laboratory providing the result should always be used in interpreting the test result.
RBC, Red blood cell.

(e.g., bilirubin). The excess serum bilirubin is unconjugated; the ultimate levels of hyperbilirubinemia depend on liver functional capacity and the rate of hemolysis; with normal livers, jaundice is rarely severe.

Hemolysis can be extravascular or intravascular:

- *Extravascular hemolysis* occurs in macrophages of the spleen (and other organs). Predisposing factors include RBC membrane injury, reduced deformability, or opsonization. The principal clinical features are anemia, splenomegaly, and jaundice; modest reductions in haptoglobin (a serum protein that binds hemoglobin) also occur.
- *Intravascular hemolysis:* RBCs can be ruptured by mechanical injury (e.g., mechanical cardiac valves), complement fixation (e.g., mismatched blood transfusion), intracellular parasites (e.g., malaria), or extracellular toxins (e.g., clostridial enzymes). Patients exhibit anemia, hemoglobinemia, hemoglobinuria, hemosiderinuria, and jaundice; there is markedly reduced serum haptoglobin. Free hemoglobin can be oxidized to methemoglobin. Both forms of the protein are excreted in the urine (imparting a brown color) or are resorbed by renal proximal tubules; iron released from hemoglobin can accumulate in tubular cells (renal hemosiderosis).

Hereditary Spherocytosis (p. 642)

Hereditary spherocytosis (HS) is due to cytoskeletal or membrane protein defects that render RBCs spheroidal and less deformable, and thus vulnerable to splenic sequestration and destruction; it is autosomal dominant in 75% of patients.

Pathogenesis (p. 642)

Insufficiency in several different proteins (spectrin, ankyrin, band 3, or band 4.2) can cause HS; all lead to reduced density of membrane skeletal components, which in turn causes reduced stability of the lipid bilayer and loss of membrane fragments as RBC age. Compound heterozygosity for two defective alleles typically causes a more severe phenotype. Reduction in surface area causes RBC to assume a spheroidal shape with diminished deformability and a propensity for being trapped and destroyed by splenic macrophages.

Morphology (p. 643)

Spherocytic RBCs are small and lack central pallor; there is reticulocytosis and marrow erythroid hyperplasia. Marked splenic congestion is seen with prominent erythrophagocytosis in the cords of Billroth.

Clinical Features (p. 643)

Diagnosis depends on family history, hematologic findings, and increased RBC osmotic fragility; the mean RBC hemoglobin concentration is increased due to cellular dehydration. Anemia, moderate splenomegaly, and jaundice are characteristic. Although the clinical course is typically stable due to compensatory increases in erythropoiesis, increased RBC turnover or diminished erythropoiesis can be problematic. Thus, *aplastic crisis* occurs when parvovirus induces transient suppression of erythropoiesis; events that increase splenic RBC destruction (e.g., infectious mononucleosis) trigger *hemolytic crisis.* Half of adults develop gallstones from chronic hyperbilirubinemia.

Hemolytic Disease Due to Red Cell Enzyme Defects: Glucose-6-Phosphate Dehydrogenase Deficiency (p. 644)

Glucose-6-phosphate dehydrogenase (G6PD) is an enzyme in the hexose monophosphate shunt that reduces nicotinamide adenine dinucleotide phosphate (NAPD) to NADPH; in turn, NADPH reduces RBC glutathione, providing protection against RBC oxidative injury. In G6PD-deficient cells, oxidant stress (e.g., due to inflammation, drugs, or foods such as fava beans) causes hemoglobin sulfhydryl cross-linking and protein denaturation. The altered hemoglobin precipitates as *Heinz bodies* that can cause direct hemolysis; in addition, the precipitated hemoglobin can attach to the inner cell membrane, reduce deformability, and increase susceptibility to splenic macrophage destruction.

G6PD deficiency is an X-linked disorder; although there are several G6PD variants, only two—G6PD⁻ and G6PD Mediterranean—lead to clinically significant hemolysis. G6PD⁻ is present in about 10% of African-American; abnormal protein folding leads to increased proteolytic degradation and thus progressive loss of G6PD in older RBCs. Because younger RBCs are unaffected, hemolytic episodes are usually self-limited. In the Mediterranean form, G6PD levels are much lower and hemolytic episodes are more severe.

Sickle Cell Disease (p. 645)

Hemoglobin is a tetrameric protein composed of two pairs of globin chains. Normal adult red cells mainly contain HbA ($\alpha_2\beta_2$) with smaller amounts of HbA$_2$ ($\alpha_2\delta_2$) and fetal hemoglobin HbF ($\alpha_2\gamma_2$).

Sickle cell disease is a hereditary hemoglobinopathy resulting from substitution of valine for glutamic acid at the sixth position of the β-globin chain; the resultant mutant hemoglobin substitutes for the normal β-globin to generate HbS. This is an autsomal recessive disorder; 8% to 10% of African Americans are heterozygous for the abnormal allele (*sickle cell trait*, which is largely asymptomatic), while 70,000 individuals in the United States are homozygous ($\alpha_2\beta_{S2}$) and have *sickle cell disease.*

Pathogenesis (p. 645)

When deoxygenated, HbS polymerizes into long, stiff chains that deform (sickle) RBCs. This, in turn, causes chronic hemolysis, microvascular occlusion, and tissue damage. Several variables affect the rate and degree of sickling:

- *Interaction of HbS with other types of hemoglobin within RBCs.* In heterozygotes, HbS constitutes only 40% of the hemoglobin with the remainder being HbA; the HbA interferes with HbS polymerization. Consequently, in heterozygotes, sickling occurs only with profound hypoxia. β-globin chains other than HbA also influence sickling. Thus, HbF also interferes with HbS polymerization, and newborns do not manifest disease complications until 5 to 6 months of age when RBC HbF content is reduced to adult levels. For the fortunate adult patient who has hereditary persistence of HbF, the sickle cell disease is considerably less severe. Another variant of hemoglobin is HbC (substituting lysine for the glutamic acid in the β-chain sixth position); in patients with both β-globin S and C alleles (HbSC), HbS constitutes 50% of the hemoglobin, and the HbSC cells have a tendency to lose salt and water, becoming dehydrated—which increases the intracellular HbS concentrations. Both factors increase the tendency of the HbS to polymerize and thus result in HbSC patients having a symptomatic (albeit milder) sickling disorder called *HbSC disease.*
- *Mean corpuscular hemoglobin concentration (MCHC):* Higher HbS concentrations increase the probability of interaction between individual HbS molecules. Thus, dehydration—which increases MCHC—facilitates sickling. Conversely, concurrent diseases that reduce MCHC (e.g., α-thalassemia) lessen sickling severity.
- *Intracellular pH:* Reduced pH reduces hemoglobin oxygen affinity, thereby increasing the proportion of deoxygenated HbS and the propensity to polymerize.
- *Microvascular transit time:* Normally, the capillary transit rate is sufficiently high that significant deoxygenation (and therefore sickling) cannot occur. Consequently, sickling is usually confined to tissues with intrinsically sluggish blood flow (e.g., spleen, bone marrow) or those involved by inflammation, where transit rates are retarded.

Although re-oxygenation depolymerizes HbS, repeated cycles of sickling eventually result in irreversible RBC damage. This happens because polymerized HbS herniates through the membrane skeleton ensheathed by only a lipid bilayer; such severe membrane derangements cause Ca^{2+} influx, protein cross-linking, and water and potassium efflux. With repeated episodes, RBCs become progressively dehydrated, dense, and rigid, and the most damaged cells eventually become end-stage, non-deformable RBCs that retain the sickle shape even when fully oxygenated. Non-deformable cells are prone to macrophage sequestration and destruction and are also intrinsically more mechanically fragile, undergoing intravascular hemolysis.

Microvascular occlusion with resultant tissue hypoxia and infarction is the most clinically important clinical aspect of sickle cell disease. The propensity to occlude small vessels is not strictly dependent on the percentage of irreversibly sickled cells in the blood; rather, it is a function of RBC stickiness (sickled RBCs express increased levels of adhesion molecules), local inflammation, and platelet aggregation. Stagnation of RBCs in inflamed vascular beds likely leads to a vicious cycle of sickling, obstruction, hypoxia, and more inflammation. Also, free hemoglobin released from ruptured RBCs binds and inactivates nitric oxide (NO)—increasing vascular tone and enhancing platelet aggregation.

Morphology (p. 646)

- *Peripheral blood* shows variable numbers of irreversibly sickled cells, reticulocytosis, and target cells due to RBC dehydration.
- In childhood, there is *splenomegaly* due to sickled cell trapping in splenic cords. By adulthood, repeated episodes of vaso-occlusion have caused progressive fibrosis and shrinkage (*autosplenectomy*).

- *Bone marrow* shows normoblastic hyperplasia. When hyperplasia is severe, expansion of the marrow can cause bone resorption; extramedullary hematopoiesis can occur.
- *Microvascular occlusions* produce damage and infarction in various tissues.

Clinical Features (p. 647)

- Chronic hemolytic anemia (hematocrits from 18% to 30%) is associated with chronic hyperbilirubinemia and a propensity for gallstones. Chronic hypoxia will cause generalized impairment of growth and development.
- *Vaso-occlusive crises* present as painful episodes of ischemic necrosis, most commonly involving bones, lungs, liver, brain, penis, and spleen. *Acute chest syndrome* is a particularly serious vaso-occlusive crisis caused by pulmonary inflammation that impedes lung vascular flow; sickling and occlusion compromises pulmonary function and potentially leads to a fatal cycle of worsening pulmonary and systemic hypoxia.
- *Aplastic crisis* due to transient suppression of erythropoiesis is triggered by parvovirus infections. *Sequestration crises* occur in children with intact spleens; massive entrapment of sickled RBCs leads to rapid splenic enlargement, hypovolemia, and occasionally shock.
- Progressive splenic fibrosis and impairment of the alternate complement pathway predispose to infections, particularly involving encapsulated organisms such as *Streptococcus pneumoniae* and *Haemophilus influenzae*.

Diagnosis is based on clinical findings, sickle cells in the peripheral blood smear, and detection of HbS by hemoglobin electrophoresis. Prenatal detection is possible through fetal DNA analysis. Hydroxyurea is a therapeutic mainstay: it increases HbF levels and also reduces white cell production (reducing inflammation). Some 90% of patients survive to age 20 years, and more than half of patients live to age 60 years.

Thalassemia Syndromes (p. 648)

Thalassemia syndromes are a heterogeneous group of inherited disorders caused by mutations that reduce α- or β-globin chain synthesis (Table 14-2). β Chains are encoded by a single gene on chromosome 11 (yielding two copies); α chains are encoded by two closely linked genes on chromosome 16 (yielding four copies). Diminished synthesis of one chain has pathologic consequences due to: low intracellular hemoglobin (hypochromia) and effects related to a relative excess of the other chain. The syndromes are most common in Mediterranean countries, parts of Africa, and Southeast Asia.

β-THALASSEMIAS (p. 648)

- *β-Thalassemias* are characterized by deficient synthesis of β-globin:
- β^0 mutations abrogate β-globin chain synthesis; most commonly these involve chain termination mutations that create premature stop codons.
- β^+ mutations lead to reduced (but detectable) β-globin synthesis; most commonly these involve aberrant RNA splicing, although some are promoter region mutations.

Molecular Pathogenesis (p. 648)

With decreased β-globin synthesis, there is reduced HbA production; the "under-hemoglobinized" RBC are hypochromic and microcytic with reduced oxygen carrying capacity. In addition, excess unbound

TABLE 14-2 Clinical and Genetic Classification of Thalassemias

Clinical Syndromes	Genotype	Clinical Features	Molecular Genetics
β-Thalassemias			
β-Thalassemia major	Homozygous β-thalassemia (β^0/β^0, β^+/β^+, β^0/β^+)	Severe; requires blood transfusions	Mainly point mutations that lead to defects in the transcription, splicing, or translation of β-globin mRNA
β-Thalassemia intermedia	Variable (β^0/β^+, β^+/β^+, β^0/β, β^+/β)	Severe but does not require regular blood transfusions	
β-Thalassemia minor	Heterozygous β-thalassemia (β^0/β, β^+/β)	Asymptomatic with mild or absent anemia; red cell abnormalities seen	
α-Thalassemias			
Silent carrier	$-/\alpha$ α/α	Asymptomatic; no red cell abnormality	Mainly gene deletions
α-Thalassemia trait	$-/-$ α/α (Asian) $-/\alpha$ $-/\alpha$ (black African, Asian)	Asymptomatic, like β-thalassemia minor	
HbH disease	$-/-$ $-/\alpha$	Severe; resembles β-thalassemia intermedia	
Hydrops fetalis	$-/-$ $-/-$	Lethal in utero without transfusions	

α chains form highly unstable aggregates that cause cell membrane damage; this leads to precursor destruction in the marrow (ineffective erythropoiesis) and splenic sequestration of mature RBCs. Severe anemia causes marked compensatory expansion of the erythropoietic marrow, ultimately encroaching on cortical bone and causing skeletal abnormalities in growing children. Ineffective erythropoiesis is also associated with excessive absorption of dietary iron; along with repeated blood transfusions this leads to severe iron overload.

Clinical Syndromes (p. 649)

Classification of β-thalassemia is based on the severity of anemia; severity is based on the genetic defect (β^+ or β^0), as well as gene dosage (homozygous or heterozygous).

- *β-Thalassemia major:* Patients with two β-thalassemia alleles (β^+/β^+, β^+/β^0, or β^0/β^0 typically have severe, transfusion-dependent anemia; the manifestations begin 6 to 9 months after birth as hemoglobin synthesis switches from HbF to HbA.

    Peripheral blood shows marked anisocytosis (variability in cell size) with many microcytic, hypochromic RBCs, target cells, and erythrocyte fragments; poorly hemoglobinized RBC precursors (normoblasts) are also common.

    There is marked expansion of the hematopoietic marrow, with erosion of existing cortical bone and subsequent new bone formation. Extramedullary hemaotopoiesis is common with splenomegaly.

    Without transfusions, death occurs at an early age from profound anemia. Blood transfusions lessen the anemia and suppress the secondary bone deformities. In multiply transfused patients, morbidity and fatality are related to cardiac failure resulting from progressive iron overload and secondary hemochromatosis; iron chelation can slow (but not prevent) these complications. Bone marrow transplantation is the only curative therapy.

- *β-Thalassemia minor:* Heterozygotes are usually asymptomatic due to sufficient β-globin synthesis.

    Peripheral blood shows minor abnormalities, including hypochromia, microcytosis, basophilic stippling, and target cells. Hemoglobin electrophoresis shows increased HbA_2 ($\alpha_2\delta_2$ hemoglobin) due to increased ratios of δ- versus β-globin synthesis.

    Recognition of β-thalassemia trait is important for genetic counseling.

- *β-Thalassemia intermedia:* Clinical consequences and severity are intermediate between the major and minor forms. These patients are genetically heterogeneous.

α-THALASSEMIAS (p. 651)

These are due to inherited defects that reduced α-globin synthesis; gene deletion is the most common genetic cause. The clinical consequences are due to imbalanced synthesis of α and non-α chains (γ chains in infancy, β and δ chains after 6 months of age). Free β chain tetramers (HbH) have extremely high oxygen (O_2) affinity and thus cause tissue hypoxia disproportionate to hemoglobin levels. In addition, HbH is prone to oxidation, leading to precipitation of intracellular protein aggregates that promote RBC sequestration by macrophages. Free γ chains form stable tetramers (HbBarts) that also bind O_2 with excessive avidity, resulting in tissue hypoxia.

    Silent carrier state: Completely asymptomatic, resulting from a single α-globin gene deletion; changes in total α-globin chain synthesis are barely detectable.

α-Thalassemia trait: Either one chromosome has both α-globin genes or each chromosome has a deletion of one gene; the clinical picture is comparable to β-thalassemia minor. Although these two genotypes are clinically identical, they differ in whether offspring are at risk for severe α-thalassemia (three or more α chains deleted).

Hemoglobin H (HbH) disease: Deletion of three α-globin genes causes marked suppression of α chain synthesis and formation of unstable HbH tetramers; clinically, it resembles β-thalassemia intermedia.

Hydrops fetalis: Deletion of all four α-globin genes. Early fetal development is permitted by embryonic ζ-chain synthesis; however, as ζ-globin ceases and the fetal $ζ_2γ_2$ tetramers are replaced by γ-globin tetramers (HbBarts), the high oxygen affinity prevents O_2 release to tissues and is not compatible with life. Intrauterine (and then life-long) transfusions can be life-saving.

Paroxysmal Nocturnal Hemoglobinuria *(p. 652)*

Paroxysmal nocturnal hemoglobinuria (PNH) is a rare X-linked hemolytic disease resulting from acquired mutations in phosphatidylinositol glycan complementation group A gene (PIGA); PIGA mutations lead to deficient expression of a family of proteins normally anchored into the cell membrane via glycosylphosphatidylinositol (GPI). Among the GPI-linked proteins affected are several that regulate complement inactivation: decay-accelerating factor (CD55), membrane inhibitor of reactive lysis (CD59), and C8-binding protein. Their deficiency renders RBCs hypersensitive to complement, which is activated spontaneously at low rates. Granulocyte and platelet GPI-linked proteins are also affected, resulting in a predisposition to thrombosis, particularly in portal, cerebral, and hepatic veins. Hemolysis is intravascular, but it is paroxysmal and nocturnal in only 25% of cases.

PNH may arise due to an autoimmune response to GPI-linked proteins on hematopoietic stem cells. In this scenario, rare clones harboring a mutated *PIGA* gene thus have a selective advantage and eventually "take over" the marrow. This pathogenic basis explains the association of PNH with aplastic anemia, a marrow failure syndrome with an autoimmune pathogenesis. In 5% to 10% of patients, PNH transforms to acute myeloid leukemia or myelodysplastic syndrome. Bone marrow transplantation can be curative.

Immunohemolytic Anemia *(p. 653)*

Immunohemolytic anemia is caused by antibodies that bind to RBCs and cause their premature destruction; classification is based on the characteristics of the responsible antibody (see later discussion). Diagnosis requires detection of antibodies and/or complement on RBCs. This is accomplished by the *direct Coombs test:* the patient's RBCs are mixed with antibodies directed against human immunoglobulin or complement, with RBC agglutination constituting a positive test. In the *indirect Coombs test,* a patient's serum is assayed for its ability to agglutinate test RBC expressing specific surface antigens.

Warm antibody type (p. 653) is the most common immunohemolytic anemia; half of the cases are idiopathic *(primary),* with the remainder being associated with other autoimmune disorders (e.g., lupus), lymphoid neoplasms, or drug hypersensitivity. Most commonly, immunoglobulin G (IgG) anti-RBC antibodies (anti-Rh in most idiopathic cases) coat the RBC and act as opsonins; erythrocytes become spheroidal due to partial macrophage phagocytosis and are eventually completely destroyed in the spleen. Splenomegaly is characteristic. Drug-induced hemolytic anemias occur through two mechanisms:

- *Antigenic drugs:* Drugs (e.g., penicillin, cephalosporins, quinidine) bind to the RBC surface; antibodies then interact with the drug or an RBC-drug complex.
- *Tolerance-breaking drugs:* Drugs (e.g., α-methyldopa) induce antibodies against intrinsic RBC antigens.

Cold agglutinin type (p. 654) anemia is caused by IgM antibodies that agglutinate RBCs at low temperatures; it accounts for 15% to 30% of immune hemolytic anemias

- *Acute* hemolysis occurs during recovery from certain infections (e.g., *Mycoplasma*, Epstein-Barr virus [EBV], or human immunodeficiency virus [HIV] infections). It is usually self-limited and rarely induces significant hemolysis.
- *Chronic* hemolysis can be idiopathic or can occur in the setting of B-cell neoplasms. Clinical symptoms result from RBC agglutination and complement fixation in vascular beds cooler than 30° C; although there is minimal complement-mediated hemolysis, the complement-coated cells are readily phagocytized in spleen, liver, and bone marrow. The hemolytic anemia is of variable severity; vascular obstruction in areas exposed to cold temperatures results in pallor, cyanosis, and Raynaud phenomenon.

Cold hemolysin type (p. 654) anemia occurs in *paroxysmal cold hemoglobinuria,* capable of causing substantial (sometimes fatal) intravascular hemolysis. The autoantibodies are IgG that bind to the P blood group antigen at low temperatures and fix complement; when the temperature is elevated, hemolysis occurs. Most cases occur in children after viral infections and are transient.

Hemolytic Anemia Resulting from Trauma to Red Cells (p. 654)

Turbulent flow and increased shear forces cause RBC fragmentation and intravascular hemolysis; peripheral blood reveals fragmented RBC *(schistocytes).* Causes include:

- Prosthetic heart valves (mechanical more than bioprosthetic valves)
- Microangiopathic hemolytic anemia with diffuse microvascular narrowing owing to fibrin or platelet deposition (e.g., disseminated intravascular coagulation, thrombotic thrombocytopenic purpura, hemolytic-uremic syndrome)

Anemias of Diminished Erythropoiesis (p. 654)

Impaired RBC production can occur due to deficiency of erythropoietin or a vital nutrient (iron, vitamin B_{12}, folate), inherited defects, neoplasia, or stem cell failure.

Megaloblastic Anemias (p. 654)

Megaloblastic anemias are most commonly due to deficiency of vitamin B_{12} or folate. These are coenzymes required for the synthesis of thymidine (and are also involved in normal methionine synthesis); in their absence, inadequate DNA synthesis causes defective nuclear maturation of rapidly proliferating cells. The resultant blockade in cell division leads to abnormally large RBCs and erythroid precursors (megaloblasts), and also affects granulocyte maturation. Neurologic complications of B_{12} deficiency (see later discussion) are attributed to abnormal myelin degradation.

Morphology (p. 655)

- Prominent peripheral blood anisocytosis with abnormally large and oval RBCs (macro-ovalocytes)
- In the marrow, erythroid precursor nuclear maturation lags behind cytoplasmic maturation; ineffective erythropoiesis is reflected by increased apoptosis with compensatory megaloblastic hyperplasia·
- Abnormal granulopoiesis with giant metamyelocytes in marrow and hypersegmented neutrophils in peripheral blood

Normal Vitamin B$_{12}$ Metabolism (p. 656)

Microorganisms are the ultimate source of vitamin B$_{12}$ (cobalamin); plants and vegetables contain little cobalamin, and most dietary cobalamin comes from animal products.

- Peptic digestion releases dietary vitamin B$_{12}$; it is bound to salivary proteins called *R binders.*
- R-B$_{12}$ complexes are digested in the duodenum by pancreatic proteases; released vitamin B$_{12}$ binds to intrinsic factor (IF), a protein secreted by parietal cells of the gastric fundus.
- IF-B$_{12}$ complexes bind to IF receptors in the distal ileum epithelium; absorbed vitamin B$_{12}$ complexes with transcobalamin II and is transported to tissues.
- 1% of ingested vitamin B$_{12}$ can be absorbed through an alternative pathway independent of intrinsic factor or the terminal ileum.

Except for strict vegans or in chronic alcoholism, most diets contain adequate cobalamin. Thus, most deficiencies in vitamin B$_{12}$ result from impaired absorption:

- Achlorhydria (in elderly individuals) impairs vitamin B$_{12}$ release from R binders
- Gastrectomy causes loss of IF
- Pernicious anemia (see the following discussion)
- Resection of the distal ileum prevents IF-B$_{12}$ absorption
- Malabsorption syndromes
- Increased requirements (e.g., pregnancy)

ANEMIAS OF VITAMIN B$_{12}$ DEFICIENCY: PERNICIOUS ANEMIA (p. 655)

Pernicious anemia is a specific form of megaloblastic anemia caused by autoimmune gastritis and attendant loss of IF production. Gastric injury is likely initiated by autoreactive T cells; secondary autoantibodies against proteins involved in B$_{12}$ uptake are not the primary cause of disease but can exacerbate the process:

- Type I antibodies (present in 75% of patients) block B$_{12}$ binding to IF
- Type II antibodies block IF or IF-B$_{12}$ binding to the ileal receptor
- Type III antibodies (i.e., 85% to 90% of patients) directed against parietal proton pump proteins affect acid secretion

Morphology (p. 658)

- Bone marrow shows megaloblastic erythroid hyperplasia, giant myelocytes and metamyelocytes, hypersegmented neutrophils, and large, multilobed nuclei in megakaryocytes
- Atrophic glossitis; the tongue is shiny, glazed, and red
- Gastric fundal atrophy with virtual absence of parietal cells and replacement by mucus-secreting goblet cells ("intestinalization")
- Central nervous system (CNS) lesions occur in 75% of cases, characterized by demyelination of dorsal and lateral spinal cord tracts

Clinical Features (p. 658)

Onset is insidious, with symptoms due to anemia and posterolateral spinal tract involvement; the latter includes spastic paresis and sensory ataxia. Diagnosis is based on the presence of megaloblastic anemia, leukopenia with hypersegmented neutrophils, low serum B_{12} levels, and elevated homocysteine and methylmalonic acid (consequences of diminished thymidine and methionine synthesis). The diagnosis is confirmed by profound reticulocytosis after parenteral B_{12} administration; serum anti-IF antibodies are highly specific for pernicious anemia. There is a significant association of pernicious anemia with other autoimmune disorders of the adrenal and thyroid glands, as well as increased risk of gastric cancer.

ANEMIA OF FOLATE DEFICIENCY (p. 658)

Folate is involved in single carbon transfers in a variety of biochemical pathways. Deficiency induces a megaloblastic anemia hematologically indistinguishable from that seen with B_{12} deficiency; notably, however, gastric atrophy and the neurologic sequelae of B_{12} deficiency do not occur. Diagnosis of folate deficiency requires demonstration of reduced serum or RBC folate levels. Deficiency occurs with:

- Inadequate intake (e.g., chronic alcoholics, very elderly, or indigents)
- Malabsorption syndromes (e.g., sprue) or diffuse infiltrative disease of the bowel (e.g., lymphoma)
- Increased demand (e.g., pregnancy, infancy, or disseminated cancer)
- Folate antagonists (e.g., methotrexate for chemotherapy)

Iron Deficiency Anemia (p. 659)

Iron deficiency is the most common nutritional disorder in the world.

Iron Metabolism (p. 659)

The normal Western diet contains 10 to 20 mg of iron daily, mostly as heme iron in animal products (the remainder is inorganic iron from vegetables); intake is usually sufficient to balance daily losses of 1 to 2 mg from sloughed skin and gastrointestinal epithelial cells. Some 15% to 20% of total body iron is in *stored form* bound to hemosiderin or ferritin; serum ferritin level is a good indicator of total iron stores. The rest of the body's iron is complexed in a number of functional proteins; 80% is contained in hemoglobin with myoglobin, catalase, and cytochromes making up the rest. Excess iron can be highly toxic, so that uptake must be carefully regulated.

Iron balance is maintained by regulating the absorption of dietary iron across the duodenal epithelium (Fig. 14-1). Heme iron enters mucosal cells directly ($\sim$20% is absorbable), whereas non-heme iron is first reduced to ferrous iron (via cytochome B) before transport; only 1% to 2% of non-heme iron is absorbed. Absorbed iron is transported across the basolateral membrane, where it is bound to plasma transferrin for distribution throughout the body; this basolateral transport requires ferriportin, a membrane transporter, and hephaestin to re-oxidize the reduced iron. The remaining intracellular iron is bound to ferritin and subsequently lost when the epithelium is sloughed during normal turnover. Iron homeostasis is regulated in large part by hepcidin, a hepatic peptide that blocks duodenal iron transepithelial transport by inducing the degradation of ferroportin. As hepcidin levels decrease (e.g., with reduced iron stores or increased erythropoiesis), ferroportin expression is increased, and iron transport into the bloodstream is enhanced.

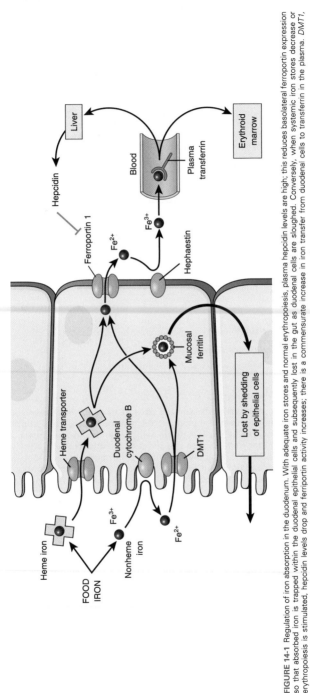

FIGURE 14-1 Regulation of iron absorption in the duodenum. With adequate iron stores and normal erythropoiesis, plasma hepcidin levels are high; this reduces basolateral ferroportin expression so that absorbed iron is trapped within the duodenal epithelial cells and subsequently lost in the gut as duodenal cells are sloughed. Conversely, when systemic iron stores decrease or erythropoiesis is stimulated, hepcidin levels drop and ferroportin activity increases; there is a commensurate increase in iron transfer from duodenal cells to transferrin in the plasma. *DMT1,* Divalent metal transporter 1.

Conversely, as stores become replete, hepcidin levels increase, ferroportin is degraded, and iron transport into the bloodstream is blocked. Hepcidin also blocks the release of iron from macrophages, an important source of iron for heme synthesis in erythropoiesis. Abnormalities in hepcidin levels lead to disturbances in iron metabolism ranging from some forms of anemia to *hemochromatosis* (systemic iron overload).

Pathogenesis (p. 661)

Negative iron balance can result from low dietary intake (rare in the United States), malabsorption, excessive demand (infancy or pregnancy), or chronic blood loss. The last is the most important cause of iron deficiency anemia in the Western world; blood loss occurs through the gastrointestinal tract (e.g., peptic ulcers, colon cancer, hemorrhoids) or the female genital tract (e.g., menstruation). Anemia occurs when iron reserves are depleted; it is accompanied by low serum iron, ferritin, and transferrin saturation levels.

Morphology (p. 661)

Whatever the cause, iron deficiency produces a *hypochromic, microcytic anemia*, with increased RBC central pallor and poikilocytosis. Marrow exhibits a mild to moderate erythroid hyperplasia, with loss of stainable iron in marrow macrophages.

Clinical Features (p. 662)

Besides the fatigue and pallor attendant with anemia, depletion of essential iron-containing enzymes can cause alopecia, koilonychia, and atrophy of the tongue and gastric mucosa. The *Plummer-Vinson triad* of hypochromic microcytic anemia, atrophic glossitis, and esophageal webs may occur.

Anemia of Chronic Disease (p. 662)

Anemia of chronic disease occurs in the setting of chronic inflammation, infections, or neoplasms; elevated interleukin-6 increases hepatic hepcidin production and reduces iron export from duodenal epithelium and macrophages (see preceding discussion). Erythropoietin production is also inappropriately low, exacerbating the anemia. Serum iron is low, but ferritin levels are high. The anemia is normocytic/normochromic or microcytic/hypochromic. Successful treatment of the underlying condition corrects the anemia; erythropoietin therapy is partially effective.

Aplastic Anemia (p. 662)

Aplastic anemia is a syndrome of chronic primary hematopoietic failure; pancytopenia affecting all lineages results.

Pathogenesis (p. 663)

Known causes fall into three broad categories:

- Toxic exposures

  Total body irradiation
  Drugs or chemicals are the most common causes of secondary aplastic anemia; marrow suppression can be dose related, predictable, and reversible (benzene, alkylating agents, and antimetabolites such as vincristine) or idiosyncratic, affecting only some exposed individuals in an unpredictable manner (chloramphenicol, chlorpromazine, and streptomycin)

- Viral infections (most commonly non-A, non-B, non-C, and non-G hepatitis)

- Inherited diseases (e.g., Fanconi anemia, defects in telomerase activity)

In idiopathic cases (65% of aplastic anemia), stem cell failure may be due to:

- A primary defect in the number or function of stem cells, in some cases due to mutagen exposure; occasionally, genetically damaged stem cells transform to myeloid neoplasms
- Suppression of antigenically altered stem cells by T-cell–mediated immune mechanisms

Morphology (p. 664)

Hypocellular marrow (hematopoietic cells are replaced by fat cells), with secondary effects due to granulocytopenia (infections) and thrombocytopenia (bleeding).

Clinical Features (p. 664)

Onset is insidious with symptoms related to the pancytopenia; splenomegaly is absent. Withdrawal of a potential inciting agent can sometimes lead to recovery; more commonly, bone marrow transplantation or immunosuppression is required.

Pure Red Cell Aplasia (p. 664)

Pure red cell aplasia is a form of marrow failure due to erythroid precursor suppression. Outside of cases associated with B19 parvovirus infections (that infect and destroy RBC precursors), the etiology is likely autoimmune; it can occur in association with drug exposures, autoimmune diseases, and neoplasms (e.g., large granular lymphocytic leukemia or thymoma). In such settings, the anemia may remit with immunosuppression, plasmapheresis, or following thymoma resection.

Other Forms of Marrow Failure (p. 665)

- *Myelophthisic anemia:* Space-occupying lesions (e.g., metastatic cancer or granulomatous disease) destroy/distort the marrow architecture and depress hematopoiesis; pancytopenia results, often with immature precursors in the peripheral blood.
- *Chronic renal failure:* This is almost invariably associated with anemia. Although multifactorial, insufficient erythropoietin production is most important; recombinant erythropoietin is usually efficacious.
- *Diffuse liver disease* (toxic, infectious, or cirrhotic): anemia is primarily due to bone marrow failure, often exacerbated by (variceal) bleeding, and folate and/or iron deficiency.

Polycythemia (p. 665)

Polycythemia denotes an abnormally high RBC count, usually with an associated increase in hemoglobin level. *Relative* increases may be caused by hemoconcentration due to dehydration (e.g., water deprivation, vomiting, or diarrhea) or due to *stress polycythemia* (also called *Gaisböck* syndrome). *Absolute increases* can be:

- *Primary* due to *polycythemia vera*, a myeloproliferative disorder in which RBC precursors proliferate in an erythropoietin-independent fashion (Chapter 13). Mutations in the erythropoietin receptor can also render its activity erythropoietin independent.
- *Secondary* due to increased erythropoietin, which may be physiologic (lung disease, high-altitude living, cyanotic heart disease) or pathophysiologic (erythropoietin-secreting tumors, such as renal cell or hepatocellular carcinomas).

Bleeding Disorders: Hemorrhagic Diatheses (p. 666)

Excessive bleeding can result from increased blood vessel fragility, platelet disorders, and/or coagulation defects. Evaluation requires laboratory investigation: prothrombin and partial thromboplastin times (and levels of specific clotting factors and anticoagulants) assess the protein components, while platelet number and function assays (e.g., bleeding time) test the cellular aspects.

Bleeding Disorders Caused by Vessel Wall Abnormalities (p. 666)

Such disorders are relatively common but usually cause only petechia and purpura without serious bleeding. Platelet counts and coagulation and bleeding times are typically normal. Causes include:

- *Infections* (e.g., meningococcus and rickettsia): Underlying mechanisms are microvascular damage (vasculitis) or disseminated intravascular coagulation (DIC).
- *Drug reactions:* These are attributed to immune complex deposition with resulting hypersensitivity vasculitis.
- *Poor vascular support:* Abnormal collagen synthesis (e.g., scurvy or Ehlers-Danlos syndrome), loss of perivascular supporting tissue (e.g., Cushing syndrome), or vascular wall amyloid deposition are included.
- *Henoch-Schönlein purpura:* This is a systemic hypersensitivity response due to immune complex deposition and characterized by purpuric rash, abdominal pain, polyarthralgia, and acute glomerulonephritis.
- *Hereditary hemorrhagic telangiectasia (Osler-Weber-Rendu syndrome):* This is an autosomal dominant disorder characterized by dilated, thin-walled vessels (often in mucous membranes of the nose and gastrointestinal tract).

Bleeding Related to Reduced Platelet Number: Thrombocytopenia (p. 667)

Thrombocytopenia is defined as counts 100,000/µL or less, but spontaneous bleeding does not occur until platelet decrease to 20,000/µL or less; counts between 20,000 and 50,000/µL can exacerbate post-traumatic hemorrhage. Most spontaneous bleeds involve small vessels of the skin and mucous membranes. Causes of thrombocytopenia include:

- *Decreased production* due to ineffective megakaryopoiesis (e.g., HIV, myelodysplastic syndromes) or due to generalized marrow disease that also compromises megakaryocyte number (e.g., aplastic anemia, disseminated cancer).
- *Decreased survival* due to increased consumption (e.g., DIC) or due to immune-mediated platelet destruction, the latter secondary to anti-platelet antibodies or immune complex deposition on platelets.
- *Sequestration* in the red pulp of enlarged spleens
- *Dilution* due to massive transfusions; prolonged storage of whole blood results in prompt subsequent platelet sequestration. Thus, while plasma volume and RBC mass are reconstituted by transfusion, the number of circulating platelets is relatively reduced.

Chronic Immune Thrombocytopenia Purpura (p. 667)

Chronic immune thrombocytopenia purpura (ITP) is caused by autoantibodies to platelets; these can be primary or can arise in the setting of certain exposures or pre-existing conditions (e.g., lupus, B-cell neoplasms, or HIV).

Pathogenesis (p. 667)

Platelet autoantibodies are usually directed toward one of two platelet antigens—the platelet membrane glycoprotein complexes IIb/IIIa or Ib/IX. Destruction of antibody-coated platelets occurs in the spleen, and splenectomy can be beneficial.

Morphology (p. 668)

The spleen is normal in size but shows sinusoidal congestion and prominent germinal centers. Bone marrow megakaryocyte numbers are increased.

Clinical Features (p. 668)

Chronic ITP is classically a disease of women younger than 40 years of age; there is often a long history of easy bruising or epistaxis. Cutaneous bleeding often takes the form of petechiae. Initial manifestations can be melena, hematuria, or heavy menses; subarachnoid or intracerebral hemorrhages are rare but serious. The bleeding time is prolonged, while prothrombin and partial thromboplastin times are normal; tests for antiplatelet antibody are not reliable. Most patients respond to glucocorticoids (inhibiting macrophage function), but some require splenectomy or immunomodulation (e.g., anti-CD20 antibody).

Acute Immune Thrombocytopenic Purpura (p. 668)

Acute ITP is mainly a self-limited disorder seen most often in children after a viral infection; platelet destruction is due to transient production of anti-platelet autoantibodies.

Drug-Induced Thrombocytopenia (p. 668)

Drug-induced thrombocytopenia occurs when drugs act as haptens on platelet proteins or participate in the formation of immune complexes that deposit on platelet surfaces; antibodies to the drugs or modified platelet molecules then cause platelet removal via macrophage ingestion.

Heparin-induced thrombocytopenia (HIT) has a distinctive pathogenesis. Type I thrombocytopenia occurs rapidly after drug administration and is due to a direct platelet-aggregating effect of heparin; it is usually of little clinical significance and spontaneously resolves. Type II thrombocytopenia, while less common, has significant potential for adverse clinical consequences. It occurs 5 to 14 days after therapy and is caused by autoantibodies directed against a complex of heparin and platelet factor 4 that activates platelets. This, in turn, leads to thrombi in arteries and veins—even in the setting of thrombocytopenia—that can be limb- and life-threatening (e.g., from pulmonary embolism of deep venous thromboses). Therapy requires heparin discontinuation and alternate anticoagulation administration (Chapter 4).

HIV-Associated Thrombocytopenia (p. 669)

HIV-associated thrombocytopenia is due to both diminished platelet production and increased destruction. Megakaryocytes express both CXCR4 and CD4 and thus can be directly infected by HIV; infected cells are prone to apoptosis and defective platelet production. HIV-mediuated dysregulation of B cells leads to anti-platelet autoantibodies that can also cause their premature destruction.

Thrombotic Microangiopathies: Thrombotic Thrombocytopenic Purpura and Hemolytic-Uremic Syndrome (p. 669)

Thrombotic thrombocytopenic purpura (TTP) and hemolytic-uremic syndrome (HUS) are related disorders within the spectrum of *thrombotic microangiopathies;* these are characterized by thrombocytopenia, microangiopathic hemolytic anemia, fever, transient neurologic deficits (in TTP), or renal failure (in HUS). Although clinically similar to DIC, activation of the protein clotting factors is not a prominent feature in the thrombotic microangiopathies; rather HUS and TTP are both caused by excessive platelet activation. Most of the clinical manifestations are due to *widespread hyaline microthrombi* in arterioles and capillaries composed of dense aggregates of platelets and fibrin.

- *TTP* is associated with inherited or acquired deficiencies in ADAMTS13, a serum metalloprotease that limits the size of von Willebrand factor multimers in the plasma. In its absence, very high molecular weight multimers accumulate that are capable of promoting platelet aggregation throughout the microcirculation. In the case of acquired TTP, patients often have antibodies directed against ADAMTS13.
- *HUS* most commonly follows gastrointestinal infections with verotoxin-producing *Escherichia coli.* Verotoxin injures endothelial cells and thereby promotes dysregulated platelet activation and aggregation.

Acquired TTP typically affects women; HUS often occurs in children and the elderly during outbreaks of food poisoning. Plasma exchange or plasmapheresis is effective in both, probably due to removal of antibodies (acquired TTP) or toxins (epidemic HUS). Endothelial injury mediated by other causes (e.g., toxic drugs, radiation) may cause chronic forms of HUS that are difficult to treat.

Bleeding Disorders Related to Defective Platelet Functions (p. 670)

These disorders are characterized by prolonged bleeding time in association with normal platelet count.

Congenital defects (Chapter 4):

- *Defective platelet adhesion,* for example, autosomal-recessive Bernard-Soulier syndrome caused by deficient platelet membrane glycoprotein complex GpIb-IX (platelet receptor for von Willebrand factor, necessary for platelet-collagen adhesion).
- *Defective platelet aggregation,* for example, Glanzmann thrombasthenia, an autosomal recessive disorder caused by a deficiency of platelet membrane glycoprotein GpIIb-IIIa, (involved in binding fibrinogen).
- *Disorders of platelet secretion* of prostaglandins and/or granule-bound ADP that promote further aggregation.

Acquired defects:

- *Aspirin* irreversibly inhibits cyclooxygenase and can suppress the synthesis of thromboxane A_2, necessary for platelet aggregation.
- *Uremia* causes defects in platelet adhesion, granule secretion, and aggregation.

Hemorrhagic Diatheses Related to Abnormalities in Clotting Factors (p. 670)

The bleeding associated with clotting factor abnormalities differs from that seen with platelet deficiencies:

- Spontaneous petechiae or purpura is uncommon; more often, bleeding manifests as large ecchymoses or hematomas after injury or as prolonged bleeding after laceration or surgery.
- Bleeding into the gastrointestinal and urinary tracts, and particularly into weight-bearing joints *(hemarthrosis)* is common.

Clotting abnormalities can be acquired or hereditary. *Acquired deficiencies* are usually associated with multiple clotting abnormalities. Thus, vitamin K deficiency results in depressed synthesis of factors II, VII, IX, and X and protein C, and liver failure of any cause can result in deficient synthesis of multiple coagulation factors. DIC also produces a deficiency of multiple coagulation factors.

Hereditary deficiencies typically affect a single clotting factor. The most common inherited disorders are hemophilia (A and B) and von Willebrand disease.

The Factor VIII–vWF Complex (p. 670)

The factor VIII–von Willebrand factor (vWF) complex is made up of two separate proteins—factor VIII and vWF; circulating factor VIII is stabilized by binding to vWF, and deficient levels of vWF thus lead to commensurate reductions in factor VIII.

Factor VIII is an essential co-factor for factor IXa activation of factor X (Chapter 4); factor VIII deficiency causes classic hemophilia *(hemophilia A; see later discussion).*

As described earlier (see TTP), circulating vWF exists as large multimers. Besides factor VIII, these multimers interact with other hemostatic proteins; most importantly, vWF mediates platelet adhesion to subendothelial matrix by bridging platelet glycoprotein Ib-IX and collagen. vWF also promotes platelet aggregation by binding to factor IIb-IIIa, particularly under high shear stress.

Von Willebrand Disease (p. 671)

Von Willebrand disease is the most common heritable bleeding disorder, affecting 1% of the United States population. It is molecularly heterogeneous with more than 20 variants; most are autosomal dominant. Symptoms are generally mild (epistaxis, excess bleeding from wounds, etc.), but can be more severe. Therapy can include desmopressin (stimulating vWF release) or infusions of plasma concentrates containing the missing factor(s).

- *Type 1* and *type 3 von Willebrand disease* are associated with reduced levels of vWF. Type 1 is autosomal dominant and most common; it is clinically mild. Type 3 is an uncommon autosomal recessive variant associated with marked vWF deficiency and a severe phenotype.
- *Type 2* is an autosomal dominant form caused by qualitative defects in vWF. Type 2A (autosomal dominant) is most common; vWF levels are normal, but the ability to form the most active high-molecular-weight multimers is defective, leading to a functional deficit. Patients have mild to moderate bleeding.

Hemophilia A (Factor VIII Deficiency) (p. 672)

Hemophilia A is the most common hereditary disease associated with life-threatening bleeding. It is an X-linked recessive disorder (thus, primarily affecting males), characterized by a reduced amount and/or activity of factor VIII. Severe disease occurs when factor VIII levels are less than 1% of normal; patients with 2% to 5% of normal levels have moderately severe disease, and those with 6% to 50% of normal levels typically have a mild phenotype. The variable deficiency in factor VIII results from different types of genetic mutations. Clinically, petechiae are characteristically absent; instead, symptomatic patients exhibit the following:

- Massive hemorrhage after trauma or operative procedures
- Spontaneous hemorrhages in regions of the body normally subject to trauma (e.g. joints); this can lead to progressive, crippling deformities

The partial thromboplastin time is prolonged (intrinsic pathway defect), and specific diagnosis is made by assay for factor VIII. Treatment consists of replacement therapy with recombinant factor VIII or factor VIII concentrates.

Hemophilia B (Christmas Disease, Factor IX Deficiency) (p. 672)

Hemophilia B is an X-linked recessive disease caused by factor IX deficiency; it is clinically indistinguishable from hemophilia A. Identification of hemophilia B requires assay of factor IX levels; treatment involves infusions of recombinant factor IX.

Disseminated Intravascular Coagulation (p. 673)

DIC is a thrombohemorrhagic disorder characterized by excessive activation of coagulation leading to formation of thrombi in the microvasculature. It is a secondary complication in a variety of diseases; DIC symptoms arise from tissue ischemia (due to the thrombosis) and/or bleeding caused by the exuberant consumption of clotting factors or activation of fibrinolytic pathways.

Pathogenesis (p. 673)

DIC is triggered by two major mechanisms: (1) release of tissue factor or thromboplastic substances into the circulation or (2) widespread endothelial cell injury (Fig. 14-2).

- *Thromboplastic substances* can be derived from a variety of sources; placenta or amniotic fluid in obstetric complications; damaged tissues following major trauma, burns, or surgery; granules of leukemic cells in acute promyelocytic leukemia; or mucus released from certain adenocarcinomas. In sepsis, bacterial endotoxins activate monocytes to release tumor necrosis factor-α, thereby increasing tissue factor expression on endothelial cell membranes while simultaneously decreasing thrombomodulin expression. This results in both activation of the clotting system and inhibition of coagulation control.
- *Endothelial injury* initiates DIC by causing tissue factor release from endothelial cells, by promoting platelet aggregation, and by activating the intrinsic coagulation pathway by exposing subendothelial connective tissue. Widespread endothelial injury can occur through antigen-antibody complex deposition (e.g., systemic lupus erythematosus), hypoxia, acidosis, temperature extremes (e.g., heatstroke, burns), or infections (e.g., meningococci, rickettsiae).

Morphology (p. 674)

Microthrombi, with infarctions and, in some cases, hemorrhages, are found in many organs and tissues. In lungs, alveolar capillary microthrombi may be associated with histology resembling acute respiratory distress syndrome. In the adrenals, massive hemorrhages due to DIC give rise to the *Waterhouse-Friderichsen syndrome* seen in meningococcemia. Similarly, *Sheehan postpartum pituitary necrosis* is a form of DIC complicating labor and delivery.

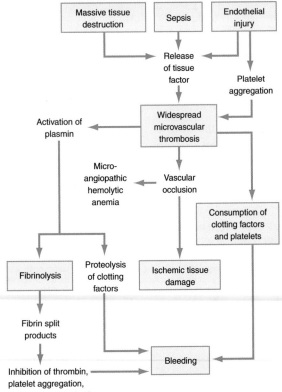

FIGURE 14-2 Pathophysiology of disseminated intravascular coagulation (DIC).

Clinical Features (p. 674)

About 50% of DIC occurs in obstetric patients with pregnancy complications; 33% occurs in the setting of carcinomatosis, with sepsis and trauma responsible for most of the remaining cases. In the setting of trauma or obstetric complications, bleeding is the dominant complication, while thrombosis is the major manifestation in malignancy. Onset can be fulminant, as in endotoxic shock or amniotic fluid embolism, or insidious, as in cases of carcinomatosis or retention of a dead fetus. Clinical manifestations include:

- Microangiopathic hemolytic anemia
- Respiratory symptoms (e.g., dyspnea, cyanosis)
- Neurologic signs and symptoms, including convulsions and coma
- Oliguria and acute renal failure
- Circulatory failure and shock

Prognosis is highly variable and is heavily impacted by the underlying disorder; the only definitive treatment is to remove the inciting cause. Depending on the clinical picture, anticoagulants (e.g., heparin), or procoagulants (fresh-frozen plasma) can be administered.

15

The Lung

Congenital Anomalies (p. 679)

- *Pulmonary hypoplasia* (small lungs) reflects defective development with diminished weight, volume, and acinar number. This is caused by abnormalities that either compress the lung or impede normal expansion *in utero* (e.g., congenital diaphragmatic hernia or oligohydramnios).
- *Foregut cysts* are formed by abnormal detachment of primitive foregut; they are typically located in the hilum or mid-mediastinum. Bronchogenic cysts, lined by bronchial-type epithelium, are most common.
- *Pulmonary sequestration* is lung tissue (lobes or segments) lacking connection to the airway system; the vascular supply usually derives from the aorta or its branches (rather than the pulmonary artery).

  Extralobar sequestrations are external to the lungs and occur anywhere in the thorax or mediastinum; they are commonly found in infants as mass lesions and often associated with other congenital anomalies.

  Intralobar sequestrations occur within the lung parenchyma; they typically occur in older children as recurrent localized infection or bronchiectasis.

Atelectasis (Collapse) (p. 679)

Atelectasis represents incomplete lung expansion, or collapse of previously inflated lung. Significant atelectasis reduces oxygenation and predisposes to infection. Acquired atelectasis is classified as:

- *Resorption atelectasis*, following complete airway obstruction and resorption of oxygen in the dependent alveoli. Causes include excessive secretions (mucus plugs), foreign body aspiration, or bronchial neoplasms. The mediastinum shifts towards the atelectatic lung.
- *Compressive atelectasis*, when the pleural space is expanded by fluid (e.g., effusions from cardiac failure or neoplasms, or blood from aneurysm rupture), or by air *(pneumothorax)*. The mediastinum shifts away from the atelectatic lung.
- *Contraction atelectasis*, when local or generalized fibrotic changes in the lung or pleura prevent full expansion.

Pulmonary Edema (p. 680)

Pulmonary edema results from either *increased hydrostatic pressure* or *increased capillary permeability* (due to endothelial or alveolar wall injury); therapy and outcome depend on the underlying etiology (Table 15-1). Regardless of cause, lungs become heavy and wet, with

TABLE 15-1   Classification and Causes of Pulmonary Edema

Hemodynamic Edema

Increased hydrostatic pressure (increased pulmonary venous pressure)
 Left-sided heart failure (common)
 Volume overload
 Pulmonary vein obstruction
Decreased oncotic pressure (less common)
 Hypoalbuminemia
 Nephrotic syndrome
 Liver disease
 Protein-losing enteropathies
Lymphatic obstruction (rare)

Edema Due to Microvascular Injury (Alveolar Injury)

Infections: pneumonia, septicemia
Inhaled gases: oxygen, smoke
Liquid aspiration: gastric contents, near-drowning
Drugs and chemicals: chemotherapeutic agents (bleomycin), other
 medications (amphotericin B), heroin, kerosene, paraquat
Shock, trauma
Radiation
Transfusion related

Edema of Undetermined Origin

High altitude
Neurogenic (central nervous system trauma)

dependent fluid accumulation. Histologically, capillaries are engorged and the alveolar spaces exhibit granular pink precipitates. With chronic congestion, the lungs become brown and firm *(brown induration)* due to interstitial fibrosis and hemosiderin-laden macrophages *("heart failure" cells)*. In addition to impairing normal respiratory function, edema predisposes to infection.

Acute Lung Injury and Acute Respiratory Distress Syndrome (Diffuse Alveolar Damage) (p. 680)

Acute lung injury (ALI) is characterized by abrupt hypoxemia and diffuse pulmonary infiltrates in the absence of cardiac failure; acute respiratory distress syndrome (ARDS) is at the severe end of the ALI spectrum. Both ALI and ARDS have inflammation-associated increases in pulmonary vascular permeability, associated with endothelial and epithelial cell death; the histologic manifestations are called *diffuse alveolar damage (DAD)*. Causes can be localized to the lungs or systemic; they include infection, trauma, toxic exposures, pancreatitis, uremia, and immune reactions. In the absence of an etiology, similar pathologic changes are called *acute interstitial pneumonia (AIP*, see following discussion).

Morphology (p. 680)

- *Acute:* Lungs are diffusely firm, red, boggy, and heavy; microscopically, there is edema, hyaline membranes (composed of necrotic epithelial debris and exuded proteins) and acute inflammation.
- *Organizing:* There is granulation tissue in response to the hyaline membranes with type II pneumocyte hyperplasia; this may resolve or progress to interstitial fibrosis. Fatal cases often have superimposed bacterial infections.

Pathogenesis (p. 681) (Fig. 15-1)

The integrity of the alveolar wall vascular/air interface is compromised by damage to capillary endothelium and/or alveolar epithelium. Regardless of the specific cause, injury occurs through an imbalance of pro- and anti-inflammatory mediators; NF-κB transcription factor activation is an important proximate event in tipping the balance toward inflammation.

- Pulmonary macrophage activation leads to the release of mediators that recruit neutrophils (e.g., interleukin-8 [IL-8]) and activate endothelium (e.g., tumor necrosis factor [TNF] and interleukin-1 [IL-1]).
- Activated neutrophils aggregate in the pulmonary vasculature and damage the epithelium by secreting oxygen-derived free radicals and lysosomal enzymes (proteases), as well as arachidonic acid metabolites that further augment neutrophil aggregation.
- The combined endothelial and epithelial assault culminates in *increased vascular permeability and loss of surfactant,* rendering alveoli stiff and resistant to expansion. There is also dysregulation of the coagulation system; procoagulants are increased while anticoagulant factors decrease.

Clinical Course (p. 682)

Dyspnea and tachypnea herald ALI, followed by cyanosis, hypoxemia, and respiratory failure refractory to oxygen therapy; chest x-ray films reveal diffuse bilateral infiltrates. The functional abnormalities are not evenly distributed; normal regions of compliance and ventilation are interspersed with consolidation and atelectasis. Poorly aerated regions continue to be perfused, leading to ventilation-perfusion mismatch and hypoxemia. Therapy involves mechanical ventilation and treatment of the underlying cause (e.g., infection); the overall mortality rate is 40%, primarily secondary to sepsis or multi-organ failure.

Acute Interstitial Pneumonia (p. 682)

Acute interstitial pneumonia is a clinicopathologic entity used to describe widespread ALI of unknown etiology, often with an aggressive course. Mortality is 50%, typically in the first 1 to 2 months after diagnosis; survivors are prone to recurrence and chronic interstitial disease.

Obstructive vs. Restrictive Pulmonary Diseases (p. 683)

Chronic, non-infectious, diffuse pulmonary disease is physiologically classified as:

- *Obstructive disease:* Increased resistance to airflow, at any level from trachea to alveoli
- *Restrictive disease:* Reduced expansion of lung parenchyma, with decreased total lung capacity, generally occurring in two general categories:

  Chest wall disorders (e.g., neuromuscular disease, obesity, pleural disease, etc.)
  Chronic interstitial and infiltrative diseases

Obstructive Pulmonary Diseases (p. 683)

The relevant entities (i.e., emphysema, chronic bronchitis, asthma, and bronchiectasis) have distinct characteristics (Table 15-2) but can also share some common elements. Emphysema and chronic

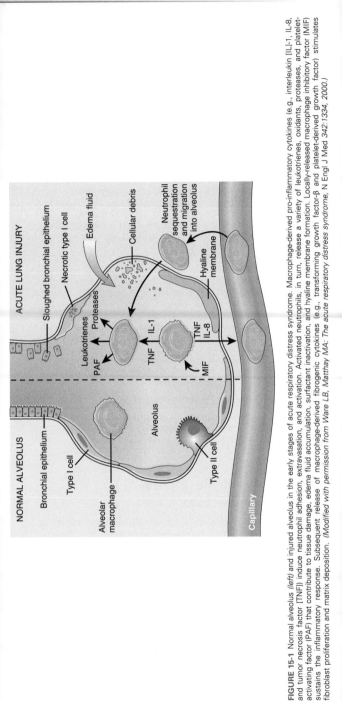

FIGURE 15-1 Normal alveolus *(left)* and injured alveolus in the early stages of acute respiratory distress syndrome. Macrophage-derived pro-inflammatory cytokines (e.g., interleukin [IL]-1, IL-8, and tumor necrosis factor [TNF]) induce neutrophil adhesion, extravasation, and activation. Activated neutrophils, in turn, release a variety of leukotrienes, oxidants, proteases, and platelet-activating factor (PAF) that contribute to tissue damage, edema fluid accumulation, surfactant inactivation, and hyaline membrane formation. Locally-released macrophage inhibitory factor (MIF) sustains the inflammatory response. Subsequent release of macrophage-derived fibrogenic cytokines (e.g., transforming growth factor-β and platelet-derived growth factor) stimulates fibroblast proliferation and matrix deposition. *(Modified with permission from Ware LB, Matthay MA: The acute respiratory distress syndrome, N Engl J Med 342:1334, 2000.)*

TABLE 15-2 Disorders Associated with Airflow Obstruction: The Spectrum of Chronic Obstructive Pulmonary Disease

Clinical Term	Anatomic Site	Major Pathologic Changes	Etiology	Signs/Symptoms
Chronic bronchitis	Bronchus	Mucous gland hyperplasia, hypersecretion	Tobacco smoke, air pollutants	Cough, sputum production
Bronchiectasis	Bronchus	Airway dilation and scarring	Persistent or severe infections	Cough, purulent sputum, fever
Asthma	Bronchus	Smooth muscle hyperplasia, excess mucus, inflammation	Immunologic or undefined causes	Episodic wheezing cough, dyspnea
Emphysema	Acinus	Airspace enlargement; wall destruction	Tobacco smoke	Dyspnea
Small airway disease, bronchiolitis	Bronchiole	Inflammatory scarring/obliteration	Tobacco smoke, air pollutants, miscellaneous	Cough, dyspnea

bronchitis are typically grouped together as *chronic obstructive pulmo-nary disease (COPD)* because many patients have overlapping features of damage (unsurprising, since cigarette smoking is often a common denominator). Asthma is usually distinguished from emphysema and chronic bronchitis by the presence of reversible bronchospasm; how-ever, asthmatic patients can develop an irreversible component. Conversely, typical COPD can also have reversible features.

Emphysema (p. 684)

Emphysema is characterized by irreversible enlargement of airspaces distal to the terminal bronchioles, accompanied by alveo-lar wall destruction with minimal fibrosis. Emphysema is classified according to its anatomic distribution (Fig. 15-2).

• Centriacinar (centrilobular) emphysema (p. 684)

Destruction and enlargement of the central or proximal parts of the respiratory unit (i.e., the acinus) sparing distal alveoli
Predominant involvement of upper lobes and apices
Occurs primarily in heavy smokers, often associated with chronic bronchitis

• Panacinar (panlobular) emphysema (p. 684)

Uniform destruction and enlargement of the acinus
Predominance in lower basal zones
Strong association with α_1-antitrypsin deficiency (Chapter 18)

• Distal acinar (paraseptal) emphysema (p. 684)

Involves mostly the distal acinus
Typically near the pleura and adjacent to fibrosis or scars

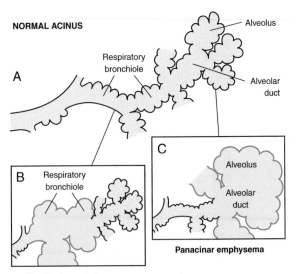

FIGURE 15-2 A, Diagram of normal structures within the acinus, the fundamental unit of the lung. A terminal bronchiole *(not shown)* is immediately proximal to the respiratory bronchiole. **B,** *Centriacinar emphysema* with dilation that initially affects the respiratory bronchioles. **C,** *Panacinar emphysema* with initial distention of the peripheral structures (alveolus and alveolar duct); the disease later extends to affect the respiratory broinchioles.

Frequently the underlying lesion in spontaneous pneumothorax

- Airspace enlargement with fibrosis (irregular emphysema) (p. 684)

  Irregular acinar involvement, associated with scarring
  Most cases are asymptomatic and clinically insignificant

Pathogenesis (p. 684)

Alveolar wall destruction in emphysema likely results from imbalances between pulmonary proteases and their inhibitors, abetted by disparities in oxidants and anti-oxidants.

- Individuals with hereditary deficiency of the major protease inhibitor (i.e., α_1-antitrypsin) have a marked propensity for developing emphysema, which is compounded by smoking.
- Tobacco smoking contributes to emphysema by:

  Recruiting and activating inflammatory cells (i.e., macrophages and neutrophils) via direct chemoattractive effects of nicotine and the induction of NF-κB transcription by oxygen free radicals
  Inducing neutrophil release of cellular proteases (i.e., elastase, proteinase 3, and cathepsin G)
  Enhancing macrophage elastase activity, which is not inhibited by α_1-antitrypsin, as well as inducing neutrophil and macrophage matrix metalloproteinase activity
  Inactivating α_1-antitrypsin (via tobacco smoke oxidants or neutrophil-derived free radicals)
  Reducing antioxidant (e.g., superoxide dismutase, glutathione) levels via the presence of abundant reactive oxygen species

- Loss of alveolar elastic tissue reduces radial traction and causes respiratory bronchiole collapse during expiration, resulting in functional obstruction.
- In addition, small airway (i.e., bronchioles less than 2 mm) inflammation (including T and B lymphocytes) causes goblet cell metaplasia with mucus plugging, as well as bronchiolar wall thickening due to fibrosis and smooth muscle hyperplasia, thereby augmenting the airway obstruction.

Morphology (p. 686)

With diffuse disease, lungs can become voluminous and overlap the heart. Microscopically, alveolar spaces are enlarged, separated by thin septa; septal capillaries are compressed and bloodless. Alveolar wall rupture can produce very large airspaces (*blebs* and *bullae*).

Clinical Course (p. 686)

Symptoms (e.g., dyspnea, wheezing, cough) manifest when a third of the pulmonary parenchyma has been lost; there may also be severe weight loss. Patients are classically barrel-chested with obvious prolonged expiration; spirometry is a key diagnostic tool. Classically, patients overventilate to compensate for loss of parenchyma and are typically well-oxygenated at rest, so-called *pink puffers*. Development of pulmonary hypertension with heart failure has a poor prognosis; death in severe emphysema is due to respiratory acidosis, right-sided heart failure, or massive pneumothorax.

Other Forms of Emphysema (p. 687)

- *Compensatory hyperinflation* of remaining lung after loss of pulmonary parenchyma (e.g., surgical lobectomy) without septal wall destruction

- *Obstructive overinflation* due to subtotal obstruction of an airway, thereby creating a ball-valve that admits air on inspiration but traps it on expiration
- *Interstitial emphysema* reflecting entry of air into connective tissue of lung, mediastinum, or subcutaneous tissues (usually due to alveolar tears)

Chronic Bronchitis (p. 687)

Chronic bronchitis is defined as persistent cough with sputum production for at least 3 months in at least 2 consecutive years but in the absence of any other identifiable cause.

Pathogenesis (p. 687)

Chronic irritation of the airways by inhaled substances (especially tobacco smoke) is the dominant pathogenic mechanism. Irritants cause:

- Mucous gland hypertrophy with mucus hypersecretion (stimulated by neutrophil proteases)
- Goblet cell metaplasia in bronchiolar epithelium, which contributes to the mucus production and small airway obstruction
- Bronchiolitis with wall thickening due to fibrosis and smooth muscle hyperplasia
- Secondary infections exacerbate the smoking-initiated injury

Morphology (p. 688)

- Hyperemia and edema of lung mucous membranes
- Mucinous secretions filling airways
- Mucous gland hyperplasia
- Bronchiolar inflammation and fibrosis
- Bronchial epithelium squamous metaplasia and dysplasia

Clinical Features (p. 688)

Beyond the defining cough and sputum production, dyspnea on exertion eventually develops. In classic cases, patients are hypoxic, cyanotic, and hypercapnic (i.e., retain carbon dioxide [CO_2]); so-called *blue bloaters*. Long-standing disease often progresses to cor pulmonale with heart failure; death can also be secondary to infection.

Asthma (p. 688)

This chronic relapsing inflammatory disorder is characterized by paroxysmal reversible bronchospasm due to smooth muscle hyper-reactivity; increased mucus production is also a feature. The incidence has increased significantly in the past four decades in the Western world. Asthma can be categorized into two major forms:

- *Atopic (allergic) asthma* is most common. It is caused by a classic type I (i.e., immunoglobulin E [IgE])-mediated hypersensitivity reaction triggered by environmental antigens (e.g,. pollen, certain foods; Chapter 6); a family history of atopy is common.
- *Nonatopic asthma* can be triggered by respiratory tract infections, chemical irritants, or drugs, usually without a family history. Airway hyperirritability is attributed to virally or chemically induced inflammation that reduces the threshold for vagal stimulation by other minor irritants.

Several pharmacologic agents can also induce asthma; non-steroidal anti-inflammatory drugs (NSAIDs) are commonly in this category. These agents inhibit cyclooxygenase (without affecting lipoxygenase activity) and tip the balance of arachidonic acid metabolism toward bronchoconstrictor leukotrienes. Occupational exposures can also mediate asthma through some combination of type I responses and direct liberation of bronchoconstrictor substances.

Pathogenesis (p. 689)

T-cell differentiation is skewed to overproduce T_H2-type cells (Chapter 6) with subsequent IgE- and eosinophil-dominated immune responses; in pre-sensitized patients, repeat antigen exposure causes (Fig. 15-3):

- Acute phase: Antigen binding to IgE-coated mast cells cause primary (e.g., leukotriene) and secondary (e.g., cytokine) mediator release. Acute-phase mediators cause bronchospasm, edema, mucus secretion, and leukocyte recruitment.
- Late phase: This is mediated by recruited leukocytes (e.g., eosinophils, lymphocytes, neutrophils, monocytes) and is characterized by persistent bronchospasm and edema, leukocytic infiltration, and epithelial damage and loss.
- Repeated bouts cause *airway remodeling* with bronchial smooth muscle and mucus gland hypertrophy and hyperplasia, increased vascularity, and increased deposition of subepithelial collagen.

Genetics of Asthma (p. 691)

Multiple susceptibility loci interact with environmental factors to produce asthma; implicated genes can affect primary or secondary immune responses, tissue remodeling, or even the patient's response to therapy. The strongest genetic associations have been made with certain human leukocyte antigen (HLA) alleles, and polymorphisms in IL-13, CD14 (the monocyte receptor for endotoxin), ADAM-33 (a matrix metalloproteinase that influences smooth muscle and fibroblast proliferation), β_2-adrenergic receptor (influencing airway reactivity), and the IL-4 receptor.

Morphology (p. 691)

Lungs are overinflated with patchy atelectasis and mucus plugging of airways. *Microscopically,* the lungs exhibit edema, bronchiolar inflammatory infiltrates with numerous eosinophils, subepithelial fibrosis, and bronchial wall smooth muscle and mucosal gland hypertrophy. Whorled mucus plugs *(Curschmann spirals)* and crystalloid eosinophil granule debris *(Charcot-Leyden crystals)* deposit in airways.

Clinical Course (p. 692)

Classic attacks last up to several hours; symptoms include chest tightness, wheezing, dyspnea, and cough. In severe episodes *(status asthmaticus)*, acute symptoms persist for days to weeks, and significant airflow obstruction can cause cyanosis and death.

Bronchiectasis (p. 692)

Bronchiectasis represents abnormal *permanent* dilation of airways due to a destructive necrotizing infection of bronchi and bronchioles; it can develop in:

- Congenital or hereditary conditions (e.g., cystic fibrosis, Kartagener syndrome, or pulmonary sequestration)
- Postinfectious state (e.g., after necrotizing bacterial, viral, or fungal pneumonia)
- Bronchial obstruction (e.g., by tumor or foreign body)
- Other chronic inflammatory states (e.g., rheumatoid arthritis, chronic graft-versus-host disease, or allergic bronchopulmonary aspergillosis)

TRIGGERING OF ASTHMA

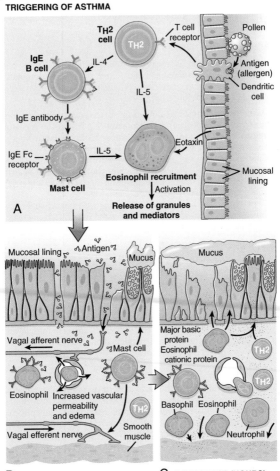

B IMMEDIATE PHASE (MINUTES)   **C LATE PHASE (HOURS)**

FIGURE 15-3 Asthma pathogenesis. A, Inhaled allergens (antigen) elicit a T$_H$2-dominated response favoring IgE production and eosinophil recruitment and activation. B, On re-exposure to antigen (Ag), an *immediate phase* reaction is triggered by Ag-induced cross-linking of IgE bound to their receptors on mast cells; mast cells then release pre-formed mediators that induce bronchospasm, increased vascular permeability, and mucus production and recruit additional inflammatory cells. C, The arrival of the various recruited leukocytes signals the *late-phase* response and a fresh round of mediator release from leukocytes, endothelium, and epithelium. Factors, especially major basic protein and eosinophil cationic protein from eosinophils, also damage the epithelium. *IL,* Interleukin.

Pathogenesis (p. 692)

Obstruction and infection are the major etiologies, and both are likely necessary for full-blown bronchiectasis. Thus, bronchial obstruction impedes normal clearing so that infections and inflammation can fester and eventually cause the requisite tissue destruction.

Morphology (p. 693)

Most severe changes occur in peripheral lower lobes; airways can be dilated up to four times the normal size. Histology shows a spectrum of mild to necrotizing acute and chronic inflammation of the larger airways with bronchiolar fibrosis.

Clinical Course (p. 693)

The presentation is marked by persistent, severe cough, fever, and abundant purulent sputum. Symptoms may be episodic and precipitated by upper respiratory tract infection; alternatively, coughing can be associated with morning rising and positional changes that drain collected pus and secretions into the bronchi. Complications include cor pulmonale, brain abscesses, and amyloidosis.

Chronic Diffuse Interstitial (Restrictive) Diseases (p. 693)

These are a heterogeneous group of disorders characterized by *inflammation and pulmonary interstitial tissue fibrosis*, particularly involving alveolar walls; many have unknown causes. The clinical and functional changes are those of *restrictive lung disease;* diffusing capacity, lung volumes, and compliance are all compromised without evidence of airway obstruction. Secondary pulmonary hypertension and cor pulmonale are long-term sequelae. Although the early stages of the different entities can often be distinguished histologically, there is substantial morphologic overlap, and most devolve to a common end-stage marked by parenchymal destruction and scarring, called *honey-comb lung.*

Fibrosing Diseases (p. 694)

Idiopathic Pulmonary Fibrosis (p. 694)

Idiopathic pulmonary fibrosis is a disorder of unknown cause *characterized by progressive pulmonary interstitial fibrosis.*

Pathogenesis (p. 694)

Repeated cycles of epithelial activation/injury by some unidentified agent are postulated to cause abnormal "wound healing," resulting in excessive fibroblast proliferation; transforming growth factor-$\beta 1$ (TGF-$\beta 1$) is the likely driver, both by inducing fibrosis and also by promoting epithelial cell apoptosis.

Morphology (p. 695)

The pathologic pattern of fibrosis is denoted *usual interstitial pneumonia (UIP);* this is non-specific and can also be seen in connective tissue disorders, chronic hypersensitivity pneumonia, and asbestosis.

- Patchy interstitial fibrosis has a characteristic subpleural and interlobular septal distribution, as well as lower lobe predominance.
- There is heterogeneity of the histologic changes; new, cellular *fibroblastic foci* with moderate inflammation coexist with older, more densely fibrotic areas.
- Destruction of the alveolar architecture leads to *honeycomb lung* with dense fibrosis and cystic spaces lined by hyperplastic type II pneumocytes or bronchiolar epithelium; arteriolar hypertensive changes are often present.

Clinical Course (p. 695)

The disease typically has an insidious onset between ages 40 and 70 years marked by dyspnea on exertion and a dry cough. The course progression is unpredictable in any given patient, but most have a gradual deterioration with hypoxemia and cyanosis despite anti-inflammatory and anti-proliferative therapies. Mean survival is 3 years or less; lung transplantation is the only definitive therapy.

Nonspecific Interstitial Pneumonia *(p. 695)*

Nonspecifc interstitial pneumonia (NSIP) is a diffusely fibrosing disease of unknown etiology, manifesting with chronic dyspnea and cough. The histologic pattern shows either moderate interstitial inflammation or interstitial fibrosis without the temporal heterogeneity seen in UIP. The prognosis for NSIP is better than for UIP.

Cryptogenic Organizing Pneumonia *(p. 696)*

Formerly called *bronchiolitis obliterans organizing pneumonia (BOOP)*, *cryptogenic organizing pneumonia (COP)* has an unknown etiology. Patients present with cough and dyspnea, with patchy subpleural or peribronchial consolidation. *Histologically*, there are loose fibrous tissue plugs (Masson bodies) within bronchioles, alveolar ducts, and alveoli, but there is no interstitial fibrosis or honeycombing. Patients can spontaneously recover, although most require steroid therapy. Notably, the same morphologic changes are seen in response to infections or inflammatory lung injury.

Pulmonary Involvement in Connective Tissue Diseases *(p. 696)*

Pulmonary involvement in connective tissue diseases (e.g., systemic lupus erythematosus, rheumatoid arthritis, and scleroderma) is common; patterns include NSIP, UIP, vascular sclerosis, organizing pneumonia, and bronchiolitis. Prognosis is variable (depending on the underlying disease) but is better than for idiopathic UIP.

Pneumoconioses *(p. 696)*

Pneumoconioses are the non-neoplastic lung responses to inhaled aerosols, including mineral dusts, organic dusts, fumes, and vapors. In general, only a small percentage of an exposed population develops a respiratory disease, suggesting a genetic predisposition in those affected.

Pathogenesis *(p. 696)*

Pneumoconiosis development depends on:

- *Amount of dust retained*: This is a function of the original concentration, duration of exposure, and effectiveness of clearance mechanisms.
- *Size, shape, and particle buoyancy*: Particles between 1 and 5 μm are the most dangerous because they can reach terminal alveoli and settle in their linings.
- *Physicochemical reactivity (toxicity) and particle solubility*: Highly soluble particles may rapidly cause toxicity; insoluble particles may persist and cause a chronic fibrosis.
- *Additional effects of other irritants* (e.g., cigarette smoking)

COAL WORKERS' PNEUMOCONIOSIS *(p. 697)*

The spectrum of pulmonary effects of carbon dust varies from asymptomatic *anthracosis* to simple *coal workers' pneumoconiosis (CWP)* without significant pulmonary dysfunction to complicated CWP or *progressive massive fibrosis (PMF)* with compromised lung function. The factors underlying the progression from simple

CWP to PMF are not understood; possibilities include the duration and magnitude of exposure, contaminants in the carbon (e.g., silicates), and the propensity of an individual's coal dust–laden macrophages to produce fibrogenic cytokines.

Morphology (p. 697)

- In *anthracosis,* inhaled carbon is taken up by alveolar and insterstitial macrophages, which then accumulate in lymphatics and lymphoid tissues.
- In *simple* CWP, 1 to 2 mm *coal macules* are composed of dust-filled macrophages; slightly larger *coal nodules* also contain delicate networks of collagen. These are located primarily adjacent to respiratory bronchioles.
- In *PMF,* large, blackened collagenous scars (often with central ischemic necrosis) replace substantial portions of the lung.

Clinical Course (p. 698)

CWP usually causes little functional decrement; PMF will develop in less than 10%, with associated respiratory insufficiency and pulmonary hypertension, and it may be progressive even without further exposures.

SILICOSIS (p. 698)

Prolonged inhalation of silica particles produces a chronic, progressive, nodular fibrosis.

Pathogenesis (p. 698)

Crystalline forms of silica (vs. amorphous forms) are most fibrogenic; ingestion by macrophages causes their activation, with release of oxidants, cytokines, and growth factors that ultimately cause fibroblast proliferation and collagen deposition. Interestingly, silica mixed with a variety of other minerals (e.g., iron) is less fibrogenic.

Morphology (p. 698)

Collagenous nodules start in the upper lung, becoming larger and more diffuse with disease progression. Lesion coalescence forms large areas of dense scar. Calcification or concomitant blackening by coal dust often occurs. Microscopically, there are hyalinized whorls of collagen with scant inflammation. Polarized light reveals birefringent silica particles.

Clinical Course (p. 699)

Dyspnea is not usually present until progressive massive fibrosis has developed; the disease can progress even after exposure ends. Silicosis is associated with increased susceptibility to tuberculosis, likely due to depressed cell-mediated immunity.

ASBESTOS-RELATED DISEASES (p. 699)

Asbestos is a family of fibrous silicates; occupational exposures are linked to:

- Localized pleural plaques and effusions or, rarely, diffuse pleural fibrosis
- Parenchymal interstitial fibrosis *(asbestosis)*
- Lung carcinoma, malignant mesothelioma, and laryngeal and other extrapulmonary neoplasms

Pathogenesis (p. 699)

Different forms of asbestos have different clinical consequences. Straight, stiff *amphiboles* reach the deep lung more readily than flexible, curved *serpentine* fibers, accounting for their greater pathogenicity; serpentine fibers are also more soluble than amphiboles and thus are gradually leached from the tissues.

- Alveolar macrophages ingest inhaled fibers, leading to their activation and production of mediators (e.g., fibrogenic cytokines and growth factors).
- Asbestos fibers can act as both tumor initiators and promoters. Some oncogenic effects are related to free radical generation, while adsorption of potentially toxic substances (e.g., tobacco smoke carcinogens) on fibers also contributes to their tumorigenicity.

Morphology (p. 700)

- *Pleural plaques* are well-circumscribed plaques of dense collagen; although they do not contain asbestos bodies (see further discussion), they rarely occur in the absence of prior asbestos exposures.
- *Asbestosis* is marked by diffuse interstitial fibrosis that is indistinguishable from similar lesions caused by other disorders (e.g., UIP) *except* for the presence of *asbestos bodies*; these are ingested fibers coated by iron-containing proteinaceous material to form characteristic beaded, dumbbell-shaped fibers. They occur in the process of attempted macrophage endocytosis; similar iron encrustation can occur with other inorganic particulates and are called *ferruginous bodies*.

Clinical Course (p. 701)

Plaques are typically asymptomatic. Dyspnea is usually the first manifestation of asbestosis, often accompanied by a productive cough; these symptoms typically occur with a lag of 10 to 20 years after exposure. With advanced pneumoconiosis, honeycombing develops, and the course may be static or can progress to respiratory failure or cor pulmonale. Asbestsosis complicated by pulmonary/pleural malignancy has a grim prognosis.

Complications of Therapies (p. 701)

- *Drug-induced lung diseases* range from acute bronchospasm (aspirin) to pneumonitis (amiodarone) to fibrosis (bleomycin).
- *Radiation-induced lung disease* occurs in 10% to 20% of patients, beginning as *acute radiation pneumonitis* and DAD 1 to 6 months after therapy; many cases resolve (especially with steroid therapy), but some progress to *chronic radiation pneumonitis* (pulmonary fibrosis).

Granulomatous Diseases (p. 701)

Sarcoidosis (p. 701)

Sarcoidosis is a systemic disease of unknown etiology, characterized by noncaseating granulomas in virtually all tissues; 90% of cases involve hilar lymph nodes or lung. Women are affected more frequently than men, with American blacks affected 10 times more often than American whites.

Pathogenesis (p. 701)

Sarcoidosis is likely a disease of disordered immune response in genetically predisposed individuals to certain environmental agents. Evidence includes:

- Association with specific HLA genotypes (e.g., HLA-A1 and HLA-B8)
- Accumulation of oligoclonal activated CD4+ T cells
- Increased T_H1 cytokine production (IL-2 and interferon-γ) causing T-cell expansion and macrophage activation

- Increased macrophage tumor necrosis factor (TNF) production leading to granuloma formation
- Cutaneous anergy to common antigens (e.g., tuberculin or candida)
- Polyclonal hypergammaglobulinemia

Morphology (p. 702)

Granulomas are characteristically noncaseating with tightly clustered epithelioid histiocytes and frequent multinucleated giant cells. *Schaumann bodies* (laminated, calcified proteinaceous concretions) and *asteroid bodies* (stellate inclusions within giant cells) commonly occur but are not pathognomonic.

- *Lungs* exhibit diffuse, scattered granulomas, forming a reticulonodular pattern on x-ray films. Pulmonary lesions tend to heal, and only residual hyalinized scars may be seen.
- *Lymph nodes* are virtually always involved, most commonly in the hilar and mediastinal regions; tonsils are involved in 25% to 33% of cases.
- *Spleen and liver* are microscopically affected in 75% of patients, although gross splenomegaly and hepatomegaly occurs in less than 20% of cases.
- *Bone marrow* involvement is seen in 20% of cases; radiologically visible lesions have a phalangeal predilection.
- *Skin* involvement occurs in 33% to 50% of patients as discrete subcutaneous nodules or erythematous scaling plaques or macules; mucous membrane lesions also occur.
- *Eyes* are affected in 20% to 50% of cases, including iritis, iridocyclitis, or choroid retinitis, often with lacrimal gland inflammation and reduced lacrimation. Concurrent *salivary gland* involvement constitutes the *Mikulicz syndrome.*

Clinical Course (p. 703)

Because of its varying severity and different patterns of organ involvement, sarcoidosis can be entirely asymptomatic and discovered only incidentally, or it can manifest as isolated cutaneous or ocular lesions, peripheral lymphadenopathy, or hepatosplenomegaly. Patients most commonly present with the insidious onset of respiratory difficulties or constitutional symptoms (e.g., fever, night sweats, weight loss).

Diagnosis is established by biopsy demonstrating noncaseating granulomas; other diseases with the same histology (e.g., tuberculosis and fungal infections) are ruled out by culture or special stains. *Sarcoidosis is a diagnosis of exclusion.*

Sarcoidosis follows an unpredictable course and can have a slowly progressive, remitting and relapsing course (with or without steroid therapy), or can spontaneously resolve. Most patients (65% to 70%) recover with no or only minimal residua; 20% have permanent lung or ocular dysfunction; and 10% to 15% of patients succumb, often to progressive pulmonary fibrosis.

Hypersensitivity Pneumonitis (p. 703)

Hypersensitivity pneumonitis is a spectrum of immunologically mediated interstitial disorders caused by inhaled dusts or antigens; as opposed to asthma, these disorders primarily affect the alveoli ("allergic alveolitis"):

- *Farmer's lung:* Actinomycete spores in hay
- *Pigeon breeder's lung:* Proteins from bird feathers or excreta
- *Humidifier* or *air-conditioner lung:* Bacteria in heated water reservoirs

Morphology (p. 703)

Histologic changes include interstitial pneumonitis and fibrosis centered on bronchioles and (in two thirds of patients) noncaseating granulomas. Early cessation of exposure to the injurious agent prevents progression to serious chronic fibrosis and honeycombing.

Clinical Features (p. 703)

The clinical manifestations are varied and include cough, dyspnea, fever, diffuse and nodular radiographic densities, and a restrictive pattern of pulmonary dysfunction.

Pulmonary Eosinophilia (p. 704)

These are diverse clinicopathologic conditions characterized by interstitial or alveolar eosinophil infiltrates:

- *Acute eosinophilic pneumonia with respiratory failure:* Unknown etiology; rapid onset of fever, dyspnea, and hypoxia, and prompt response to corticosteroids
- *Simple pulmonary eosinophilia (Loeffler syndrome):* Uncertain etiology: transient infiltrates with prominent eosinophilia in blood and lung
- *Tropical eosinophilia:* Caused by microfilariae
- *Secondary eosinophilia:* Induced by infections, hypersensitivity, asthma, or allergic bronchopulmonary aspergillosis
- *Idiopathic chronic eosinophilic pneumonia:* Unknown etiology; it is manifested by focal lung consolidation with extensive lymphocyte and eosinophil infiltration, and is steroid responsive.

Smoking-Related Interstitial Diseases (p. 704)

Desquamative Interstitial Pneumonia (p. 704)

Desquamative interstitial pneumonia (DIP) is characterized by an insidious onset of dyspnea and dry cough; histology reveals abundant *intra-alveolar* dusty brown (smokers') macrophages with mild interstitial inflammation and minimal fibrosis. Emphysema is often present. Steroid therapy or smoking cessation yields improvement.

Respiratory Bronchiolitis–Associated Interstitial Lung Disease (p. 704)

Respiratory bronchiolitis–associated interstitial lung disease causes gradual usually mild dyspnea and cough; histology reveals patchy *bronchiolar* accumulations of smokers' macrophages with peribronchiolar inflammation and mild fibrosis. Smoking cessation yields improvement.

Pulmonary Alveolar Proteinosis (p. 705)

Pulmonary alveolar proteinosis (PAP) is a rare entity characterized by surfactant accumulation in alveoli and bronchioles; there are three distinct classes with different pathogenesis but similar histology:

- *Acquired PAP* accounts for 90% of cases. Autoantibodies against granulocyte-macrophage colony stimulating factor (GM-CSF) lead to functional GM-CSF deficiency and to impaired surfactant clearance by pulmonary macrophages.
- *Congenital PAP* occurs in newborns and is rapidly fatal; it is caused by a number of mutations involved in either GM-CSF production or signaling or in surfactant synthesis and transport.
- *Secondary PAP* follows exposure to irritating dusts or chemicals, or it occurs in immunocompromised individuals.

PAP is characterized *clinically* by respiratory difficulty, cough, and abundant sputum often containing chunks of gelatinous material. *Histologically,* there is dense, amorphous, periodic acid–Schiff (PAS)-positive, lipid-laden protein exudates filling alveolar spaces. Patients are at risk for developing secondary infections.

Diseases of Vascular Origin (p. 706)

Pulmonary Embolism, Hemorrhage, and Infarction (p. 706; see also Chapter 4)

Pulmonary artery occlusions are almost always embolic; *in situ* thromboses are rare but can occur with pulmonary hypertension, pulmonary atherosclerosis, and heart failure. Deep leg veins are the source of more than 95% of pulmonary emboli (PE), and the prevalence of PE correlates with predisposition to leg thrombosis.

The pathophysiologic response and clinical significance of PE depend on the extent of pulmonary arterial obstruction, size of occluded vessel(s), number of emboli, overall status of the cardiovascular system, and release of vasoactive factors from platelets at the site of thrombosis. Emboli cause *respiratory compromise* due to lack of perfusion of ventilated lung and *hemodynamic compromise* due to increased pulmonary arterial resistance.

Clinical Course (p. 707)

Large emboli impact in the major pulmonary arteries or astride the pulmonary artery bifurcation *(saddle embolus)* and can cause sudden death due to *electromechanical dissociation* (no blood in the pulmonary circulation) or acute *cor pulmonale* (right-sided heart failure). Multiple or recurrent small to medium emboli can have the same effect, although more commonly these are clinically silent, or only cause transient chest pain and/or hemoptysis from pulmonary hemorrhage. Only 10% of PE cause infarction; this occurs in patients with compromised pulmonary circulation (cardiac failure) and manifests as peripheral wedge-shaped hemorrhagic areas of necrosis. Uncommonly, multiple, small PE (overt or covert) produce pulmonary hypertension, vascular sclerosis, and chronic cor pulmonale.

Pulmonary Hypertension (p. 707)

Pulmonary hypertension (PH) occurs when the pulmonary pressure reaches 25% of systemic levels. Causes include:

- Chronic obstructive or interstitial lung disease
- Congenital or acquired heart disease with left-sided heart failure
- Recurrent PE
- Connective tissue diseases
- Obstructive sleep apnea
- Idiopathic or familial forms of PH (rare)

Pathogenesis (p. 707)

The *familial form of PH* is caused by mutations in the *bone morphogenetic protein receptor type 2 (BMPR2)* signaling pathway. In vascular smooth muscle cells (SMCs), BMPR2 signaling inhibits proliferation and favors apoptosis; defective signaling therefore results in SMC hyperplasia and increased vascular resistance. The phenotype is also influenced by environmental triggers or by modifier genes that affect vascular tone (e.g., endothelin, prostacyclin, nitric oxide, and angiotensin-converting enzyme activities).

The *secondary forms of PH* are attributed to endothelial dysfunction that increase vascular tone, promote thrombosis, or increase the production of cytokines that promote SMC proliferation and/or matrix synthesis.

Morphology (p. 708)

- Atherosclerosis in the pulmonary artery and major branches
- Medial hypertrophy of muscular and elastic arteries
- Right ventricular hypertrophy
- *Plexiform lesions* (tufts within capillary channels creating a vascular plexus) represent the severe end of the spectrum of changes; they are most prominent in primary pulmonary hypertension and with some congenital cardiovascular anomalies.
- Numerous organized thrombi suggest recurrent pulmonary thromboembolism as an etiology

Clinical Course (p. 709)

Clinical signs and symptoms in all forms of PH become evident only with advanced disease. *Idiopathic PH* occurs most often in women between 20 and 40 years old; it generally progresses to severe respiratory insufficiency, decompensated cor pulmonale (often with superimposed thromboembolism and pneumonia), and death within 2 to 5 years. Therapy includes vasodilators and lung transplantation.

Diffuse Pulmonary Hemorrhage Syndromes (p. 709)

Goodpasture Syndrome (p. 709)

Goodpasture syndrome is caused by autoantibodies directed against the non-collagenous domain of the collagen IV α3 chain; these cause basement membrane destruction in renal glomeruli and pulmonary alveoli, giving rise to rapidly progressive glomerulonephritis (Chapter 20) and necrotizing hemorrhagic interstitial pneumonitis. Most cases occur in people in adolescence or in their twenties with a male predominance; the vast majority are smokers. Histology of the lung reveals focal alveolar wall necrosis with intra-alveolar hemorrhage and hemosiderin-laden macrophages; immunofluorescence shows linear immunoglobulin deposition along septal basement membranes. Hemoptysis is a typical presenting feature, followed by symptoms of glomerulonephritis; uremia is the most common cause of death. Therapy involves plasmapheresis and immunosuppression.

Idiopathic Pulmonary Hemosiderosis (p. 710)

Idiopathic pulmonary hemosiderosis is a rare disease of children characterized by intermittent diffuse alveolar hemorrhage; it presents with cough and hemoptysis. Although the cause is unknown, a favorable response to immunosuppression suggests an immunologic basis.

Wegener Granulomatosis (p. 710)

Wegener granulomatosis is an autoimmune disease typically presenting with hemoptysis (Chapter 11); diagnostically important features are capillaritis and scattered, poorly formed granulomata.

Pulmonary Infections (p. 710)

Pulmonary infections occur when lung or systemic defenses are impaired. Pulmonary defenses include nasal, tracheobronchial, and alveolar mechanisms to filter, neutralize, and clear inhaled organisms and particles. These can be compromised by:

- Decreased cough reflex leading to aspiration (e.g., coma, anesthesia, neuromuscular disorders)
- Injury to mucociliary apparatus (e.g., cigarette smoking, viral infection, genetic defects)

- Secretion accumulation (e.g., cystic fibrosis, chronic bronchitis)
- Decreased phagocytic or bactericidal function of alveolar macrophages (e.g., tobacco smoke, oxygen toxicity)
- Edema or congestion (e.g., congestive heart failure)

Pneumonias are broadly defined as any infection of the lung parenchyma; these are classified by the specific etiologic agent or the clinical setting (Table 15-3). Additional points:

- One type of pneumonia (e.g., viral) often predisposes to another type (e.g., bacterial) due to compromise of systemic or specific pulmonary defenses.
- Although most pneumonias begin via the respiratory tract, hematogenous spread from other sites can occur.
- Many patients with chronic diseases develop terminal infections when hospitalized *(nosocomial infections);* this is due to a combination of antibiotic resistance, invasive procedures, equipment contamination, and a greater chance for exposure.

Community-Acquired Acute Pneumonias (p. 711)

These pneumonias can be bacterial or viral; predisposing conditions include extremes of age, chronic disease (e.g., COPD), immune deficiencies, and lack of splenic function.

- *Streptococcus pneumoniae,* or *pneumococcus,* is the most common cause of community-acquired pneumonia.
- *Haemophilus influenzae* can cause life-threatening lower respiratory tract infections and meningitis in children and is a common cause of pneumonia in adults, especially those with COPD. It is a pleomorphic Gram-negative organism that colonizes the pharynx, occurring as encapsulated and unencapsulated forms; type b (of serotypes a through f) is the most common *encapsulated* cause of severe invasive disease although infection by unencapsulated forms is increasing. Virulence factors include adhesive pili, a factor that dysregulates ciliary beating, and a protease that degrades IgA.
- *Moraxella catarrhalis* causes bacterial pneumonia, especially in the elderly; it exacerbates COPD and is a common cause of pediatric otitis media.
- *Staphylococcus aureus* pneumonia often complicates viral illnesses and has a high risk of abscess formation and empyema. Intravenous (IV) drug abusers are at high risk of staphylococcal pneumonia in association with endocarditis.
- *Klebsiella pneumoniae* is the most common cause of Gram-negative pneumonia; it afflicts debilitated individuals, especially chronic alcoholics.
- *Pseudomonas aeruginosa* is a common cause of nosocomial infections with a propensity to invade blood vessels and spread systemically; it is also common in cystic fibrosis and neutropenic patients.
- *Legionella pneumophilia* is the agent of Legionnaires' disease and Pontiac fever. It flourishes in artificial aquatic environments such as water-cooling towers and spreads through aerosolization; infection causes severe pneumonia in the immunocompromised patient.

Morphology (p. 712)

Bacterial infections, caused by various Gram-positive or Gram-negative organisms, occur in overlapping morphologic patterns—*bronchopneumonia* and *lobar pneumonia.* Depending on bacterial virulence and host resistance, the same organism can cause bronchopneumonia, lobar pneumonia, or something intermediate.

TABLE 15-3 The Pneumonia Syndromes

Community-Acquired Acute Pneumonia

Streptococcus pneumoniae
Haemophilus influenzae
Moraxella catarrhalis
Staphylococcus aureus
Legionella pneumophila
Enterobacteriaceae *(Klebsiella pneumoniae)* and *Pseudomonas* spp.

Community-Acquired Atypical Pneumonia

Mycoplasma pneumoniae
Chlamydia spp. *(C. pneumoniae, C. psittaci, C. trachomatis)*
Coxiella burnetti (Q fever)
Viruses: respiratory syncytial virus, parainfluenzavirus (children);
   influenzavirus A and B (adults); adenovirus (military recruits); SARS*
   coronavirus

Nosocomial Pneumonia

Gram-negative rods belonging to Enterobacteriaceae *(Klebsiella* spp.,
   Serratia marcescens, Escherichia coli) and Pseudomonas spp.
Staphylococcus aureus (usually penicillin-resistant)

Aspiration Pneumonia

Anaerobic oral flora *(Bacteroides, Prevotella, Fusobacterium,
   Peptostreptococcus),* admixed with aerobic bacteria *(Streptococcus
   pneumoniae, Staphylococcus aureus, Haemophilas influenzae, and
   Pseudomonas aeruginosa)*

Chronic Pneumonia

Nocardia
Actinomyces
Granulomatous*: Mycobacterium tuberculosis* and atypical mycobacteria,
   Histoplasma capsulatum, Coccidioides immitis, Blastomyces dermatitidis

Necrotizing Pneumonia and Lung Abscess

Anaerobic bacteria (extremely common), with or without mixed aerobic
   infection
Staphylococcus aureus, Klebsiella pneumoniae, Streptococcus pyogenes,
   and type 3 pneumococcus (uncommon)

Pneumonia in the Immunocompromised Host

Cytomegalovirus
Pneumocystis jiroveci
Mycobacterium avium-intracellulare
Invasive aspergillosis
Invasive candidiasis
"Usual" bacterial, viral, and fungal organisms (listed above)

SARS, Severe acute respiratory syndrome.

- *Lobar pneumonia involves essentially an entire lobe:* Four stages of inflammatory response are classically described: (1) initial *congestion* due to vascular engorgement and alveolar transudates, (2) *red hepatization* marking a stage of massive neutrophilic exudation with hemorrhage (grossly resembling liver), (3) *gray hepatization* characterized by red cell disintegration but persistence of fibrinopurulent exudates, (4) *resolution* marked by progressive enzymatic digestion of the exudates and macrophage resorption of the debris, or fibroblast ingrowth. Exudate resolution usually restores normal lung structure and function, but organization with fibrous scarring can occur.
- *Bronchopneumonia is marked by patchy exudative consolidation of lung parenchyma.* Grossly, the lungs exhibit focal areas of palpable consolidation. Histologically, there is acute (neutrophilic)

suppurative exudation filling bronchi, bronchioles, and alveoli; this will also eventually resolve.
- Involvement of the pleura *(pleuritis)* can resolve or result in fibrous thickening and adhesions. Expansion of infection into the pleural space causes a fibrinopurulent *empyema*.

Clinical Course (p. 714)

Symptoms include high fever, rigors, and productive cough, occasionally with hemoptysis; a friction rub and pleuritic chest pain herald pleural involvement. The clinical picture is markedly changed by antibiotic administration. Complications include abscess formation and systemic dissemination causing endocarditis, meningitis, suppurative arthritis, or metastatic abscesses.

Community-Acquired Atypical (Viral and Mycoplasmal) Pneumonias (p. 714)

Infections by viruses or certain non-viral organisms (e.g., *Mycoplasma pneumoniae* or *Chlamydia pneumonieae*) range from relatively mild upper respiratory tract involvements (e.g., the common cold) to severe lower respiratory tract disease. The common pathogenic mechanism is attachment of organisms to epithelial cells followed by cellular necrosis and inflammation. In alveoli, this may cause fluid transudation; in upper airways, loss of the normal mucociliary clearance of the respiratory epithelium predisposes to secondary bacterial infection.

Morphology (p. 714)

- Patchy or lobar areas of congestion appear *without* the consolidation of bacterial pneumonias (hence the term *atypical pneumonia*).
- Interstitial pneumonitis occurs with widened, edematous alveolar walls with mononuclear inflammation.
- *Hyaline membranes* reflect DAD.
- In some viral infections, characteristic cytopathic changes occur (Chapter 8).

Influenza Infections (p. 715)

Influenza is a single-stranded RNA virus composed of eight strands bound by a nucleoprotein that determines the type of the virus (i.e., A, B, or C). Type A influenza viruses infect humans, pigs, horses, and birds and are the major cause of influenza epidemics through viral mutations. Types B and C do not mutate; consequently, childhood infections result in largely life-long antibody-mediated protection against future disease.

The influenza virus surface is a lipid bilayer studded with viral hemagglutinin (in human-tropic viruses, these are H1, H2, or H3) and viral neuraminidase (i.e., N1 or N2) that determine the virus subtype; antibodies to these molecules prevent future infections to the particular viral strain. Clearing an established infection requires cytotoxic T cells and innate immune responses (including a macrophage anti-influenza protein *Mx1*).

Epidemics occur when viruses acquire mutations in their hemagglutinin or neuraminidase proteins that allow escape from most host antibodies *(antigenic drift)*. Pandemics occur when these proteins are replaced altogether by recombination of RNA segments with those of animal viruses *(antigenic shift)*.

The particular pathogenicity of the avian H5N1 virus (60% human mortality) derives from its ability to spread throughout the body and not be confined to lung; the tropism of the avian H5 hemagglutinin derives from its ability to be cleaved (and activated) by diverse tissue proteases, whereas the more common hemagglutinins are only cleaved in the lung.

Human Metapneumovirus (p. 716)

Human metapneumovirus (MPV) is a paramyxovirus discovered in 2001; it causes bronchiolitis and pneumonia in the very young, the very old, and the immunocompromised; it is responsible for 5% to 10% of hospitalizations and up to 20% of pediatric out-patient visits for acute respiratory tract infections.

Severe Acute Respiratory Syndrome (p. 716)

Severe acute respiratory syndrome (SARS) is a coronavirus first identified in China in November 2002. Nearly 30% of upper respiratory tract infections are due to coronaviruses, but SARS differs in its ability to infect the lower respiratory tree and spread systemically.

SARS is transmitted primarily through infected respiratory secretions; after a 2- to 10-day incubation, there is a dry cough, malaise, myalgias, and fever. One third of patients recover; the remainder progress to severe respiratory disease, and nearly 10% die. In fatal cases, the lungs show DAD with multinucleated giant cells; virus can be visualized by electron microscopy.

Aspiration Pneumonia (p. 716)

Aspiration pneumonia occurs in markedly debilitated or unconscious patients; it results in partly chemical (gastric acid) and partly bacterial (mixed oral flora) pneumonia. The pneumonia is often necrotizing and pursues a fulminant course; lung abscess is a common complication.

Lung Abscess (p. 716)

This is an infection marked by localized suppurative necrosis of lung tissue.

Pathogenesis (p. 716)

Commonly involved are staphylococci, streptococci, numerous Gram-negative species, and anaerobes. Mixed infections are frequent, reflecting aspiration of oral contents as a common etiology. Abscesses can be due to:

- Aspiration of infective material (e.g., oropharyngeal procedures or secondary to diminished consciousness); aspiration abscesses are more common in the right lung, reflecting the more vertical right bronchus
- Antecedent primary bacterial infection
- Septic emboli from infected thrombi or right-sided endocarditis
- Obstructive tumors (10% to 15% of abscesses).
- Direct traumatic punctures or spread of infection from adjacent organs

Morphology (p. 717)

Abscesses may be single or multiple and vary from microscopic to large cavities. They contain variable mixtures of pus and air, depending on available drainage through airways. Chronic abscesses are often surrounded by a reactive fibrous wall.

Clinical Course (p. 717)

Complications include extension into the pleural cavity, hemorrhage, septic embolization, and secondary amyloidosis.

Chronic Pneumonia (p. 717)

Chronic pneumonia is typically a localized granulomatous inflammation in immunocompetent patients, with or without regional lymph node involvement. In the immunocompromised host, the infection may become disseminated. Tuberculosis is described in Chapter 8; the following are fungal causes. Most are asymptomatic and result in only limited granulomatous disease; however, immunocompromise can cause fulminant, widespread dissemination.

Histoplasmosis *(p. 717)*

Histoplasmosis is an intracellular parasite of macrophages; it is endemic along the Ohio and Mississippi Rivers and in the Caribbean basin. Infection by *Histoplasma capsulatum* produces granulomas with coagulative necrosis that subsequently undergo fibrosis and concentric calcification. Silver stain identifies the 3-5 μ thin-walled cyst of the fungus, which can persist for years.

Blastomycosis *(p. 718)*

Blastomycosis occurs in the central and southeastern United States, Canada, Mexico, the Middle East, Africa, and India. It can occur as pulmonary, disseminated, and (rarely) primary cutaneous forms. *Blastomyces dermatidis* is a 5-15 μ, thick-walled yeast that divides by broad-based budding; it causes suppurative granulomas.

Coccidioidomycosis *(p. 719)*

Coccidioidomycosis is endemic in the southwest and western United States and Mexico, where more than 80% of the population have a delayed-type hypersensitivity response to the organism. *Coccidioides immitis* causes lesions varying from pyogenic to granulomatous; silver stains demonstrate a 20-60 μ, thick-walled spherule containing small endospores.

Pneumonia in the Immunocompromised Host *(p. 719)*

Opportunistic infections rarely cause infection in normal hosts but can cause life-threatening pneumonias in the immunocompromised host. Often, more than one agent is involved. *Pseudomonas*, mycobacteria, *Legionella*, and *Listeria* are the more common bacterial agents; CMV and herpesviruses are the more common viruses; and *Pneumocystis, Candida,* and *Aspergillus* are the most common fungi.

Pulmonary Disease in Human Immunodeficiency Virus Infection *(p. 719)*

- In these patients pulmonary disease may be due to more than one cause and symptoms may be atypical.
- The absolute CD4+ T-cell count can define the risk of infection with specific organisms:

  More than 200/μL: bacteria, including tuberculosis
  50 to 200/μL: *Pneumocystis*
  Less than 50/μL: CMV and *Mycobacterium avium* complex

- In addition to opportunistic infections, "common" bacterial pathogens also cause severe disease.
- Malignancies (e.g., Kaposi sarcoma, lymphoma, lung cancer) also cause pulmonary disease.

Lung Transplantation *(p. 720)*

Lung transplantation is typically performed in otherwise healthy patients for emphysema, idiopathic pulmonary fibrosis, cystic fibrosis, and primary pulmonary hypertension; in most cases, single-lung transplants are performed. Complications include:

- Infections (similar to those in other immunocompromised patients)
- Acute rejection (vascular and airway mononuclear cell infiltrates)
- Chronic rejection with variable fibrotic occlusion of small airways *(bronchiolitis obliterans).*

1-, 5-, and 10-year survival rates are 78%, 50%, and 26% respectively.

Tumors (p. 721)

Carcinomas (p. 721)

Carcinomas constitute 90% to 95% of lung tumors; they are the most common cause of cancer death in both men and women.

Pathogenesis (p. 721)

Pathogenesis involves a stepwise accumulation of genetic abnormalities; 10 to 20 mutations have occurred by the time a tumor is clinically apparent. Contributory factors:

- *Tobacco smoking* is the most important etiologic factor, correlating with amount and duration of smoking. Women have a higher susceptibility to tobacco carcinogens than do men. Cessation of smoking reduces risk after 10 years, but never to control levels. *Secondhand smoke* causes 3000 cases of lung cancer annually. Tobacco smoke contains more than 1200 compounds, many of which are potential carcinogens.
- *Environmental exposures* include radiation (e.g., radon, uranium), air pollution (particulates), and occupational inhaled substances (e.g., nickel, chromates, arsenic). Asbestos increases risk of cancer five-fold (with a latency of 10 to 30 years); when combined with smoking, the risk is 50- to 90-fold greater.
- *Genetic mechanisms* include mutations in dominant oncogenes (*c-MYC, K-RAS, EGFR,* and *HER-2/neu*) and loss of tumor-suppressor genes (e.g., *p53, RB,* and *p16[INK4a]*); m-TOR pathway molecules are mutated in up to 30% of lung cancers, and c-KIT (a receptor tyrosine kinase) and telomerase activities are also often increased.
- *Precursor lesions* (notably, these do not necessarily progress to malignancy) include:

  Squamous dysplasia and carcinoma *in situ*
  Atypical adenomatous hyperplasia
  Diffuse idiopathic pulmonary neuroendocrine cell hyperplasia

Classification (p. 723)

Lung carcinomas are classified by their predominant histologic appearance (see later discussion). However, the most relevant clinical and therapeutic grouping is *small cell carcinomas* (almost always metastatic with high initial responses to radiation and chemotherapy) vs. *non–small cell carcinomas* (less often metastatic, less responsive).

Morphology (p. 723)

- *Adenocarcinoma* is the most common lung cancer (37% of male and 47% of female lung cancers). It typically presents as a peripheral mass with characteristic microscopic gland formation, usually producing mucin, and an adjacent desmoplastic response. These grow more slowly than squamous cell carcinomas but tend to metastasize earlier.
- *Bronchioloalveolar carcinoma* is a less common form of adenocarcinoma arising in the terminal bronchioloalveolar regions. Grossly, there may be single or multiple nodules or a diffuse, pneumonia-like tumor consolidation. Histologically, there are distinctive tall, columnar, often mucin-producing tumor cells arrayed along preserved alveolar septa and forming papillary projections. Clinically, these occur equally in men and women and are not usually associated with smoking. Prognosis is relatively

favorable after solitary nodule resection but dismal in diffuse disease.

- *Squamous cell carcinoma* (32% of male and 25% of female lung cancers) has the closest correlation with smoking. Most arise in or near the lung hilus. Microscopically, they vary from well-differentiated keratinizing neoplasms to wildly anaplastic tumors.
- *Small cell carcinoma* (14% of male and 18% of female lung cancers) is the most malignant of lung cancers and usually occurs as a central or hilar tumor. It is strongly associated with cigarette smoking. The characteristic microscopic features include nests or clusters of small cells with little cytoplasm and without squamous or glandular differentiation. Ultrastructurally, the cancer cells exhibit neurosecretory granules, and immunohistochemical stains usually demonstrate neuroendocrine markers. These tumors most often produce *paraneoplastic syndromes* (see later discussion).
- *Large cell carcinoma* (18% of male and 10% of female lung cancers) probably represents poorly differentiated squamous cell carcinomas or adenocarcinomas.

Clinical Course (p. 727)

Presenting symptoms for lung carcinoma include cough, weight loss, chest pain, and dyspnea. Adrenal, brain, liver, and bone are favored metastatic sites. Small cell carcinoma has almost always metastasized by the time of diagnosis, precluding surgical intervention; although it is responsive to chemotherapy, it ultimately recurs. Other types show overall disappointing responses to chemotherapy. Outcome depends on stage at presentation; the overall 5-year survival rate is 15% although surgical resection of solitary tumors (a minority of patients) has a better survival rate (48%).

Secondary pathologies related to lung neoplasm include partial airway obstruction with distal emphysema and/or post-obstructive pneumonia and bronchiectasis; total obstruction with atelectasis; and obstruction of the superior vena cava with impaired head and upper extremity drainage *(superior vena cava syndrome)*. Tumors can also invade neural structures around the trachea, including the cervical sympathetic plexus, giving rise to the *Horner syndrome* (ptosis, miosis, and anhidrosis); these are called *Pancoast tumors.*

Paraneoplastic syndromes associated with lung carcinoma (1% to 10% of tumors) result from release of:

- Antidiuretic hormone (syndrome of inappropriate antidiuretic hormone)
- Adrenocorticotropic hormone (ACTH; Cushing syndrome)
- Parathormone, parathyroid hormone–related peptide, or prostaglandin E (hypercalcemia)
- Calcitonin (hypocalcemia)
- Gonadotropins (gynecomastia)
- Serotonin (carcinoid syndrome)

Other paraneoplastic syndromes include Lambert-Eaton myasthenic syndrome (due to autoantibody formation), peripheral neuropathy, acanthosis nigricans, and hypertrophic pulmonary osteoarthropathy (finger clubbing).

Neuroendocrine Proliferations and Tumors (p. 729)

Tumorlets are small benign hyperplastic nests of neuroendocrine cells, typically seen adjacent to chronic inflammation or scarring. *Carcinoid tumors* exhibiting neuroendocrine differentiation constitute 1% to

5% of all lung tumors. These are low-grade malignancies that are subclassified as *typical* or *atypical* depending on the absence or presence, respectively, of *p53* mutations or abnormalities in *BCL2* and *BAX* expression.

Morphology (p. 729)

Grossly, the tumors are usually intrabronchial, highly vascular, polypoid masses less than 3 to 4 cm. Microscopically, there are nests and cords of uniform, small, round cells resembling intestinal carcinoids. Atypical carcinoids exhibit increased numbers of mitoses, greater pleomorphism, and a propensity for lymphatic invasion. Neurosecretory granules are seen ultrastructurally, and neuroendocrine differentiation is confirmed by immunostaining for neuron-specific enolase, serotonin, calcitonin, or bombesin.

Clinical Features (p. 730)

Manifestations relate to intrabronchial obstruction, capacity to metastasize, and the production of vasoactive amines, causing flushing, diarrhea, and cyanosis. Most follow a relatively benign course with 10-year survivals of 87% for typical carcinoids; atypical carcinoids have somewhat poorer survivals (56% at 5 years and 35% at 10 years).

Miscellaneous Tumors (p. 730)

Hamartomas are relatively common, benign, nodular neoplasms composed of cartilage and other mesenchymal tissues (e.g., fat, blood vessels, fibrous tissue).

Mediastinal tumors arise from local structures or may represent metastatic disease (Table 15-4); they can invade or compress the lungs. These are discussed elsewhere in appropriate chapters.

Metastatic Tumors (p. 730)

Secondary involvement of the lung by metastatic tumor is common and can occur via direct extension from contiguous organs or via lymphatics or hematogenous routes. Patterns of disease include discrete masses or nodules, and growth within peribronchial lymphatics.

TABLE 15-4 Mediastinal Tumors and Other Masses

Superior Mediastinum

Lymphoma
Thymoma
Thyroid lesions
Metastatic carcinoma
Parathyroid tumors

Anterior Mediastinum

Thymoma
Teratoma
Lymphoma
Thyroid lesions
Parathyroid tumors

Posterior Mediastinum

Neurogenic tumors (schwannoma, neurofibroma)
Lymphoma
Gastroenteric hernia

Middle Mediastinum

Bronchogenic cyst
Pericardial cyst
Lymphoma

Pleura (p. 731)

Most pleural lesions are secondary to underlying lung disease.

Pleural Effusion (p. 731)

Accumulations of transudate (hydrothorax) or serous exudate can occur with:

- Increased hydrostatic pressure (e.g., heart failure)
- Increased vascular permeability (e.g., pneumonia)
- Decreased oncotic pressure (e.g., nephrotic syndrome)
- Increased negative intrapleural pressure (e.g., atelectasis)
- Decreased lymphatic drainage (e.g., carcinomatosis)

Inflammatory Pleural Effusions (p. 731)

- *Serofibrinous pleuritis* reflects pulmonary inflammation, for example, tuberculosis, pneumonia, infarcts, abscesses, or systemic diseases (e.g., rheumatoid arthritis, uremia).
- *Suppurative pleuritis* (empyema) usually reflects pleural space infection, leading to pus accumulation.
- *Hemorrhagic pleuritis* occurs with bleeding disorders, neoplastic involvement, and certain rickettsial diseases.

Organization of these exudates with dense fibrous adhesions can affect lung expansion.

Noninflammatory Pleural Effusions (p. 732)

Other pleural fluid accumulations include *hydrothorax* (most commonly due to heart failure, but also renal or hepatic failure); *hemothorax* (a fatal complication of a ruptured aortic aneurysm); and *chylothorax* (a collection of milky lymph fluid, usually due to neoplastic lymphatic obstruction).

Pneumothorax (p. 732)

Pneumothorax refers to air or gas in the pleural cavity, usually with associated ipsilateral lung deflation; it can be traumatic (e.g., after rib fractures that puncture the lung) or spontaneous, occurring after peripheral apical bleb rupture. *Tension pneumothorax* occurs when a defect between airways and pleura acts as a one-way valve, admitting air during inspiration but failing to release it during expiration. The progressively increasing pleural pressure compresses the contralateral lung and mediastinal structures and represents a serious, potentially fatal complication.

Pleural Tumors (p. 732)

Most common pleural tumors are metastases from lung, breast, ovaries, or other organs; malignant effusions often contain cytologically detectable tumor cells.

Solitary Fibrous Tumor (p. 732)

These noninvasive, fibrosing, rarely malignant tumors are composed of spindle cells resembling fibroblasts; they also occur in other sites and are not related to asbestos exposure. Resection is usually curative.

Malignant Mesothelioma (p. 733)

This uncommon tumor of mesothelial cells occurs most often in the pleura (less frequently in the peritoneum or other sites). It is associated with asbestos exposure in 90% of cases; only 20% of these patients have pulmonary asbestosis. The lifetime risk in heavily exposed individuals is 7% to 10%, with a latency period between exposure and tumor development of 25 to 45 years.

Notably, among asbestos workers, *carcinoma remains the most common lung tumor.*

Morphology (p. 733)

Tumor spreads diffusely over the lung surface and fissures, forming an encasing sheath. Microscopic patterns are *epithelioid* (60%), *sarcomatoid* (20%), and mixed *(biphasic)* (20%) tumors.

* *Epithelioid pattern* shows epithelium-like cells forming tubules and papillary projections resembling adenocarcinomas. Antigenic (calretinin, WT-1 and CK5/6 positivity) and ultrastructural (long, slender microvilli) features allow distinction from adenocarcinomas (MOC31 and BG8 positivity and short, plump microvilli).
* *Sarcomatoid pattern* shows malignant, spindle-shaped cells resembling fibrosarcoma.

Clinical Course (p. 734)

Patients present with chest pain, dyspnea, and recurrent pleural effusion. Mesotheliomas are highly malignant tumors that invade the lung and can metastasize widely. Few patients survive longer than 2 years.

16

Head and Neck

ORAL CAVITY (p. 740)

Teeth and Supporting Structures (p. 740)

Caries (Tooth Decay) (p. 740)

Caries represents focal tooth degradation due to mineral dissolution; it occurs through acids released by oral bacteria during sugar fermentation. Caries is the most common reason for tooth loss before age 35 years.

Gingivitis (p. 740)

Gingivitis is soft tissue inflammation of the squamous mucosa and soft tissues around teeth, with erythema, edema, bleeding, and gingival degeneration. Inadequate oral hygiene leads to accumulation of *dental plaque* (a biofilm of bacteria, salivary proteins, and desquamated epithelial cells), with subsequent mineralization (*tartar*); plaque bacteria cause caries and plaque build-up below the gumline leads to gingivitis.

Periodontitis (p. 741)

Periodontitis is inflammation of tooth-supporting structures (e.g., periodontal ligaments, alveolar bone, and cementum); it can progress to complete destruction of the periodontal ligament and alveolar bone, with tooth loss. As opposed to facultative Gram-positive colonization of typical plaque, periodontitis-associated plaque contains anaerobic and microaerophilic Gram-negative flora. While typically occurring in isolation, periodontal disease can also occur in several systemic diseases, especially those affecting immunologic function. Periodontal infections can also underlie systemic diseases (e.g., infective endocarditis and brain abscesses).

Inflammatory/Reactive Tumor-Like Lesions (p. 741)

Fibrous Proliferative Lesions (p. 741)

These are benign reactive lesions, usually cured by surgical excision.

- *Irritation fibromas* (61% of reactive lesions) typically occur along the "bite line"; these are nodules of fibrous tissue covered by squamous mucosa.
- *Pyogenic granulomas* (12%) are rapidly growing, highly vascular lesions similar to granulation tissue. Common in children or during pregnancy, they can regress (particularly after pregnancy),

undergo fibrous maturation, or develop into peripheral ossifying fibromas.

- *Peripheral ossifying fibromas* (22%) can arise from pyogenic granulomas, although most have unknown etiologies. With a 15% to 20% recurrence rate, surgical excision to the periosteum is the treatment of choice.
- *Peripheral giant cell granulomas* are composed of multinucleated foreign body–like giant cells separated by fibroangiomatous stroma.

Apthous Ulcers (Canker Sores) (p. 742)

Apthous ulcers affect up to 40% of the U.S. population; they can have a familial predilection, and recurrent ulcers may be associated with sprue and inflammatory bowel disease. Lesions are painful, shallow, hyperemic ulcerations initially infiltrated by mononuclear inflammatory cells; secondary bacterial infection recruits neutrophils.

Glossitis (p. 742)

Glossitis implies tongue inflammation, but it is also applied to the "beefy-red" tongues of certain deficiency states associated with papilla atrophy and mucosal thinning, exposing the underlying vasculature. Such changes occur in sprue and in vitamin B_{12}, riboflavin, niacin, iron, or pyridoxine deficiencies.

Infections (p. 742)

Normal oral mucosa resists infection by competitive suppression from low-virulence commensal organisms, high levels of immunoglobulin A, the antibacterial properties of saliva, and dilution from ingested food and liquids. Alteration in these defenses (e.g., due to immunodeficiency or antibiotic therapy) contributes to infections.

Herpes Simplex Virus Infections (p. 742)

Herpes simplex virus-1 and -2 (HSV-1 and -2) infections classically cause "cold sores" with minimal morbidity; 10% to 20% of primary infections present as *acute herpetic gingivostomatitis* with diffuse oral vesicles and ulceration, lymphadenopathy, and fever.

Morphology (p. 742)

Lesions consist of vesicles, large bullae, or shallow ulcerations. Histologically, there is intra- and intercellular edema *(acantholysis),* eosinophilic intranuclear inclusions, and multinucleated giant cells (visualized by microscopic examination of vesicular fluid, called a *Tzanck test).* Vesicles heal spontaneously in 3 to 4 weeks, but virus treks along regional nerves and becomes doermant in local ganglia; reactivation (e.g., driven by trauma, infection, or immune suppression) occurs with crops of small vesicles that clear in 4 to 6 days.

Oral Candidiasis (Thrush) (p. 743)

Oral candidiasis can present as erythematous or hyperplastic lesions, but it classically manifests as superficial gray-white inflammatory membranes composed of fibrinosuppurative exudates containing fungus. It occurs with broad-spectrum antibiotics, diabetes, neutropenia, or immunodeficiency.

Oral Manifestations of Systemic Disease (p. 743)

Characteristic oral lesions occur in:

- Infections (e.g., scarlet fever, measles, and infectious mononucleosis)
- Dermatologic conditions (e.g., lichen planus and erythema multiforme)

- Hematologic disorders (e.g., pancytopenias and leukemias, especially *monocytic leukemia*)
- Melanotic pigmentations of Addison disease and pregnancy
- Fibrous gingival enlargement of chronic phenytoin (Dilantin) ingestion
- Telangiectasias of *Rendu-Osler-Weber syndrome*

Hairy Leukoplakia (p. 743)

Hairy leukoplakia is a distinctive oral lesion seen in immunocompromised patients (80% are human immunodeficiency virus [HIV] infected). Caused by Epstein-Barr virus (EBV), the lesions are white patches of hyperkeratosis on tongue lateral borders; superimposed candidal infections can augment the "hairiness."

Tumors and Precancerous Lesions (p. 744)

Leukoplakia and Erythroplakia (p. 744)

Tobacco use is the most common antecedent.

- *Leukoplakia* signifies a white plaque on the oral mucosa that cannot be removed by scraping and cannot be classified as another disease entity. Lesions vary from benign epithelial thickenings to highly atypical dysplasia verging on *carcinoma in situ*. Leukoplakia occurs in 3% of individuals; 5% to 25% of lesions are premalignant. Thus, until proved otherwise, leukoplakia should be considered precancerous.
- *Erythroplakia* is a red, velvety, relatively flat lesion; it is less common than leukoplakia but more ominous because the epithelium is markedly atypical and has greater risk of malignant transformation.

Squamous Cell Carcinoma (p. 745)

Squamous cell carcinoma constitutes 95% of oral cancers, with 45,000 new cases annually in the United States; overall 5-year survival is 50%, varying depending on stage (i.e., early-stage = 80%; late-stage = 19%). The high rate of second primaries (3% to 7% per year) suggests "field cancerization" due to diffuse mucosal exposure to carcinogens.

Pathogenesis (p.746)

Pathogenesis is multifactorial. Tobacco and alcohol are the most common associations, although 50% of oropharyngeal cancers harbor ongogenic variants of human papillomavirus (HPV). Patients with HPV-positive tumors do better than those without. Other risk factors:

- Familial associations, related to genomic instability
- Actinic radiation (sunlight)
- Pipe smoking
- Betel nut and paan chewing (India and Asia)

Molecular Biology (p. 746)

Development of malignancy is a multistage process; although heterogeneous, a general pathway is:

- *p16* inactivation leads to loss of an inhibitor of cyclin-dependent kinase and progression to hyperplasia/hyperkeratosis
- *p53* mutations lead to progression to dysplasia
- Gross genomic alterations and/or deletions (4q, 6p, 8p, 11q, 13q, or 14q) predict progression to malignancy
- Cyclin D1 overexpression causes constitutively active cell cycle progression

Morphology (p. 747)

Tumors occur most commonly in the ventral tongue, mouth floor, lower lip, soft palate, and gingiva; lesions can be raised, firm, ulcerated, or verrucous. Histologically, they are typical squamous carcinomas of variable differentiation; the degree of differentiation does not predict clinical behavior. Tumors need not progress to full-thickness squamous cell *carcinoma in situ* before invading the underlying stroma. Local infiltration precedes metastasis; common metastatic sites are cervical lymph nodes, lungs, liver, and bones.

Odontogenic Cysts and Tumors (p. 748)

Epithelium-lined cysts in the mandible and maxilla derive from odontogenic remnants; they may be developmental or inflammatory.

- *Dentigerous cysts* originate near crowns of unerupted teeth and may result from dental follicle degeneration. They are most often associated with impacted third molars. These are unilocular lesions lined by stratified squamous epithelium, with associated chronic inflammation. Complete removal is curative.
- *Odontogenic keratocysts (OKCs)* are potentially aggressive; treatment requires complete resection (recurrence rates of 60% for partial resection). They occur most commonly in the posterior mandible of males who are 10 to 40 years old and are unilocular or multilocular lesions typically lined by parakeratinized stratified squamous. Patients with multiple OKCs merit evaluation for nevoid basal cell carcinoma syndrome *(Gorlin syndrome),* related to *PTCH* tumor-suppressor gene mutations (Chapter 25).
- *Periapical cysts* are inflammatory lesions found at tooth apices; these develop from long-standing pulpitis due to caries or tooth trauma. Persistent chronic inflammation leads to granulation tissue and proliferation of quiescent rests of odontogenic epithelium.
- *Odontogenic tumors* demonstrate diverse histology and clinical behavior. Some are true neoplasms (both benign and malignant); others are hamartomas.
- *Ameloblastoma* is a true neoplasm arising from odontogenic epithelium and shows *no* ectomesenchymal differentiation. It is typically cystic, slow growing, and locally invasive, but it often has an indolent course.
- *Odontoma* is the most common odontogenic tumor. It is likely a hamartoma, arising from epithelium with extensive enamel and dentin deposition.

UPPER AIRWAYS (p. 749)

Nose (p. 749)

Inflammations (p. 749)

Infectious rhinitis (p. 749) or "common cold" is caused by adeno-, echo-, and rhinoviruses. There is erythematous and edematous nasal mucosa with profuse catarrhal discharge; bacterial superinfection can induce mucopurulent exudates.

Allergic rhinitis (p. 749) or "hay fever" affects 20% of individuals; it is an immunoglobulin E (IgE)-mediated immune reaction (Chapter 6) with mucosal edema and erythema, as well as eosinophil-rich infiltrates.

Nasal polyps (p. 749) occur with recurrent rhinitis; these are edematous mucosa infiltrated by neutrophils, eosinophils, and plasma cells. When multiple or large, they obstruct the airway and impair sinus drainage, necessitating removal. Most are *not* due to atopy, and only 0.5% of atopic patients develop polyps.

Chronic rhinitis (p. 749) is the sequela to chronic acute rhinitis. There is superficial mucosal ulceration with variable inflammatory infiltrates that can extend into the sinuses.

Sinusitis (p. 750) is commonly preceded by acute or chronic rhinitis (edema impairs sinus drainage); maxillary sinusitis can occur by extension of a periapical tooth infection. *Kartagener syndrome* is a triad of *sinusitis, bronchiectasis,* and *situs inversus* due to congenitally defective ciliary action. Offending organisms are oral commensals, although diabetics can develop fungal sinusitis (e.g., *mucormycosis*). Although most commonly uncomfortable rather than serious, infections can spread into the orbit or surrounding bone to cause osteomyelitis or dural venous sinus thrombophlebitis.

Necrotizing Lesions of the Nose and Upper Airways (p. 750)

- Spreading fungal infections
- Wegener granulomatosis (Chapter 11)
- *Lethal midline granuloma,* a lymphoma of natural killer cells infected with EBV (Chapter 14), often complicated by ulceration and bacterial superinfection. Radiotherapy can control localized disease, but spread into the cranial vault, or necrosis with infection and sepsis, can be fatal.

Nasopharynx (p. 750)

Inflammations (p. 750)

Pharyngitis and *tonsillitis* are frequent concomitants of viral upper respiratory infections; there is mucosal edema and erythema with reactive lymphoid hyperplasia. Bacterial superinfection exacerbates the process, particularly in immunocompromised individuals or children without protective immunity.

Tumors of the Nose, Sinuses, and Nasopharynx (p. 751)

Nasopharyngeal angiofibroma (p. 751) is a highly vascularized benign tumor occurring in adolescent boys; serious bleeding can complicate surgical resection.

Sinonasal (Schneiderian) papilloma (p. 751) is a benign neoplasm of squamous or columnar epithelium. The *inverted papilloma* form is locally aggressive, and complete excision is required to prevent recurrence with potential invasion into the orbit or cranial vault.

Olfactory neuroblastoma (esthesioneuroblastoma) (p. 751) is an uncommon, highly malignant tumor composed of neuroendocrine cells.

Nasopharyngeal carcinoma (p. 751) is characterized by a distinctive geographic distribution, close anatomic relationship to lymphoid tissue, and association with EBV infection. It classically occurs in Africa (in children) and southern China (in adults). Tumors may be keratinizing or non-keratinizing squamous cell carcinomas or undifferentiated carcinomas with abundant lymphocytic infiltrate. The lesions are often clinically occult for extended periods; 70% have nodal metastases at initial presentation. Most are sensitive to radiotherapy with 50% to 70% 3-year survival rates.

Larynx (p. 752)

Inflammations (p. 752)

Laryngitis can be caused by allergic, viral, bacterial, or chemical injury. In children, *Haemophilus influenzae* laryngoepiglottitis can be life-threatening due to airway obstruction from rapid-onset severe mucosal edema; the inspiratory stridor it produces is called *croup*. The most common form of adult laryngitis is caused by heavy smoking, and predisposes to squamous epithelial metaplasia and carcinoma.

Reactive Nodules (Vocal Cord Nodules and Polyps) (p. 752)

Reactive nodules occur most often in heavy smokers (unilateral) or singers (*singer's nodules;* bilateral); these are small (millimeters), smooth, rounded excrescences on true vocal cords. These are myxoid, occasionally vascular, connective tissue covered by (occasionally hyperplastic) squamous epithelium. Although a cause of progressive hoarseness, malignant transformation is rare.

Squamous Papilloma and Papillomatosis (p. 752)

Squamous papillomas are 1 cm (or less) benign squamous epithelium-lined lesions, usually on the true vocal cords; in children, they may be multiple *(juvenile laryngeal papillomatosis)* and can spontaneously regress at puberty. Lesions are caused by HPV types 6 and 11; they frequently recur, but cancerous transformation is rare.

Carcinoma of the Larynx (p. 753)

Squamous cell carcinoma accounts for 95% of laryngeal cancers; usually occurring on the vocal cords, these can also develop on the epiglottis or pyriform sinuses. They present as persistent hoarseness but later can produce pain, dysphagia, and hemoptysis. Tobacco smoke is the major cause, although alcohol is also a risk factor; up to the point of frank malignancy, changes typically regress after smoking cessation. HPV, radiation, and asbestos exposure can also contribute. With surgery and radiation, more than 65% of patients are cured.

Morphology (p. 753)

Epithelial changes range from *hyperplasia* and *atypical hyperplasia* to *dysplasia, carcinoma in situ,* and invasive cancer. The likelihood of developing overt carcinoma is proportional to the atypia seen at first diagnosis.

EARS (p. 754)

The most common aural disorders (in descending order of frequency):

- Acute and chronic *otitis* (most often middle ear and mastoid), occasionally leading to a *cholesteatoma*
- Symptomatic *otosclerosis*
- *Polyps*
- *Labyrinthitis*
- *Carcinomas* (mostly external ear)
- *Paragangliomas* (mostly middle ear)

Inflammatory Lesions (p. 754)

- *Acute otitis media* occurs mostly in infants and children. These are typically viral with serous exudates, but they can have superimposed bacterial infections with suppuration; typical organisms are *Streptococcus pneumoniae, H. influenzae,* and β-hemolytic streptococci. *Chronic disease* is usually caused by *Pseudomonas, Staphylococcus,* or a fungus. In diabetics, otitis media due to *P. aeruginosa* is especially aggressive and can cause destructive necrotizing lesions.
- *Cholesteatomas* are associated with chronic otitis media; they are 1 to 4 cm cystic lesions with surrounding chronic inflammation, lined by keratinizing squamous epithelium and filled with amorphous debris, occasionally containing cholesterol spicules.

Otosclerosis (p. 754)

Otosclerosis is *abnormal bone deposition* in the middle ear, hampering stapes footplate mobility. Bone growth occurs through uncoupling of normal resorption and formation, although the cause is obscure; most cases are familial with an autosomal dominant predilection and variable penetrance. The process is slowly progressive, eventually causing marked hearing loss.

NECK (p. 754)

Branchial Cyst (Cervical Lymphoepithelial Cyst) (p. 755)

Branchial cysts are 2- to 5-cm benign lesions with fibrous walls lined by stratified squamous or pseudostratified columnar epithelium accompanied by lymphocytic infiltrates or reactive lymphoid tissue. They arise on the anterolateral neck typically from branchial arch remnants; similar lesions can occur in the parotid gland or beneath the tongue.

Thyroglossal Duct Cyst (p. 755)

These cysts arise from remnants of the developmental tract of the embryonic thyroid anlage; thus, they can occur anywhere from the base of the tongue to the anterior neck. Cysts are 1 to 4 cm, lined by squamous or respiratory epithelium, with walls that can exhibit lymphoid aggregates and/or thyroid tissue.

Paraganglioma (Carotid Body Tumor)
(p. 755)

These are slow-growing tumors typically occurring in individuals 50 to 70 years old; they arise in extra-adrenal paraganglia—either paravertebral or, more commonly, around the great vessels, including the *carotid bodies.* Paragangliomas consist of nests *(zellballen)* of polygonal neuroendocrine cells enclosed by fibrous trabeculae and elongated sustentacular cells. Sporadic forms are typically single; familial forms (i.e., in multiple endocrine neoplasia 2 syndrome) (Chapter 24) are usually multiple and bilateral. Carotid body paragangliomas recur after excision in half of cases and can be fatal due to infiltrative growth.

SALIVARY GLANDS (p. 756)

Xerostomia (p. 756)

Xerostomia (i.e., dry mouth) is due to lack of salivary secretions; it can occur in autoimmune inflammation and fibrosis (e.g., *Sjögren syndrome;* Chapter 6), or may be a complication of radiation therapy or a wide variety of pharmacologic agents.

Presentations range from oral dryness, to tongue fissuring and ulceration with papillary atrophy, to concomitant inflammatory salivary gland enlargement (Sjögren syndrome). Complications include increased caries, candidiasis, and difficulties with swallowing and speaking.

Inflammation (Sialadenitis) (p. 756)

Sialadenitis may be traumatic, viral (*mumps* is most common), bacterial, or autoimmune (e.g., *Sjögren syndrome;* Chapter 6).

Mucoceles (p. 756) are the most common salivary gland lesions; they result from ductal blockage or rupture with saliva leakage into surrounding stroma. Most often on the lower lip, they typically result from trauma; lesions fluctuate in size, particularly in association with meals. Incomplete excision can result in recurrence. A *ranula* refers specifically to a mucocele of the sublingual gland.

Sialolithiasis (p. 756) is salivary gland ductal obstruction caused by stones (due to periductal edema and/or impacted food debris); *nonspecific sialadenitis* (p. 756) with painful salivary gland enlargement and purulent discharge typically follows ductal obstruction. Dehydration and decreased secretory function predispose to secondary infection by *S. aureus* or *Streptococcus viridans.*

Neoplasms (p. 757)

There are 30 benign and malignant tumors of salivary glands (Table 16-1). Parotids account for 65% to 80% (15% to 30% are malignant); 10% occur in the submandibular glands (40% malignant), with the remainder being in the minor salivary glands (70% to 90% malignant).

TABLE 16-1 Histologic Classification and Approximate Incidence of Benign and Malignant Tumors of the Salivary Glands

Benign	Malignant
Pleomorphic adenoma (50%) (mixed tumor)	Mucoepidermoid carcinoma (15%)
Warthin tumor (5% to 10%)	Adenocarcinoma (NOS) (10%)
Oncocytoma (1%)	Acinic cell carcinoma (5%)
Other adenomas (5% to 10%)	Adenoid cystic carcinoma (5%)
Basal cell adenoma	Malignant mixed tumor (3% to 5%)
Canalicular adenoma	Squamous cell carcinoma (1%)
Ductal papillomas	Other carcinomas (2%)

NOS, Not otherwise specified.
Data from Ellis GL, Auclair PL: *Tumors of the salivary glands. Atlas of tumor pathology,* Third Series. Washington, DC, 1996, Armed Forces Institute of Pathology.

Pleomorphic Adenoma (p. 757)

These are benign tumors exhibiting mixed epithelial and mesenchymal differentiation; they constitute 60% of all parotid tumors, and lesser percentages in other salivary glands. Tumors are painless, slow-growing, mobile, discrete masses, with epithelial nests dispersed in a variable matrix of myxoid, hyaline, chondroid, or osseous differentiation.

Recurrence rates approach 25% if not well excised. Malignant transformation (usually as adenocarcinoma or undifferentiated carcinoma) occurs in 10% of tumors of more than 15 years of duration. Malignant transformation is associated with 30% to 50% 5-year mortality.

Warthin Tumor (Papillary Cystadenoma Lymphomatosum) (p. 759)

A benign tumor of unknown histogenesis found almost exclusively in the parotid; 10% are multifocal and 10% are bilateral. The tumor is 8 times more common in smokers. It is well encapsulated, consisting of glandular spaces lined by a double layer of epithelial cells atop a dense lymphoid stroma.

Mucoepidermoid Carcinoma (p. 759)

Mucoepidermoid carcinoma is the most common primary malignant salivary tumor, constituting 15% of all salivary gland neoplasms. Up to 8 cm in size, these lack well-defined capsules. Histologically, there are cords, sheets, or cystic arrangements of squamous, mucous, or intermediate cells with mucus-filled vacuoles. Low-grade tumors can invade locally with 15% recurrence rates; high-grade tumors have 25% recurrence rates and 50% 5-year survival rates.

Other Salivary Gland Tumors (p. 760)

- *Adenoid cystic carcinoma* is relatively uncommon; half occur in minor salivary glands. Histologically, tumor cells are small with scant cytoplasm; they are arrayed in tubular or cribriform patterns with intercellular spaces filled with excess basement membrane–like material. Although slow-growing, they are stubbornly recurrent and invasive, eventually becoming metastatic. Five-year survival rates are 60% to 70%.
- *Acinic cell tumors* constitute 2% to 3% of all salivary gland tumors and arise most commonly in the parotid glands; tumor cells resemble normal salivary serous acinar cells. Clinical behavior is dependent on cellular pleomorphism; 10% to 15% metastasize to lymph nodes, and the 5-year survival rate is 90%.

17

The Gastrointestinal Tract

CONGENITAL ABNORMALITIES (p. 764)

Atresia, Fistulae, and Duplications (p. 764)

When present in the esophagus, these various defects usually present shortly after birth with regurgitation during feeding; prompt surgical correction is important. Esophageal atresia is also associated with congenital heart defects, genitourinary malformations, and neurologic disorders.

- *Atresia:* In esophageal atresia, a portion of the conduit is replaced by a thin, noncanalized cord, with blind pouches above and below the atretic segment. *Imperforate anus* is the most common form of congenital intestinal atresia, caused by failure of the cloacal membrane to involute.
- *Fistula:* A connection between the esophagus and the trachea or a mainstem bronchus; swallowed material or gastric fluids can enter the respiratory tract.
- *Stenosis:* An incomplete form of atresia; the lumen is reduced by a fibrous thickened wall; this can be congenital or result from inflammatory scarring (e.g., due to chronic reflux, irradiation, or scleroderma).
- *Congenital duplication cysts:* Cystic masses with redundant smooth muscle layers; they can occur throughout the gastrointestinal tract.

Diaphragmatic Hernia, Omphalocele, and Gastroschisis (p. 765)

- *Diaphragmatic* hernia occurs when incomplete formation of the diaphragm allows cephalad displacement of abdominal viscera; when hernia is substantial, subsequent pulmonary hypoplasia is incompatible with post-natal life.
- *Omphalocele* occurs when abdominal musculature is incomplete and the viscera herniate into the ventral membranous sac; 40% are associated with other birth defects.
- *Gastroschisis* is similar to omphalocele except that all layers of the abdominal wall (from peritoneum to skin) fail to develop.

Ectopia (p. 765)

Ectopic tissues are common in the gastrointestinal tract. The most common site for *gastric mucosa* ectopia is the proximal esophagus, leading to dysphagia and esophagitis; it can also occur in the small bowel or colon, presenting with occult blood loss or peptic ulceration.

Pancreatic heterotopia occurs in esophagus and stomach; in the pylorus, it can cause inflammation, scarring, and obstruction.

Meckel Diverticulum (p. 765)

A *true diverticulum* is a blind pouch leading off the alimentary tract, lined by mucosa and including all three layers of the bowel wall, *mucosa, submucosa,* and *muscularis propria.* Meckel diverticula—the most common (2% of the population)—result from persistence of the vitelline duct (connecting yolk sac and gut lumen), leaving a solitary outpouching within 85 cm of the ileocecal valve; the male to female ratio is 2:1. Heterotopic gastric mucosa or pancreatic tissue can be present; the former can cause peptic ulceration.

Pyloric Stenosis (p. 766)

Congenital hypertrophic pyloric stenosis occurs in roughly 1 in 500 births, with a male to female ratio of 4:1; there is a complex polygeneic inheritance and associations with Turner syndrome and trisomy 18. Patients classically present with regurgitation and projectile vomiting within 3 weeks of birth; there is externally visible peristalsis and a palpable firm ovoid mass. Full-thickness, muscle-splitting incision *(myotomy)* is curative.

Acquired pyloric stenosis is a complication of chronic antral gastritis, peptic ulcers close to the pylorus, and malignancy.

Hirschsprung Disease (p. 766)

Also known as *congenital aganglionic megacolon,* this disorder results from arrested migration of neural crest cells into the gut, yielding an aganglionic segment lacking peristaltic contractions; there is functional obstruction and progressive dilation and hypertrophy of unaffected proximal colon. It occurs in roughly 1 in 5000 live births. The rectum is always affected; proximal involvement is more variable.

Pathogenesis (p. 766)

There is a genetic component in most cases. Heterozygous loss-of-function mutations in the RET tyrosine kinase receptor accounts for 15% of sporadic cases and the majority of familial cases; more than seven other genes involved in enteric neurodevelopment have been identified. Penetrance is incomplete, influenced by sex-linked factors (males are four times more commonly affected) and other genetic and environmental modifiers.

Clinical Features (p. 767)

Hirschsprung disease presents with neonatal failure to pass meconium or abdominal distention with severely distended *megacolon* (up to 20 cm in diameter); patients risk perforation, sepsis, or enterocolitis with fluid derangement.

Acquired megacolon may occur in Chagas disease, bowel obstruction, inflammatory bowel disease, and psychosomatic disorders; only in Chagas are ganglia actually lost.

ESOPHAGUS (p. 767)

Esophageal Obstruction (p. 767)

A number of esophageal lesions can cause dysphagia (difficulty swallowing), especially with solid foods. Stenosis was described previously.

- *Spasm* can be short- or long-lived and focal or diffuse; *diffuse esophageal spasm* causes functional obstruction; increased wall stress can cause diverticula to form.
- *Diverticula* can contain one or more wall layers; if sufficiently large they can accumulate enough food to present as a mass with food regurgitation:

    Zenker (pharyngeoesophageal) diverticulum occurs immediately above the upper esophageal sphincter
    Traction diverticulum occurs at the esophageal mid-point
    Epiphrenic diverticulum occurs immediately above the lower esophageal sphincter

- *Mucosal webs* are ledgelike protrusions of fibrovascular tissue and overlying epithelium; they are most common in the upper esophagus, and typically occur in women older than 40 years. A constellation of webs, iron deficiency anemia, glossitis, and cheilosis is called the *Plummer-Vinson syndrome* (also called *Paterson-Brown-Kelly syndrome*)
- *Esophageal rings (Schatzki rings)* are similar to webs but are circumferential and thicker; they include mucosa, submucosa, and occasionally hypertrophic muscularis propria. Above the gastroesophageal junction, they are called *A rings* and have squamous epithelium; when located at the squamocolumnar junction, they are *B rings* and can have gastric cardia-type mucosa.

Achalasia (p. 768)

Achalasia is a triad of incomplete relaxation of the lower esophageal sphincter (LES), increased LES tone (due to cholinergic signaling), and esophageal aperistalsis. *Primary achalasia* is idiopathic and results from failure of distal esophageal neurons to induce LES relaxation during swallowing (normally driven by nitric oxide and vasoactive intestinal peptide signaling); it can also happen with degenerative changes in neural innervation. *Secondary achalasia* occurs with Chagas disease *(Trypanosoma cruzi)*, disorders of the vagal dorsal motor nuclei (e.g., polio, surgical ablation), diabetic autonomic neuropathy, and infiltrative disorders (e.g., malignancy, amyloidosis, sarcoidosis). Treatment involves myotomy, balloon dilation, and/or botulinum toxin injection to inhibit LES cholinergic neurons.

Esophagitis (p. 768)

Lacerations (p. 768)

Mallory-Weiss tears are longitudinal lacerations (millimeters to centimeters in length) at the gastroesophageal junction associated with excessive vomiting—often in the setting of alcohol intoxication. Normally, a reflex relaxation of the LES precedes the anti-peristaltic wave associated with vomiting; with prolonged vomiting, this relaxation fails, resulting in esophageal stretching and tearing. Patients typically present with hematemesis; up to 10% of upper gastrointestinal bleeding is associated with such tears. Lacerations are not usually fatal; healing tends to be prompt.

Chemical and Infectious Esophagitis (p. 768)

The esophageal squamous epithelium can be damaged by a variety of agents: alcohol, corrosive acids or alkalis, excessively hot fluids, and heavy smoking. Pills that lodge and dissolve in the esophagus can also cause esophagitis; irradiation, chemotherapy, or graft-versus-host disease (GVHD) are iatrogenic etiologies. Occasionally, the esophagus is involved by systemic desquamative disorders (e.g., pemphigoid, epidermolysis bullosa) or Crohn disease. Infections occur more frequently in immunocompromised hosts; these include *Herpes simplex virus (HSV)*, cytomegalovirus (CMV), or fungal organisms (most commonly *Candida*).

Pain and dysphagia are the chief symptoms; in severe and/or chronic cases, hemorrhage, stricture, or perforation can result.

Morphology (p. 768)

The morphology depends on the etiology.

- Dense neutrophilic infiltrates are most common, although chemical injury may initially cause outright necrosis without inflammation.
- Any epithelial ulceration is accompanied by granulation tissue and eventually fibrosis.
- *Candidiasis*, when severe, is associated with adherent grey-white *pseudomembranes* composed of densely matted fungal hyphae and inflammatory cells.
- Herpes viruses typically cause punched-out ulcers, whereas CMV presents with shallower ulcerations with characteristic viral inclusions.
- Lesions associated with esophageal GVHD or blistering disorders resemble their counterparts in skin (Chapter 25).

Reflux Esophagitis (p. 769)

Reflux of gastric contents is the foremost cause of esophagitis; the clinical condition is called *gastroesophageal reflux disease (GERD)*.

Pathogenesis (p. 769)

Reflux of gastric juices is the major source of mucosal injury; in severe cases, duodenal bile reflux can exacerbate the damage. Reflux is caused by decreased LES tone and/or increased abdominal pressure and can be exacerbated by alcohol, tobacco use, obesity, central nervous system (CNS) depressants, pregnancy, delayed gastric emptying, or increased gastric volume. *Hiatal hernia* is also a cause of GERD it occurs when the diaphragmatic crura are separated and the stomach protrudes into the thorax. Hiatal hernias can be congenital or acquired; less than 10% are symptomatic.

Morphology (p. 769)

- Hyperemia and edema
- Basal zone hyperplasia (exceeding 20% of the epithelium) and thinning of superficial epithelial layers
- Neutrophil and/or eosinophil infiltration

Clinical Features (p. 769)

GERD is most common in adults older than 40 years; symptoms include dysphagia, heartburn, and regurgitation of gastric contents into the mouth. Complications of long-standing reflux include ulceration, hematemesis, melena, stricture, or Barrett esophagus. Symptomatic relief (with reduced mucosal damage) is obtained with proton pump inhibitors and/or H_2 histamine receptor antagonists.

Eosinophilic Esophagitis (p. 770)

Adults present with food impaction and dysphagia; children present with feeding intolerance and GERD-like symptoms. The cardinal histologic feature is large numbers of intraepithelial eosinophils. Most patients have one of several atopic disorders (e.g., atopic dermatitis, asthma, etc.), and therapy for their esophageal disorder involves dietary restriction and/or steroids.

Barrett Esophagus (p. 770)

Barrett esophagus is a complication of chronic GERD characterized by *intestinal metaplasia within the esophageal squamous mucosa*. It occurs in an estimated 10% of individuals with chronic

GERD; the typical patient is a white man between ages 40 and 60 years. Barrett esophagus confers an increased risk of esophageal adenocarcinoma; pre-invasive *dysplasia* is detected each year in 0.2% to 2% of patients with Barrett esophagus.

Morphology (p. 770)

- *Gross:* Patches of red, velvety mucosa extend up from the gastro-esophageal junction.
- *Microscopic:* Intestinal-type columnar epithelium, particularly mucin-secreting goblet cells, is required for the diagnosis. When present, *dysplasia* is classified as low or high grade. Intramucosal carcinoma is characterized by neoplastic cell invasion into the lamina propria.

Clinical Features (p. 771)

Diagnosis requires both gross (endoscopic) and biopsy confirmation; once identified, a periodic surveillance endoscopy is performed to look for dysplasia or frank malignancy. Multifocal high-grade dysplasia (with a high risk for progression) or carcinoma typically requires esophagectomy, although newer modalities (e.g., laser ablation, photodynamic therapy) are also used.

Esophageal Varices (p. 771)

Pathogenesis (p. 771)

Severe portal hypertension induces collateral bypass channels between the portal and caval circulations (Chapter 18). These lead to congested subepithelial and submucosal veins in the distal esophagus *(varices)*. In Western societies, alcoholic cirrhosis is the most common cause (90% of cirrhotic patients develop varices); worldwide, hepatic schistosomiasis is the second most common cause.

Morphology (p. 771)

Tortuous dilated veins are present in the distal esophageal and proximal gastric submucosa; there is irregular luminal protrusion of overlying mucosa with superficial ulceration, inflammation, or adherent blood clots.

Clinical Features (p. 771)

Varices are clinically silent until they rupture with catastrophic hematemesis; causes of rupture include inflammatory erosion, increased venous pressure, and increased hydrostatic pressure associated with vomiting. Bleeding can be treated with sclerotherapy, balloon tamponade, or band ligation. Up to half of such patients die with their first bleed either due to exsanguination or following hepatic coma; in survivors, there is a 50% chance of recurrence within a year with the same mortality rate.

Esophageal Tumors (p. 772)

Adenocarcinoma (p. 772)

Esophageal adenocarcinomas largely evolve from dysplastic changes in Barrett mucosa; they occur most frequently in white men (i.e., 7:1 male to female ratio) and account for half of all esophageal cancers in the United States.

Pathogenesis (p. 772)

There is a stepwise accumulation of genetic and epigenetic alterations from Barrett esophagus to adenocarcinoma. Chromosomal and *p53* abnormalities occur early; additional changes include amplification of *c-ERB-B2* and *cyclin D1* and E *genes* and mutations in *Rb* and the *p16/INK4a* cyclin-dependent kinase inhibitor.

Morphology (p. 772)

- *Grossly:* Lesions range from exophytic nodules to excavated and deeply infiltrative masses, mostly in the distal third of the esophagus.
- *Microscopically:* Tumors typically produce mucin and form glands, often with intestinal-type morphology; diffusely infiltrative signet ring tumors are less common, and the histology rarely reveals adenosquamous or small poorly differentiated cells.

Clinical Features (p. 772)

Although occasionally found during evaluation for GERD or surveillance for Barrett esophagus, esophageal adenocarcinomas typically present with dysphagia, weight loss, hematemesis, chest pain, or vomiting. Because most tumors are detected at advanced stages, the 5-year survival rate is less than 25%.

Squamous Cell Carcinoma (p. 773)

In the United States, esophageal squamous cell carcinoma typically occurs in adults older than 45 years, in men four times more frequently than women, and in blacks six times more frequently than whites. Risk factors include alcohol and tobacco use, caustic esophageal injury, achalasia, Plummer-Vinson syndrome, and frequent consumption of scalding hot beverages. There is considerable geographic variability, with highest incidences in Iran, central China, Hong Kong, Brazil, and South Africa.

Pathogenesis (p. 773)

The pathogenesis is multifactorial; environment and diet contribute synergistically, modified by genetic factors. Alcohol and tobacco synergize to increase risk, and they contribute to the majority of cancers in the United States. Nutritional deficiencies, as well as polycyclic hydrocarbons, nitrosamines, other mutagenic compounds (e.g., from fungal contaminants), and human papillomavirus (HPV) all likely contribute to the geographic variation in incidence.

Morphology (p. 773)

Half of esophageal squamous cell cancers occur in the middle third of the esophagus.

- They typically begin as *in situ* gray-white, plaque-like mucosal thickenings.
- Lesions can subsequently expand as exophytic lesions, ulcerate, or become diffusely infiltrative with wall thickening and luminal stenosis.
- A rich submucosal lymphatic network promotes circumferential and longitudinal spread. Tumors can invade deeply into adjacent mediastinal structures.
- Most tumors are moderately to well differentiated; less common variants are verrucous, spindle, and basaloid squamous cell carcinomas.

Clinical Features (p. 774)

Onset is insidious and symptom onset is late; patients develop dysphagia, obstruction, weight loss, hemorrhage, sepsis secondary to ulceration, or respiratory fistulae with aspiration. Superficial carcinomas have a 5-year survival rate of 75%, but the overall 5-year survival rate is 9%.

Uncommon Esophageal Tumors (p. 774)

- Benign tumors are usually mesenchymal in origin and arise in the esophageal wall; leiomyomas are most common, but fibromas, lipomas, hemangiomas, neurofibromas, and lymphangiomas also occur.
- Benign tumors can also take the form of mucosal polyps (e.g., *fibrovascular polyps, pedunculated lipomas,* and *squamous papillomas*); occasionally, HPV-associated *condylomas* occur. Masses of inflamed granulation tissue can grow either as *inflammatory polyps* or as invasive *inflammatory pseudotumors.*

STOMACH (p. 774)

Acute Gastritis (p. 774)

Acute gastritis is a transient mucosal inflammatory process; it can be asymptomatic or cause varying degrees of pain, nausea, and vomiting. Severe cases exhibit ulceration with hemorrhage presenting as hematemesis or melena.

Pathogenesis (p. 774)

Acute gastritis occurs when one or more of the mechanisms that protect gastric mucosa from the acidic environment is overwhelmed or defective (Fig. 17-1). Increased acid production with back diffusion, decreased bicarbonate or mucin production, or direct mucosal damage can all be pathogenic. Thus, chronic use of nonsteroidal anti-inflammatory drugs (NSAIDs) reduces bicarbonate production and interferes with the cytoprotective action of prostaglandins (these inhibit acid production, promote mucin synthesis, and increase vascular perfusion); excessive alcohol consumption and heavy smoking can be directly toxic, and ischemia and shock secondarily injure the mucosa.

Morphology (p. 775)

- *Grossly:* There is moderate edema and hyperemia, occasionally with hemorrhage *(acute hemorrhagic erosive gastritis).*
- *Microscopically:* Neutrophils invade the epithelium, with superficial epithelial sloughing *(erosion)* and a fibrinous luminal exudate.

Acute Gastric Ulceration (p. 775)

Acute gastric ulceration refers to focal, acute mucosal defects. These commonly occur as a complication of NSAID use or as a consequence of severe physiologic stress:

- *Stress ulcers* occur after shock, sepsis, or severe trauma.
- *Curling ulcers* occur in the proximal duodenum and are associated with burns or trauma.
- *Cushing* ulcers are gastric, duodenal, and esophageal ulcers arising in patients with intracranial disease; they have a high risk of perforation.

Pathogenesis (p. 775)

NSAID-associated ulcer mechanisms are described earlier. Lesions associated with brain injury are attributed to direct vagal stimulation causing gastric acid hypersecretion. Systemic acidosis, hypoxia, and reduced splanchnic blood flow are contributory in the other forms of ulcers.

Morphology (p. 776)

Ulcers are usually smaller than 1 cm in diameter, multiple, and shallow; they may be found anywhere in the stomach. The ulcer base is brown (blood), while the adjacent mucosa is normal.

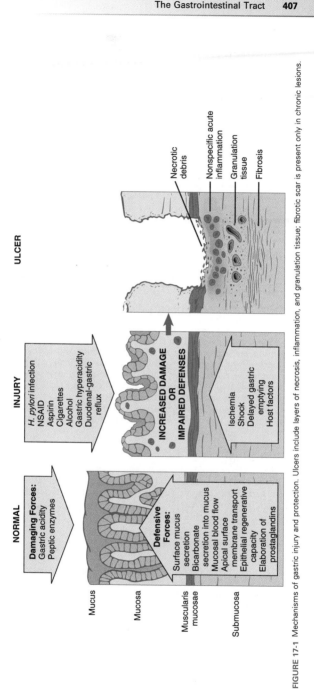

FIGURE 17-1 Mechanisms of gastric injury and protection. Ulcers include layers of necrosis, inflammation, and granulation tissue; fibrotic scar is present only in chronic lesions.

Clinical Features (p. 776)

Most critically ill patients have some evidence of gastric mucosal injury; 10% to 15% have bleeding and 1% to 4% have blood loss sufficient to warrant transfusion, while up to 5% of ulcers can perforate. After removal of the injurious factors, healing with complete re-epithelialization is the norm. The single most important determinant of outcome is the *ability to correct the underlying conditions.*

Chronic Gastritis (p. 776)

Chronic gastritis is characterized by ongoing mucosal inflammation with mucosal atrophy; it provides a substrate in which dysplasia (and carcinoma) can arise. Compared to acute gastritis, the symptoms are usually less severe but are more persistent. Causes include *Helicobacter pylori* infection (most common), alcohol, tobacco, psychological stress, and caffeine; autoimmune gastritis (10% of cases) is the most common cause in the absence of *H. pylori.*

Helicobacter Pylori Gastritis (p. 776)

Epidemiology (p. 776)

Although *H. pylori* is a widely prevalent gastric infection (colonization rates from 10% to 80% of the population), a much smaller percentage of those infected actually develop gastritis. Nevertheless, *H. pylori* infection is the most common cause of chronic gastritis; organisms are present in up to 90% of individuals with disease. Humans are the only host—spread is via fecal-oral, oral-oral, or environmental routes; consequently, lower socioeconomic status and crowding lead to higher colonization rates. A related organism, *Helicobacter heilmannii,* can infect humans as well as cats, dogs, pigs, and non-human primates; recognition of this organism in a human host is an indication for treatment of a household pet to eliminate a reservoir.

Pathogenesis (p. 777)

H. pylori induces predominantly an antral gastritis, characterized by increased acid production and disruption of the normal mucosal protection mechanisms (see Fig. 17-1). Virulence factors in *H. pylori* infections include:

- *Motility* via flagella
- *Urease production* buffering gastric acid
- Bacterial *adhesins* to bind surface epithelial cells
- *Toxins* (e.g., cagA and vacA cytotoxins)

Over time, the initial antral gastritis progresses to *multifocal atrophic gastritis* (i.e., mucosal atrophy with reduced acid production) and intestinal metaplasia. Host-pathogen interactions influence whether gastritis results from the initial infection; for example, polymorphisms in interleukin-1β (IL-1β) and tumor necrosis factor (TNF) genes correlate with the development of chronic disease.

Morphology (p. 777)

- *Grossly:* Infected mucosa is erythematous and coarse to nodular.
- *Microscopically: H. pylori* are typically found in the antrum; gastric biopsy usually demonstrates organisms concentrated in the superficial mucus overlying surface and neck epithelium. There

are variable numbers of intraepithelial and lumenal neutrophils (forming *pit abscesses*), and the lamina propria contains abundant plasma cells, macrophages, and lymphocytes
- Long-standing gastritis is associated with diffuse mucosal atrophy, with prominent lymphoid aggregates occasionally with germinal centers.

Clinical Features (p. 778)

H. pylori can be diagnosed by antibody serologic test, urea breath test, bacterial culture, direct bacterial visualization in gastric biopsy, or DNA-based tests. *H. pylori* infection is a risk factor for peptic ulcer disease, gastric adenocarcinoma, and gastric lymphoma.

Autoimmune Gastritis (p. 778)

This form of gastritis typically spares the antrum and is associated with *hypergastrinemia*.

Pathogenesis (p. 778)

CD4+ T cell-mediated autoimmune destruction of parietal cells is the major pathogenic mechanism; there are also circulating and gastric-secreted antibodies to parietal cells and intrinsic factor, but these are probably only secondary manifestations of disease and not causal. Parietal cell cytotoxicity leads in turn to defective gastric acid secretion *(achlorhydria)* that triggers hypergastrinemia, and antral G-cell hyperplasia. Reduced intrinsic factor production impedes B_{12} absorption and causes pernicious anemia. Secondary bystander damage to chief cells reduces the pepsinogen I production.

Morphology (p. 779)

Rugal folds are lost and there is diffuse mucosal damage of the acid-producing parietal cells, primarily in the body and fundus. The inflammatory infiltrate is predominantly lymphocytes, macrophages, and plasma cells; lymphoid aggregates can be present.

Clinical Features (p. 779)

Autoantibodies are detected early in the course; progression to gastric atrophy occurs over 20 to 30 years. Patients present with symptoms referable to anemia; B_{12} deficiency can also manifest with atrophic glossitis, malabsorption, peripheral neuropathy, spinal cord lesions, and cerebral dysfunction. A strong genetic underpinning is suggested by the observation that autoimmune gastritis is often associated with other autoimmune diseases such as Hashimoto thyroiditis, type 1 diabetes, and Addison disease; 20% of relatives of affected patients also have autoimmune gastritis.

Uncommon Forms of Gastritis (p. 779)

- *Reactive gastropathy* (p. 779) is a group of disorders marked by edema, glandular hyperplasia, and regenerative changes; it is caused by chemical injury including NSAID use or bile reflux.
- *Eosinophilic gastritis* (p. 780) is characterized by heavy eosinophilic infiltration of the mucosa or submucosa; it can be infectious, due to allergy to ingested material, or part of a systemic collagen-vascular disease (e.g., scleroderma).
- *Lymphocytic gastritis* (p. 780) is an idiopathic disorder predominantly affecting women; 40% of cases are associated with celiac disease (see later discussion). There is marked accumulation of intraepithelial CD8+ T cells.

- *Granulomatous gastritis* (p. 780) is a diverse group of diseases sharing the presence of granulomas; sarcoid, Crohn disease, and infections are causes.

Complications of Chronic Gastritis (p. 780)

Peptic Ulcer Disease (p. 780)

Peptic ulcer disease (PUD) typically occurs in the first portion of the duodenum or the antrum (4:1 ratio). The most common causes are *H. pylori*–induced hyperchlorhydric chronic gastritis (85% to 100% of duodenal ulcers and 65% of gastric ulcers) and NSAID use. In the United States, the life-time risk of PUD is 10% for males and 4% for females.

Pathogenesis (p. 780)

PUD results from imbalances in mucosal damage and defenses (see Fig. 17-1). Hyperacidity in PUD can be caused by infection, parietal cell hyperplasia, excessive secretory response, or increased gastrin production (e.g., secondary to hypercalcemia, or produced by a tumor). NSAIDs and steroids block the normal prostagladin cytoprotective effects (discussed previously), and cigarette smoking impairs mucosal blood flow and healing.

Morphology (p. 780)

Most ulcers are solitary.

- *Grossly:* There is a sharply punched-out defect with overhanging mucosal borders and smooth, clean ulcer bases.
- *Microscopically:* There are thin layers of fibrinoid debris with underlying inflammation merging into granulation tissue and deep scarring. The surrounding mucosa usually exhibits chronic gastritis.

Clinical Features (p. 781)

- Classic symptoms include epigastric gnawing, burning, or aching pain, worse at night and 1 to 3 hours after meals. Nausea, vomiting, bloating, belching, and weight loss can also occur.
- Complications include anemia, hemorrhage, perforation, and obstruction. Malignant transformation is rare and is related to underlying gastritis. Treatment is focused on *H. pylori* eradication, as well as neutralization or reduced production of gastric acid.

Dysplasia (p. 781)

Long-standing, chronic gastritis exposes epithelium to inflammation-related free radical damage and proliferative stimuli. Over time, the combination can lead to the accumulation of genetic alterations resulting in carcinoma; pre-invasive *in situ* lesions can be recognized histologically as *dysplasia*.

Hypertrophic Gastropathies (p. 782)

These are uncommon conditions featuring giant enlargement of gastric rugal folds due to epithelial hyperplasia; they are linked to excessive growth factor production.

Ménétrier Disease (p. 782)

There is diffuse foveolar cell hyperplasia, with a protein-losing enteropathy that causes systemic hypoproteinemia. It is caused by overexpression of transforming growth factor-α (TGF-α). Risk of gastric adenocarcinoma is increased.

Zollinger-Ellison Syndrome (p. 782)

This is caused by gastrin-secreting tumors *(gastrinomas)* typically in the small bowel or pancreas. Patients classically present with multiple duodenal ulcers and/or chronic diarrhea. Elevated gastrin levels induce a marked (up to five-fold) increase in gastric parietal cells, as well as more modest increases in mucous neck cells and gastric endocrine cells. Gastrinomas are sporadic in 75% of patients; in the remainder, they are associated with multiple endocrine neoplasia, type I. Some 60% to 90% of gastrinomas are malignant.

Gastric Polyps and Tumors (p. 783)

Polyps are nodules or masses that project above the level of the surrounding mucosa; they can result from epithelial or stromal hyperplasia, inflammation, ectopia, or neoplasia.

Inflammatory and Hyperplastic Polyps (p. 783)

Hyperplastic or *inflammatory polyps* constitute 75% of gastric polyps. They are most common between ages 50 and 60 years, and they typically arise in association with chronic gastritis. The majority are less than 1 cm and are frequently multiple; they typically have a smooth surface, occasionally with superficial erosions, and histologically show irregular, cystically dilated and elongated glands with variable amounts of acute and chronic inflammation. Risk of dysplasia increases with size; polyps more than 1.5 cm should be resected.

Fundic Gland Polyps (p. 783)

Fundic gland polyps occur sporadically (typically in women older than 50 years) or in the setting of familial adenomatous polyposis (FAP); their incidence is also increased by proton pump inhibitors and the consequent increased gastrin secretion. They are single or multiple, smooth, well-circumscribed lesions composed of irregular, cystically dilated glands with minimal inflammation.

Gastric Adenoma (p. 784)

Gastric adenomas comprise 10% of gastric polyps. These almost always occur on a background of FAP or chronic gastritis with atrophy and intestinal metaplasia; the male to female ratio is 3:1 and the incidence increases with age. Usually solitary and less than 2 cm, gastric adenomas all exhibit some degree of dysplasia; 30% can harbor carcinoma, and lesions more than 2 cm are particularly concerning.

Gastric Adenocarcinoma (p. 784)

Adenocarcinomas constitute more than 90% of gastric malignancies; they are divided into *intestinal* and *diffuse* forms with different risk factors, genetic perturbations, and clinical and pathologic presentations (see following discussion).

Epidemiology (p. 784)

Worldwide distribution is widely variable; the incidence in Japan, Chile, Costa Rica, and Eastern Europe is 20-fold greater than in North America and northern Europe. The United States incidence decreased 85% in the 20th century (mostly due to decreases in the intestinal form that is associated with atrophic gastritis); gastric carcinoma now constitutes less than 2.5% of all cancer deaths in the United States. The epidemiology suggests a role for environmental factors (e.g., *H. pylori* infections). Diet also influences risk;

thus decreased consumption of carcinogens (e.g., *N*-nitroso compounds and benzo[a]pyrene, associated with some forms of food preservation) and increased intake of antioxidants in fruits and green leafy vegetables reduce gastric cancer incidence. Conversely, *partial gastrectomy* (e.g., for PUD) increases the risk by permitting bile reflux and the development of chronic gastritis.

Pathogenesis (p. 785)

Loss of intercellular adhesion is a key step in oncogenesis, particularly of *diffuse gastric cancer*. Thus, germline mutations in the *CDH1* gene encoding E-cadherin are associated with familial gastric carcinomas and also occur in 50% of sporadic lesions. *Intestinal-type gastric cancers* are associated with FAP, mutations in proteins that associate with E-cadherin (e.g., β-catenin), microsatellite instability, and hypermethylation of *TGFβRII, BAX, IGFRII,* and *p16/INK4a*. In both types of gastric cancer associated with *H. pylori* infections, immune response gene polymorphisms influence risk; *p53* mutations are also present in the majority of sporadic cancers of both types.

Morphology (p. 785)

Gastric cancers involve the antrum more than the lesser curvature more than the greater curvature.

- Tumors with *intestinal morphology* tend to form bulky exophytic tumors composed of glandular structures. These develop from precursor lesions including flat dysplasia and adenomas.
- Tumors with a *diffuse infiltrative* pattern of growth tend to be composed of *signet-ring cells* (intracellular mucin vacuoles push the nucleus to the periphery) that are discohesive and do not form glands; these also tend to induce a fibrous desmoplastic response. There are no identified precursor lesions. The gross correlate to these tumors is a rigid, thickened gastric wall termed *linitus plastica* (literally "leather bottle").

Clinical Features (p. 786)

Gastric carcinoma is an insidious disease; early symptoms resemble those for chronic gastritis (i.e., dysphagia, dyspepsia, and nausea). Advanced stages announce themselves with weight loss, anorexia, altered bowel habits, anemia, and hemorrhage. Prognosis critically depends on *depth of invasion* and the *extent of nodal or distant metastases*. After surgical resection, the 5-year survival of early gastric cancer is more than 90%, even with nodal spread; in comparison, advanced gastric cancer has a 5-year survival of less than 20%. Overall, 5-year survival in the United States is 30%.

Lymphoma (p. 786)

Extra-nodal lymphomas can arise in any tissue, but they do so most commonly in the gastrointesinal tract and especially the stomach. Patients typically present with dyspepsia and epigastric pain; hematemesis, melena, or weight loss can also occur. *Gastrointestinal lymphomas* (also called *m*ucosa-*a*ssociated *l*ymphoid *t*issue or *MALTomas*) constitute 5% of gastric malignancies; most are marginal zone B-cell lymphomas. A smaller fraction of primary gastrointestinal lymphomas are large B-cell lymphomas.

Pathogenesis (p. 786)

Extranodal marginal B-cell lymphomas arise at sites of chronic inflammation. In the stomach, this is typically associated with chronic *H. pylori* infection; interestingly, antibiotic treatment can induce tumor regression. Antibiotic-resistant tumors often harbor a t(11;18) translocation; t(1;14) and t(14;18) translocations are less common but are predictive for response failure. The t(11;18) translocation links the apoptosis inhibitor 2 gene (*API2* on chromosome 11) with the mutated in MALT lymphoma gene (*MLT* on chromosome 18); the t(14;18) translocation increases MLT expression, while t(1:14) increases BCL-10 expression. Each of the translocations leads to constitutive NF-κB transcription factor activation, promoting B-cell growth and survival. With time, these MALTomas can transform into the more aggressive diffuse large B-cell lymphomas, often associated with inactivation of *p53* and/or *p16* tumor suppressor genes.

Morphology (p. 787)

Microscopically: There is a dense infiltrate of atypical lymphocytes in the lamina propria; focal invasion of the mucosal epithelium forms diagnostic *lymphoepithelial lesions.* Markers are as described for other mature B-cell tumors (Chapter 13).

Carcinoid Tumor (p. 787)

Carcinoid *(carcinoma-like)* tumors arise from diffusely distributed endocrine cells. Most arise in the gut (lungs are second in frequency) and 40% occur in the small intestine; the cells of origin in the gastrointestinal tract are responsible for hormone secretion that coordinates gastrointestinal function.

Morphology (p. 787)

These are well-differentiated neuroendocrine carcinomas.

- *Grossly:* Carcinoids are yellow-tan intramural or submucosal masses forming small polypoid lesions. An intense desmoplastic response makes them firm and can cause bowel obstruction.
- *Microscopically:* The tumors range from islands to sheets of uniform cohesive cells with scant granular cytoplasm and oval, stippled nuclei; cells are typically positive for neuroendocrine markers (e.g., chromogranin A and synaptophysin).

Clinical Features (p. 788)

Peak incidence is in the sixth decade. Carcinoids are usually indolent, slow-growing malignancies, and symptoms are largely a function of the hormones produced. Thus, gastrin synthesis causes Zollinger-Ellison syndrome, while ileal tumors systemically secrete vasoactive products that manifest with cutaneous flushing, bronchospasm, increased bowel motility, and right-sided cardiac valve thickening *(carcinoid syndrome).* Carcinoid syndrome occurs in 10% or less of patients with gastrointestinal carcinoid due to hepatic catabolism of the secreted products; presence of the syndrome is therefore usually associated with bulky hepatic metastatic disease.

The most important prognostic factor for gastrointestinal carcinoid is the primary site of the tumor:

- Foregut tumors (esophagus, stomach, and duodenum) rarely metastasize and are cured by resection
- Midgut carcinoids (jejunum and ileum) are usually multiple and aggressive.
- Hindgut tumors (appendix and colon) are usually found only incidentally.

  Appendiceal carcinoids are usually found at the tip, are less than 2 cm, and are usually benign.
  Colonic carcinoids can be large and can metastasize.
  Rectal carcinoids can secrete polypeptide hormones and/or cause pain, but they usually do not metastasize.

Gastrointestinal Stromal Tumor (p. 789)

Gastrointestinal stromal tumor (GIST) is the most common gastro-intestinal mesenchymal tumor; more than half are in the stomach.

Epidemiology (p. 789)

Peak age of GIST diagnosis is approximately age 60 years; incidence is increased in patients with neurofibromatosis type I, and in children (usually girls) with *Carney triad,* a non-hereditary syndrome with GIST, paragangliomas, and pulmonary chondromas.

Pathogenesis (p. 789)

GISTs appear to arise from the interstitial cells of Cajal (pacemakers for gut peristalsis) in the muscularis propria. Approximately 75% to 80% of all GISTs contain *oncogenic gain-of-function mutations in the gene coding for the tyrosine kinase c-KIT* (c-KIT is the stem cell factor receptor); 8% have activating *platelet-derived growth factor receptor-α* (PDGFRA) mutations. Constitutive tyrosine kinase activity leads to downstream activation of *RAS* and PI3K/AKT pathways promoting tumor cell proliferation and survival.

Morphology (p. 790)

- *Grossly:* GISTs are usually solitary, well-circumscribed fleshy masses; they can grow as large as 30 cm.
- *Microscopically:* Tumors are classified as either *epithelioid* (i.e., plump and cohesive cells) or *spindle cell type; c-KIT* expression is the most useful diagnostic marker.

Clinical Features (p. 790)

Symptoms are usually related to mass effects or blood loss. Surgical resection is the primary treatment for localized gastric GIST. Metastases are rare when tumors are less than 5 cm but common when more than 10 cm. These typically take the form of peritoneal serosal nodules or liver implants; spread outside the abdomen is uncommon. Tumors not amenable to resection can be treated with *imatinib,* a tyrosine kinase inhibitor that inhibits *c-KIT* and PDGFRA.

SMALL INTESTINE AND COLON (p. 790)

Due to their roles in nutrient and water transport and their inter-face with diverse food and microbial antigens, the intestines are unsurprisingly involved by an array of malabsorption, infectious, inflammatory, and neoplastic processes.

Intestinal Obstruction (p. 790)

Tumors and infarctions account for 10% to 15% of obstructions; 80% are attributable to the following four entities (Fig. 17-2):

Hernias (p. 790)

Peritoneal wall defects permit peritoneal sac protrusion *(hernia sac)* in which bowel segments can be trapped *(external herniation).* Subsequent vascular stasis and edema lead to *incarceration;* vascular compromise leads to *strangulation.* Locations include the femoral and inguinal canals, umbilicus, and surgical scars.

Adhesions (p. 790)

Adhesions are residua of localized peritoneal inflammation *(peritonitis)* following surgery, infection, endometriosis, or radiation;

Herniation   **Adhesions**

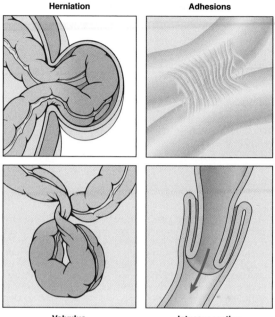

Volvulus   **Intussusception**

FIGURE 17-2 Causes of intestinal obstruction.

healing leads to fibrous bridging between viscera. Congenital adhesions also rarely occur. Complications include *internal herniation* (within the peritoneal cavity), obstruction, and strangulation.

Volvulus (p. 791)

Volvulus is complete twisting of a bowel loop about its mesenteric vascular base, leading to vascular and luminal obstruction with infarction. Volvulus occurs most often in redundant loops of sigmoid colon; cecum and small bowel are involved less frequently.

Intussusception (p. 791)

Intussusception occurs when an intestinal segment (usually small bowel) telescopes into the immediately distal segment. Peristalsis propels the invaginated segment, along with its attached mesentery, potentially resulting in obstruction, vessel compression, and infarction. In *infants and children*, intussusception is usually spontaneous or can be associated with rotaviral infection. In older individuals, the point of traction is usually a tumor.

Ischemic Bowel Disease (p. 791)

The abundant collateral supply throughout much of the gastrointestinal tract usually allows the bowel to tolerate slowly progressive loss of blood supply. In comparison, abrupt compromise of any major vessel can cause infarction of several meters of intestine. *Watershed zones* between major vessel branches (e.g., the splenic flexure between superior and inferior mesenteric artery circulations) are most vulnerable. Damage ranges from mucosal infarction to transmural infarction. Because they are at the end of the capillary network, the epithelial cells at the tips of villi are more susceptible to ischemia than are the crypt epithelial cells.

Important causes of ischemia are atherosclerosis, aortic aneurysm, hypercoagulable states, embolization, and vasculitis; hypoperfusion can also be associated with cardiac failure, shock, dehydration, or vasoconstrictive drugs. Mesenteric venous obstruction or thrombosis due to hypercoagulability, masses, or cirrhosis can also cause ischemic disease.

Pathogenesis (p. 792)

An initial *hypoxic injury* occurs at the onset of vascular compromise, although intestinal epithelium is relatively resistant to transient hypoxia; however, subsequent reperfusion leads to an influx of inflammatory cells and mediators (Chapter 1), which cause the majority of damage.

Morphology (p. 792)

- *Mucosal infarction:* Patchy mucosal hemorrhage occurs, but with normal serosa.
- *Mural infarction:* Complete mucosal necrosis occurs with variable necrosis of submucosa and muscularis propria. Distribution is typically segmental, without serositis.
- *Transmural infarction:* Involved bowel segments are usually hemorrhagic and there is associated serositis. Coagulative necrosis of the muscularis propria with perforation develops within 1 to 4 days.
- *Microscopically:* There is atrophy and sloughing of surface epithelium, but preserved crypts can be hyperproliferative. The extent of inflammation and edema depends on the duration of injury. Superimposed bacterial infection can induce pseudomembrane formation.
- Chronic vascular insufficiency results in fibrosis of the lamina propria and occasionally stricture formation.

Clinical Features (p. 793)

Typically occurring in older individuals with coexisting cardiac or vascular disease, ischemic bowel presents with severe abdominal pain, bloody diarrhea or gross melena, abdominal rigidity, nausea, and vomiting. Patients can progress to shock within hours, and mortality can exceed 50%.

Angiodysplasia (p. 793)

Lesions of *angiodysplasia* are tortuous, ectatic dilations of mucosal or submucosal veins occurring in approximately 1% of the population; most common in the cecum or ascending colon (usually after age 60), angiodysplasia accounts for 20% of major episodes of lower gastrointestinal bleeding. Lesions are attributed to partial, intermittent venous occlusion; the cecal/right colonic predilection derives from the greater wall tension in those locations owing to their larger diameter.

Malabsorption and Diarrhea (p. 793)

Malabsorption is characterized by defective absorption of fats, fat- and water-soluble vitamins, proteins, carbohydrates, electrolytes, minerals, and water. General symptoms are diarrhea, flatus, abdominal pain, and muscle wasting; a classic hallmark is *steatorrhea* characterized by excessive fecal fat and greasy, malodorous stools. Clinical consequences (due to various deficiencies) include:

- Anemia and mucositis (pyridoxine, folate, or B_{12})
- Bleeding (vitamin K)

- Osteopenia and tetany (calcium, magnesium, vitamin D)
- Peripheral neuropathy (vitamin A or B_{12})

The most common causes of malabsorption in the United States are celiac disease, pancreatic insufficiency, and Crohn disease (Table 17-1). The pathogenesis involves disturbance(s) in:

- *Intraluminal digestion:* Emulsification and initial enzymatic break-down
- *Terminal digestion:* Hydrolysis within the enterocyte brush border
- *Transepithelial transport* through enterocytes
- *Lymphatic transport* of absorbed lipids

Diarrhea is defined as increased stool mass, frequency, or fluidity, usually exceeding 200 g per day. Severe cases can exceed 14 L per day and can be fatal without fluid restoration. Painful, bloody, small-volume diarrhea is called *dysentery*. General categories include:

- *Secretory:* Isotonic with plasma, and persists during fasting
- *Osmotic:* Unabsorbed luminal solutes (e.g., due to lactase deficiency) increase osmotic pull of fluid; stool can be 50 mOsm or more hyperosmolar relative to plasma; abates with fasting
- *Malabsorptive:* As described previously; abates on fasting
- *Exudative:* Due to inflammatory disease; purulent, bloody stools persist during fasting

Celiac Disease (p. 795)

Also called *gluten-sensitive enteropathy* or *celiac sprue*, celiac disease is an immune-mediated diarrheal disorder triggered by ingestion of gluten-containing foods (e.g., derived from wheat, oat, rye, or barley) in genetically predisposed individuals. In whites of European descent, the prevalence is 0.5% to 1%.

Pathogenesis (p. 795)

Sprue results from a gluten-mediated, delayed-type hypersensitivity, specifically directed against a 33 amino acid α-*gliadin* polypeptide resistant to digestive enzymes.

- Gliadin induces epithelial IL-15 expression with local activation and proliferation of CD8+ cytotoxic cells that can drive enterocyte apoptosis.
- Easier gliadin access to the underlying tissue permits increased deamidation by transglutaminase.
- Deamidated peptide binds to specific MHC on antigen presenting cells in susceptible individuals (expressing HLA-DQ2 or HLA-DQ8), which leads to CD4+ T cell activation and cytokine-mediated epithelial damage.
- Additional factors that influence disease susceptibility include polymorphisms of genes that affect immune regulation and epithelial polarity.

Morphology (p. 795)

Diffusely flattened (atrophic) villi and elongated regenerative crypts are associated with intraepithelial CD8+ T cells and exuberant lamina propria chronic inflammation. Severity is greatest in the more proximal intestine.

Clinical Features (p. 796)

Celiac disease occurs in infants to middle-aged people who present with diarrhea, flatulence, weight loss, and the effects of anemia. The most sensitive serologic test assesses the presence of immunoglobulin A (IgA) antibodies to tissue transglutaminase, or IgA or IgG to deamidated gliadin.

TABLE 17-1 Defects in Malabsorptive and Diarrheal Disease

Disease	Intraluminal Digestion	Terminal Digestion	Transepithelial Transport	Lymphatic Transport
Celiac disease		+	+	
Tropical sprue		+	+	
Chronic pancreatitis	+			
Cystic fibrosis	+			
Primary bile acid malabsorption	+		+	
Carcinoid syndrome			+	
Autoimmune enteropathy		+	+	
Disaccharidase deficiency		+		
Whipple disease				+
Abetalipoproteinemia			+	
Viral gastroenteritis		+	+	
Bacterial gastroenteritis		+	+	
Parasitic gastroenteritis		+	+	
Inflammatory bowel disease	+	+	+	

+ indicates that the process is abnormal in the disease indicated. Other processes are not affected.

- Celiac disease is often (10% of patients) associated with the pruritic, blistering skin disorder *dermatitis herpetiformis.* Lymphocytic gastritis or colitis is also more common.
- Besides iron and vitamin deficiencies, there is increased risk of *enteropathy-associated T-cell lymphoma,* and small intestinal adenocarcinoma.
- Celiac disease usually responds to gluten withdrawal.

Tropical Sprue (p. 796)

This malabsorption syndrome occurs almost exclusively in people inhabiting or visiting tropical climes. The histology is similar to celiac disease, although the distal small bowel is most severely affected. An infectious etiology is implicated, and broad-spectrum antibiotics aid recovery.

Autoimmune Enteropathy (p. 796)

This is an X-linked disorder of children characterized by a persistent auto-immune–driven diarrhea. A severe familial form (*i*mmune dysregulation, *p*olyendocrinopathy, *e*nteropathy, and *X*-linked [IPEX]) is due to germline mutations in the *FOXP3* gene, a transcription factor responsible for the differentiation of CD4+ regulatory T cells. Autoantibodies to a variety of gastrointestinal epithelial cell types may be present.

Lactase (Disaccharidase) Deficiency (p. 797)

Lactase is an apical membrane disaccharidase of surface absorptive cells. With *lactase deficiency,* undigested and unabsorbed lactose exerts an osmotic pull, causing diarrhea and malabsorption; bacterial fermentation of lactose can also cause abdominal distention and flatus. Histologically, the mucosal is unremarkable.

- A rare congenital autosomal recessive form is due to mutations in the lactase gene.
- The acquired form is caused by down-regulation of lactase gene expression; it is common in Native American, African-American, and Chinese populations.

Abetalipoproteinemia (p. 797)

Abetalipoproteinemia is a rare autosomal recessive disease caused by inability of lipids to egress absorptive epithelial cells. The underlying defect is a mutation in the *microsomal triglyceride transfer protein (MTP)* responsible for lipoprotein and fatty acid export from mucosal cells. Affected infants present with failure to thrive, diarrhea, and steatorrhea, as well as complete absence of all lipoproteins containing apolipoprotein B (although the apolipoprotein B gene is unaffected). Failure to absorb essential fatty acids leads to deficiencies of fat-soluble vitamins as well as lipid membrane defects.

- Increased enterocyte triglyceride stores manifest as *lipid vacuolation.*
- Altered erythrocyte lipid membranes manifest as acanthocytes *(burr cells).*

Infectious Enterocolitis (p. 797)

The symptoms of enterocolitis run the gamut from urgency to diarrhea to incontinence and from perianal discomfort to abdominal pain; the outcomes can include dehydration, malabsorption, or hemorrhage. Half of all deaths worldwide that occur before age 5 years are due to infectious enterocolitis; in developing countries, more than 12,000 children die *daily* as a consequence. Bacterial infections are frequently responsible, but the most common pathogens vary with geography, age, nutrition, and host immune status (see later discussion); pediatric infectious diarrhea is often caused by enteric viruses.

Cholera (p. 797)

Cholera is caused by *Vibrio cholerae*, Gram-negative bacteria typically transmitted by drinking contaminated water; humans, shellfish, and plankton are the only reservoirs.

Pathogenesis (p. 797)

Vibrio organisms are non-invasive, although flagellar proteins are important for epithelial attachment and efficient bacterial colonization; mucosal biopsies show normal histology. *V. cholerae* causes diarrhea by production of a *cholera toxin* that is internalized after binding enterocyte surface G_{M1} gangliosides:

- The *toxin A subunit* is processed in the endoplasmic reticulum to a fragment that enters the cytosol.
- The toxin A fragment interacts with *ADP ribosylation factors* to activate the G protein $G_{s\alpha}$.
- Activated $G_{s\alpha}$ stimulates adenylate cyclase.
- The resulting surge in cytosolic cAMP opens the cystic fibrosis transmembrane conductance regulator (CFTR) and releases chloride ions into the lumen.
- Luminal chloride causes secretion of bicarbonate and sodium, with obligate water, leading to massive diarrhea.

Clinical Features (p. 799)

Only a minority of patients develop severe diarrhea; in those unfortunate patients, up to a liter per hour of "rice water"-like stool can be produced. Without treatment, the mortality is 50% due to dehydration, hypotension, and shock; however, most can be saved with timely rehydration.

Campylobacter Enterocolitis (p. 799)

Campylobacter jejuni is a Gram-negative organism; it is the most common bacterial enteric pathogen in developed countries and an important cause of "traveler's diarrhea." Transmission is often through ingestion of poorly cooked chicken, but water or milk contamination can occur.

Pathogenesis (p. 799)

The major virulence factors are flagellar motility, adherence molecules to facilitate colonization, cytotoxins and a cholera toxin–like enterotoxin. Infections can also result in extra-intestinal complications such as reactive arthritis, erythema nodosum, and Guillain-Barré syndrome.

Clinical Features (p. 800)

Diagnosis is primarily through stool cultures; biopsies show only non-specific neutrophilic colitis with variable epithelial damage. Diarrhea is typically watery; dysentery, associated with invasive strains, occurs in 15% of cases. Antibiotic therapy is usually not required; patients can shed bacteria for a month after symptoms resolve.

Shigellosis (p. 800)

Shigella is a non-encapsulated Gram-negative bacillius; it is a facultative anaerobe and one of the most common causes of bloody diarrhea. Humans are the only reservoir; fecal-oral transmission is accomplished with as few as several hundred microbes. Most infections and deaths occur in children younger than 5 years; in endemic areas *Shigella* causes 10% of pediatric diarrhea and 75% of diarrhea-related deaths.

Pathogenesis (p. 800)

Organisms are highly resistant to gastric acidity; they are taken up by intestinal M cells, escape into the lamina propria, and are ingested by macrophages that then undergo apoptosis. The subsequent inflammation and release of Shiga toxin causes epithelial damage that facilitates even greater bacterial access.

Morphology (p. 800)

The mucosa is hemorrhagic and ulcerated, often with pseudomembranes.

Clinical Features (p. 800)

Shigella is typically a self-limited diarrhea of about 6 days. Initially, watery diarrhea becomes dysenteric in half of patients; fever and abdominal pain can persist after the diarrhea ceases. Diagnosis requires stool cultures; antibiotics can shorten the clinical course and reduce the duration of bacterial shedding.

Salmonellosis (p. 801)

Salmonella is a Gram-negative bacillus; *S. typhi* and *S. paratyphi* cause *typhoid fever* (see next section) while nontyphoid *Salmonella* infection is usually due to *S. enteritides*. Transmission is through contaminated food; children and the elderly are most commonly affected.

Pathogenesis (p. 801)

Virulence factors include a *type III secretion system* that transfers bacterial proteins into M cells and enterocytes and facilitates bacterial uptake and growth in phagosomes; some strains also express a virulence factor that prevents TLR4 activation. Mucosal T_H17 responses limit infection to the colon but can cause secondary injury.

Clinical Features (p. 801)

Symptoms and pathologic appearances are similar to other enteric pathogens; diagnosis requires stool cultures. Most infections are self-limited (exceptions are immunocompromised hosts) and last about a week; antibiotics are not recommended since they prolong the carrier state and do not shorten the duration of diarrhea.

Typhoid Fever (p. 801)

In endemic areas, children and adolescents are most affected; infection is also strongly related to travel in India, Mexico, Phillipines, and other less-developed countries. Humans are the only reservoir, and transmission is most commonly through contaminated food and water. Gallbladder colonization can be associated with gallstones and a chronic carrier state.

Pathogenesis (p. 801)

Organisms are resistant to gastric acid; they invade M cells and are subsequently engulfed by mononuclear cells in the mucosal lymphoid tissues. Bacteria then disseminate widely via lymphatics and blood vessels, causing systemic macrophage and lymph node hyperplasia.

Morphology (p. 801)

- Infection causes marked expansion of Peyer's patches and draining nodes.
- Acute and chronic inflammatory cell recruitment to the lamina propria is associated with necrotic debris and overlying mucosal ulceration.
- The liver shows focal hepatocyte necrosis with macrophage aggregates, called *typhoid nodules.*

Clinical Features (p. 801)

An initial dysentery is followed by bacteremia (90% of patients), fever, and abdominal pain that can persist for 2 weeks without antibiotic treatment *(typhoid fever).* Systemic dissemination can cause extraintestinal complications including: encephalopathy, meningitis, endocarditis, myocarditis, pneumonia, and cholecystitis. Patients with sickle cell disease are prone to osteomyelitis.

Yersinia (p. 802)

Gastrointestinal *Yersinia* infections are caused by *Yersinia enterocolitica* and *Yersinia pseudotuberculosis.* These infections typically occur through ingestion of contaminated pork, milk, or water; *Yersinia pestis,* the agent of bubonic plague, is described in Chapter 8.

Pathogenesis (p. 802)

Yersinia invade M cells, using bacterial *adhesions* to bind to host cell β1 integrins. A bacterial iron uptake system increases *Yersinia* virulence and systemic dissemination; hence, patients with hemolytic anemia or hemochromatosis are more likely to become septic and die.

Morphology (p. 802)

Yersinia preferentially invades ileum, appendix, and the right colon; organisms proliferate in lymph nodes, resulting in regional nodal hyperplasia; also, overlying mucosal can become hemorrhagic and ulcerated.

Clinical Features (p. 802)

Abdominal pain, fever, and diarrhea can occur (mimicking appendicitis). Extra-intestinal manifestations (e.g., pharyngitis, arthralgia, and erythema nodosum) are common, and post-infectious complications include sterile arthritis, Reiter syndrome, myocarditis, glomerulonephritis, and throiditis.

Escherichia Coli (p. 802)

Escherichia coli are Gram-negative bacilli that colonize the normal gastrointestinal tract; most are non-pathogenic but a subset (classified by morphology, *in vitro* characteristics, and pathogenesis) cause disease:

- *Enterotoxigenic E. coli* (p. 802) are spread in contaminated food or water, and are the chief cause of traveler's diarrhea. They produce a heat-stable toxin that increases intracellular cGMP or a heat-labile cholera-like toxin that increases intracellular cAMP; both cause chloride and water secretion and inhibit epithelial fluid absorption, leading to a non-inflammatory watery diarrhea.
- *Enterohemorrhagic E. coli* (p. 802) are spread in contaminated meat, milk, and vegetables and produce a shiga-like toxin; clinical symptoms and morphology resemble infections with *Shigella dysenteriae.* There are two major serotypes: O157:H7 and non-O157:H7; the former is more likely to cause large outbreaks, dysentery, and hemolytic uremic syndrome.

- *Enteroinvasive E. coli* (p. 802) are bacteriologically akin to *Shigella*. Although not toxin-producing, they invade epithelial cells and cause an acute, self-limited colitis.
- *Enteroaggregative E. coli* (p. 802) attach to epithelium by adherence fimbriae, aided by a bacterial *dispersin* that neutralizes the negative surface charge of lipopolysaccharide. They produce a shiga-like toxin but typically cause only a non-bloody diarrhea.

Pseudomembranous Colitis (p. 803)

Pseudomembranous colitis (PMC) is characterized by *formation of adherent inflammatory pseudomembranes overlying sites of mucosal injury;* it is classically caused by overgrowth (and toxin production) by *Clostridium difficile* after competing bowel organisms have been eliminated by antibiotics; *Salmonella, C. perfringens,* or *S. aureus* can also cause PMC

Morphology (p. 803)

There is epithelial denudation with plaquelike adhesion of fibrinopurulent necrotic, gray-yellow debris and mucus. The pseudomembrane is not specific and can form with any severe mucosal injury (e.g., ischemia or necrotizing infections).

Clinical Features (p. 803)

C. difficile is prevalent in hospitals; 30% of hospitalized patients can be colonized (*vs.* 3% of the general population). Patients present with fever, leukocytosis, crampy abdominal pain, and watery diarrhea; toxin detection in stool yields the definitive diagnosis, and metronidazole or vancomycin are generally effective therapies.

Whipple Disease (p. 803)

This is a rare, systemic condition caused by the Gram-positive actinomycete *Tropheryma whippelii*. Patients present with *diarrhea, weight loss, and malabsorption*. Extra-intestinal manifestations (due to bacterial spread) include arthritis, fever, and lymphadenopathy, as well as neurologic, cardiac, or pulmonary disease.

Morphology (p. 803)

- *Grossly:* There is marked villous expansion in the small bowel, imparting a shaggy appearance to the mucosal surface.
- *Microscopically:* The characteristic feature is a dense accumulation of distended foamy macrophages in small intestine lamina propria; these cells are stuffed with PAS-positive bacteria within lysosomes.
- Similarly laden macrophages are present in lymphatics, lymph nodes, joints, and the brain.
- Active inflammation is largely absent.

Viral Gastroenteritis (p. 804)

Norovirus (p. 804)

Previously called *Norwalk-like virus,* this is a single-stranded RNA virus; it accounts for half of all gastroenteritis outbreaks worldwide. Local outbreaks are due to contaminated food or water, but person-to-person transmission underlies most sporadic infections. Patients develop a self-limited watery diarrhea, often with abdominal pain, nausea, and vomiting. Biopsy morphology is non-specific.

Rotavirus (p. 804)

An encapsulated, segmented, double-stranded RNA virus, rotavirus is the most common cause of severe childhood diarrhea (infecting 140 million and causing 1 million deaths worldwide annually). It is readily spread between individuals; the minimal infective inoculum is 10 particles. Rotavirus selectively infects and destroys mature small intestine enterocytes, and the epithelium is repopulated with immature secretory cells; thus, a net secretion of water and electrolytes is compounded by malabsorption and an osmotic diarrhea.

Adenovirus (p. 805)

Adenovirus is the second most common cause of pediatric diarrhea; patients present with a self-limited diarrhea, vomiting, and abdominal pain. The histologic findings are non-specific.

Parasitic Enterocolitis (p. 805)

Parasitic and protozoal infections collectively affect over half of the world's population on a chronic or recurrent basis. Common organisms include:

- *Ascaris lumbricoides* (p. 805): This worm infects more than a billion individuals worldwide; fecal-oral transmission is followed by an intestine-liver-lung-intestine life cycle. Systemically disseminated larvae can cause hepatic abscesses or pneumonitis; adult worm masses induce an eosinophil-rich inflammation that can physically obstruct the intestine or biliary tract. Diagnosis is made by detecting eggs in the stool.
- *Strongyloides* (p. 805): Stongyloides larvae in fecally contaminated soil penetrate unbroken skin, migrate to the lungs (where they cause inflammation), and then mature into adult worms in the gastrointestinal tract. Released eggs can hatch in the intestine, and luminal larvae can penetrate the mucosa, causing an auto-infection. *Strongyloides* typically incite strong eosinophil responses.
- *Necator duodenale and Ancylostoma duodenale (hookworms)* (p. 806): These infect more than a billion people worldwide. The life cycle begins with larval penetration through skin and subsequent maturation in the lung; after migration up the trachea, they are swallowed. Worms then attach to duodenal mucosa and extract blood, causing mucosal damage and iron deficiency anemia.
- *Enterobius vermicularis (pinworms)* (p. 806): Transmission is principally fecal-oral. Because pinworms do not invade host tissues, and their entire life-cycle transpires in the intestinal lumen, they rarely cause serious illness. Classically, adult worms migrate at night to the anal orifice, where eggs are deposited, causing intense irritation and pruritus.
- *Trichuris trichiura (whipworms)* (p. 806): This worm primarily infects children. Although there is no tissue invasion, heavy infestations can cause bloody diarrhea and rectal prolapse.
- *Schistosomiasis* (p. 806): Adult worms can reside within mesenteric veins; trapped eggs in the mucosa and submucosa induce a granulomatous response with bleeding and obstruction.
- *Intestinal cestodes (tapeworms)* (p. 806): Infections occur by ingesting raw or undercooked fish, pork, or other contaminated meats. Parasites reside within the lumen without tissue invasion; a scolex attaches to the mucosa, and proglottids contain eggs that are shed in the feces.
- *Entamoeba histolytica* (p. 806): Transmission is fecal-oral. Infection occurs by ingesting acid-resistant cysts; released trophozoites colonize colonic epithelium and reproduce under anaerobic conditions. Dysentery results when amoebae induce colonic epithelial apoptosis to invade into the lamina propria and attract neutrophils. Subsequent damage yields a classic

flask-shaped ulcer with a narrow neck and broad base. Amoebae can also embolize to the liver, producing abscesses in more than 40% of infected individuals. Metronidazole therapy targets the organism-specific enzyme pyruvate oxidoreductase.

- *Giardia lamblia* (p. 806): This is a flagellated protozoan and the most common pathogenic parasitic infection in humans. *Giardia* cysts are ingested from fecally contaminated water or food; duodenal trophozoites exhibit characteristic morphology (pear-shaped and binucleate). *Giardia* does not invade the tissue, but it secretes products that damage the microvillus brush border and causes malabsorption. Secretory IgA and mucosal IL-6 are important for clearance; thus, immunocompromised individuals are often severely affected. *Giardia* can also persist for prolonged durations in immunocompetent hosts through continuous modification of their major surface antigen.

- *Cryptosporidium* (p. 807): This causes a self-limited diarrhea in immunocompetent hosts, but it can cause chronic diarrhea in immunocompromised individuals. Contaminated drinking water is the most common means of transmission. As few as 10 encysted oocytes can cause disease; stomach acid activates proteases that release motile sporozoites, which are subsequently internalized by absorptive enterocytes. Sodium malabsorption, chloride secretion, and increased epithelial permeability are responsible for the ensuing watery diarrhea.

Irritable Bowel Syndrome (p. 807)

Irritable bowel syndrome (IBS) is characterized by chronic, relapsing abdominal pain, bloating, and changes in stool frequency or form; it is most common in women between the ages of 20 and 40 years. IBS results from interplay of psychologic stressors, diet, and abnormal gastrointesinal motility, perhaps via disruption of signaling in the brain-gut axis.

Inflammatory Bowel Disease (p. 807)

Inflammatory bowel disease (IBD) results from inappropriate mucosal immune responses to normal gut flora; it comprises two disorders (Table 17-2):

- *Ulcerative colitis (UC)*—severe ulcerating inflammation extending into the mucosa and submucosa, and limited to the colon and rectum.
- *Crohn disease (CD;* also called *regional enteritis)*—typically transmural inflammation, occurring anywhere in the gastrointestinal tract.

Epidemiology (p. 807)

IBD is more common in women, typically during adolescence and in their twenties. It is also more common in developed countries, consistent with the *hygiene hypothesis*, that is, reduced frequency of enteric infections results in inadequate development of mucosal immune regulation.

Pathogenesis (p. 808)

IBD results from *a combination of defects in host interactions with gastrointestinal flora, intestinal epithelial dysfunction, and aberrant mucosal immunity.* The current prevailing model is that transepithelial flux of microbes activates innate and adaptive immune responses. In a susceptible host, subsequent TNF release and other inflammatory signals increase the permeability

TABLE 17-2 Features that Differ between Crohn Disease and Ulcerative Colitis

Feature	Crohn Disease	Ulcerative Colitis
Macroscopic		
Bowel region	Ileum $\pm$ colon	Colon only
Distribution	Skip lesions	Diffuse
Stricture	Yes	Rare
Wall appearance	Thick	Thin
Microscopic		
Inflammation	Transmural	Limited to mucosa
Pseudopolyps	Moderate	Marked
Ulcers	Deep, knife-like	Superficial, broad based
Lymphoid reaction	Marked	Moderate
Fibrosis	Marked	Mild to none
Serositis	Marked	Mild to none
Granulomas	Yes ($\sim$35%)	No
Fistulae/sinuses	Yes	No
Clinical		
Perianal fistula	Yes (in colonic disease)	No
Fat/vitamin malabsorption	Yes	No
Malignant potential	With colonic involvement	Yes
Recurrence after surgery	Common	No
Toxic megacolon	No	Yes

Note: All features may not be present in a single case.

of tight junctions. These events establish a self-amplifying cycle of microbial influx and host immune responses that ultimately culminate in IBD.

- *Genetics:* There is familial clustering, and concordance of monzygotic twins is 50% for CD and 16% for UC. *NOD2* (nucleotide oligomerization binding domain 2) polymorphisms are linked to CD (albeit not absolutely); the gene encodes a protein that binds to intracellular bacterial peptidoglycans and subsequently activates NF-κB. Disease-associated *NOD2* variants are less effective at recognizing and combating microbes, which then enter the lamina propria and trigger greater inflammatory responses. Additional genes uncovered by genome-wide association studies are also related to microbial recognition and/or regulating subsequent immune responses.

- *Mucosal immune responses:*

  In CD, helper T cells are polarized to produce T_H1 cytokines (Chapter 6); T_H17 cells may also be contributory, and polymorphisms in the IL-23 receptor (regulating T_H17 cell development) may be protective.

  In UC, helper T cells tend to be polarized to produce T_H2 cytokines; polymorphisms near the IL-10 gene have been linked to UC.

- *Epithelial defects:* Barrier dysfunction, including defects in epithelial tight junctions, transporter genes, and polymorphisms in extracellular matrix proteins or metalloproteinases are associated with IBD.

- *Microbiota*: The composition of the gastrointestinal flora, and in particular those organisms that populate the intestinal mucus layer may influence pathogenesis by affecting innate and adaptive immune responses; antibiotics can be helpful in managing IBD.

Crohn Disease (p. 810) (See Table 17-2.)

Morphology (p. 810)

CD involves the small intestine alone in 40% of cases, the small intestine and colon in 30%, and colon alone in 30%; other areas of the gastrointestinal tract are uncommonly involved.

- *Grossly:*

    Skip lesions—separate, sharply delineated disease areas with granular and inflamed serosa and adherent *creeping* mesenteric fat; the bowel wall is thick and rubbery and often strictured.

    Punched-out mucosal *aphthous* ulcers, coalescing into axially oriented serpentine ulcers

    Sparing of interspersed mucosa can give a *cobblestone appearance* with diseased tissue depressed relative to normal mucosa; fissures and fistula tracts are also common.

- *Microscopically:*

    Mucosal inflammation and ulceration with intraepithelial neutrophils and crypt abscesses

    Chronic mucosal damage with villus blunting, atrophy, pseudopyloric or Paneth cell metaplasia, and architectural disarray

    Transmural inflammation with lymphoid aggregates in submucosa, muscle wall, and subserosal fat

    Noncaseating granulomas, which occur throughout the gut, even in uninvolved segments (but are seen in only 35% of patients)

Clinical Features (p. 811)

Patients present with intermittent attacks of diarrhea, fever, and abdominal pain; asymptomatic periods can last for weeks to months.

- Depending on the segment affected, extensive CD can lead to malabsorption and malnutrition, loss of albumin (protein-losing enteropathy), iron-deficiency anemia, and/or B_{12} deficiency.
- Fibrotic strictures or fistulas to adjacent viscera, abdominal and perineal skin, bladder, or vagina typically require surgical resection; disease often recurs at the anastomosis with 40% of patients requiring additional surgery within a decade.
- Extra-intestinal manifestations include migratory polyarthritis, sacroiliitis, ankylosing spondylitis, erythema nodosum, uveitis, cholangitis, amyloidosis.
- There is increased risk of colonic adenocarcinoma in patients with long-standing colon involvement.

Ulcerative Colitis (p. 811)

Morphology (p. 811)

UC is a disease of continuity with no *skip* lesions, involving the rectum and extending proximally in retrograde fashion to involve the entire colon (pancolitis); the distal ileum may also show some inflammation (*backwash ileitis*).

- *Grossly:* Mucosa is reddened, granular, and friable with inflammatory *pseudopolyps,* and easy bleeding; there can be extensive ulceration or atrophic and flattened mucosa.
- *Microscopically:* Mucosal inflammation is similar to CD but is generally limited to the mucosa; there are crypt abscesses, ulceration, chronic mucosal damage, glandular architectural distortion, and atrophy but *no* fissures, aphthous ulcers, or granulomas.

Clinical Features (p. 812)

Patients present with intermittent attacks of bloody mucoid diarrhea and abdominal pain that can persist for days to months before subsiding. Although half of patients have clinically mild disease, most patients relapse within 10 years, and up to 30% of patients require a colectomy within 3 years to control symptoms.

- *Extra-intestinal manifestations* include migratory polyarthritis, sacroiliitis, ankylosing spondylitis, uveitis, cholangitis and primary sclerosing cholangitis (up to 7.5% of patients), and skin lesions.
- There is increased *risk of colonic adenocarcinoma* (see later discussion).

Colitis-Associated Neoplasia (p. 813)

Risk of malignancy in IBD:

- Increases sharply 8 to 10 years after disease onset
- Is greater with pancolitis versus left-sided only disease
- Increases with the severity and duration of active inflammation

Patients with long-standing disease are followed by biopsy surveillance; dysplasia is classified histologically as low or high grade, and it can be multifocal.

Other Causes of Chronic Colitis (p. 813)

Diversion Colitis (p. 813)

Diversion colitis occurs in the blind distal colonic segment created after surgery that diverts the fecal stream to an ostomy site. Lack of short-chain fatty acids and other nutrients and changes in the flora of the segment are implicated. There is mucosal erythema and friability with lymphoplasmacytic inflammation, as well as a characteristic lymphoid follicular hyperplasia.

Microscopic Colitis (p. 814)

Patients (typically middle-aged women) present with chronic watery diarrhea and abdominal pain. Endoscopic findings are grossly normal, hence the designation *microscopic colitis.* There are two forms:

- *Collagenous colitis* is characterized by dense submucosal band-like collagen with mixed inflammation in the lamina propria.
- *Lymphocytic colitis* is characterized by a prominent intraepithelial infiltrate of lymphocytes without the band-like collagen; it is associated with autoimmune diseases and sprue.

Sigmoid Diverticulitis (p. 814)

Acquired *colonic pseudodiverticular outpouchings (diverticulosis)* are uncommon in patients younger than 30 years but occur in 50% of Western populations older than 60 years.

Pathogenesis (p. 814)

Focal bowel wall weakness (at sites of penetrating blood vessels) allows mucosal outpouching when there is *increased intraluminal pressure* (e.g., with constipation and exaggerated peristaltic contractions).

Morphology (p. 815)

Multiple flasklike outpouchings that are 0.5 to 1 cm in diameter; more common in the distal colon.

- These occur where the vasculature penetrates the inner circular layer of the muscularis propria at the taeniae coli.
- The diverticulum wall is lined by mucosa and submucosa without significant muscularis propria, although the muscularis between diverticuli is hypertrophic.
- Obstruction of diverticuli leads to inflammation producing *diverticulitis* with tissue damage and increased pressure, these can perforate.

Clinical Features (p. 815)

Diverticular disease is usually asymptomatic but may be associated with cramping, abdominal discomfort, and constipation. Diverticulitis can result in pericolic abscesses, sinus tracts, and peritonitis. Even without perforation, diverticulitis can cause fibrotic thickening and stricture formation.

Polyps (p. 815)

Masses that protrude into the gut lumen can be pedunculated or sessile, and can be non-neoplastic or neoplastic.

Inflammatory Polyps (p. 815)

These result from recurrent cycles of injury and healing; there is lamina propria fibromuscular hyperplasia, mixed inflammatory cell infiltrates, and mucosal erosion and/or hyperplasia.

Hamartomatous Polyps (p. 816)

Hamartomatous polyps (tumor-like growths of tissues normally present at the site) are important to recognize because they usually occur in the setting of various genetic or acquired syndromes (Table 17-3).

- *Juvenile polyps* (p. 816) are focal hamartomatous malformations of small intestine and colon mucosa; most occur in children younger than 5 years and involve the rectum. Mutations in *SMAD4* and *BMPR1A* genes involved in TGF-β signaling are implicated in some cases. Polyps are typically single, large (1 to 3 cm), rounded, and pedunculated with cystically dilated glands and abundant lamina propria.
- The *juvenile polyposis syndrome* is a rare autosomal dominant disorder characterized by up to 100 hamartomatous polyps. Patients may require colectomy to limit bleeding due to polyp ulceration, and pulmonary arteriovenous malformations are a known extra-intestinal manifestation. There is also an increased risk of colonic adenocarcinoma.
- *Peutz-Jeghers syndrome* (p. 817) is a rare autosomal dominant syndrome (median age of onset is 11 years) associated with *multiple gastrointestinal hamartomatous polyps and mucocutaneous hyperprigmentation*. In half of patients, there is a heterozygous loss-of-function mutation in the *LKB1/STK11* gene encoding a kinase that regulates cell polarization and growth.

TABLE 17-3 Gastrointestinal Polyposis Syndromes

Syndrome	Mean Age at Presentation (yr)	Mutated Gene	Gastrointestinal Lesions	Selected Extra-Gastrointestinal Manifestations
Peutz–Jeghers syndrome	10-15	*LKB1/STK11*	Arborizing polyps; Small intestine > colon > stomach; colonic adenocarcinoma	Skin macules; increased risk of thyroid, breast, lung, pancreas, gonadal, and bladder cancers
Juvenile polyposis	<5	*SMAD4, BMPR1A*	Juvenile polyps; risk of gastric, small intestinal, colonic, and pancreatic adenocarcinoma	Pulmonary arteriovenous malformations, digital clubbing
Cowden syndrome, Bannayan-Ruvalcaba-Riley syndrome	<15	*PTEN*	Hamartomatous polyps, lipomas, ganglioneuromas, inflammatory polyps, risk of colon cancer	Benign skin tumors, benign and malignant thyroid and breast lesions
Cronkhite-Canada syndrome	>50	Nonhereditary	Hamartomatous colon polyps, crypt dilation and edema in nonpolypoid mucosa	Nail atrophy, hair loss, abnormal skin pigmentation, cachexia, and anemia
Tuberous sclerosis		*TSC1, TSC2*	Hamartomatous polyps (rectal)	Facial angiofibroma, cortical tubers, renal angiomyolipoma
Familial adenomatous polyposis (FAP)				
Classic FAP	10-15	*APC, MUTYH*	Multiple adenomas	Congenital RPE hypertrophy
Attenuated FAP	40-50	*APC, MUTYH*	Multiple adenomas	
Gardner syndrome	10-15	*APC, MUTYH*	Multiple adenomas	Osteomas, desmoids, skin cysts
Turcot syndrome	10-15	*APC, MUTYH*	Multiple adenomas	CNS tumors, medulloblastoma

CNS, Central nervous system; *RPE*, retinal pigmented epithelium.

- The polyps (small bowel more than colon and stomach) are large, pedunculated, and lobulated with arborizing smooth muscle surrounding normal abundant glands; they can initiate intussusception. The hyperpigmentation takes the form of macules around the mouth, eyes, nostrils, buccal mucosa, palms, and genital and perianal regions. Recognition of the syndrome is important since these patients have increased risk of several cancers including colon, pancreas, breast, lung, gonads, and uterus.
- *Cowden syndrome and Bannayan-Ruvalcaba-Riley syndrome* (p. 818) are autosomal dominant hamartomatous polyp syndromes associated with loss-of-function mutations in *PTEN*, encoding a phosphatase that inhibits signaling through the PI3K/AKT pathway.

    - *Cowden syndrome* is characterized by gastrointestinal polyps, macrocephaly, and benign skin tumors; patients are at increased risk of breast, thyroid, and endometrial cancers.
    - *Bannayan-Ruvalcaba-Riley syndrome* patients have similar manifestations as for Cowden syndrome, but they also have mental deficiency and developmental delays, while their risk of malignancy is less.

- *Cronkhite-Canada syndrome* (p. 818) is a rare *non-hereditary* syndrome of unknown etiology; it develops in individuals older than 50 years. Patients present with cachexia, diarrhea, and abdominal pain, as well as nail atrophy, hair loss, and skin pigmentation changes. Patients have polyps throughout the gastrointestinal tract that histologically resemble juvenile polyps. Despite nutritional support, there is 50% mortality.

Hyperplastic Polyps (p. 818)

These polyps result from decreased epithelial turnover with delayed shedding; they have no malignant potential. These are usually smaller than 5 mm and are composed of well-formed mature, albeit crowded, glands.

Neoplastic Polyps (p. 819)

Colonic adenomas are benign polyp precursors to the majority of colorectal carcinomas; they are characterized by the presence of epithelial dysplasia. The incidence of adenomas approaches 50% by age 50 years, but it should be emphasized that the majority do *not* progress to malignancy. Most are clinically silent, although large specimens can cause anemia through occult bleeding or rarely, protein and potassium losses cause hypoproteinenic hypokalemia.

Risk of malignancy is correlated to size (i.e,. polyps more than 4 cm have a 40% risk harboring cancer) and severity of dysplasia.

Morphology (p. 819)

Ademomas range from 0.3 to 10 cm and can be pedunculated or sessile. Dysplastic changes include hyperplasia, nuclear hyperchromasia, and loss of polarity. Adenomas are classified based on architecture (*tubular, tubulovillous,* and *villous*), although these have little clinical significance.

- In *sessile serrated adenomas* the full gland length exhibits serrated architecture; despite malignant potential, they *do not* have the typical dysplastic changes seen in other adenomas.
- *Intramucosal carcinoma* occurs when dysplastic cells invade the lamina propria or muscularis mucosa. Such polyps have little metastatic potential since colonic mucosa lack lymphatic channels.

- Polyps with *invasive adenocarcinoma* are malignant and have metastatic potential because they have crossed into submucosa and can access lymphatics.

Familial Syndromes (p. 820)

Several syndromes characterized by colonic polyps and increased rates of colon cancer have enlightened our understanding of the pathogenesis of sporadic colon cancers (Table 17-4).

Familial Adenomatous Polyposis (p. 820)

FAP is an autosomal dominant disorder caused by mutations of the *adenomatous polposis coli (APC)* gene. Patients in adolescence characteristically develop more than 100 colonic adenomatous polyps; if untreated, colorectal carcinoma will develop in 100% by age 30 years. Although prophylactic colectomy eliminates the risk of colon cancer, these patients also develop adenomas in the stomach and ampulla of Vater. AFP variants include:

- *Gardner syndrome* exhibits multiple osteomas (e.g., mandible, skull, long bones), epidermal cysts, fibromatosis (i.e., desmoid tumors), abnormal dentition (i.e., impacted teeth), and increased incidence of duodenal and thyroid cancers.
- *Turcot syndrome* is rarer; besides adenomas, patients develop medulloblastomas.

Some FAP patients without *APC* loss have mutations of the base-excision repair gene *MUTYH*. Moreover, some *APC* and *MUTYH* mutations give rise to attenuated forms of FAP, characterized by delayed polyp development and the appearance of colon carcinoma after age 50 years.

Hereditary Non-Polyposis Colorectal Cancer (p. 821)

Also known as *Lynch syndrome, hereditary non-polyposis colorectal cancer (HNPCC)* is caused by mutations in genes encoding proteins responsible for the detection, excision, and repair of DNA replication errors (Chapter 7). The majority of cases involve mismatch repair genes *MSH2* and *MLH1*; patients inherit one defective copy and, when the second is lost by mutation or epigenetic silencing, mutations accrue at rates up to 1000 times normal, mostly in regions of microsatellite repeats, which leads to *microsatellite instability*.

TABLE 17-4 **Common Patterns of Sporadic and Familial Colorectal Neoplasia**

Etiology	Molecular Defect	Target Gene(s)	Transmission
Familial adenomatous polyposis (70% of FAP)	APC/WNT pathway	APC	Autosomal dominant
Familial adenomatous polyposis (<10% of FAP)	DNA mismatch repair	MUTYH	None, recessive
Hereditary nonpolyposis colorectal cancer	DNA mismatch repair	MSH2, MLH1	Autosomal dominant
Sporadic colon cancer (80%)	APC/WNT pathway	APC	None
Sporadic colon cancer (10% to 15%)	DNA mismatch repair	MSH2, MLH1	None

Adenocarcinoma (p. 822)

Colonic adenocarcinoma is the most common GI malignancy and constitutes 15% of all cancer-related deaths in the United States; it is a major cause of morbidity and mortality worldwide.

Epidemiology (p. 822)

Dietary factors influence risk; increased rates of colorectal cancer are seen with reduced vegetable fiber intake and increased levels of refined carbohydrates and fat. These may influence the composition of gastrointestinal flora, as well as the synthesis of carcinogenic by-products that remain in prolonged contact with intestinal mucosa due to diminished stool bulk. Diminished antioxidants (e.g., vitamins A, C, and E) can also influence malignant potential. NSAIDs have a protective effect, potentially related to inhibition of the formation of prostaglandin E_2 that promotes epithelial proliferation.

Pathogenesis (p. 823)

Multiple genetic and epigenetic events contribute to colorectal carcinogenesis (Figure 17-3). No single event or sequence of events is requisite, but a multi-hit genetic mechanism appears to be operative.

- *APC/β-catenin pathway* associated with the WNT signaling pathway (Chapter 7) adenoma-carcinoma sequence. *APC is a key negative regulator of β-catenin*; APC protein normally binds to and promotes β-catenin degradation. With loss of APC, β-catenin accumulates and translocates to the nucleus, where it activates a cassette of genes that promote proliferation.
- *Microsatellite instability* associated with defects in DNA mismatch repair; mutations result in increased proliferation and diminished apoptosis.
- Late *K-RAS* and *p53* mutations promote growth and prevent apoptosis.
- *SMAD* mutations reduce TGF-β signaling and thus promote cell cycle progression.
- *Telomerase* re-activation prevents cellular senescence.

Morphology (p. 824)

Tumors are roughly equally distributed along the colon.

- *Grossly:* Polypoid, exophytic masses are characteristic in the cecum and right colon; annular masses with *"napkin-ring"* obstruction are characteristic of the distal colon. Both forms penetrate the bowel wall over the course of many years.
- *Microscopically:* Tumors are typically composed of tall columnar cells resembling adenomatous neoplastic epithelium but with invasion into the submucosa, muscularis propria, or beyond; a minority produce copious extracellular mucin.
- Carcinomas can also be poorly differentiated solid tumors without gland formation. Less commonly, foci of neuroendocrine differentiation, signet-ring features, or squamous differentiation occur.
- Invasive tumors characteristically incite a strong *desmoplastic response.*

Clinical Features (p. 825)

Colorectal carcinoma develops insidiously and may go undetected for long periods. Fatigue, weakness, iron deficiency anemia, abdominal discomfort, progressive bowel obstruction, and liver enlargement (metastases) eventually occur. *Prognosis varies with the stage of disease at diagnosis;* 5-year survival rates are related to the depth of tumor penetration and lymph node involvement,

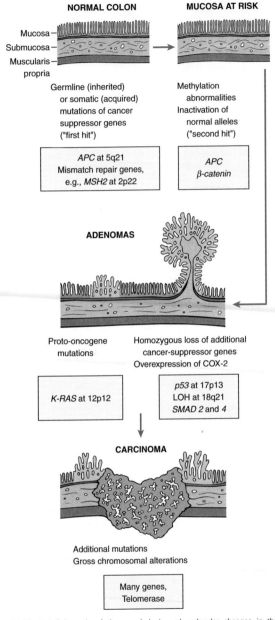

FIGURE 17-3 Schematic of the morphologic and molecular changes in the adenoma-carcinoma sequence. As a first "hit," patients may be born with a mutant allele of the tumor suppressor "gatekeeper" gene *APC* or may have an early loss of one normal copy; loss of the remaining normal *APC* copy becomes the "second hit." Subsequent mutations in the *K-RAS* oncogene, losses involving *SMAD 2* and *4*, and inactivation of *p53* lead to the emergence of carcinoma, in which other mutations can accrue. Although presented sequentially, *it is the accumulation of mutations rather than their specific order that is most important.* *COX-2*, Cyclooxygenase-2.

and range from almost 100% for lesions limited to the mucosa to 44% for extensively invasive tumors; distal metastasis reduces 5-year survival to 8%. Currently, only surgery can be curative.

Hemorrhoids (p. 826)

Hemorrhoids are variceal dilations of anal and perianal submucosal venous plexi; they affect 5% of adults. Hemorrhoids are causally associated with constipation (straining at stool), venous stasis during pregnancy, and cirrhosis (portal hypertension). *External hemorrhoids* occur with ectasia of the inferior hemorrhoidal plexus below the anorectal line; *internal hemorrhoids* are due to ectasia of the superior hemorrhoidal plexus above the anorectal line. Secondary thrombosis (with recanalization), strangulation, or ulceration with fissure formation can occur.

Acute Appendicitis (p. 826)

Acute appendicitis is the most common acute abdominal condition requiring surgery; the lifetime risk is 7%.

Pathogenesis (p. 827)

Some 50% to 80% of appendicitis cases are associated with obstruction of the appendiceal lumen by a fecalith, tumor, or worms *(Oxyuriasis vermicularis)* causing increased intraluminal pressure. This is followed by ischemia—exacerbated by edema and exudate—and bacterial invasion.

Morphology (p. 827)

- *Early acute appendicitis* exhibits a scant appendiceal neutrophil exudate with subserosal congestion and perivascular neutrophil emigration; the serosa is dull, granular, and red.
- *Advanced acute appendicitis (acute suppurative appendicitis)* involves more severe neutrophilic infiltration with fibrinopurulent serosal exudate, luminal abscess formation, ulceration, and suppurative necrosis. This can progress to *acute gangrenous appendicitis*, followed by perforation.

Clinical Features (p. 827)

Acute appendicitis can occur at any age, but it mainly affects adolescents and young adults. Classically, there is periumbilical pain migrating to the right lower quadrant, nausea and/or vomiting, abdominal tenderness, mild fever, and leukocytosis. Other mimics for appendicitis include enterocolitis, mesenteric lymphadenitis, systemic viral infection, acute salpingitis, ectopic pregnancy, mittelschmerz, and Meckel diverticulitis. Complications include pyelophlebitis, portal vein thrombosis, liver abscess, and bacteremia.

Tumors of the Appendix (p. 828)

- *Carcinoid* is the most common tumor of the appendix (see earlier discussion).
- *Mucocele* reflects dilation of the appendiceal lumen by mucinous secretions; it can be due to innocuous obstruction with inspissated mucus, mucin-secreting adenomas, or adenocarcinoma.
- *Mucinous cystadenocarcinoma* is indistinguishable from cystadenomas except for *appendiceal wall invasion by neoplastic cells and peritoneal implants.* The peritoneum becomes distended with tenacious, semisolid, mucin-producing anaplastic adenocarcinoma cells, designated *pseudomyxoma peritonei;* it is ultimately fatal.

PERITONEAL CAVITY (p. 828)

Inflammatory Disease (p. 828)

Peritonitis can result from bacterial infection or chemical irritation; the latter can be caused by:

- Leakage of bile or pancreatic enzymes *(sterile peritonitis)*
- Perforation of the biliary system or abdominal viscera usually complicated by bacterial superinfection
- *Acute hemorrhagic pancreatitis;* bowel wall damage can lead to secondary bacterial peritonitis
- *Foreign* material, inducing granulomas and scarring
- *Endometriosis* (ectopic endometrial implants) or ruptured *dermoid cysts*

Peritoneal Infection (p. 828)

Bacterial peritonitis results when gastrointestinal tract bacteria are released into the abdominal cavity—usually after bowel perforation (e.g., due to appendicitis, peptic ulcer, cholecystitis, diverticulitis, and intestinal ischemia); acute salpingitis, abdominal trauma, or peritoneal dialysis are other potential bacterial sources.

Spontaneous bacterial peritonitis develops without an obvious source of contamination; it occurs in the setting of ascites (e.g., nephrotic syndrome or cirrhosis).

Morphology (p. 828)

Peritoneal membranes become dull and gray, followed by exudation and frank suppuration; localized abscesses can develop, although the inflammation tends to remain superficial.

Sclerosing Retroperitonitis (p. 829)

Also known as *Ormond disease,* this disorder is characterized by a dense fibrosis of retroperitoneal tissues; it is likely a primary inflammatory process.

Tumors (p. 829)

Tumors may be primary or secondary; virtually all are malignant.

- *Primary* tumors are rare; they include *mesothelioma* (similar to pleural or pericardial mesotheliomas) and *desmoplastic small round cell tumor.* The latter has a characteristic t(11;22) translocation yielding a fusion of genes associated with Ewing sarcoma and Wilms tumor *(EWS-WT1);* the tumor morphologically resembles a Ewing sarcoma.
- *Secondary* tumors are common and can derive from any cancer; ovarian and pancreatic adenocarcinomas are most common.

18

Liver and Biliary Tract

THE LIVER (p. 834)

General Features of Hepatic Disease (p. 835)

Although the liver is vulnerable to a host of insults, the most common primary diseases in the United States are viral hepatitis, alcohol-related liver disease, nonalcoholic fatty liver disease, and hepatocellular carcinoma. The liver is also secondarily affected by common disorders such as congestive heart failure and metastatic cancer. Although injury may be apparent through laboratory testing (Table 18-1), an enormous functional hepatic reserve typically masks the clinical impact of early damage. Most liver disease is insidious with symptoms of decompensation developing over weeks to years. Nevertheless, disrupted bile flow or progressive disease can be life-threatening; liver failure accounts for roughly 1% of deaths in the United States.

Patterns of Hepatic Injury (p. 835)

Hepatic responses to injury constitute a fairly limited repertoire:

- Hepatocyte degeneration
- Intracellular accumulations
- Hepatocyte necrosis and apoptosis
- Inflammation
- Regeneration
- Fibrosis

Hepatic Failure (p. 835)

Hepatic failure occurs when greater than 80% to 90% of hepatic function is lost; the mortality rate is approximately 80%. While occasionally caused by massive acute destruction *(fulminant hepatic failure)*, it is more commonly a consequence of successive waves of injury or progressive chronic damage. Patients with marginal hepatic function can also be tipped into frank failure when intercurrent disease places a greater demand on hepatic function.

Causes of liver failure include:

- *Acute liver failure* (defined as liver illness associated with encephalopathy within 6 months of initial diagnosis): Caused by hepatic necrosis attributable to drug or toxin (e.g., mushroom poisoning) injury, viral hepatitis, or autoimmune damage.
- *Chronic liver disease* (most common cause of failure): The endpoint of relentless chronic hepatitis ending in *cirrhosis*

TABLE 18-1 Laboratory Evaluation of Liver Disease	
Test Category	**Serum Measurement***
Hepatocyte integrity	Cytosolic hepatocellular enzymes[†] *Serum aspartate aminotransferase (AST)* *Serum alanine aminotransferase (ALT)* Serum lactate dehydrogenase (LDH)

Biliary excretory function	Substances normally secreted in bile[†]
	 Serum bilirubin
	     Total: unconjugated plus conjugated
	     Direct: conjugated only
	     Delta: covalently linked to albumin
	 Urine bilirubin
	 Serum bile acids
	 Plasma membrane enzymes (from damage to bile canaliculus)[†]
	 Serum alkaline phosphatase
	 Serum γ-glutamyl transpeptidase
	 Serum 5'-nucleotidase

Hepatocyte function	Proteins secreted into the blood *Serum albumin*[‡] *Prothrombin time*[†] (factors V, VII, X, prothrombin, fibrinogen) Hepatocyte metabolism Serum ammonia[†] Aminopyrine breath test (hepatic demethylation)[‡] Galactose elimination (intravenous injection)[‡]

*The most common tests are in italics.
[†]An elevation implicates liver disease.
[‡]A decrease implicates liver disease.

- *Hepatic dysfunction without overt necrosis:* Viable hepatocytes unable to perform normal metabolic functions (e.g., tetracycline toxicity)

Clinical Features (p. 836)

The manifestations of liver failure—reflecting the loss of normal hepatocyte function— are the same regardless of etiology.

- Jaundice
- Hypoalbuminemia with systemic edema
- Hyperammonemia (see later discussion)
- *Fetor hepaticus,* an odor related to mercaptan formation
- Hyperestrogenemia due to impaired estrogen metabolism with palmar erythema, spider angiomata, hypogonadism, and gynecomastia

Complications include:

- Coagulopathy (inadequate hepatic synthesis of clotting factors)
- Multiple organ failure
- *Hepatic encephalopathy,* a life-threatening disorder of CNS and neuromuscular transmission; it is caused by porto-systemic shunting and loss of hepatocellular function. Resulting excess ammonia in the blood impairs neuronal function and causes brain edema, leading to disturbances in consciousness (confusion to coma), limb rigidity, hyperreflexia, and asterixis.
- *Hepatorenal syndrome,* causing renal failure; the etiology is decreased renal perfusion pressure, followed by renal vasoconstriction, with sodium retention and impaired free-water

excretion. The incidence is 8% per year in patients with cirrhosis and ascites; prognosis is poor.

- *Hepatopulmonary syndrome,* presenting with hypoxia. The likely cause is intrapulmonary vascular dilation (due to increased nitric oxide) and functional shunting of blood from pulmonary arteries to veins; altered blood flow causes ventilation-perfusion mismatch.

Cirrhosis (p. 837)

Cirrhosis is the twelfth leading cause of death in the United States. The most common causes worldwide are alcohol abuse, viral hepatitis, and non-alcoholic steatohepatitis, with biliary disease and hemochromatosis being less frequent. In 20% of cases, an etiology cannot be ascertained *(cryptogenic cirrhosis)*. There are three morphologic characteristics of cirrhosis:

- *Bridging fibrosis* linking portal tracts to each other and to central veins
- *Parenchymal nodules* resulting from hepatocyte regeneration when encircled by fibrosis
- Disruption of hepatic parenchymal architecture

Pathogenesis (p. 837)

The central features are hepatocyte death, extracellular matrix (ECM) deposition, and vascular reorganization. Interstitial collagen (types I and III), which is normally concentrated in portal tracts and around central veins, becomes extensively deposited in the space of Disse. Sinusoidal endothelium loses its fenestrations, and the vascular architecture is further disrupted by liver damage and fibrosis; new vascular channels bypass the parenchyma by shunting blood directly from the portal triads to the central veins. Throughout, the surviving hepatocytes are stimulated to regenerate, doing so as spherical nodules within the fibrous septa.

Although portal fibroblasts also contribute collagen, the predominant source of fibrosis is the proliferation and activation of hepatic *stellate cells;* driven by increased expression of platelet-derived growth factor receptor β, these stellate cells become highly fibrogenic and myofibroblast-like. Besides increased collagen synthesis, these cells are contractile and can increase intrahepatic vascular resistance. Stellate cells and portal fibroblasts are activated by:

- Proinflammatory cytokines (e.g., tumor necrosis factor-α [TNF-α] and interleukin-1β [IL-1β] from chronic inflammation)
- Cytokines (e.g. transforming growth factor-β [TGF-β]) released by endogenous cells (e.g., Kupffer cells, endothelial cells, hepatocytes, bile duct epithelium)
- Disruption of the ECM
- Direct toxin stimulation

Clinical Features (p. 838)

Cirrhosis can be clinically silent until far advanced (i.e., 40% of patients); it ultimately presents with anorexia, weight loss, weakness, and debilitation. Overt hepatic failure can be precipitated by intercurrent infection or gastrointestinal hemorrhage. Death is caused by:

- Progressive liver failure (as discussed previously)
- Complications of portal hypertension (see later discussion)
- Hepatocellular carcinoma (see later discussion)

Portal Hypertension (p. 838)

Portal hypertension results from a combination of increased flow into the portal circulation and/or increased resistance to portal blood flow; causes are:

- *Prehepatic:* Thrombosis, portal vein narrowing, increased splanchnic arterial circulation, or massive splenomegaly with increased splenic vein blood flow
- *Intrahepatic:* Cirrhosis (most common), schistosomiasis, massive fatty change, granulomatous disease, or nodular regenerative hyperplasia
- *Posthepatic:* Right-sided heart failure, constrictive pericarditis, or hepatic vein obstruction

Major clinical consequences of portal hypertension are:

- *Ascites* (p. 839), a collection of excess serous fluid in the peritoneal cavity; most often a consequence of cirrhosis, the pathogenesis involves:

  Hepatic sinusoidal hypertension (exacerbated by hypoalbuminemia)
  Percolation of hepatic lymph into the peritoneal cavity
  Splanchnic vasodilation causing systemic hypotension that triggers vasoconstrictor responses (e.g., renin-angiotensin), with renal retention of sodium and water and subsequent intestinal capillary transudation

- *Portosystemic shunts* (p. 839), which arise as portal pressures rise; flow is reversed from the portal into the systemic circulation where there are shared capillary beds:

  Esophagogastric varices (most significant), which occur in 40% of patients with advanced cirrhosis; these rupture and can cause massive hematemesis; each bleed has a 30% mortality.
  Rectum (hemorrhoids).
  Falciform ligament and umbilicus *(caput medusa).*

- *Splenomegaly* (p. 839), caused by long-standing congestion; can cause thrombocytopenia (or even pancytopenia) due to hypersplenism.

Jaundice and Cholestasis (p. 839)

Excess bilirubin (the end product of heme degradation) leads to *jaundice* and *icterus* (yellow skin and sclera discoloration, respectively); common causes are bilirubin overproduction, hepatitis, and bile outflow obstruction. *Cholestasis* denotes retention of all bile solutes including bilirubin, bile salts, and cholesterol.

Bilirubin and Bile Formation (p. 839)

The degradation of heme (more than 85% is derived from hemoglobin) throughout the body progresses from biliverdin to bilirubin; the latter is bound to albumin and delivered to the liver. After carrier-mediated uptake, bilirubin is conjugated with 1 to 2 molecules of glucuronic acid by the hepatic endoplasmic transferase UGT1A1. The resulting water-soluble bilirubin glucuronides are excreted in the bile and subsequently deconjugated by gut bacteria and degraded to urobilinogens that are primarily fecally eliminated; 20% of urobilinogens are resorbed and recycled to the liver, with a small fraction excreted in the urine.

Bile acids are water-soluble modifications of cholesterol (mostly cholic acid and chenodeoxycholic acid) that act as detergents to solubilize dietary and biliary lipids. Bile salts (bile acids conjugated to taurine or glycine) constitute two thirds of bile organic compounds. More than 95% of bile acids and salts are reabsorbed from the gut and recirculate back to the liver *(enterohepatic circulation).*

Pathophysiology of Jaudice (p. 840)

Jaundice occurs when bilirubin production exceeds hepatic uptake, conjugation, and/or excretion. Excess production or diminished uptake and/or conjugation causes *unconjugated hyperbilirubinemia;* defective excretion (intrahepatic or bile flow related) causes mostly *conjugated hyperbilirubinemia.*

- *Unconjugated bilirubin* is virtually insoluble in water; it normally circulates tightly bound to albumin and cannot be excreted in urine. A small amount of unconjugated bilirubin circulates as a free anion that can diffuse into tissues (especially neonatal brain), and cause injury; this unbound fraction can increase with severe hemolysis, or when drugs displace bilirubin from albumin.
- *Conjugated bilirubin* is water-soluble, non-toxic, and only loosely bound to albumin; excess conjugated bilirubin can be renally excreted

Neonatal Jaundice (p. 841)

Because hepatic metabolic machinery does not mature until roughly 2 weeks of age, almost every newborn develops transient, mild unconjugated hyperbilirubinemia. This can be exacerbated by breast-feeding due to bilirubin-deconjugating enzymes in breast milk.

Hereditary Hyperbilirubinemias (p. 841)

- *Unconjugated hyperbilirubinemia*

  Crigler-Najjar syndrome type I (autosomal recessive): Total absence of UGT1A1 causes jaundice with high serum levels of unconjugated bilirubin and a histologically normal liver. Without liver transplantation, fatal neurologic damage *(kernicterus)* will ensue.

  Crigler-Najjar syndrome type II (autosomal dominant): Less severe UGT1A1 deficiency. Although kernicterus can occur, the condition is not usually lethal.

  Gilbert syndrome (autosomal recessive): Mild, fluctuating unconjugated hyperbilirubinemia, with 30% reduction in UGT1A1 activity attributable in most cases to a mutation that affects gene transcription. Affecting 6% to 10% of the population, the hyperbilirubinemia (and jaundice) may be exacerbated by infection, stenuous exercise, or fasting.

- *Conjugated hyperbilirubinemia:*

  Dubin-Johnson syndrome (autosomal recessive): Defective hepatocyte secretion of bilirubin conjugates due to absent multidrug resistance protein 2 (MDR2), a camalicular protein responsible for bilirubin glucuronide transport. The liver is brown, with accumulated pigment granules (polymers of epinephrine metabolites, *not* bilirubin pigment). Patients are jaundiced but have normal life expectancy.

  Rotor syndrome (autosomal recessive): Defective hepatocellular bilirubin uptake or excretion. The liver is not pigmented; patients are jaundiced but have normal life spans.

Cholestasis (p. 842)

Cholestasis denotes impaired bile formation or flow, leading to the accumulation of intrahepatic bile pigments. Cholestasis can be extrahepatic (due to duct obstruction) or intrahepatic (due to hepatocellular dysfunction or canalicular obstruction). Consequences include jaundice, *pruritus* from bile salt retention, *xanthomas* (skin accumulations of cholesterol), and intestinal malabsorption. Serum alkaline phosphatase and γ-glutamyl transpeptidase (GGT) are characteristically elevated.

Morphology (p. 842)

Whether intra- or extrahepatic cholestasis, bile pigment accumulates within the hepatic parenchyma, leading to dilated bile canaliculi and hepatocyte degeneration.

- Obstruction also leads to distended proliferating bile ducts in the portal tracts, with edema and periductular neutrophils.
- Prolonged obstruction can cause extensive hepatocyte injury with the formation of bile lakes, *portal tract fibrosis*, and eventually cirrhosis.

Progressive familial intrahepatic cholestasis (PFIC) (p. 843) is a heterogeneous group of autosomal recessive disorders caused by mutations in one of three adenosine triphosphate (ATP)-dependent transporter proteins:

- PFIC-1 *(Byler disease)* involves mutations in the *ATP8B1* gene, resulting in impaired bile secretion; cholestasis begins in infancy and relentlessly progresses to liver failure before adulthood. There is no damage to the canaliculi or biliary tree; thus, GGT levels are normal and portal tracts do not exhibit bile duct proliferation.

Benign recurrent intrahepatic cholestasis is a milder form of PFIC-1 (affecting the same gene) with only intermittent attacks of cholestasis and without progression to chronic liver disease.

- PFIC-2 involves mutations in the *ABCB11* gene coding for the hepatocyte canalicular *bile salt export pump;* besides cholestasis, patients exhibit extreme pruritus, growth failure, and progression to cirrhosis in the first decade. GGT levels are normal.
- PFIC-3 is caused by mutations in the *ABCB4* gene; this encodes the MDR3 protein responsible for biliary phosphatidylcholine secretion. Serum GGT levels are high because the biliary epithelium is damaged by the full detergent action of bile salts.

Infectious Disorders (p. 843)

Viral Hepatitis (p. 843)

Several systemic viral infections can involve the liver (e.g., Epstein-Barr virus [EBV], cytomegalovirus, and yellow fever virus). Less commonly—usually in children and immunosuppressed individuals—rubella, adenovirus, enterovirus, and herpesvirus also cause hepatic infections. Nevertheless, unless specified, the term *viral hepatitis refers only to infection of the liver by the hepatotropic viruses A, B, C, D, or E.* All produce similar clinical and morphologic patterns of acute hepatitis, but they vary in their routes of transmission and potential to induce carrier states or chronic disease (Table 18-2).

Hepatitis A Virus (p. 844)

Hepatitis A virus (HAV) is a single-stranded RNA virus that causes a benign, self-limited disease; fulminant HAV is rare (fatality rate less than 0.1%). It is not directly cytopathic; hepatocyte damage is due to CD8+ T cell responses. HAV accounts for 25% of acute hepatitis worldwide; it has a fecal-oral route of spread. Acute infection is marked by anti-HAV immunoglobulin M (IgM) in serum; IgG appears as IgM declines (within a few months) and persists for years, conferring long-term immunity. An effective vaccine is available.

Hepatitis B Virus (p. 845)

Hepatitis B virus (HBV) can cause (Fig. 18-1):

- Acute, self-limited hepatitis
- Non-progressive chronic hepatitis

TABLE 18-2   The Hepatic Viruses

Feature	Hepatitis A	Hepatitis B	Hepatitis C	Hepatitis D	Hepatitis E
Type of virus	ssRNA	Partially dsDNA	ssRNA	Circular defective ssRNA	ssRNA
Viral family	Hepatovirus; related to picornavirus	Hepadnavirus	Flaviridae	Subviral particle in Deltaviridae family	Calicivirus
Route of transmission	Fecal-oral (contaminated food or water)	Parenteral, sexual contact, perinatal	Parenteral; intranasal cocaine use is a risk factor	Parenteral	Fecal-oral
Mean incubation period	2 to 4 weeks	1 to 4 months	7 to 8 weeks	Same as HBV	4 to 5 weeks
Frequency of chronic liver disease	Never	10%	~80%	5% (co-infection); ≤70% for superinfection	Never
Diagnosis	Detection of serum IgM antibodies	Detection of HBsAg or antibody to HBcAg	PCR for HCV RNA; third-generation ELISA for antibody detection	Detection of IgM and IgG antibodies; HDV RNA serum; HDAg in liver	PCR for HEV RNA; detection of serum IgM and IgG antibodies

dsDNA, Double-stranded DNA; *ELISA*, enzyme-linked immunosorbent assay; *HBcAg*, hepatitis B core antigen; *HBsAg*, hepatitis B surface antigen; *HBV*, hepatitis B virus; *HCV*, hepatitis C virus; *HDAg*, hepatitis D antigen; *HDV*, hepatitis D virus; *HEV*, hepatitis E virus; *IV*, intravenous; *PCR*, polymerase chain reaction; *ssRNA*, single stranded RNA.

Data from Washington K: Inflammatory and infectious diseases of the liver. In Iacobuzio-Donahue CA, Montgomery EA (eds): *Gastrointestinal and liver pathology*, Philadelphia, 2005, Churchill Livingstone.

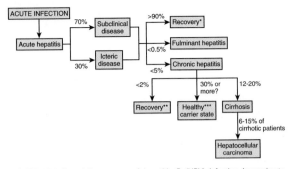

FIGURE 18-1 Potential outcomes of hepatitis B (HBV) infection (approximate frequencies in the United States). *Recovery from acute hepatitis refers to complete recovery, or latent infections with maintained T cell responses. **Recovery from chronic hepatitis is indicated by a negative hepatitis B surface antigen (HBsAg) test. *** Healthy carrier state is reflected by persistent HBsAg positivity, hepatitis B e antigen (HBeAg) negativity, and HBV DNA less than 10^5 copies/mL, with normal serum aspartate aminotransferase (AST) and serum alanine aminotransferase (ALT) levels and minimal inflammation and necrosis on liver biopsy.

- Progressive chronic disease culminating in cirrhosis (and increased risk of hepatocellular carcinoma)
- Fulminant hepatitis with massive liver necrosis
- Asymptomatic carrier state

The host immune response to the virus is the major determinant of the outcome of infection. Innate immunity is protective during the initial phases of infection, and strong responses by virus-specific CD4+ and CD8+ interferon (IFN)-γ–producing cells is associated with resolution. Antibodies prevent subsequent re-infection and form the basis of effective vaccines. HBV is not cytopathic; rather, hepatocyte killing is mediated by cytotoxic CD8+ T lymphocytes directed against virus-infected cells. Viral DNA sequences can also integrate into host genomes, constituting a pathway for cancer development.

HBV is a circular, partially double-stranded DNA virus; mature virus exists as a spherical *Dane particle* with an outer surface protein and lipid envelope encasing an electron-dense core. There are eight viral genotypes with distinct global distributions. The HBV genome has four open reading frames:

- Nucleocapsid core antigen (HBcAg), plus a longer polypeptide transcript (HBeAg) that is secreted into the bloodstream.
- Hepatitis B surface antigen (HBsAg) envelope glycoproteins (large, middle, and small); infected hepatocytes can synthesize and secrete massive quantities of noninfective HBsAg (mostly small HBsAg).
- Polymerase with both DNA polymerase and reverse transcriptase activity; viral replication occurs through an intermediate RNA template: DNA → RNA → DNA.
- Hbx protein, a transcriptional transactivator of host and viral genes, necessary for viral replication.

HBsAg appears before symptoms (anorexia, fever, jaundice), peak during overt disease, and it declines over months. HBeAg and HBV DNA appear soon after HBsAg and before disease onset; HBeAg is detectable in serum during viral replication although some mutant strains do not produce it. HBeAg usually declines within weeks; persistence suggests progression to chronic disease.

IgM anti-HBcAg is usually the first antibody to appear, followed shortly by anti-HBeAg and IgG anti-HBcAg. Anti-HBsAg signifies the end of acute disease and persists for years, conferring immunity. A chronic carrier is defined by the presence of HBsAg in serum for 6 months.

More than 2 billion people worldwide have been infected, and 400 million have chronic infections; there are 46,000 new cases annually in the United States. The mode of transmission varies geographically; in high-prevalence areas (i.e., Africa, Asia), transmission during childbirth accounts for 90%. In intermediate-prevalence regions (i.e., southern and eastern Europe), horizontal transmission in childhood by minor cuts or breaks in mucus membranes is most common. In low-prevalence areas (i.e., United States and western Europe), intravenous (IV) drug abuse and unprotected intercourse (hetero- or homosexual) are the major modes of transmission.

Hepatitis C Virus (p. 847)

Hepatitis C virus (HCV) is a single-stranded RNA enveloped virus. Low fidelity of the HCV RNA polymerase causes substantial genomic variability and constitutes a major obstacle to vaccine development; indeed, any given individual can harbor a population of related but divergent *quasispecies*. Viral replication begins with translation of a single polypeptide that is processed into nucleocapsid protein, envelope proteins, and seven nonstructural proteins; the E2 envelope protein is a target of several anti-HCV antibodies, but it is also the most variable region of the genome, allowing escape from otherwise neutralizing titers. Thus, anti-HCV antibodies do not confer protection, and a characteristic feature of HCV infection is repeated bouts of damage. *As opposed to HBV, progression to chronic disease occurs in most (80% to 85%) HCV-infected patients, and cirrhosis occurs in 20% to 30%.* Like HBV, hepatocellular damage is immune-mediated, although the cellular immune responses are largely unable to completely eradicate HCV infections.

In the United States, 4.1 million individuals are infected (accounting for half of the U.S. burden of chronic liver disease); the incidence is declining as a result of blood supply screening. Primary risk groups are intravenous drug abusers and individuals with multiple sexual partners. HCV RNA is detectable in blood for 1 to 3 weeks during active infection coincident with transaminase elevations; anti-HCV antibodies occur in only 50% to 70% of patients in the acute setting, although 90% of patients with chronic disease eventually develop such antibodies. Chronic HCV infection is potentially curable; treatment includes IFN-γ and ribovarin.

Hepatitis D Virus (p. 848)

Hepatitis D virus (HDV) is a defective RNA virus that can replicate and cause infection only when encapsulated by HBsAg. Thus, *HDV infection can develop only when there is concomitant HBV infection. Acute co-infection* by HDV and HBV leads to hepatitis that ranges from mild to fulminant, but chronicity rarely develops. In comparison, HDV *superinfection* of an unrecognized HBV carrier or in a patient with chronic HBV leads to eruption of acute hepatitis, with frequent conversion to chronic disease and cirrhosis (see Table 18-2). There is a high prevalence (20% to 40%) of HDV in Africa, the Middle East, Italy, and the Amazon basin; it is uncommon in the United States, Southeast Asia, and China.

HDV is composed of a *Dane-like particle* with an HBV envelope; HDV produces only one protein, which forms part of an internal polypeptide assembly, called the *delta antigen,* associated with a small, circular, single-stranded RNA. Viral replication requires host RNA polymerase activity.

HDV RNA appears in blood and liver before and during early acute symptomatic infection. IgM anti-HDV indicates recent HDV exposure; IgM anti-HBcAg suggests acute HBV co-infection while serum HBsAg implies a superinfection. Vaccination against HBV can prevent HDV infection.

Hepatitis E Virus *(p. 849)*

Hepatitis E virus (HEV) is a non-enveloped, single-stranded RNA virus; it is an enterically transmitted water-borne infection with several animal reservoirs (e.g., monkeys, cats, pigs, and dogs). HEV epidemics have occurred in Asia, Mexico, and Africa; HEV is also endemic in India, where 30% to 60% of cases of acute hepatitis are HEV related. Although HEV is typically a self-limiting disease with no tendency to chronicity, *there is a high rate (i.e., 20%) of fatal fulminant hepatitis in pregnant women* (see Table 18-2). HEV antigen is found in hepatocytes during active infection, and virions and RNA can be detected in stool and serum before symptom onset. The subsequent development of IgG anti-HEV confers long-lived protection against re-infection.

Hepatitis G Virus *(p. 849)*

Hepatitis G virus (HGV) a non-pathogenic RNA virus (similar to HCV) present in 1% to 4% of United States blood donors; it is not hepatotropic and does not cause transaminase elevations but rather replicates in marrow and spleen.

Clinicopathologic Syndromes of Viral Hepatitis *(p. 850)*

Infection by any of the hepatotropic viruses can be asymptomatic or symptomatic; a fulminant course is uncommon.

- *Acute asymptomatic infection with recovery* (p. 850): Patients are identified only incidentally based on elevated transaminases, or by anti-viral antibody titers. HAV and HBV infections are frequently sub-clinical.
- *Acute symptomatic infection with recovery* (p. 850): Acute symptomatic infections are all similar, with a variable incubation period, asymptomatic pre-icteric phase, symptomatic icteric phase, and convalescence. Peak infectivity occurs during the last asymptomatic days of the incubation period and the early days of acute symptoms.
- *Chronic hepatitis* (p. 850): This is defined as symptomatic disease (e.g., fatigue, malaise, jaundice) with biochemical or serologic evidence of ongoing hepatic damage for more than 6 months. HCV frequently progresses to chronic hepatitis while HBV and HDV do so less commonly; HAV and HEV do not cause chronic disease. Age at the time of infection is the best predictor of developing chronicity; younger patients are more likely to develop chronic hepatitis, and maternal-fetal transmission confers substantial risk. Besides ongoing liver injury and the risk of cirrhosis and/or hepatocellular carcinoma, immune complex disease (due to circulating antibody-antigen complexes) may develop with vasculitis and glomerulonephritis; 35% of chronic hepatitis C patients develop cryoglobulinemia.
- *The carrier state* (p. 850): A *carrier* harbors and can transmit hepatitis but has no manifest symptoms. This includes patients with chronic disease but few or no symptoms and those with few or no adverse effects *(healthy carriers)*; for HBV, healthy carriers lack HBeAg, but have anti-HBeAg, normal serum

aminotransferase levels, low serum HBV DNA, and a liver biopsy without significant necrosis or inflammation. In the United States, less than 1% of adult HBV infections produce a carrier state; in contrast, more than 90% of HBV infections acquired early in life in endemic areas result in carrier states.

- *HIV and chronic viral hepatitis* (p. 850): Similar transmission modes and risks result in frequent HIV and hepatitis virus co-infections; 10% of HIV patients are infected with HBV and 30% with HCV, often resulting in more aggressive liver disease. Chronic hepatitis is a major cause of morbidity and mortality in HIV-infected patients, and liver disease is the second most common cause of death in AIDS.

Morphology of Acute and Chronic Hepatitis (p. 851)

Most of the morphologic changes are shared by all the hepatotropic viruses; these features are largely non-specific and can be mimicked by drug reactions or autoimmune liver disease. Nevertheless, a few histologic changes can suggest a specific virus: in HBV, infected hepatocytes can show a finely granular "ground glass" cytoplasm packed with HBsAg; in HCV, there are often portal lymphoid aggregates, bile duct reactive changes, and lobular regions of macrovesicular steatosis.

Acute hepatitis:

- Injured hepatocytes are eosinophilic and rounded with shrunken or fragmented nuclei *(apoptosis)*, or are swollen *(ballooning degeneration)*. In severe hepatitis, confluent damage causes *bridging necrosis* between portal and central regions of adjacent lobules. Cholestasis can occur.
- There is Kupffer cell hyperplasia, and macrophage aggregates mark the site of hepatocyte loss. Portal tracts exhibit mononuclear cell inflammation, often with spillover into the adjacent parenchyma associated with periportal apoptosis *(interface hepatitis)*.

Chronic hepatitis:

- Histologic changes range from exceedingly mild to severe to cirrhosis.
- In mild disease, the inflammatory infiltrates are limited to portal tracts.
- Progressive disease is marked by extension of chronic inflammation from portal tracts with *interface hepatitis;* linking of portal-portal and portal-central regions constitutes *bridging necrosis.*
- Continued loss of hepatocytes results in fibrous septum formation; associated hepatocyte regeneration results in cirrhosis.

Fulminant hepatic failure (p. 853) is defined by hepatic insufficiency with hepatic encephalopathy occurring within 2 to 3 weeks after symptom onset. Viral hepatitis (HBV more than HAV much more than HCV and other viruses) is the cause in 12% of cases of fulminant liver failure; more than half of the cases of fulminant hepatic failure are due to drug or chemical toxicity, and 15% have unknown causes. In HBV-induced fulminant hepatitis, there is massive hepatocyte apoptosis. Mortality rate is 80% without transplantation and 35% with transplantation.

Morphology of Fulminant Hepatitis (p. 853)

The entire liver, or just portions, may be involved; in massive disease, the liver is shrunken. Affected areas are soft and muddy-red or bile-stained. Entire lobules are destroyed, leaving cellular debris and a collapsed reticulin network; inflammation may be minimal. With substantial destruction, regeneration is disorderly with scarring that produces a coarsely lobulated pattern of cirrhosis.

Bacterial, Parasitic, and Helminthic Infections (p. 854)

- Extrahepatic infections (especially sepsis) can induce hepatic inflammation and varying degrees of cholestasis; this is related to Kupffer cell and endothelial cell production of cytokines in response to circulating endotoxin.
- Biliary obstruction and intra-biliary bacterial proliferation can cause a severe acute inflammatory response (ascending cholangitis).
- Parasitic infections (e.g., amebic, echinococcal, malarial, or helminthic organisms) are common causes of hepatic abscesses in developing countries (Chapter 8).
- Abscesses occurring in developed countries are rare and are usually bacterial or candidal; sources are intra-abdominal (via portal vein), systemic (via arterial supply), biliary tree, direct extension, and penetrating injuries. Abscesses are associated with fever, right upper quadrant pain, tender hepatomegaly, and possibly jaundice. Mortality rate ranges from 30% to 90%; survival is improved by early recognition. Rupture of echinoccal cysts can precipitate systemic spread of the organism with severe immune-mediated shock

Morphology (p. 854)

Histologic features are those seen in any abscess; parasitic fragments or fungal organisms may be identifiable. Echinococcal infections develop characteristic cystic structures with laminated (and often calcified) walls; hooklets and intact organisms can often be identified.

Autoimmune Hepatitis (p. 855)

Autoimmune hepatitis (AIH) is a chronic, progressive hepatitis attributed to T-cell–mediated autoimmunity (cytotoxic T cells, and T-cell production of IFN-γ); AIH can be triggered by viral infections or drugs, or it may be a component of other autoimmune disorders (e.g., rheumatoid arthritis, Sjögren syndrome, or ulcerative colitis). The entire histologic spectrum of hepatitis can be seen in AIH, but clusters of periportal plasma cells is characteristic.

There is a female predominance (78% of cases), with elevated serum IgG levels but no serum markers of viral infection. AIH is classified on the basis of the patterns of autoantibodies (in the United States, type 1 is much more common):

- Type 1 AIH shows autoantibodies to nuclear, smooth muscle, actin, and soluble liver antigen/liver-pancreas antigens; it is associated with the HLA-DR3 haplotype.
- Type 2 AIH exhibits autoantibodies directed against the liver kidney microsome-1 and liver cytosol-1 antigens.

Acute onset of symptoms of liver failure occurs in 40% of patients; symptomatic patients tend to show substantial liver destruction and scarring at the time of diagnosis. Untreated, 6-month mortality can reach 40%, and 40% of survivors will develop cirrhosis. Immunosuppression is a mainstay of therapy, with transplantation for end-stage disease; AIH recurs in 22% to 42% of transplants.

Drug- and Toxin-Induced Liver Disease (p. 856)

Damage from toxin or drug should be considered in the differential diagnosis of any form of liver disease (e.g., hepatocyte necrosis, hepatitis, cholestasis, fibrosis, or insidious onset of liver dysfunction)

TABLE 18-3   Patterns of Injury in Drug- and Toxin-Induced Hepatic Injury

Pattern of Injury	Examples of Associated Agents
Cholestatsis	Contraceptive and anabolic steroids; estrogen replacement therapy
Cholestatic hepatitis	Numerous antibiotics; phenothiazines
Hepatocellular necrosis	Methyldopa, phenytoin acetaminophen, halothane isoniazid, phenytoin
Steatosis	Ethanol, methotrexate, corticosteroids, total parenteral nutrition
Steatohepatitis	Amiodarone, ethanol
Fibrosis and cirrhosis	Methotrexate, isoniazid, enalapril
Granulomas	Sulfonamides, numerous other agents
Vascular lesions	High-dose chemotherapy, bush teas, oral contraceptives, numerous other agents, anabolic steroids, tamoxifen
Neoplasms	Oral contraceptives, anabolic steroids Thorotrast, vinyl chloride

Data from Washington K: Metabolic and toxic conditions of the liver. In Iacobuzio-Donahue CA, Montgomery EA (eds): *Gastrointestinal and liver pathology*, Philadelphia, 2005, Churchill Livingstone.

(Table 18-3). Injury due to drugs or toxins can be immediate or develop over weeks to months; mechanisms include direct toxicity, hepatic conversion to an active toxin, or immune-mediated injury.

Some compounds are predictably toxic, whereas others can idiosyncratically cause injury. Thus, *acetaminophen* in sufficiently high doses is uniformly hepatotoxic; indeed, it is the leading cause of drug-induced acute liver failure. Conversely, *Reye syndrome* is a rare, but potentially fatal, syndrome of mitochondrial dysfunction, characterized by massive microvesicular steatosis; it occurs unpredictably in children receiving aspirin for febrile illness.

Alcoholic Liver Disease (p. 857)

Alcoholic liver disease (ALD) is the leading cause of liver pathology in most Western countries; it affects more than 2 million Americans and causes 27,000 deaths annually. There are three (overlapping) forms:

Morphology (p. 857)

- *Hepatic steatosis (fatty liver)* is marked by microvesicular lipid droplets within hepatocytes and can occur with even moderate alcohol intake. With chronic alcohol intake, lipid accumulates in *macrovesicular* droplets, displacing the nucleus. The liver becomes enlarged, soft, greasy, and yellow. There is little to no fibrosis (at least initially) and the condition is reversible.
- *Alcoholic hepatitis* is characterized by ballooning degeneration and hepatocyte necrosis. There is also *Mallory body* formation (intracellular eosinophilic aggregates of intermediate filaments), *neutrophilic reaction* to degenerating hepatocytes, portal and periportal mononuclear inflammation, and *fibrosis*.

- *Alcoholic cirrhosis* is the final and largely irreversible outcome. The liver is transformed from fatty and enlarged to brown, shrunken, and nonfatty. Regenerative nodules can be prominent or obliterated by dense fibrous scar. End-stage alcoholic cirrhosis resembles cirrhosis of virtually any other cause.

Pathogenesis (p. 858)

- Only 10% to 15% of alcoholics develop cirrhosis, suggesting other factors in the development and severity of ALD:

    Gender: Women are more susceptible to alcohol-related damage. This is partly related to gender-related alcohol pharmacokinetics and metabolism; however, estrogen also increases gut permeability to endotoxin, with subsequent Kupffer cell activation and increased pro-inflammatory cytokine production.

    Ethnicity: African-Americans have higher cirrhosis rates than white Americans, independent of alcohol consumption levels.

    Genetics: Polymorphisms in metabolizing enzymes (e.g., aldehyde dehydrogenase) or cytokine promoters are associated with higher frequencies of alcoholic cirrhosis.

    Co-morbid disease: Iron overload or viral hepatitis increases the severity of ALD.

- *Steatosis* results from:

    Impaired lipoprotein assembly and secretion
    Increased peripheral catabolism of fat
    Shunting of substrates away from catabolism and toward lipid biosynthesis.

- The injury in *alcoholic hepatitis* results from:

    Acetaldehyde generated from alcohol catabolism inducing lipid peroxidation and acetaldehyde-protein adduct formation.

    Induction of cytochrome P-450 generating reactive oxygen species (ROS) and augmenting catabolism of other drugs to form potentially toxic metabolites.

    Impaired metabolism of methionine resulting in reduced glutathione levels that are normally protective for oxidative injury.

    Alcohol becoming a *caloric food source,* resulting in malnutrition and vitamin deficiency.

    Alcohol-mediated release of bacterial endotoxin from the gastrointestinal tract causing increasing inflammatory responses.

- *Cirrhosis* is the result of collagen deposition by perisinusoidal stellate cells (described previously). Hepatic blood flow is also deranged by the result of progressive fibrosis, as well as alcohol-induced release of vasoconstrictive *endothelins* from sinusoidal endothelial cells.

Clinical Features (p. 859)

- *Hepatic steatosis* is associated with hepatomegaly, as well as mild elevations of serum bilirubin and alkaline phosphatase. Abstention and adequate diet are sufficient treatments.
- *Alcoholic hepatitis* usually manifests acutely after a bout of heavy drinking; manifestations range from minimal to fulminant hepatic failure and include malaise, anorexia, and tender hepatomegaly. Bilirubin and alkaline phosphatase are elevated, accompanied by neutrophilic leukocytosis. Each bout incurs 10% to 20% mortality, and repeated incidents lead to cirrhosis in a third of patients. Typically, adequate nutrition and abstention leads to a slow resolution; occasionally, the hepatitis persists and progresses to cirrhosis.

- *Alcoholic cirrhosis* is irreversible; its manifestations are similar to any other form of cirrhosis.

   Proximate causes of death are hepatic coma, massive gastrointestinal hemorrhage, intercurrent infection, hepatorenal syndrome, and hepatocellular carcinoma.

Metabolic Liver Disease (p. 860)

Nonalcoholic Fatty Liver Disease (p. 860)

Nonalcoholic fatty liver disease (NAFLD) is a group of conditions characterized by hepatic steatosis in the absence of heavy alcohol consumption. The rising incidence (30% of Americans) is attributed to the increasing prevalence of obesity; 70% of overweight individuals have some form of NAFLD. At the most pathologic end of this group, *nonalcoholic steatohepatitis (NASH)* presents with steatosis plus hepatocyte damage and inflammation; it progresses to cirrhosis in 10% to 20% of cases. NASH is also strongly associated with the metabolic syndrome of dyslipidemia, hyperinsulinemia, and insulin resistance.

Pathogenesis (p. 860)

NAFLD is probably a consequence of hepatocyte fat accumulation and increased hepatic oxidative stress, leading to increased lipid peroxidation and ROS generation.

Morphology (p. 860)

Hepatocytes are filled with fat vacuoles in the absence of inflammatory infiltration (steatosis), or with inflammatory infiltrates (steatohepatitis).Varying degrees of fibrosis are present.

Clinical Features (p. 860)

Patients with simple steatosis are generally asymptomatic. With NASH, individuals can be symptom free although many report fatigue, malaise, and/or right upper quadrant discomfort; serum transaminase levels are elevated. Because of the association between NASH and the metabolic syndrome, cardiovascular disease is a frequent cause of morbidity and mortality. Treatment is therefore targeted at correcting the associated obesity, hyperlipidemia, and insulin resistance.

Hemochromatosis (p. 861)

Hemochromatosis is characterized by excessive iron accumulation in the parenchymal cells of various organs, particularly liver and pancreas.

- *Hereditary hemochromatosis (primary hemochromatosis)* is a homozygous recessive heritable disorder caused by excessive iron absorption.
- *Hemosiderosis (secondary hemochromatosis)* denotes disorders associated with parenteral iron administration (e.g., repetitive transfusions, ineffective erythropoiesis, increased iron intake, or chronic liver disease).

Pathogenesis (p. 862)

Tissue damage in hemochromatiosis is attributed to direct iron toxicity, presumably via free radical formation with lipid peroxidation, stimulation of collagen formation by hepatocyte stellate cells, and/or iron- and ROS-DNA interactions.

   Total body iron content is regulated by intestinal absorption (Chapter 14). *Hepcidin* exerts the greatest effect by controlling the expression of ferroportin, an iron efflux channel on intestinal epithelium and macrophages; *hepcidin lowers plasma iron, while hepcidin deficiency causes iron overload.* Other proteins involved in iron metabolism (e.g., hemojuvelin, transferrin receptor 2, and HFE) do so largely by modulating hepcidin levels.

The adult form of hemochromatosis is almost always caused by mutations of the *HFE* gene on the short arm of chromosome 6, close to the HLA locus. The most common mutation (more than 70% of patients) is a cysteine-to-tyrosine substitution at amino acid 282 (C282Y) that inactivates HFE and reduces hepcidin expression. The frequency of C282Y heterozygosity is 11% (homozygosity occurs with a frequency of 0.45%). However, disease penetrance is low and the genetic condition alone does not invariably lead to hemochromatosis.

Morphology (p. 862)

Iron (demonstrated by Prussian blue histologic reaction or atomic absorption analysis) accumulates as hemosiderin in various tissues—in decreasing order of severity: liver, pancreas, myocardium, endocrine glands, joints, and skin. Cirrhosis and pancreatic fibrosis are the chief additional morphologic changes.

Clinical Features (p. 863)   *Arthropathy of 2nd & 3rd joint*

Fully developed cases of hemochromatosis uniformly exhibit micronodular cirrhosis; diabetes mellitus and skin pigmentation occur in 75% to 80% of these individuals. Iron accumulation is life-long, but the injury caused by excessive iron is gradual, so that symptoms usually appear after age 40 years. Men predominate (6:1) owing to physiologic iron loss in women (e.g., menstruation, pregnancy) that delays the iron accumulation.

Death can result from cirrhosis (and/or hepatocellular carcinoma) and cardiac involvement. Regular phlebotomy is sufficient treatment; early diagnosis can therefore enable normal life expectancy, and screening of genetic probands is therefore important.

Wilson Disease (p. 863)

This autosomal recessive disorder is caused by mutations of the *ATP7B* gene coding for a canalicular copper-transporting ATPase; copper absorption and delivery to the liver is normal, but copper excretion into the bile is reduced, copper is not incorporated into ceruloplasmin, and ceruloplasmin secretion into the blood is inhibited. This causes copper accumulation in the liver, which results in hepatic injury through ROS generation. In addition, spillover into the circulation of non–ceruloplasmin–bound copper causes hemolysis and pathology in other sites, especially the cornea and brain.

Morphology (p. 864)

Liver damage ranges from minor to severe, manifested by fatty change, acute and chronic hepatitis (with Mallory bodies), cirrhosis, and/or (rarely) massive necrosis. Central nervous system (CNS) toxicity predominantly affects the basal ganglia, with atrophy and even cavitation. Nearly all patients with neurologic involvement develop eye lesions, called *Kayser-Fleischer rings*—green-brown copper deposits in Desçemet's membrane of the corneal limbus.

Clinical Features (p. 864)

Age at onset and clinical presentation are extremely variable; acute or chronic liver disease before age 40 years is the most common initial manifestation. Neuropsychiatric disorders also occur, including mild behavioral changes, frank psychosis, and Parkinson-like symptoms. The biochemical diagnosis is based on decreased serum ceruloplasmin, *increased hepatic copper content,* and increased urinary copper excretion. *Serum copper levels are of no diagnostic value.* Copper chelation is standard therapy; liver transplantation may be necessary.

α_1-Antitrypsin Deficiency (p. 864)

α_1-Antitrypsin (α_1-AT) deficiency is an autosomal recessive disorder marked by very low serum levels of this protease inhibitor (Pi); deficiency leads primarily to emphysema (Chapter 15) and hepatic disease (cholestasis or cirrhosis).

Pathogenesis (p. 865)

α_1-AT is synthesized primarily by hepatocytes. The gene is extremely polymorphic with more than 75 isoforms designated alphabetically based on gel migration mobilities; the most common genotype (more than 90% of people) is designated PiMM. Most mutations result in no or only moderate reductions in α_1-AT levels and have no clinical manifestations. However, PiZZ homozygotes (the most common disease genotype) have circulating α_1-AT levels below 10% of normal. This occurs because PiZ has a single glutamic acid to lysine substitution, resulting in protein misfolding and preventing egress from the endoplasmic reticulum. This triggers the endoplasmic reticulum (ER) stress response, including autophagy, mitochondrial dysfunction, and pro-inflammatory nuclear factor κB (NF-κB) activation, all causing hepatocyte damage. Additional genetic or environmental factors modify the pathogenesis, since only 10% to 15% of PiZZ homozygotes develop overt liver disease.

Morphology (p. 865)

α_1-AT deficiency is characterized by periodic acid–Schiff (PAS)-positive (diastase-resistant) cytoplasmic globules in periportal hepatocytes. Hepatic manifestations range from cholestasis to hepatitis to cirrhosis.

Clinical Features (p. 866)

Neonatal hepatitis with cholestatic jaundice occurs in 10% to 20% of newborns with α_1-AT deficiency; later presentation may be attributable to acute hepatitis or complications of cirrhosis. Hepatocellular carcinoma develops in 2% to 3% of PiZZ homozygous adults. Smoking accentuates lung emphysematous damage. Treatment is liver transplantation.

Neonatal Cholestasis (p. 866)

Neonatal cholestasis (prolonged conjugated hyperbilirubinemia) affects 1 in 2500 live births; infants present with jaundice, dark urine, light stools, and hepatomegaly. The major causes are cholangiopathies (20% of cases; primarily biliary atresia) and a variety of disorders collectively referred to as *neonatal hepatitis* (although not all are inflammatory). No cause is identified in half the cases; α_1-AT deficiency is responsible for 15%, with neonatal infections, toxic exposures, and metabolic diseases (e.g., Niemann-Pick) rounding out the list. Establishing an etiology is important since biliary atresia requires surgical intervention.

Morphology (p. 866)

There is hepatocyte death and lobular disarray, hepatocyte giant cell formation, prominent cholestasis, portal tract inflammation, and extramedullary hematopoiesis. Bile duct proliferation can help distinguish biliary atresia from the other causes of neonatal cholestasis.

Intrahepatic Biliary Tract Disease (p. 866)

These disorders are summarized in Table 18-4.

Secondary Biliary Cirrhosis (p. 867)

This condition arises from uncorrected obstruction of the extrahepatic biliary tree. The most common causes are cholelithiasis (stones), malignancies of the biliary tree or pancreatic head, and strictures from previous surgical procedures; biliary atresia, cystic fibrosis, and choledochal cysts occur in children and are overall less common. Prolonged cholestasis leads to inflammation (described previously), which in turn induces periportal fibrosis and eventually cirrhosis. Subtotal obstruction can promote secondary bacterial infection *(ascending cholangitis)* that aggravates the inflammatory injury.

Primary Biliary Cirrhosis (p. 867)

Primary biliary cirrhosis (PBC) is an autoimmune destructive disorder of the intrahepatic biliary tree leading to portal inflammation and progressing over decades to cirrhosis; it is primarily a disease of middle-aged women.

Morphology (p. 868)

Lesions exhibit varying degrees of severity throughout the liver.

- Dense chronic portal tract inflammation with focal non-caseating granulomas is associated with interlobular bile duct destruction and generalized cholestasis.
- Intrahepatic biliary obstruction leads to progressive secondary upstream damage, with ductular proliferation, as well as inflammation and necrosis of periportal hepatocytes.
- At end stage, PBC is indistinguishable from other forms of cirrhosis.

Clinical Features (p. 868)

Onset is insidious with pruritus, hepatomegaly, jaundice, and xanthomas (from retained cholesterol); with progression to cirrhosis, variceal bleeding and encephalopathy often occur. Serum alkaline phosphatase and cholesterol levels are increased; *antimitochondrial antibodies are highly characteristic of PBC and are elevated in 90% to 95% of patients.* Patients can have extrahepatic autoimmune manifestations (e.g., Sjögren syndrome, scleroderma, thyroiditis, Raynaud phenomenon, and membranous glomerulonephritis). Liver failure is the major cause of mortality, followed by variceal bleeding and intercurrent infections; patients have an increased risk of hepatocellular carcinoma.

Primary Sclerosing Cholangitis (p. 869)

Primary sclerosing cholangitis (PSC) is chronic cholestatic disease distinguished by inflammation and obliterative fibrosis of both the extrahepatic and intrahepatic biliary tree; dilation of the preserved segments yields a characteristic "beading" of injected radiologic contrast material. Patients with PSC also typically have ulcerative colitis (70% of patients); that association and the presence of circulating autoantibodies (antinuclear antibody, anti–smooth muscle antibody, rheumatoid factor and an atypical perinuclear-antineutrophil cytoplasmic antibody against a nuclear envelope protein) all suggest an autoimmune-mediated pathogenesis.

Morphology (p. 869)

Bile ducts exhibit periductular inflammation and concentric (onion-skin) fibrosis, with progressive atrophy and eventual

TABLE 18-4   Distinguishing Features of the Major Intrahepatic Bile Duct Disorders

	Secondary Biliary Cirrhosis	Primary Biliary Cirrhosis	Primary Sclerosing Cholangitis
Etiology	Extrahepatic bile duct obstruction: biliary atresia, gallstones, stricture, carcinoma of pancreatic head	Possibly autoimmune	Unknown, possibly autoimmune; 50% to 70% associated with inflammatory bowel disease
Sex predilection	None	Female to male, 6:1	Female to male, 1:2
Symptoms and signs	Pruritus, jaundice, malaise, dark urine, light stools, hepatosplenomegaly	Same as secondary biliary cirrhosis; insidious onset	Same as secondary biliary cirrhosis; insidious onset
Laboratory findings	Conjugated hyperbilirubinemia, increased serum alkaline phosphatase, bile acids, cholesterol	Same as secondary biliary cirrhosis, plus elevated serum IgM autoantibodies (especially M2 form of anti-mitochondrial antibody)	Same as secondary biliary cirrhosis, plus elevated serum IgM, hypergammaglobulinemia
Important pathologic findings before cirrhosis develops	Prominent bile stasis in bile ducts, bile ductular proliferation with surrounding neutrophils, portal tract edema	Dense lymphocytic infiltrate in portal tracts with granulomatous destruction of bile ducts	Periductal portal tracts fibrosis, segmental stenosis of extrahepatic and intrahepatic bile ducts

IgM, Immunoglobulin M.

luminal obliteration; obstruction culminates in biliary cirrhosis and hepatic failure.

Clinical Features (p. 869)

PSC is most common in middle-aged men. It follows a protracted course (i.e., 5 to 15 years); severe disease is associated with weight loss, ascites, variceal bleeding, and encephalopathy. There is an increased incidence of chronic pancreatitis and hepatocellular carcinoma; 7% of patients develop cholangiocarcinoma. Liver transplantation is the definitive therapy for end-stage disease.

Anomalies of the Biliary Trees (Including Liver Cysts) (p. 869)

These are heterogeneous lesions; they may be found only incidentally or can present as hepatosplenomegaly and portal hypertension. The first four are associated with polycystic kidney disease due to mutations in *PKD1* (Chapter 20).

- *Von Meyenberg complexes* (*"bile duct hamartomas"*; p. 869) are small clusters of dilated bile ducts or cysts within a fibrous stroma; they are extremely common but usually clinically insignificant.
- *Polycystic liver disease* (p. 869) manifests as a handful to hundreds of biliary epithelium-lined lesions. A form *not* associated with polycystic kidney disease is caused by mutations in *PRKCSH*, a gene encoding the protein hepatocystin, a substrate for protein kinase C.
- *Congenital hepatic fibrosis* (p. 870) is caused by incomplete involution of embryonic ductal structures with ensuing portal tract fibrosis, which can cause portal hypertension. This disorder is strongly associated with mutations in the *PKHD1* gene that cause the autosomal recessive forms of polycystic kidney disease.
- *Caroli disease* (p. 870) manifests as segmental dilation of larger ducts of intrahepatic biliary tree with associated bile inspissation; it is frequently complicated by cholelithiasis and hepatic abscesses, with an increased risk of cholangiocarcinoma.
- *Alagille syndrome* (*syndromatic paucity of bile ducts; arteriohepatic dysplasia*) (p. 870) is a rare autosomal dominant disorder characterized by absence of intrahepatic bile ducts. It is caused by mutations in the Jagged 1 (a cell surface protein)-Notch signaling pathway involved in the development of many organ systems. Besides chronic cholestasis, patients often also have extrahepatic anomalies including peculiar facies, and vertebral and cardiovascular defects.

Circulatory Disorders (p. 870)

Impaired Blood Flow into the Liver (p. 870)

Hepatic Artery Compromise (p. 870)

Infarction is rare due to the dual hepatic blood supply; however, thrombosis or compression of intrahepatic arterial branches can infrequently result in localized pale infarct, occasionally made hemorrhagic by portal blood suffusion.

Portal Vein Obstruction and Thrombosis (p. 871)

Manifestations of extrahepatic portal vein obstruction can range from insidious and well tolerated to catastrophic and potentially lethal (e.g., due to variceal bleeding). Causes include neonatal umbilical vein infection intra-abdominal sepsis causing pylephlebitis in the splanchnic circulation, acquired or heritable coagulopathies, trauma, pancreatic lesions that initiate splenic vein thromboses, and cirrhosis.

Impaired Blood Flow through the Liver (p. 871)

Cirrhosis is the most important cause. Sinusoidal occlusion can also be caused by disseminated intravascular coagulation (DIC) (e.g., eclampsia), sickle cell disease, metastatic tumors, and sarcoidosis.

Passive Congestion and Centrilobular Necrosis (p. 872)

Systemic hypoperfusion (e.g., shock) leads to hepatocyte necrosis around the central vein *(centrilobular necrosis)*. With superimposed passive congestion (e.g., right-sided heart failure or constrictive pericarditis), there is hemorrhage as well, producing *centrilobular hemorrhagic necrosis,* with the liver taking on a variegated mottled appearance *(nutmeg liver)*. Protracted right-sided heart failure causes chronic passive congestion and pericentral fibrosis *(cardiac sclerosis)*, eventually culminating in cirrhosis.

Peliosis Hepatitis (p. 872)

Peliosis hepatis is a reversible hepatic sinusoid dilation associated with several disorders including malignancy, acquired immunodeficiency syndrome (AIDS), tuberculosis, and post-transplant immunosuppression. It also occurs with exposure to anabolic steroids (rarely oral contraceptives and danazol). The etiology is unknown.

Hepatic Venous Outflow Obstruction (p. 872)

Hepatic Vein Thrombosis and Inferior Vena Cava Thrombosis (p. 872)

Budd-Chiari syndrome occurs when two or more major hepatic veins are obstructed; hepatic damage is a consequence of increased intrahepatic blood pressure. Hepatic vein thrombosis occurs in the setting of primary myeloproliferative disorders (e.g., polycythemia vera), heritable coagulopathies, pregnancy, anti-phospholipid antibody syndrome, paroxysmal nocturnal hemoglobinuria, and intra-abdominal cancers. A membranous inferior vena cava valve can also cause hepatic venous obstruction.

The mortality of untreated acute hepatic vein thrombosis is high; prompt surgical porto-systemic shunting improves the prognosis. Subacute or chronic cases are considerably less lethal but can develop superimposed fibrosis.

Sinusoidal Obstruction Syndrome (Veno-Occlusive Disease) (p. 873)

Veno-occlusive disease (VOD), originally described in Jamaican drinkers of pyrrolizidine alkaloid–containing bush tea, now occurs primarily as a consequence of toxic injury to sinusoidal endothelium by chemotherapy; mortality approaches 30%. Patients present with tender hepatomegaly, ascites, weight gain, and jaundice.

Morphology (p. 873)

VOD is characterized by patchy obliteration of smaller hepatic vein radicles by endothelial swelling and collagen deposition. Acute VOD shows centrilobular congestion with hepatocellular necrosis, while progressive disease exhibits venule lumen obliteration with dense perivenular fibrosis and hemosiderin deposition.

Hepatic Complications of Organ or Bone Marrow Transplantation (p. 874)

Graft-Versus-Host Disease and Liver Rejection (p. 874)

- Graft-versus-host disease (GVHD) occurs in the setting of bone marrow or stem cell transplantation and is characterized by *direct lymphocyte attack on liver cells, particularly bile duct epithelium.*

  Acute GVHD is characterized by hepatitis (parenchymal inflammation and hepatocyte necrosis), chronic vascular inflammation and intimal proliferation *(endothelialitis),* and *bile duct destruction.*

  Chronic GVHD exhibits portal tract inflammation, bile duct destruction (or complete loss), and fibrosis.

- *Acute rejection* of liver allografts exhibits portal tract inflammation (frequently including eosinophils), bile duct damage, and endothelialitis. *Chronic rejection,* occurring months or years after transplantation, is characterized by bile duct loss and arteriopathy, with eventual graft failure.

Hepatic Disease Associated with Pregnancy (p. 874)

Abnormal liver tests occur in 3% to 5% of pregnancies. Viral hepatitis is the most common cause of jaundice in pregnancy; with the exception of hepatitis E (which has 10% to 20% mortality rates in pregnancy), these infections are not typically influenced by pregnancy. Rarely (0.1%), pregnancies cause direct hepatic complications that are usually non-fatal (e.g., acute fatty liver of pregnancy and intrahepatic cholestasis of pregnancy).

Preeclampsia and Eclampsia (p. 874)

Preeclampsia affects 3% to 5% of pregnancies; it is characterized by hypertension, proteinuria, peripheral edema, coagulation abnormalities, and varying degrees of DIC. With onset of hyperreflexia and convulsion, the condition is called *eclampsia;* severe cases can require termination of the pregnancy. The *HELLP* syndrome (*h*emolysis, *e*levated *l*iver enzymes, and *l*ow *p*latelets) can be the primary manifestation of preeclampsia.

Morphology (p. 875)

Grossly: There are small, red, hemorrhagic patches with occasional yellow-white areas of infarction.
Microscopically: There is periportal sinusoidal fibrin deposition, periportal necrosis, and hemorrhage. Coalescence of bleeding can form hepatic hematomas capable of fatal rupture.

Acute Fatty Liver of Pregnancy (p. 875)

Acute fatty liver of pregnancy (AFLP) is a rare entity (1 in 13,000 deliveries) that can present along a spectrum from subclinical hepatocyte dysfunction to hepatic failure, coma, and death. Mitochondrial dysfunction is generally implicated; in particular, congenital fetal deficiency in long-chain 3-hydroxyacyl coenzyme A dehydrogenase results in toxic levels of fetal metabolites that can cause maternal hepatotoxicity. Microscopically, there is *microvesicular steatosis;* in severe cases, portal inflammation and hepatocyte drop-out and lobular disarray can occur. Definitive treatment is termination of pregnancy.

Intrahepatic Cholestasis of Pregnancy (p. 875)

Intrahepatic cholestasis of pregnancy (ICP) is attributed to the altered hormonal state of pregnancy; it is characterized by pruritus and jaundice in the third trimester, with mild cholestasis. While generally benign, pruritus can be severe, and maternal gallstones or malabsorption can also occur.

Nodules and Tumors (p. 875)

Nodular Hyperplasias (p. 875)

Nodular hyperplasias are solitary or multiple benign hepatocellular nodules in the absence of cirrhosis; the putative cause is focal hepatic vascular obliteration, with compensatory hypertrophy of adjacent well-vascularized lobules.

- *Focal nodular hyperplasia* occurs in young to middle-aged adults, and it is an irregular, unencapsulated mass containing a central stellate fibrous scar.
- *Nodular regenerative hyperplasia* is a diffuse nodular transformation of the liver *without fibrosis,* occurring as a consequence of conditions affecting intrahepatic blood flow, for example, in solid-organ transplants (especially kidney), bone marrow transplants, and vasculitis.

Benign Neoplasms (p. 876)

- *Cavernous hemangiomas* are the most common benign liver tumors; they are identical to blood vessel tumors seen in other locations (Chapter 11).
- *Hepatic adenomas* (p. 877) are benign hepatocyte neoplasms up to 30cm in diameter; they occur commonly in young women, usually associated with oral contraceptive use. Mutations in β-catenin and in the transcription factor HNF1α are frequently associated. Adenomas are composed of sheets of hepatocytes containing arteries and veins, although *portal tracts with bile ducts are absent.* Adenomas can rarely rupture with massive hemorrhage, and infrequently harbor hepatocellular carcinoma.

Malignant Tumors (p. 877)

- In the United States, the vast majority of tumors involving the liver are *metastatic.*
- *Hepatocellular carcinoma* is the most common *primary* liver cancer; cholangiocarcinomas are much less common.
- *Angiosarcomas* of the liver resemble those occurring elsewhere. Interestingly, liver angiosarcomas can be associated with exposure to vinyl chloride, arsenic, or Thorotrast (a contrast agent used in the 1950s).

Hepatoblastoma (p. 877)

Hepatoblastoma is the most common liver tumor of early childhood. A characteristic feature is activation of the Wnt/β-catenin signaling pathway; hepatoblastomas are also associated with familial polyposis syndrome and Beckwith-Wiedemann syndrome.

- The *epithelial type* vaguely recapitulates liver development.
- The *mixed epithelial and mesenchymal type* contains foci of mesenchymal differentiation including osteoid, cartilage, or striated muscle.

Hepatoblastomas are usually fatal if untreated, but resection and chemotherapy yield 80% 5-year survival rates.

Hepatocellular Carcinoma (p. 878)

Hepatocellular carcinoma (HCC) occurs most commonly in developing countries with high rates of HBV infection; it is the third most common cause of cancer deaths worldwide. The male to female ratio is 2.4:1.

Pathogenesis (p.878)

HCC usually arises in the background of chronic liver disease. The four major etiologic factors are chronic viral infection (HBV or HCV), chronic alcoholism, NASH, and food contaminants (e.g., aflatoxins); lesser causes include hemochromatosis, tyrosinemia, and α_1-antitrypsin deficiency. Chronic inflammation is associated with genotoxic products, cytokine production, and hepatocyte regeneration; such changes—along with an underlying genetic susceptibility—presumably underlie tumorigenesis. In addition, the high co-incidence of HCC with HBV and HCV infections suggests that viral factors can also contribute:

* In *HBV-related malignancy,* key events appear to be integration of HBV DNA into the host genome (potentially inducing proto-oncogene activation) and the presence of certain viral proteins (e.g., X protein, a transcriptional activator of multiple genes).
* Since HCV is an RNA virus, host DNA is not disrupted, and no oncogenic proteins are produced; nevertheless, HCV core and NS5A viral proteins may participate in HCC onset.

Of note, in high-prevalence regions, where HBV transmission is more often vertical from mother to neonate, cirrhosis is absent in up to half of cases, and carcinoma presentation is typically between ages 20 and 40 years.

Morphology (p. 879)

HCC can present as a solitary mass, as multifocal nodules, or as a diffusely infiltrative cancer with massive liver enlargement, frequently in a background of cirrhosis; intrahepatic spread and vascular invasion are common. Histologically, lesions may range from well differentiated to highly anaplastic and undifferentiated.

* A distinctive variant is *fibrolamellar carcinoma.* Constituting 5% of HCC, it usually occurs as a single scirrhous, hard tumor occurring in 20- to 40-year-olds *in the absence of chronic liver disease.* The cells are well-differentiated cells in cords or nests separated by dense lamellar collagen bundles.

Clinical Features (p. 879)

Features include hepatomegaly, right upper quadrant pain, weight loss, and elevated serum α-fetoprotein. Prognosis depends on the resectability of the tumor; mortality is secondary to cachexia, gastrointestinal or esophageal variceal bleeding, liver failure with hepatic coma, or tumor rupture and fatal hemorrhage.

Cholangiocarcinoma (p. 880)

Cholangiocarcinoma (CCA) arises from elements of the intra- and extrahepatic biliary tree; 50% to 60% are perihilar (called *Klatskin tumors*), 20% to 30% are distal, and 10% are intrahepatic. CCA accounts for 3% of cancer deaths in the United States and 7.6% of cancer deaths worldwide. Clinical outlook is dismal because CCA is rarely resectable at diagnosis.

Pathogenesis (p. 881)

Although most cases arise without antecedent risk conditions, CCA can be associated with PSC, congenital fibropolycystic lesions, HCV infection, and Thorotrast administration. In Southeast Asia, protracted biliary tree parasitic infection by *Opisthorchis sinensis* is a major risk factor. A number of genetic alterations are associated with CCA including IL-6 over-expression causing AKT activation and increased production of the anti-apoptotic protein MCL-1; *p53* expression is decreased in 40% of cases.

Morphology (p. 880)

Cholangiocarcinoma can manifest as a single large mass or as multifocal nodules, or it can be diffusely infiltrative. In contrast to HCC, CAA is typically pale since biliary epithelium does not secrete bilirubin pigment. Microscopically, there are variably differentiated bile duct elements that resemble adenocarcinomas elsewhere in the alimentary tract; most CAAs are markedly desmoplastic with dense collagenous stroma. Mixed variants of *hepatocellular-cholangiocarcinoma* can also rarely occur.

Metastatic Tumors (p. 881)

Any cancer in the body—including those of the blood-forming elements—can spread to the liver; colon, breast, lung, and pancreas primaries are most common. Typically, multiple implants are present, with massive hepatic enlargement. Large implants tend to have defective vascular supplies and become centrally necrotic. Massive involvement of the liver is usually present before hepatic failure develops.

THE BILIARY TRACT (p. 882)

Congenital Anomalies (p. 882)

The gallbladder can be congenitally absent or exist in aberrant locations (e.g., embedded in hepatic substance); other variants include a folded fundus *(phrygian cap)* or a duplicated or bilobed gallbladder. There can be agenesis of the common or hepatic bile ducts, or hypoplastic narrowing of the biliary channels.

Disorders of the Gallbladder (p. 882)

Cholelithiasis (Gallstones) (p. 882)

Gallstones afflict 10% to 20% of adult populations in developed countries; 90% of calculi are *cholesterol stones* (more than 50% cholesterol monohydrate), with the remainder being pigmented (bilirubin calcium salts). The vast majority of stones remain asymptomatic for decades.

Risk factors for cholesterol gallstones relate to increased hepatic cholesterol uptake or synthesis or to increased biliary cholesterol secretion (p. 882):

- Native Americans: there is 75% prevalence among Hopi, Navajo, and Pima groups
- Industrialized countries
- Increasing age, female more than male (2:1 ratio)
- Estrogenic influences including oral contraception and pregnancy
- Obesity, metabolic syndromes, hypercholesterolemia, and rapid weight loss
- Gallbladder stasis, as in spinal cord injury

- Hereditable conditions related to hepatic biliary transport; the D19H variant of the ATP-binding cassette transporter encoded by the *ABCG5* and *ABG2* genes accounts for roughly 10% of the risk for cholesterol gallstone formation.

Pathogenesis (p. 883)

- *Cholesterol stones* (p. 883): When cholesterol concentrations exceed the solubilizing capacity of bile salts *(supersaturation)*, cholesterol nucleates into solid cholesterol monohydrate crystals. Four conditions must occur to form cholesterol stones:

  Bile must be supersaturated with cholesterol.
  Gallbladder hypomotility promotes crystal nucleation.
  Cholesterol nucleation in bile is accelerated. Nucleation is promoted by microprecipitates of calcium salts (inorganic or bilirubin salts).
  Mucus hypersecretion in the gallbladder traps the crystals, permitting their aggregation into stones.

- *Pigment stones* (p. 883): Pigment stones form in the setting of unconjugated bilirubin *(most commonly due to chronic hemolytic conditions)* and precipitation of calcium bilirubin salts. In underdeveloped countries, pigmented stones are often formed because biliary infections (e.g., with *Escherichia coli, Ascaris lumbricoides,* or *Opisthorchis sinensis*) promote bilirubin glucuronide deconjugation.

Morphology (p. 884)

- *Cholesterol stones* arise exclusively in the gallbladder, and are classically hard and pale yellow; bilirubin salts can impart a black color. When composed predominantly of cholesterol, they are radiolucent; calcium carbonate deposition in 10% to 20% of stones is sufficient to render them radiopaque. Single stones are ovoid; multiple stones tend to be faceted.
- *Pigmented stones* can be black (sterile gallbladder bile) or brown (with infection); both are soft and usually multiple, and 50% to 75% of pigmented stones are radiopaque.

Clinical Features (p. 884)

Roughly 70% to 80% of gallstone patients are asymptomatic throughout life; patients with stones become symptomatic at the rate of 1% to 4% per year, with risk diminishing over time. *Symptoms* include spasmodic, *colicky* pain due to passing stones in the bile ducts (smaller stones cause symptoms more commonly than do large stones). Associated gallbladder inflammation *(cholecystitis)* generates right upper abdominal pain. More severe complications include empyema, perforation, fistulas, biliary tree inflammation *(cholangitis),* obstructive cholestasis or pancreatitis, and erosion of a gallstone into adjacent bowel *(gallstone ileus)*. Clear mucinous secretions in an obstructed gallbladder distend the gallbladder *(mucocele)*. There is also increased risk for gallbladder carcinoma.

Cholecystitis (p. 885)

Acute cholecystitis (p. 885): *Acute cholecystitis is an acute inflammation of the gallbladder precipitated most frequently by gallstone obstruction.* The 10% of cases without gallstone obstruction usually occur in severely ill patients.

Pathogenesis (p. 885)

- *Acute calculous cholecystitis* (*with* gallstones) is initiated by chemical irritation of the gallbladder by retained bile acids; there is subsequent release of inflammatory mediators (lysolecithin, prostaglandins), and the gallbladder develops dysmotility. In severe cases, distention and increased luminal pressures compromise mucosal blood flow, causing ischemia; bacterial contamination can be a late complication

- *Acute acalculous cholecystitis* results from ischemia due to diminished flow in the end arterial cystic artery circulation; it occurs in the setting of sepsis with hypotension and multiorgan failure, immunosuppression, major trauma or burns, diabetes mellitus, or infections.

Morphology (p. 885)

In acute cholecystitis, there is an enlarged, tense, bright-red to blotchy green-black gallbladder with a serosal fibrinous exudate. Luminal contents range from turbid to purulent. In severe cases, the gallbladder is transformed into a green-black necrotic organ *(gangrenous cholecystitis)* with multiple perforations. In milder cases, there is only gallbladder wall edema and hyperemia.

Clinical Features (p. 885)

Acute cholecystitis may be mild and intermittent or may be a surgical emergency. *Symptoms* include right upper quadrant or epigastric pain, fever, anorexia, tachycardia, diaphoresis, and nausea and vomiting. Jaundice suggests common bile duct obstruction.

Self-limited attacks subside over several days; overall mortality rate is less than 1%. In severely ill patients with acalculous cholecystitis, symptoms may not be evident due to the co-morbid conditions, and the mortality rate is higher.

Chronic Cholecystitis (p. 885)

Chronic cholecystitis can be a consequence of repeated bouts of acute cholecystitis, but it often develops without antecedent attacks. Although gallstones are usually present (90%), they may not play a direct role in initiating inflammation. Rather, chronic bile supersaturation with cholesterol permits cholesterol suffusion of the gallbladder wall and initiation of inflammation and gallbladder dysmotility. Patient populations and symptoms are the same as for acute choleccystitis.

Morphology (p. 886)

Gallbladders can be contracted (from fibrosis), normal in size, or enlarged (from obstruction). The wall is variably thickened and gray-white. The mucosa is generally preserved but may be atrophied. Cholesterol-laden macrophages in the lamina propria are common *(cholesterolosis)* and gallstones are frequent. Inflammation is variable with occasional mucosal outpouchings *(Rokitansky-Aschoff sinuses)*. Rarely, there is mural dystrophic calcification *(porcelain gallbladder)* or a fibrosed, nodular gallbladder with marked histiocytic inflammation *(xanthogranulomatous cholecystitis)*.

Clinical Features (p. 886)

Recurrent attacks of steady or colicky epigastric or right upper quadrant pain occur. Complications are the same as for acute cholecystitis, including bacterial superinfection, gallbladder perforation, and abscess formation or peritonitis, as well as the formation of biliary-enteric fistulas.

Disorders of the Extrahepatic Bile Ducts (p. 887)

Choledocholithiasis and Ascending Cholangitis (p. 887)

Choledocholithiasis refers to stones within the biliary tree; it occurs in 10% of patients with cholelithiasis. In western nations, almost all stones are gallbladder derived and are cholesterol; in Asia, they usually arise in the biliary tree and are pigmented. *Symptoms* are due to obstruction, pancreatitis, cholangitis, hepatic abscess, secondary biliary cirrhosis, and acute calculous cholecystitis.

Cholangitis refers to bile duct bacterial infection; it usually occurs in the setting of choledocholithiasis. Infections are typically due to enteric bacteria entering the biliary tract through the sphincter of Oddi. Patients present with fever, abdominal pain, and jaundice; sepsis can be a fatal complication.

Biliary Atresia (p. 887)

Biliary atresia is a cause of a third of neonatal cholestasis and is defined as extrahepatic biliary tree obstruction within the first 3 months of life; it occurs in 1 out of 12,000 live births. It is the single most frequent cause of death from liver disease in early childhood and accounts for the majority of children referred for liver transplantation.

Pathogenesis (p. 887)

- The severe early *fetal form* (20% of cases) is due to aberrant intrauterine development of the biliary tree and is frequently associated with other anomalies.
- The *perinatal form,* presumed secondary to viral infections and/ or autoimmunity, results from post-natal destruction of a normal biliary tree.

Morphology (p. 887)

In both forms, there is inflammation and fibrosing stricture of the extrahepatic biliary tree, progressing into the intrahepatic biliary system. The liver shows florid features of duct obstruction:

- Marked bile duct proliferation
- Portal tract edema
- Fibrosis progressing to cirrhosis within 6 months

In the early severe form, aberrant intrahepatic biliary morphology is evident at the time of initial diagnosis, with severe paucity of intrahepatic bile ducts. Most (90%) have atresia that extends above the porta hepatis and are not amenable to surgical correction.

Clinical Features (p. 887)

Neonatal cholestasis is seen in an infant of normal birth weight and postnatal weight gain. If untreated (liver transplantation), death occurs within 2 years of birth.

Choledochal Cysts (p. 887)

These congenital dilations of the common bile duct occur most often in children younger than 10 years with nonspecific symptoms of jaundice and recurrent colicky abdominal pain; the female to male ratio is 3:1 to 4:1. The cysts predispose to stone formation, stenosis and stricture, pancreatitis, obstructive biliary complications, and bile duct carcinoma in the adult.

Tumors (p. 888)

The primary neoplasms of the gallbladder are epithelial; malignant varieties were discussed previously under CCA. *Adenomas* are benign neoplasms similar to adenomas elsewhere in the gastrointestinal tract. *Inflammatory polyps* are sessile mucosal projections containing chronic inflammation and lipid-laden macrophages. *Adenomyosis* of the gallbladder is characterized by muscle hyperplasia.

Carcinoma of the Gallbladder (p. 888)

Carcinoma of the gallbladder is slightly more common in women, typically occurring in women older than 70 years. Gallstones coexist in 95% of U.S. patients; chronic gallbladder inflammation (with or without stones) is a critical risk factor. Gallstones are less common in Asian populations, where pyogenic and parasitic disease dominate as causes.

Morphology (p. 888)

Tumors may be *infiltrating,* with diffuse gallbladder thickening and induration, or they may be *exophytic*—growing into the lumen as an irregular, cauliflower-like mass. Most gallbladder carcinomas are adenocarcinomas; the histologic appearance can vary from papillary to infiltrating and can range from moderately differentiated to undifferentiated. Rarely, there are squamous, adenosquamous, carcinoid, or mesenchymal variants. Tumors spread by local invasion of the liver, extension to cystic duct and portohepatic lymph nodes, and metastatic seeding of peritoneum, viscera, and lungs.

Clinical Features (p. 889)

Symptoms are insidious and indistinguishable from those caused by cholelithiasis. Tumors are usually unresectable when discovered.

19

The Pancreas

Congenital Anomalies (p. 892)

Agenesis (p. 892)

Complete congenital absence is associated with other severe malformations that are usually incompatible with life.

Pancreas Divisum (p. 892)

This is the most common of pancreatic congenital anomalies (3% to 10% incidence). Failure of the ventral and dorsal fetal duct systems to fuse causes the bulk of pancreatic secretions to drain through the smaller minor papilla (rather than the large-caliber papilla of Vater); the relative stenosis predisposes to chronic pancreatitis.

Annular Pancreas (p. 893)

A bandlike ring of normal pancreatic tissue completely encircles the second portion of the duodenum, and can cause duodenal obstruction.

Ectopic Pancreas (p. 893)

Pancreatic parenchyma in an abnormal location is common (2% incidence); sites include stomach, duodenum, jejunum, Meckel diverticulum, and ileum. These are typically submucosal, can be single or multiple, and measure several millimeters to a few centimeters. While mostly asymptomatic, they can cause inflammation and pain or, rarely, mucosal bleeding.

Pancreatitis (p. 893)

By definition, *acute pancreatitis* is reversible if the inciting stimulus is withdrawn; *chronic pancreatitis* is defined by irreversible damage to the exocrine parenchyma.

Acute Pancreatitis (p. 893)

Acute pancreatitis is reversible parenchymal damage associated with inflammation; 80% of cases are associated with biliary tract disease (mostly gallstones) or alcoholism (Table 19-1). In 10% to 20% of cases, there are no known associated processes *(idiopathic),* although many have a genetic basis.

Hereditary pancreatitis (p. 893) is characterized by recurrent bouts of pancreatitis typically beginning in childhood. Most cases have autosomal dominant mutations in the cationic trypsinogen gene *(PRSS1),* rendering activated trypsin resistant to its own self-inactivation. Others have inactivating autosomal recessive mutations in the serine protease inhibitor Kazal type 1 gene *(SPINK1);* altered proteins fail to inhibit trypsin activity.

TABLE 19-1 Etiologic Factors in Acute Pancreatitis

Metabolic

Alcoholism
Hyperlipoproteinemia
Hypercalcemia
Drugs (e.g., azathioprine)

Genetic

Mutations in the cationic trypsinogen (*PRSS1*) and trypsin inhibitor
  (*SPINK1*) genes

Mechanical

Gallstones
Trauma
Iatrogenic injury
  Operative injury
  Endoscopic procedures with dye injection

Vascular

Shock
Atheroembolism
Vasculitis

Infectious

Mumps

Morphology (p. 894)

Acute pancreatitis can range from mild interstitial edema and
inflammation to extensive necrosis and hemorrhage. Basic features
include:

- Vascular leakage causing edema
- Necrosis of regional fat by lipolytic enzymes
- Acute inflammation
- Proteolytic destruction of the pancreatic substance
- Vascular injury with subsequent interstitial hemorrhage

Mild (acute interstitial) pancreatitis shows only edema, fat necrosis,
and acute inflammation these. *Acute necrotizing pancreatitis* exhibits
gray-white parenchymal necrosis and chalky white fat necrosis. In acute
hemorrhagic pancreatitis, there is patchy red-black hemorrhage
interspersed with fat necrosis.

Pathogenesis (p. 894)

Pancreatitis results from parenchymal autodigestion by activated
pancreatic enzymes; in particular, inappropriate activation of trypsinogen is a key triggering event.

- Pancreas normally secretes amylase and lipase in their active
  forms, while proteases, elastase, and phospholipase are secreted
  as proenzymes requiring proteolytic cleavage by trypsin in the
  duodenum. Trypsin, itself, is normally activated by duodenal
  enteropeptidase.
- In acute pancreatitis, inappropriate activation of trypsin in the
  pancreas leads to conversion of proenzymes to active enzymes
  and prekallikrein to kallikrein, activating the kinin system and
  clotting.
- The net result is pancreatic inflammation and thrombosis with
  tissue proteolysis, lipolysis, and hemorrhage.

Mechanisms underlying pancreatic enzyme activation:

- *Pancreatic duct obstruction:* Gallstones or sludge in the ampulla of Vater obstruct the duct, leading to accumulation of enzyme-rich fluid. Lipase in this fluid (synthesized in activated form) causes fat necrosis, with subsequent parenchymal release of pro-inflammatory cytokines. The resulting inflammation and interstitial edema compromises vascular flow, adding ischemia to the ongoing parenchymal injury.
- *Primary acinar cell injury:* May be due to damage by viruses (mumps), drugs, trauma, or ischemia.
- *Defective intracellular transport of proenzymes:* Exocrine enzymes are misdirected toward lysosomes rather than toward secretion; lysosomal hydrolysis of the proenzymes causes enzyme activation and release.
- *Alcohol:* has a direct toxic effect on pancreatic acinar cells. It also causes functional obstruction by contracting the sphincter at the ampulla of Vater and increasing pancreatic protein secretion, leading to inspissated protein plugs that block small ducts.

Clinical Features (p. 895)

Patients typically present with abdominal pain, nausea, and anorexia, along with elevated plasma levels of pancreatic enzymes (amylase and lipase). Full-blown acute pancreatitis is a medical emergency presenting with acute abdomen (intense abdominal pain), peripheral vascular collapse, and shock from explosive activation of the systemic inflammatory response. Death (5% of patients) can occur from shock, acute respiratory distress syndrome, or acute renal failure.

Laboratory findings include marked serum amylase (and later, lipase) elevations; glycosuria occurs occasionally. Hypocalcemia results from precipitation of calcium soaps in the fat necrosis. In roughly half of cases, the necrotic debris becomes secondarily infected.

Treatment involves restricting oral intake to "rest" the pancreas, and providing analgesia, nutrition, and volume support. The pancreas can return to normal function if the acute pancreatitis resolves. Possible sequelae include sterile *pancreatic abscesses* from tissue liquefaction, and *pancreatic pseudocysts*—localized collections of necrotic, hemorrhagic material rich in pancreatic enzymes.

Chronic Pancreatitis (p. 896)

Chronic pancreatitis is defined as inflammation with *irreversible parenchymal destruction and fibrosis;* in late stages, the endocrine parenchyma is also destroyed. Causes overlap with those of acute pancreatitis but long-term alcohol abuse is most common. Also implicated are ductal obstruction by pseudocysts, tumors, or calculi, pancreas divisum, hereditary pancreatitis (see preceding discussion), and *CFTR* gene mutations; the latter decrease ductal cell bicarbonate secretion and thereby promote protein plugging.

Pathogenesis (p. 896)

Most patients with recurrent bouts of acute pancreatitis develop chronic pancreatitis. Proposed events include:

- *Ductal obstruction by concretion:* When protein concentrations in secretions increase there is a propensity for ductal plugging; such plugs are particularly prominent in alcoholic chronic pancreatitis, and can calcify.
- *Toxic effects:* Toxins, including alcohol and its metabolites, may be directly injurious.
- *Oxidative stress:* This occurs from alcohol-induced oxygen-derived free radicals.

Morphology (p. 896)

There is replacement of pancreatic acinar tissue by dense fibrous connective tissue, with relative sparing of the islets of Langerhans, and variable dilation of the pancreatic ducts. The pancreas is hard with focal calcification.

Lymphoplasmacytic sclerosing pancreatitis (autoimmune pancreatitis) is a distinct form characterized by mixed inflammatory cell infiltrates, venulitis, and IgG$_4$-producing plasma cells; it responds to steroid therapy.

Clinical Features (p. 897)

Chronic pancreatitis can be silent or can be heralded by recurrent attacks of pain and/or jaundice. Episodes can be precipitated by alcohol abuse, overeating (increasing pancreatic demand) and opiates (or other drugs) that increase the tone of the sphincter of Oddi. Late complications relate primarily to the loss of exocrine and endocrine function:

- Malabsorption
- Diabetes mellitus
- Pseudocysts

The long-term outlook is poor, with mortality rates of 50% within 20 to 25 years.

Non-Neoplastic Cysts (p. 898)

Congenital Cysts (p. 898)

Congenital cysts are caused by anomalous development of the pancreatic ducts; in *congenital polycystic disease,* they frequently coexist with kidney and liver cysts. In *von Hippel-Lindau disease* (Chapter 28), pancreatic cysts and angiomas of the central nervous system (CNS) are seen. They are usually unilocular and thin-walled with a cuboidal epithelial lining.

Pseudocysts (p. 898)

Pseudocysts are collections of necrotic-hemorrhagic material rich in pancreatic enzymes; formed by walling off areas of fat necrosis, they account for 75% of pancreatic cysts. They are not lined by epithelium (thus, "pseudocysts"), rather they are encircled by fibrosed granulation tissue. They occur after bouts of acute pancreatitis or following trauma. While many spontaneously resolve, they can become secondarily infected or compress adjacent structures.

Neoplasms (p. 898)

Neoplasms of the pancreas are broadly grouped as cystic or solid.

Cystic Neoplasms (p. 899)

Cystic tumors constitute less than 5% of pancreatic neoplasms; they typically occur as painless, slow-growing masses.

- *Serous cystadenoma:* Typically seen in women older than 60 years; these are usually solitary, well-circumscribed nodules with a central stellate scar. They are composed of numerous 1- to 3-mm cysts lined by a glycogen-rich cuboidal epithelium and containing serous, watery fluid. These are almost always benign and resection is curative.
- *Mucinous cystic neoplasm:* These multiloculated cystic neoplasms are filled with thick mucinous material; the cysts are lined by mucin-producing columnar cells within a dense stroma. Almost

95% occur in women, and most arise as slow-growing painless masses in the body or tail of the gland. One third of these lesions harbor an invasive adenocarcinoma.

- *Intraductal papillary mucinous neoplasm (IPMN):* These are intraductal mucin-producing neoplasms, more common in men than women. Most arise in the head of the gland, and 10% to 20% are multifocal. They differ from mucinous cystic neoplasms by lacking an associated dense stroma and by involving a larger pancreatic duct, but they have a similar malignant potential.
- *Solid-pseudopapillary tumor:* These round and well-circumscribed neoplasms have solid and cystic regions; they occur mainly in young women and cause abdominal discomfort due to their large size. These tumors are associated with activating mutations of β-catenin. Although some are locally aggressive, complete resection is usually curative.

Pancreatic Carcinoma (p. 900)

Pancreatic cancer is an *infiltrating ductal adenocarcinoma*; it is the fourth leading cause of cancer deaths in the United States.

Precursors to Pancreatic Cancer (p. 900)

There is a progression from non-neoplastic epithelium to small ductal non-invasive lesions, to invasive carcinoma. The precursor lesions are called pancreatic intraepithelial neoplasms (PanINs); these show characteristic genetic and epigenetic alterations, as well as dramatic telomere shortening that may predispose to additional progressive chromosomal aberrations.

Molecular Carcinogenesis (p. 900)

Multiple genes are altered in pancreatic cancer; the gene expression patterns are distinct from those in other malignancies (Table 19-2):

- *KRAS* (p. 900) is the most frequently altered oncogene in pancreatic cancer (90% of cases), resulting in a constitutively active protein and increased Fos and Jun transcription factor activation.

TABLE 19-2   Molecular Alterations in Invasive Pancreatic Adenocarcinoma

Gene	Chromosomal Region	Percentage of Carcinoma with Genetic Alteration
KRAS	12p	90
p16/CDKN2A	9p	95
TP53	17p	50-70
SMAD4	18q	55
AKT2	19q	10-20
MYB	6q	10
NCOA3/AIB1	20q	10
BRCA2	13q	7-10
GATA-6	18q	10
STK11	19p	5
MAP2K4/MKK4	17p	5
TGFβ-R1	9q	2
TGFβ-R2	3p	2
RB1	13q	5

- *CDKN2A (p16)* (p. 900) is inactivated in 95% of cases, resulting in loss of an important cell cycle checkpoint.
- *SMAD4* (p. 900) is a tumor suppressor gene that is inactivated in more than half of pancreatic cancers; it encodes a protein critical for TGF-β receptor signal transduction.
- *p53* (p. 900) inactivation leads to loss of a cell cycle checkpoint and loss of a protein that induces apoptosis and cell senescence.

Pathogenesis (p. 901)

About 80% of cases occur in individuals between the ages of 60 and 80 years; smoking increases the risk roughly two-fold. Chronic pancreatitis, consumption of a diet rich in fats, a family history of pancreatic cancer (e.g., *BRCA2* mutations account for 10% of pancreatic cancer in Ashkenazi Jews), and diabetes mellitus impose a modestly increased risk.

Morphology (p. 902)

Some 60% of pancreatic cancers arise in the head of the gland, 15% occur in the body, 5% occur in the tail, and 20% diffusely involve the organ. These are typically highly invasive and elicit an intense host scarring response (desmoplasia). Most carcinomas in the head of the pancreas obstruct the distal common bile duct, leading to jaundice; conversely, cancers of the body and tail can remain clinically silent for long periods of time and are often large or widely metastatic when initially discovered. Extensive perineural and vascular invasion are common.

Microscopically, the neoplastic cells form more or less differentiated glandular patterns resembling ductal epithelium. Less common histologic variants include:

- *Adenosquamous carcinoma* with both squamous and glandular differentiation.
- *Undifferentiated carcinoma* containing prominent multinucleated osteoclast-like giant cells.

Clinical Features (p. 903)

Weight loss and pain are typical presenting symptoms; obstructive jaundice develops with tumors in the head of the gland. Metastases are common, and more than 80% of pancreatic adenocarcinomas are unresectable at presentation; massive liver metastasis frequently develops. The outlook is dismal: first-year mortality rate exceeds 80% and the 5-year survival rate is less than 5%. Migratory thrombophlebitis (*Trousseau syndrome*; Chapter 4) can occur with pancreatic neoplasms (as well as other adenocarcinomas).

Acinar Cell Carcinoma (p. 903)

These tumors exhibit acinar cell differentiation, with zymogen granules and the production of exocrine enzymes (e.g., trypsin); lipase release causes metastatic fat necrosis in 15% of patients.

Pancreatoblastoma (p. 903)

These are rare malignant tumors, primarily seen in childhood; microscopically, there are squamous islands admixed with acinar cells.

20

The Kidney

Renal diseases can be categorized based on the four basic anatomic compartments affected:

- Glomeruli (often immunologically mediated injury)
- Tubules (frequently toxic or infectious injury)
- Interstitium
- Blood vessels

Many disorders affect more than one structure; the anatomic interdependence of these compartments means that damage to one usually secondarily affects the others. Whatever the initial insult, all forms of *chronic renal disease* ultimately destroy all four kidney elements, culminating in end-stage disease.

Clinical Manifestations of Renal Diseases (p. 906)

DEFINITIONS

Azotemia is elevation of the blood urea nitrogen (BUN) and creatinine levels, largely due to decreased glomerular filtration rate (GFR).

Prerenal azotemia occurs with kidney hypoperfusion (e.g., with congestive heart failure, shock, volume depletion, or hemorrhage).

Postrenal azotemia occurs when urinary outflow is obstructed after exiting the kidney.

Uremia is the constellation of clinical signs and symptoms associated with azotemia; these include metabolic, hematologic, endocrine, gastrointestinal, neural, and cardiovascular effects.

Renal diseases typically manifest as clinically-recognizable syndromes (Table 20-1):

Nephritic syndrome is characterized by hematuria, mild to moderate proteinuria, and hypertension and is due to glomerular injury.

Rapidly progressive glomerulonephritis is a nephritic syndrome with a rapid (i.e., hours to days) decline in GFR.

Nephrotic syndrome is characterized by more than 3.5 g/day proteinuria, hypoalbuminemia, edema, hyperlipidemia, and lipiduria and is also due to glomerular injury.

Asymptomatic hematuria or proteinuria is usually a manifestation of mild glomerular injury.

Renal tubular defects—due to disorders of tubules and/or interstitium—manifest with polyuria and electrolyte abnormalities.

Urinary tract infections can affect the kidney *(pyelonephritis)* or bladder *(cystitis);* there is pyuria and bacteriuria, but symptoms are variable.

Nephrolithiasis, or calculi (stones) in the urinary space, is manifested by renal colic and hematuria.

TABLE 20-1 The Glomerular Syndromes	
Syndrome	**Clinical Features**
Acute nephritic syndrome	Hematuria, azotemia, variable proteinuria, oliguria, edema, and hypertension
Rapidly progressive glomerulonephritis	Acute nephritis, proteinuria, and acute renal failure
Nephrotic syndrome	>3.5 g/day proteinuria, hypoalbuminemia, hyperlipidemia, lipiduria
Chronic renal failure	Azotemia → uremia progressing for years
Asymptomatic hematuria or proteinuria	Glomerular hematuria; subnephrotic proteinuria

Renal Failure (p. 907)

- *Acute renal failure* is manifested by new-onset oliguria or anuria with azotemia; it can result from injury to any kidney anatomic compartment.
- *Chronic renal failure* is characterized by prolonged uremia and is the end stage of all chronic renal diseases.

Renal failure broadly progresses through four stages based on GFR and clinical manifestations:

Diminished renal reserve (up to about 50% of normal GFR); patients are asymptomatic, and BUN/creatinine levels are normal, but additional renal injury can precipitate azotemia.

Renal insufficiency (20% to 50% of normal GFR); azotemia formally occurs, often with anemia and hypertension; decreased concentrating ability can cause polyuria. Additional injury can precipitate uremia.

Chronic renal failure (less than 20% of normal GFR); patients develop edema, metabolic acidosis, and hyperkalemia, often with overt uremia.

End-stage renal disease (less than 5% of normal GFR).

Glomerular Diseases (p. 907)

- *Primary glomerulonephritis (GN):* Kidney is the principal organ involved.
- *Secondary glomerular disease:* Kidney is damaged by a systemic disease (e.g., hypertension, vasculitis, diabetes, amyloidosis).

Clinical manifestations and glomerular histologic changes can be similar in primary and secondary forms of injury.

Pathogenesis of Glomerular Injury (p. 911)

Although non-immune factors can initiate GN or influence its progression, *immune mechanisms underlie most forms of glomerular injury.* Thus, immunoglobulin deposition—either directly or as antigen-antibody complexes—along with activated complement and/or recruited inflammatory cells are found in the glomeruli of the majority of GN patients (Fig. 20-1).

Immune Complex Deposition Involving Intrinsic and In Situ Renal Antigens (p. 912)

Antibodies can react directly with intrinsic matrix or cellular (endothelial, mesangial, or epithelial) antigens or with circulating antigens that have been "trapped" in the glomerulus.

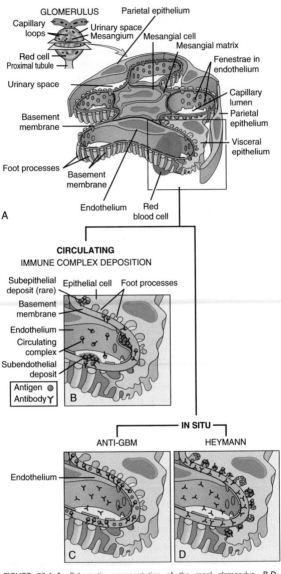

GLOMERULUS

Capillary loops
Red cell
Proximal tubule

Parietal epithelium
Urinary space
Mesangium — Mesangial cell
Mesangial matrix
Fenestrae in endothelium
Capillary lumen
Parietal epithelium
Visceral epithelium

Urinary space
Basement membrane
Foot processes
Basement membrane
Endothelium — Red blood cell

A

CIRCULATING
IMMUNE COMPLEX DEPOSITION

Subepithelial deposit (rare) — Epithelial cell — Foot processes
Basement membrane
Endothelium
Circulating complex
Subendothelial deposit

Antigen ●
Antibody Y

B

IN SITU

ANTI-GBM   HEYMANN

Endothelium

C   D

FIGURE 20-1 **A,** Schematic representation of the renal glomerulus. **B-D,** Antibody-mediated glomerular injury can result either from deposition of circulating immune complexes **(B)** or more commonly, from *in situ* formation of complexes exemplified by anti-GBM (anti-glomerular basement membrane) disease **(C)** or Heymann nephritis **(D).**

Heymann nephritis (p. 912) is an experimental rat model of GN that involves immunization with renal tubular proteins (see Fig. 20-1, *D*); immunized animals develop antibodies to a *megalin* protein antigen expressed on visceral epithelial cells. Antibody binding to megalin results in complement activation and shedding of the immune complexes to form *subepithelial deposits;* this is reflected as a *granular* pattern of immunofluorescence staining for immunoglobulin (Ig) and activated complement. The lesion morphology and the pathogenesis of the renal damage closely model human membranous GN, although the human equivalent of the Heymann antigen is not known.

Antibodies against planted antigens (p. 912) cause similar pathology. Circulating molecules can localize to the kidney by interaction with various intrinsic components of the glomerulus; cationic molecules (DNA, nucleosomes, microbial products, drugs, and aggregated proteins including immune complexes) all have affinity for the anionic glomerular basement membrane (GBM) and can become trapped. Antibodies that bind to these planted antigens often induce a discrete, granular pattern of Ig and complement immunofluorescence staining (see Fig. 20-1, *B*).

Anti-GBM antibody-induced glomerulonephritis (p. 912) is an autoimmune disease in which antibodies are directed against intrinsic fixed antigens of the GBM; the classic anti-GBM disorder is *Goodpasture syndrome,* where the autoantibody binds the noncollagenous domain of the α3 chain of type IV collagen. Such autoantibodies typically yield a *linear* immunofluorescence staining pattern (see Fig. 20-1, *C*).

Circulating Immune Complex Glomerulonephritis (p. 912)

Glomerular injury is caused by the trapping of circulating antigen-antibody complexes within glomeruli, followed by the activation of complement and inflammatory cells bearing Fc receptors. Antigens can be endogenous (e.g., double-stranded DNA in systemic lupus erythematosus [SLE]) or exogenous (e.g., infectious agents) but in most cases are not known. Immune complex deposits can be subendothelial, subepithelial, or mesangial, and immunofluorescence staining shows a granular pattern (see Fig. 20-1, *A*); the site of localization in the glomerulus depends on the charge and size of the immune complexes, as well as glomerular hemodynamics and mesangial function.

Cell-Mediated Immunity in Glomerulonephritis (p. 915)

While antibody-mediated mechanisms underlie many forms of GN, sensitized T cells are increasingly recognized as important contributors; for example, direct cytotoxicity or released cytokines may cause foot process effacement or epithelial detachment, leading to proteinuria.

Mediators of Glomerular Injury (p. 915)

Activated complement fragments are chemotactic, and Ig localized in glomeruli interacts with Fc-receptor-bearing cells; activated T cells also secrete a host of chemokines that recruit cellular effectors. Injury ensues through the following mechanisms (see also Chapter 6):

Cells:

- *Neutrophils and monocytes* release proteases, oxygen-derived free radicals, and arachidonic acid metabolites.
- *Macrophages, lymphocytes, and natural killer (NK) cells* release cytokines, cytotoxic cell mediators, and growth factors.
- *Platelets* aggregate and release eicosanoids and growth factors.
- *Resident glomerular cells (particularly mesangial cells)* produce cytokines, growth factors, chemokines, oxygen free radicals, eicosanoids, and endothelin.

Soluble mediators (p. 915):

- *C5b-C9* (membrane attack complex) causes cell lysis and induces mesangial cell activation.
- *Eicosanoids, nitric oxide, and endothelin* affect vascular flow.
- *Cytokines (especially interleukin-1 [IL-1]* and *tumor necrosis factor [TNF])* and *chemokines* (e.g., CCL5) influence inflammatory cell adhesion and recruitment.
- *Platelet-derived growth factor* influences mesangial cell proliferation; *transforming growth factor-β* and *fibroblast growth factor* affect matrix deposition; and *vascular endothelial growth factor* maintains endothelial integrity and regulates capillary permeability.
- *Coagulation proteins,* especially fibrin, can stimulate parietal epithelial cell proliferation *(crescent formation).*

Mechanisms of Progression in Glomerular Diseases (p. 916)

Regardless of etiology, once GFR is reduced to 30% to 50% of normal, progression to end-stage renal failure proceeds at a relatively constant rate. There are two major features of progressive renal damage:

Focal Segmental Glomerulosclerosis (p. 916)

Focal segmental glomerulosclerosis (FSGS) is initiated as an *adaptive change* in the relatively unaffected glomeruli of diseased kidneys. *Compensatory hypertrophy* of the remaining glomeruli putatively preserves renal function; however, proteinuria and segmental glomerulosclerosis soon develop, followed by total glomerular scarring and uremia. Glomerular hypertrophy is driven by *hemodynamic changes,* including increased glomerular blood flow, filtration, and transcapillary pressure *(glomerular hypertension),* often with systemic hypertension. In this setting, endothelial and epithelial injury lead to protein accumulation, followed by macrophage recruitment, mesangial cell activation, and increased matrix synthesis. This is compounded by the fact that mature visceral epithelial cells (podocytes) cannot proliferate after injury, and loss leads either to abnormal stretching of neighbors to compensate or uncovered (leaky) basement membrane. Ultimately, a vicious cycle of glomerular scarring supervenes; as glomeruli sclerose and drop out, the remaining glomeruli undergo the same compensatory changes that will ultimately result in *their* fibrosis.

Tubulointerstitial Fibrosis (p. 917)

Tubulointerstitial injury is a component of many forms of acute and chronic GN; indeed, renal function generally correlates better with the extent of tubulointerstitial damage than with the severity of glomerular injury. Tubulointerstitial injury results from ischemia (diminished perfusion downstream of sclerotic glomeruli or damaged capillaries) and inflammation in the surrounding interstitium. Proteinuria also causes direct injury to and activation of tubular cells. In turn, activated tubular cells elaborate proinflammatory cytokines and growth factors that drive interstitial fibrosis.

Table 20-2 summarizes the main clinical and pathologic features of the major forms of primary glomerulopathies.

Nephritic Syndrome (p. 917)

Acute Proliferative (Poststreptococcal, Postinfectious) Glomerulonephritis (p. 917)

Acute proliferative (poststreptococcal, postinfectious) glomerulonephritis (PSGN) is an immune complex–mediated disorder caused by the deposition of antigen-antibody complexes containing proteins derived from certain bacterial infections.

TABLE 20-2 Summary of Major Primary Glomerulonephrides

Disease	Most Frequent Clinical Presentation	Pathogenesis	Glomerular Pathology		
			Light Microscopy	Fluorescence Microscopy	Electron Microscopy
Poststreptococcal glomerulonephritis	Acute nephritis	Antibody mediated; circulating or planted antigen	Diffuse proliferation; leukocytic infiltration	Granular IgG and C3 in GBM and mesangium	Subepithelial humps
Goodpasture syndrome	Rapidly progressive glomerulonephritis	Anti-GBM COL4-A3 antigen	Proliferation; crescents	Linear IgG and C3; fibrin in crescents	No deposits; GBM disruptions; fibrin
Membranous glomerulopathy	Nephrotic syndrome	In situ antibody-mediated; antigen unknown	Diffuse capillary wall thickening	Granular IgG and C3; diffuse	Subepithelial deposits
Minimal change disease	Nephrotic syndrome	Unknown, loss of glomerular polyanion; podocyte injury	Normal; lipid in tubules	Negative	Loss of foot processes; no deposits
Focal segmental glomerulosclerosis	Nephrotic syndrome; non-nephrotic proteinuria	Unknown, ablation nephropathy plasma factor(?); podocyte injury	Focal and segmental sclerosis and hyalinosis	Focal; IgM and C3	Loss of foot processes; epithelial denudation
Membranoproliferative glomerulonephritis (MPGN) type I	Nephrotic syndrome	Immune complex	Mesangial proliferation; basement membrane thickening; splitting	IgG + C3; C1q + C4	Subendothelial deposits

Continued

TABLE 20-2 Summary of Major Primary Glomerulonephritides—cont'd

Disease	Most Frequent Clinical Presentation	Pathogenesis	Glomerular Pathology		
			Light Microscopy	Fluorescence Microscopy	Electron Microscopy
Dense deposit disease (MPGN type II)	Hematuria Chronic renal failure	Autoantibody; alternative complement pathway	Mesangial proliferation; basement membrane thickening; splitting	C3 ± IgG; no C1q or C4	Dense deposits
IgA nephropathy	Recurrent hematuria or proteinuria	Unknown; see text	Focal proliferative glomerulonephritis; mesangial widening	IgA +/− IgG, IgM, and C3 in mesangium	Mesangial and paramesangial dense deposits
Chronic glomerulonephritis	Chronic renal failure	Variable	Hyalinized glomeruli	Granular or negative	

GBM, Glomerular basement membrane.

Morphology (p. 918)

- There is *diffuse* GN with *global* hypercellularity due to neutrophil and monocyte infiltration, as well as endothelial, mesangial, and epithelial cell proliferation.
- Immunofluorescence shows granular mesangial and GBM IgG, IgM, and C3 deposition.
- Electron microscopy (EM) shows subepithelial, *humplike* deposits.

Clinical Course (p. 919)

Patients present with *nephritic syndrome* 1 to 4 weeks after a pharyngeal or cutaneous streptococcal infection (other infections can do this as well); only certain strains (i.e., types 1, 4, and 12) of group A β-hemolytic streptococci are nephritogenic, likely associated with expression of certain cationic proteins. Anti-streptococcal antibody titers are elevated and serum complement C3 concentrations are decreased. More than 95% of children recover quickly; less than 1% develop a rapidly progressive disease with the remainder progressing to chronic renal failure. Only 60% of adults with PSGN recover quickly; the remainder develop rapidly progressive disease, chronic renal failure, or delayed (but eventual) resolution.

Rapidly Progressive (Crescentic) Glomerulonephritis (p. 920)

Rapidly progressive (crescentic) glomerulonephritis (RPGN) is characterized clinically by a rapid, progressive renal decline. RPGN is divided into three broad groups based on immunologic findings; in each group, diseases can be associated with known disorders, although roughly 50% are idiopathic (Table 20-3).

Pathogenesis (p. 920)

- *Type I RPGN* (20% of RPGN) *is an anti-GBM disease* characterized by linear IgG (and C3) GBM deposits. In some cases, the anti-GBM antibodies cross-react with pulmonary alveolar basement membranes to produce pulmonary hemorrhages *(Goodpasture syndrome)*. The reason for autoantibody formation is unknown, although a high prevalence of certain HLA haplotypes suggests a genetic predilection; solvent exposures or virus infections have been implicated as the inciting trigger in susceptible hosts.

TABLE 20-3   Rapidly Progressive Glomerulonephritis

Type I RPGN (Anti-GBM Antibody)
Renal limited
Goodpasture syndrome

Type II RPGN (Immune Complex)
Idiopathic
Postinfectious
Systemic lupus erythematosus
Henoch-Schönlein purpura (IgA)
Others

Type III RPGN (Pauci-Immune)
ANCA-associated
Idiopathic
Wegener granulomatosis
Microscopic polyarteritis nodosa/microscopic polyangiitis

ANCA, Antineutrophil cytoplasmic antibody; *GBM,* glomerular basement membrane; *RPGN,* rapidly progressive glomerulonephritis.

- *Type II RPGN* (25% of RPGN) *is an immune complex–mediated disease.* It can be a complication of any of the immune complex nephritides, including postinfectious GN. Immunofluorescence shows characteristic granular staining; besides crescent formation, there is often glomerular cellular proliferation.
- *Type III RPGN (pauci-immune type)* (more than 50% of RPGN) is characterized by the absence of anti-GBM antibodies or immune complexes. Instead, patients typically have circulating *antineutrophil cytoplasmic antibody (ANCA)*, associated with a systemic vasculitis (Chapter 11). In idiopathic cases, more than 90% of patients have elevated ANCA titers. It is not yet clear that the ANCAs are causal in any of the type III RPGN.

Morphology (p. 921)

- RPGN histology is characterized by distinctive *crescents* formed by parietal cell proliferation and inflammatory cell migration into Bowman space. With time, crescents can undergo sclerosis.
- Immunofluorescence reveals linear staining in anti-GBM disease, granular deposits in immune complex disease, and little to no staining for pauci-immune disease.
- EM in RPGN classically exhibits distinct *ruptures in the GBM;* subepithelial electron-dense deposits can also occur in type II disease.

Clinical Course (p. 921)

All forms of RPGN typically present with hematuria, red cell casts, moderate proteinuria, and variable hypertension and edema. In Goodpasture syndrome, the course may be dominated by recurrent hemoptysis. Serum analyses for anti-GBM, antinuclear antibodies, and ANCA are diagnostically helpful. Renal involvement is usually progressive over the course of a few weeks, culminating in severe oliguria. Functional recovery can occur with intensive plasmapheresis combined with steroids and cytotoxic agents.

Nephrotic Syndrome (p. 921)

Nephrotic syndrome is characterized by excessive glomerular permeability to plasma proteins (proteinuria more than 3.5 g per day). Depending on the lesions, the proteinuria can be highly selective, for example, primarily low-molecular-weight proteins (chiefly albumin). With more severe injury, nonselective proteinuria includes higher-molecular-weight proteins in addition to albumin. Heavy proteinuria leads to hypoalbuminemia, decreased colloid osmotic pressure, and systemic edema. There are also *sodium and water retention, hyperlipidemia, lipiduria, vulnerability to infection, and thrombotic complications* (the last resulting from loss of serum anticoagulants and antiplasmins). The diseases causing nephrotic syndrome are listed in Table 20-4.

Membranous Nephropathy (p. 922)

Membranous nephropathy (MGN) is a common cause of adult nephrotic syndrome; it is idiopathic in 85% of patients, while the remainder occurs in association with malignancy, SLE, drug exposures (e.g., nonsteroidal anti-inflammatory drugs [NSAIDs], penicillamine, captopril), infections, or autoimmune disorders (e.g., thyroiditis).

Pathogenesis (p. 923)

MGN is a form of chronic immune complex–mediated disease. Antibodies can be against self-antigens (e.g., SLE) or exogenous proteins (e.g., infections) or haptens (e.g., drugs); lesions are

TABLE 20-4   Causes of Nephrotic Syndrome

Disease	Prevalence (%)*	
	Children	Adults
Primary Glomerular Disease		
Membranous glomerulopathy	5	30
Minimal-change disease	65	10
Focal segmental glomerulosclerosis	10	35
Membranoproliferative glomerulonephritides	10	10
Other proliferative glomerulonephritides (focal, "pure mesangial," IgA nephropathy)	10	15
Systemic Diseases		
Diabetes mellitus		
Amyloidosis		
Systemic lupus erythematosus		
Drugs (nonsteroidal anti-inflammatory, penicillamine, "street heroin")		
Infections (malaria, syphilis, hepatitis B and C, acquired immunodeficiency syndrome)		
Malignant disease (carcinoma, lymphoma)		
Miscellaneous (bee-sting allergy, hereditary nephritis)		

*Approximate prevalence of primary disease = 95% in children, 60% in adults. Approximate prevalence of systemic disease = 5% in children, 40% in adults.

similar to those seen in Heymann nephritis. Capillary leakiness results from complement activation that, in turn, activates epithelial and mesangial cells to liberate damaging proteases and oxidants.

Morphology (p. 923)

- By light microscopy, there is diffuse thickening of the capillary wall (hence the term *membranous*). Tubular epithelial cells contain protein reabsorption droplets, and there is interstitial chronic inflammation. With progressive disease, glomeruli sclerose.
- Immunofluorescence reveals diffuse GBM granular staining for immunoglobulin and complement.
- EM shows *subepithelial* GBM deposits, which eventually incorporate into the GBM and assume an intramembranous location.

Clinical Features (p. 923)

MGN usually manifests by insidious onset of nephrotic syndrome; hypertension and/or hematuria also occur in 15% to 35% of cases. The course of disease is variable but usually indolent. Proteinuria persists in 60% of patients, but only 10% die or progress to renal failure in 10 years; 40% eventually progress to renal insufficiency. Secondary causes of membranous GN should be excluded in any new case.

Minimal-Change Disease (p. 923)

Minimal-change disease (MCD) is the major cause of nephrotic syndrome in children, with a peak incidence between ages 2 and 6 years. The disease occasionally follows a respiratory infection or routine immunization, but it is also associated with atopic disorders and Hodgkin lymphoma (and other lymphomas and leukemias).

Pathogenesis (p. 925)

The current favored hypothesis is that MCD results from immune dysfunction and elaboration of one or more circulating cytokines that affect visceral epithelial cells; this causes loss of glomerular polyanions that form part of the normal permeability barrier and results in increased leakiness.

Morphology (p. 925)

- *Light microscopy* shows normal glomeruli (hence *minimal change*).
- *Immunofluorescence* shows no immune deposits.
- *EM* reveals diffuse effacement of the foot processes ("fusion") of visceral epithelial cells.

Clinical Features (p. 926)

The most characteristic feature of this condition is the dramatic response to corticosteroid therapy. Despite the heavy proteinuria (mostly albumin), the long-term prognosis is excellent.

Focal Segmental Glomerulosclerosis (p. 926)

Focal segmental glomerulosclerosis (FSGS) occurs:

- As a primary (idiopathic) disorder
- Secondary to other known disorders (e.g., heroin abuse, HIV infection, sickle cell disease, obesity)
- After glomerular necrosis due to other causes (e.g., IgA nephropathy)
- As an adaptive response to loss of renal tissue (e.g., chronic reflux, analgesic abuse, or unilateral renal agenesis)
- Secondary to mutations of proteins that maintain the glomerular filtration barrier; for example, podocyte proteins (e.g., podocin and α-actinin), or slit diaphragm proteins (e.g., nephrin)

Pathogenesis (p. 926)

The primary glomerular lesion in all FSGS is *visceral epithelial damage* (effacement or detachment) in affected glomerular segments. It is controversial whether idiopathic FSGS is part of a pathologic continuum with MCD. In other cases, a circulating cytokine(s) or genetic defects of the slit diaphragm complex are implicated. The ensuing glomerular sclerosis and hyalinosis stem from entrapment of plasma proteins and increased matrix synthesis.

Morphology (p. 926)

- *Light microscopy is characterized by sclerosis* of some, but not all, glomeruli (thus, *focal*); in affected glomeruli, only a portion of the capillary tuft is involved (thus, *segmental*).
- *Immunofluorescence* can show IgM and C3 in sclerotic areas or mesangium.
- *EM* (in both sclerotic and non-sclerotic areas) reveals diffuse foot process effacement with focal epithelial detachment.

Clinical Course (p. 928)

Besides proteinuria, which is relatively non-selective, FSGS patients often present with hematuria, reduced GFR, and hypertension. Idiopathic FSGS responds variably to steroids, and progression to chronic renal failure occurs in more than 20%; FSGS recurs in 25% to 50% of renal allograft recipients; proteinuria can occur within 24 hours of transplantation, emphasizing the potential role of circulating factors.

Human immunodeficiency virus (HIV)-associated nephropathy (p. 928) often manifests as a severe *collapsing glomerulopathy variant* of FSGS. There is retraction and/or collapse of the entire glomerular tuft and striking cystic dilation of tubular segments with associated inflammation and fibrosis. Proliferation and hypertrophy of glomerular visceral epithelium is associated with *endothelial tubuloreticular inclusions* (visualized by EM) caused by interferon-α-induced changes in the endoplasmic reticulum. The cause is HIV infection of tubular and glomerular cells and podocyte expression of HIV gene products *vpr* and *nef.*

Membranoproliferative Glomerulonephritis (p. 928)

Membranoproliferative glomerulonephritis (MPGN) accounts for 10% to 20% of nephrotic syndrome; it can be idiopathic or secondary to another disorder or agent.

Pathogenesis (p. 928)

MPGN is categorized into two forms:

* *Type I* (most common) is likely a consequence of antigen-antibody complex deposition and complement activation; the antigens in the complexes can originate from infection (e.g., hepatitis B or C, endocarditis, HIV), SLE, or malignancy, but in most cases the source is unknown. Type I MPGN can also be idiopathic.
* *Type II (dense-deposit disease)* is due to activation of the alternate complement pathway; most such patients have *C3 nephritic factor* in the serum, an autoantibody against C3 convertase that stabilizes its proteolytic activity.

Morphology (p. 929)

* *Light microscopy:* The adjective *membranoproliferative* reflects both thickened capillary loops and glomerular cell proliferation. Glomeruli appear "lobular" due to mesangial proliferation; the capillary walls often have a *double-contour* appearance due to interposition of cellular elements (mesangial, endothelial, or leukocyte) between reduplicated capillary basement membranes.
* *Immunofluorescence:*

  Type I: Occasional granular subepithelial and mesangial immunoglobulin and C3, C1q, and C4 deposits

  Type II: Irregular granular or linear deposits of C3 on either side of the GBM with occasional circular mesangial deposits; IgG, C1q, and C4 are absent

* *EM:*

  Type I: *Subendothelial* electron-dense deposits

  Type II: Characteristic laminar, ribbon-like electron-dense deposits in the GBM proper

Clinical Features (p. 929)

Most patients present in adolescence or young adulthood with nephrotic syndrome, occasionally with hematuria. Although steroids may slow the progression, about 50% of patients develop chronic renal failure within 10 years. There is a high recurrence rate in transplant recipients, particularly in patients with type II disease.

Isolated Urinary Abnormalities (p. 929)

IgA Nephropathy (Berger Disease) (p. 929)

IgA nephropathy (Berger disease) is probably the most common type of glomerulonephritis worldwide and is a major cause of recurrent glomerular hematuria.

Pathogenesis (p. 930)

Genetic or acquired defects in immune regulation are implicated; these result in increased mucosal IgA secretion (only IgA1 isotypes are nephritogenic) in response to ingested or inhaled antigens. Increased systemic IgA or qualitative alterations in the IgA molecule leads to augmented deposition in the mesangium and subsequent activation of the alternate complement pathway. IgA nephropathy occurs with increased frequency in patients with celiac disease (Chapter 17) or with liver pathology (due to diminished IgA clearance capacity); similar IgA deposits occur in *Henoch-Schönlein purpura* (see later discussion).

Morphology (p. 931)

- *Light microscopy:* Glomeruli can appear nearly normal, showing only subtle mesangial hypercellularity, or can have focal proliferative or sclerotic lesions.
- *Immunofluorescence:* IgA, C3, and properdin deposition is typical.
- *EM:* Electron-dense deposits in the mesangium.

Clinical Features (p. 931)

Patients typically present with gross hematuria following a respiratory, gastrointestinal, or urinary infection. The hematuria typically lasts for several days, then subsides, only to recur. Chronic renal failure develops in 15% to 40% over a period of 20 years. Older age of onset, heavy proteinuria, hypertension, crescents, and vascular sclerosis portend a poorer prognosis. Recurrence of IgA deposits is common in allografts, and 15% re-develop clinical disease.

Alport Syndrome (p. 931)

Hereditary nephritis is a heterogeneous group of renal diseases associated with glomerular injury. *Alport syndrome* is the best characterized of this group; it is manifested by hematuria progressing to chronic renal failure, associated with nerve deafness, lens dislocation, cataracts, and corneal dystrophy.

Pathogenesis (p. 932)

Disease manifestations are due to defective assembly of type IV collagen in the GBM, normally composed of a trimeric complex of $\alpha 3$, $\alpha 4$, and $\alpha 5$ subunits. The X-linked form (i.e., 85% of cases) is due to mutations in the $\alpha 5$ chain; autosomal forms are due to mutations in the $\alpha 3$ or $\alpha 4$ subunits. Abnormal type IV collagen affects the function of GBM, eye lens, and cochlea.

Morphology (p. 932)

Early lesions are only detectable by EM; there is diffuse GBM thinning, and interstitial cells are stuffed with fats and mucopolysaccharides. With disease progression, morphologic features of FSGS, tubular atrophy, and interstitial fibrosis supervene. In fully developed disease, there is irregularly thickened GBM with pronounced splitting of the lamina densa, often with a basket-weave appearance.

Thin Basement Membrane Lesion (Benign Familial Hematuria) (p. 932)

Thin basement membrane lesion (i.e., benign familial hematuria) is a fairly common entity manifesting as familial asymptomatic hematuria. Although proteinuria can be present, renal function is normal, and the prognosis is excellent; ocular abnormalities and hearing loss also do not occur. The disorder is due to mutations in the type IV collagen $\alpha 3$ or $\alpha 4$ chains, resulting in the GBM being only 150 to 250 nm thick (normal is 300 to 400 nm).

Chronic Glomerulonephritis (p. 932)

Chronic GN is the common end stage of a number of different entities; some arise without clear antecedent. Of the entities previously described, the following are the percentages that progress to chronic GN:

- Poststreptococcal GN (1% to 2%)
- RPGN (90%)
- Membranous GN (30% to 50%)
- FSGS (50% to 80%)
- MPGN (50%)
- IgA nephropathy (30% to 50%)

Morphology (p. 933)

- *Grossly:* The kidneys are symmetrically contracted with diffusely granular surfaces and a thinned cortex.
- *Microscopically:* Glomeruli are completely effaced by hyalinized connective tissue, making it impossible to identify the cause of the antecedent lesion; there is marked tubular atrophy. Associated hypertension leads to marked arteriolar sclerosis.
- *Dialysis changes:* These changes include arterial intimal thickening, acquired cystic changes, and calcium urate crystal deposition.

Clinical Course (p. 933)

Patients with chronic end-stage GN frequently develop hypertension; other secondary manifestations of uremia include pericarditis, uremic gastroenteritis, and secondary hyperparathyroidism with nephrocalcinosis and renal osteodystrophy.

Glomerular Lesions Associated with Systemic Diseases (p. 933)

Henoch-Schönlein Purpura (p. 934) Seen after SNYf infctn

Henoch-Schönlein purpura can occur at any age but typically presents in children between the ages of 3 and 8 years; findings include purpuric skin lesions (due to a vasculitis), abdominal symptoms (e.g., pain, vomiting, bleeding), arthralgia, and GN with some combination of hematuria, nephritic syndrome, and/or nephrotic syndrome. Glomerular lesions vary from focal mesangial proliferation to crescentic GN but are always associated with *mesangial IgA deposition.* Although the course is variable, the overall prognosis is usually excellent; recurrent hematuria can persist for years.

Bacterial Endocarditis–Associated Glomerulonephritis (p. 934)

Bacterial endocarditis–associated glomerulonephritis is due to immune complex (bacterial antigens and host antibodies) deposition. Presentations typically involve hematuria, although nephritic syndrome and even RPGN can occur. Renal lesions fall on a morphologic continuum from focal necrotizing GN to diffuse GN, to crescentic GN; immunofluorescence and EM studies show granular immune complex deposition.

Diabetic Nephropathy (p. 934)

Diabetic nephropathy leading to end-stage renal failure occurs in 40% of type 1 and type 2 diabetics. It is most commonly marked by glomerular disease leading to proteinuria, with or without nephrotic syndrome. However, diabetes also causes *hyalinizing arteriolar sclerosis,* increases the susceptibility to *pyelonephritis* and *papillary necrosis,* and causes a host of *tubular lesions.* The morphologic changes include:

- Capillary basement membrane thickening
- Diffuse mesangial sclerosis
- Nodular glomerulosclerosis (Kimmelstiel-Wilson disease)

Pathogenesis (p. 934)

Hyperglycemia and insulin deficiency lead to biochemical alterations in GBM, largely through the *non-enzymatic glycation* of proteins. Subsequent hemodynamic changes result in increased GFR, glomerular capillary pressure, and *glomerular hypertrophy,* which culminate in glomerulosclerosis (as discussed previously).

Amyloidosis (p. 935)

Amyloid (of any type) deposited in glomeruli and in vessel walls produces heavy proteinuria. Eventually, end-stage renal disease occurs.

Other Systemic Disorders (p. 935)

Goodpasture syndrome, polyarteritis nodosa, allergic vasculitis, and *Wegener granulomatosis* all produce similar forms of GN ranging from focal segmental necrotizing GN to crescentic GN. *Essential mixed cryoglobulinemia* can induce cutaneous vasculitis, synovitis, and MPGN. *Plasma cell dyscrasias* can be associated with amyloidosis, deposition of monoclonal Ig or light chains in the GBM, or a distinctive nodular GN (*light-chain deposition disease* ascribed to the deposition of non-fibrillar light chains).

Tubular and Interstitial Diseases (p. 935)

Acute Kidney Injury (Acute Tubular Necrosis) (p. 935)

Acute kidney injury (AKI) is synonymous with *acute tubular necrosis (ATN)* but is the increasingly favored term. AKI is the most common cause of acute renal failure and accounts for 50% of acute renal failure in hospitalized patients; it is characterized by renal tubular epithelial cell injury. Causes include:

- *Ischemia* occurring in a variety of clinical settings (e.g., shock, circulatory collapse, dehydration, malignant hypertension, vasculitis and hypercoagulable states)
- *Direct toxic injury* (e.g., drugs, radiocontrast dyes, myoglobin, hemoglobin, and radiation)
- *Acute tubulointerstitial nephritis* occurring most commonly as a hypersensitivity response to drugs
- *Urinary obstruction* due to tumors, prostatic hypertrophy, calculi, or blood clots

Pathogenesis (p. 936)

Reversible and irreversible tubular damage are the primary events leading to diminished renal function. Tubular epithelial cells are particularly sensitive to ischemia (high metabolic demand) and toxins (active transport system for ions and organic acids and capacity for drug concentration) (Fig. 20-2):

- Arteriolar vasoconstriction (with feedback involving the renin-angiotensin system and endothelial dysfunction) leads to increased endothelin and decreased nitric oxide (NO) and prostacyclin.
- Tubular obstruction by necrotic and apoptotic epithelial cells and proteinaceous material.

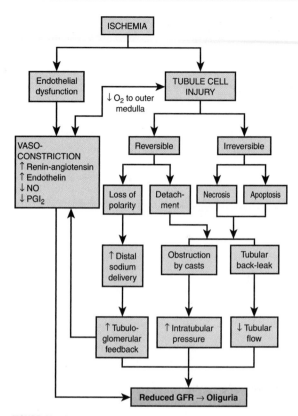

FIGURE 20-2 Pathogenic mechanisms in ischemic acute kidney injury. *GFR*, Glomerular filtration rate; *NO*, nitric oxide; *PGI₂*, prostacyclin.

- Back-leak of tubular fluids.
- Glomerular ultrafiltration is also directly affected by ischemia and toxins (attributed to mesangial contraction).

Morphology (p. 937)

Findings can be microscopically subtle:

Ischemic AKI: Patchy tubular necrosis with lesser degrees of tubular cell injury involves the proximal tubule straight segments and thick ascending loop of Henle.

Nephrotoxic AKI: Variable degrees of tubular injury and necrosis, mostly in proximal tubules; other tubular segments can be affected.

In all forms, distal tubules and collecting ducts contain cellular and protein casts, and there is interstitial edema with a variable inflammatory infiltrate. The recovery phase shows epithelial regeneration (i.e., tubular cells with hyperchromatic nuclei and mitotic figures).

Clinical Course (p. 938)

The clinical course of AKI is highly variable, but it classically proceeds through three stages:

- *Initiation phase (up to 36 hours):* Dominated by the inciting event; there is a slight decline in urine output and a rise in BUN.

- *Maintenance phase:* This phase is marked by oliguria (40 to 400 mL/day), salt and water overload, hyperkalemia, metabolic acidosis, and rising BUN.
- *Recovery phase:* This phase is heralded by rising urine volumes (up to 3 L/day) with water, sodium, and especially potassium losses (hypokalemia becomes a concern). Eventually, renal tubular function is restored and the concentrating ability improves.
- Prognosis depends in part on the cause; it is *good* (i.e., more than 95% survival) in most cases of nephrotoxic AKI, but it is poor (i.e., more than 50% mortality) for AKI secondary to overwhelming sepsis or other causes of multi-organ failure.

Tubulointerstitial Nephritis (p. 938)

These disorders have diverse causes and pathogenic mechanisms; they are distinguished from glomerular diseases by the absence of the hallmarks of nephritic or nephrotic syndrome and by the features of tubular dysfunction (e.g., impaired urine-concentrating ability [polyuria], salt wasting, and metabolic acidosis).

Pyelonephritis and Urinary Tract Infection (p. 939)

Urinary tract infection (UTI) denotes infection of the bladder *(cystitis)*, the urethra or ureter, the kidneys *(pyelonephritis)*, or all of these. The most common organisms are the normal Gram-negative bacilli inhabitants of the gastrointestinal tract. UTIs are much more common in women, due to the shorter urethra, hormonal changes affecting mucosal bacterial adherence, and the absence of prostatic fluid antibacterial compounds; other UTI risk factors include long-term catheterization, vesicoureteral reflux, pregnancy, diabetes mellitus, immunosuppression, and lower urinary tract obstructions from congenital defects, benign prostatic hypertrophy, tumors, or calculi. *Hematogenous spread* of bacteria to the renal parenchyma occurs much less commonly.

Pathogenesis (p. 939)

In either gender, pyelonephritis is most commonly the result of *ascending infection* from the bladder. The typical sequence of events is:

- Colonization of the distal urethra and introitus (females) through expression of adherence molecules (*adhesins* on pili).
- Multiplication of bacteria in the bladder, facilitated by adhesion virulence factors and urinary tract obstruction or stasis.
- Vesicoureteral reflux through an incompetent vesicoureteral orifice, allowing retrograde seeding of the renal pelvis and renal papillae. Vesicoureteral reflux is most often due to congenital defects in the intravesicular portion of the ureter (1% to 2% of otherwise normal individuals) and may be accentuated by cystitis.
- Intrarenal reflux through open papillae to renal tissue.

UTIs can be clinically silent, that is, asymptomatic bacteriuria with or without *pyuria* (leukocytes in the urine). More often, UTIs cause dysuria and frequency, and in pyelonephritis (see later discussion) they cause flank pain, fever, and urine leukocyte *casts*.

Acute Pyelonephritis (p. 941)

Acute pyelonephritis is marked by patchy, suppurative inflammation, tubular necrosis, and intratubular neutrophil casts.

Morphology (p. 941)

More advanced changes include abscesses, *papillary necrosis* (especially in diabetics and in those with obstruction), *pyonephrosis* (pelvis filled with pus), *perinephric abscesses*, and eventually renal scars with fibrotic deformation of the cortex and underlying calyx and pelvis.

Clinical Features (p. 942)

Uncomplicated pyelonephritis follows a benign course with antibiotic therapy but can recur or progress in the presence of vesicoureteral reflux, obstruction, immunocompromise, diabetes, and other conditions.

An emerging viral etiology for renal infections in kidney allografts is *polyomavirus*. Latent infections (common in the general population) get reactivated in immunocompromised hosts; these cause tubular epithelial infections and associated inflammation that can result in allograft failure in 1% to 5% of infected patients *(polyomavirus nephropathy)*.

Chronic Pyelonephritis and Reflux Nephropathy *(p. 942)*

Chronic pyelonephritis (CPN) is characterized by *tubulointerstitial inflammation, renal scarring, and dilated, deformed calyces*. It can be divided into two forms.

- *Reflux nephropathy* (p. 942) is most common. It begins in childhood, as a result of infections superimposed on congenital vesicoureteral reflux and intrarenal reflux; it can be unilateral or bilateral.
- *Chronic obstructive pyelonephritis* (p. 942) occurs when chronic obstruction (e.g., with hydronephrosis) predisposes the kidney to infections; the effects of chronic obstruction also contribute to parenchymal atrophy.

Morphology (p. 943)

Both major types of CPN are associated with broad scars, deformed calyces, and significant tubulointerstitial inflammation and fibrosis. Secondary FSGS (due to loss of glomerular mass) and vascular hypertensive changes can also be present.

Clinical Features (p. 943)

Both forms of CPN can manifest with the symptoms of acute pyelonephritis or can have a silent, insidious onset, sometimes presenting only very late in their course with hypertension or evidence of renal dysfunction in the absence of persisting infection. The development of proteinuria and FSGS is a poor prognostic sign.

Tubulointerstitial Nephritis Induced by Drugs and Toxins *(p. 944)*

- *Acute drug-induced interstitial nephritis* (p. 944) results from an idiosyncratic hypersensitivity reaction to a variety of drugs; it begins roughly 2 weeks after exposure with the offending agent(s) acting as immunizing haptens. Drugs covalently bind to tubular cellular or matrix components and induce antibody (IgE) and T-cell–mediated immune reactions.

Morphology (p. 945)

Biopsy exhibits edema, patchy tubular necrosis, and tubulointerstitial infiltrates, with variable combinations of lymphocytes, histiocytes, eosinophils, neutrophils, plasma cells, and occasionally well-formed granulomas.

Clinical Features (p. 945)

Fever, eosinophilia, skin rash, hematuria, mild proteinuria, sterile pyuria, azotemia, and acute renal failure are all variably present. Drug withdrawal usually leads to full recovery.

- *Analgesic nephropathy* (p. 945) is usually caused by excessive intake of phenacetin-containing analgesic *mixtures;* ingestion of aspirin, phenacetin, or acetaminophen in isolation rarely causes disease.

Pathogenesis (p. 945)

Papillary necrosis occurs as a consequence of direct toxicity and ischemia. Phenacetin and its acetaminophen metabolite deplete tubular cells of glutathione and then induce the formation of oxidative metabolites; aspirin contributes by inhibiting the formation of vasodilatory prostaglandins.

Morphology (p. 945)

Analgesic nephropathy is characterized by chronic tubulointerstitial nephritis with papillary necrosis.

Clinical Features (p. 946)

Early manifestations include polyuria (inability to concentrate urine) and increased stone formation due to tubular acidosis. Anemia, gastrointestinal symptoms, and hypertension are common, and urinary tract infections complicate 50% of cases. Papillary necrosis can be diagnosed radiologically, but it is not specific for analgesic nephropathy (other etiologies: diabetes mellitus, sickle cell disease, and urinary tract obstruction). There is an increased risk of transitional cell carcinoma of the renal pelvis.

- *Nephropathy associated with NSAIDs* (p. 946) is due to a combination of:

  Decreased synthesis of vasodilatory prostaglandins
  Hypersensitivity interstitial nephritis (see preceding discussion)
  Cytokine elaboration leading to podocyte foot process effacement
  Membranous nephropathy of uncertain etiology

Other Tubulointerstitial Diseases (p. 947)

- *Urate nephropathy* (p. 947): This can cause acute or chronic renal failure, depending on the tempo of uric acid deposition.

  Acute urate nephropathy occurs when uric acid crystals precipitate in tubules and collecting ducts, leading to obstruction. This is typically a consequence of tumor cell lysis following chemotherapy for hematologic malignancy.
  Chronic urate nephropathy occurs with more prolonged hyperuricemia (e.g., with gout). The acidic environment of the collecting system leads to deposition of monosodium urate, ultimately obstructing the tubules (with cortical atrophy) or forming *tophi* consisting of foreign body giant cells and fibrosis.
  Hyperuricemia also leads to *nephrolithiasis*; uric acid stones are present in 22% of patients with gout and 42% of patients with secondary hyperuricemia.

- *Hypercalcemia and nephrocalcinosis* (p. 947): Disorders associated with hypercalcemia induce renal calcium deposition (nephrocalcinosis) and calcium stone formation. Both can cause renal failure through tubular obstruction; nephrocalcinosis can also cause renal insufficiency through direct tubular epithelial effects. Calcium phosphate deposition can also be a consequence of consuming high quantities of phosphate solutions (e.g., for colonoscopic bowel preps).

- *Light-chain cast nephropathy* ("myeloma kidney") (p. 948): Renal insufficiency occurs in 50% of patients with multiple myeloma. Several factors contribute:

  Bence Jones proteinuria and cast nephropathy: Some light chains are directly toxic to epithelial cells. In addition, under acidic conditions, Bence Jones proteins combine with *Tamm-Horsfall* urinary glycoprotein to form large casts that obstruct the tubular lumens and induce a peritubular inflammatory reaction *(cast nephropathy)*. Bence Jones proteinuria occurs in 70% of patients with myeloma.

Amyloidosis: This occurs in 6% to 24% of myeloma patients.

Light-chain deposition disease: This occurs when light chains deposit in GBM or mesangium, causing a glomerulopathy, or in tubular basement membranes, causing a tubulointerstitial nephritis.

Hypercalcemia and hyperuricemia: These are common features of myeloma.

Vascular Diseases (p. 949)

Nearly all kidney diseases and many systemic disorders secondarily affect the renal vasculature. Hypertension, in particular, affects renal vessels; conversely, any vascular changes tend to amplify the hypertension.

Benign Nephrosclerosis (p. 949)

Benign nephrosclerosis denotes the kidney pathology associated with renal arteriolar sclerosis. The arteriolar lumena are stenosed by wall thickening and hyalinization from deposition of insudated proteins and increased basement membrane matrix synthesis. Larger muscular arteries show *fibroelastic hyperplasia*, with both medial and intimal thickening. *The vascular lesions cause diffuse ischemic atrophy of nephrons; as a result, the kidneys are relatively small and exhibit diffuse granular surfaces due to scarring and contraction of individual glomeruli.*

Benign nephrosclerosis rarely causes renal failure but can cause mild proteinuria. Progression to renal failure is correlated to the severity of hypertension, the presence of co-morbid disease (e.g., diabetes), and African origin.

Malignant Hypertension and Accelerated Nephrosclerosis (p. 949)

Malignant nephrosclerosis is associated with accelerated hypertension. While this can occur in previously normotensive people, most cases are superimposed on preexisting benign essential hypertension (1% to 5% of such patients), chronic renal disease (particularly GN or reflux nephropathy), or scleroderma.

Pathogenesis (p. 950)

Following an initial vascular insult (e.g., long-standing benign hypertension, arteritis, coagulopathy, etc.), endothelial injury, platelet deposition, and increased vascular permeability lead to *fibrinoid necrosis* and intravascular thrombosis. These cause renal ischemia, with stimulation of the renin-angiotensin and other vasoconstrictive systems (e.g., endothelin), as well as aldosterone-driven salt (and water) retention, perpetuating an ever-increasing cycle of escalating blood pressures.

Morphology (p. 950)

Pathologic changes include fibrinoid necrosis of arterioles, hyperplastic arteriopathy (onion-skinning), necrotizing glomerulitis, and a glomerular thrombotic microangiopathy.

Clinical Features (p. 951)

Patients have systolic pressures more than 200 mm Hg and diastolic blood pressures more than 120 mm Hg; there is also proteinuria, hematuria, papilledema, encephalopathy, cardiovascular abnormalities, and eventually renal failure. Plasma renin, angiotensin, and aldosterone levels are all increased. With prompt anti-hypertensive intervention, 75% of patients survive 5 years, and half recover pre-crisis renal function.

Renal Artery Stenosis (p. 951)

Unilateral renal artery stenosis accounts for 2% to 5% of patients with renal hypertension; the vascular narrowing induces excessive renin secretion by the involved kidney. Obstructive *atheromatous plaque* at the renal artery take-off underlies 70% of cases; the remainder is caused by *fibromuscular dysplasia*. The latter is a heterogeneous group of disorders, usually occurring in young women (between ages 20 and 40 years), and characterized by non-arteriosclerotic *intimal, medial,* or *adventitial* hyperplasia. Revascularization surgery cures 70% to 80% of cases if performed before arteriolosclerosis develops in the contralateral kidney.

Thrombotic Microangiopathies (p. 952)

This group of diseases has overlapping clinical manifestations (e.g., microangiopathic hemolytic anemia, thrombocytopenia, renal failure, and manifestations of intravascular coagulation) (Chapter 14). *Endothelial injury* with *platelet activation and aggregation* are shared pathogenic mechanisms; they lead to increased leukocyte adhesion, increased endothelin, decreased NO production (favoring vasoconstriction), and endothelial lysis. *Hemolytic-uremic syndrome (HUS)* is largely due to endothelial injury, whereas platelet activation underlies *thrombotic thrombocytopenic purpura (TTP)*.

- *Typical (childhood) HUS* is associated with consumption of food contaminated with bacteria (e.g., *E. coli* strain O157:H7) that synthesize Shiga-like toxins.
- *Atypical HUS* is associated with mutations of complement-regulatory proteins, antiphospholipid antibodies, contraceptives, complications of pregnancy, certain drugs, radiation, and scleroderma.
- *TTP* is caused by inherited or acquired deficiencies of ADAMTS13, a plasma metalloproteinase that regulates von Willebrand factor (vWF) function.

Morphology (p. 953)

Although they have diverse causes, these disorders are characterized morphologically by thromboses in the interlobular arteries, afferent arterioles, and glomeruli, together with necrosis and thickening of the vessel walls. The morphologic changes are similar to those in malignant hypertension, but the changes can precede the development of hypertension or be seen in its absence.

Other Vascular Disorders (p. 954)

Atheroembolic Renal Disease (p. 954)

Cholesterol crystals and debris embolize from atheromatous plaques after manipulation of severely diseased aortas (e.g., during aortic cannulation). They lodge in intrarenal vessels, causing arterial narrowing and focal ischemic injury. Rarely, renal function becomes compromised.

Sickle-Cell Disease Nephropathy (p. 954)

This occurs in both sickle cell heterozygotes and homozygotes; accelerated sickling in the hypertonic, hypoxic renal medulla leads to vascular occlusion with hematuria, diminished concentrating ability, and even proteinuria. Patchy *papillary necrosis* with cortical scarring can also result.

Diffuse Cortical Necrosis (p. 954)

This is an uncommon but potentially fatal complication of obstetric emergency (e.g., abruptio placenta), septic shock, or extensive surgery. Patients develop diffuse glomerular and arteriolar microthrombi (morphologically akin to disseminated intravascular coagulopathy) leading to renal necrosis. The etiology is unknown.

Renal Infarcts (p. 955)

Renal infarcts are common occurrences because kidneys receive 25% of cardiac output (and a substantial number of any systemic atheroemboli) and because of their "end organ" arterial blood supply without significant collateral circulation. Left atrial or ventricle mural thrombi (secondary to atrial fibrillation or myocardial infarction) are a major source of emboli, followed by left-sided valvular vegetations, aortic aneurysms, and aortic atherosclerosis. Most renal infarcts are asymptomatic but can cause pain and/or hematuria. Large infarcts of one kidney can cause hypertension.

Congenital Anomalies (p. 955)

Approximately 10% of newborns have potentially significant malformations of the urinary system; renal dysplasias and hypoplasias account for 20% of pediatric chronic renal failure. Most arise from acquired developmental defects rather than as hereditable lesions.

- *Agenesis of the kidney* (p. 955): *Bilateral* absence of renal development is incompatible with life. *Unilateral* agenesis is associated with compensatory hypertrophy of the remaining kidney; with time, the hypertrophied kidney can develop glomerulosclerosis and renal failure.
- *Hypoplasia* (p. 955): This refers to failure to develop to normal size, usually as a unilateral defect. A truly hypoplastic kidney shows no scars and possesses a reduced number (i.e., 6 or fewer) of renal lobes and pyramids.
- *Ectopic kidneys* (p. 955): These lie either just above the pelvic brim or sometimes within the pelvis. Kinking or tortuosity of the ureters may cause urinary obstruction, predisposing to bacterial infection.
- *Horseshoe kidneys* (p. 955): These result from renal fusion—upper poles in 10% of cases, and lower poles in 90%—producing a U-shaped structure continuous across the midline and anterior to the aorta and inferior vena cava.

Multicystic Renal Dysplasia (p. 955)

This is a sporadic disorder resulting from abnormal metanephric differentiation; it can be unilateral or bilateral. Affected kidneys are enlarged and multicystic with abnormal lobar organization; histologically, there are immature ducts surrounded by undifferentiated mesenchyme, often with cartilage formation. Most cases are associated with obstructive abnormalities of the ureter and lower urinary tract.

Cystic Diseases of the Kidney (p. 956)

Table 20-5 summarizes the genetics, pathologic findings, and clinical consequences of the various cystic diseases.

TABLE 20-5 Summary of Renal Cystic Diseases

	Inheritance	Pathologic Features	Clinical Features or Complications	Typical Outcome	Diagrammatic Representation
Adult polycystic kidney disease	Autosomal dominant	Large multicystic kidneys, liver cysts, berry aneurysms	Hematuria, flank pain, urinary tract infection, renal stones, hypertension	Chronic renal failure beginning at age 40-60 years	
Childhood polycystic kidney disease	Autosomal recessive	Enlarged, cystic kidneys at birth	Hepatic fibrosis	Variable, death in infancy or childhood	
Medullary sponge kidney	None	Medullary cysts on excretory urography	Hematuria, urinary tract infection, recurrent renal stones	Benign	
Familial juvenile nephronophthisis	Autosomal recessive	Corticomedullary cysts, shrunken kidneys	Salt wasting, polyuria, growth retardation, anemia	Progressive renal failure beginning in childhood	
Adult-onset medullary cystic disease	Autosomal dominant	Corticomedullary cysts, shrunken kidneys	Salt wasting, polyuria	Chronic renal failure beginning in adulthood	
Simple cysts	None	Single or multiple cysts in normal-sized kidneys	Microscopic hematuria	Benign	
Acquired renal cystic disease	None	Cystic degeneration in end-stage kidney disease	Hemorrhage, erythrocytosis, neoplasia	Dependence on dialysis	

Autosomal Dominant (Adult) Polycystic Kidney Disease (p. 956)

Autosomal dominant (adult) polycystic kidney disease (ADPKD) occurs in 1 of every 400 to 1000 persons and accounts for 5% to 10% of chronic renal failure; it has high penetrance and is universally bilateral.

Pathogenesis (p. 956)

ADPKD is caused in most cases by mutations in one of two genes:

- *PKD1* mutations (chromosome 16p13.3) account for about 85% of cases. *PKD1* encodes *polycystin 1*, a large (460 kD) protein that localizes to tubular epithelial cells and has domains that are usually involved in cell-cell and cell-matrix interactions.
- *PKD2* mutations (4q21) are responsible for most of the remaining cases. *PKD2* encodes *polycystin 2*, a cation channel; mutations disrupt the regulation of intracellular calcium.

The current pathogenic hypothesis for ADPKD revolves around the sensing and transduction of mechanical signals. Thus, a single apical non-motile primary cilium in tubular epithelial cells functions as a mechanosensor to monitor changes in fluid flow and shear stress, while intercellular junctional complexes and focal adhesions monitor forces between cells and extracellular matrix. In response to external forces, these sensors regulate ion flux that, in turn, modulates cell polarity and proliferation. Polycystin 1 and 2 are both localized to the primary cilium and potentially form a complex that regulates intracellular calcium in response to fluid flow. Mutated proteins could conceivably affect intracellular second messengers and thereby influence proliferation, apoptosis, ECM interactions, and secretory function, leading to the progressive formation of tubular cysts.

Morphology (p. 958)

Kidneys are massively enlarged and composed almost entirely of cysts up to 3 to 4 cm in diameter. Cysts arise anywhere along the nephron and compress adjacent parenchyma. In late disease, there is interstitial inflammation and fibrosis.

Clinical Features (p. 958)

Although most patients are asymptomatic until renal insufficiency supervenes, cystic dilation or hemorrhage can cause pain and/or hematuria, and hypertension, polyuria, and proteinuria also occur. For *PKD1* mutations, renal failure is present in 35% by age 50 years, 70% by age 60 years, and 95% by age 70 years; the corresponding figures for *PKD2* mutations are 5%, 15%, and 45%. Progression is accentuated in the presence of hypertension. Roughly 40% of patients have scattered liver biliary cysts *(polycystic liver disease),* and *mitral valve prolapse* occurs in 20% to 25%. About 40% of patients die of hypertensive or coronary heart disease, 25% of infections, 15% from ruptured *berry aneurysms* in the circle of Willis (causing subarachnoid hemorrhages) or hypertensive brain hemorrhage, and the rest of other causes.

Autosomal Recessive (Childhood) Polycystic Kidney Disease (p. 959)

Autosomal recessive (childhood) polycystic kidney disease (ARPKD) is genetically distinct from ADPKD; it is categorized by age of presentation *(perinatal* through *juvenile)* and the presence of associated hepatic lesions. In most cases, the disease is caused by mutations of *PKHD1* (chromosome 6p21-p23), encoding for *fibrocystin,* a large transmembrane protein that localizes to the primary cilium of tubular epithelial cells. Kidneys are enlarged by multiple, cylindrically dilated collecting ducts oriented at right angles to the cortex and filling both the cortex and medulla. The liver almost always has cysts and proliferating bile ducts; in the infantile and juvenile forms patients develop *congenital hepatic fibrosis.*

Cystic Diseases of Renal Medulla *(p. 959)*

Medullary Sponge Kidney *(p. 959)*

Medullary sponge kidney presents in adults with multiple cystic dilations in the medullary collecting ducts. Although typically an innocuous lesion discovered incidentally by radiographic studies, it can predispose to renal calculi.

Nephronophthisis and Adult-Onset Medullary Cystic Disease *(p. 959)*

These constitute a family of progressive renal disorders characterized by small medullary cysts typically concentrated at the corticomedullary junction. There are four variants:

• Sporadic, nonfamilial (20%)
• Familial juvenile nephronophthisis (50%); autosomal recessive
• Renal-retinal dysplasia (15%); autosomal recessive
• Adult-onset medullary cystic disease (15%); autosomal dominant

Affected children present with polyuria, sodium wasting, and tubular acidosis, followed by progression to renal failure over 5 to 10 years. These disorders should be strongly considered in children with otherwise unexplained chronic renal failure, a positive family history, and chronic tubulointerstitial nephritis on biopsy.

Pathogenesis *(p. 960)*

At least seven gene loci have been identified; *NPH1, NPH2,* and *NPH3* underlie the juvenile form of nephronophthisis. The gene products of *NPH1* and *NPH3* are called *nephrocystins* and are associated with the primary cilia; *NHP2* codes for *inversin,* which mediates right-left embryologic patterning. Initial injury to the distal tubules with basement membrane disruption leads to chronic progressive tubular atrophy and interstitial fibrosis.

Acquired (Dialysis-Associated) Cystic Disease *(p. 960)*

End-stage kidneys of patients undergoing prolonged renal dialysis develop multiple cortical and medullary cysts due to obstruction from calculi and/or interstitial fibrosis. The cysts often contain calcium oxalate crystals and are commonly lined by atypical, hyperplastic epithelium that can undergo malignant transformation.

Simple Cysts *(p. 960)*

Single or multiple cysts of the cortex (rarely medulla) are lined by low cuboidal epithelium and can range from 1 to 10 cm in size; they are common lesions. They have smooth walls and are filled with clear serous fluid; occasionally, hemorrhage can cause flank pain, and calcification with irregular contours can mimic renal carcinoma.

Urinary Tract Obstruction (Obstructive Uropathy) *(p. 960)*

Obstruction increases susceptibility to infection and stone formation, and unrelieved obstruction almost always leads to permanent renal atrophy. *Hydronephrosis is the term for pelvis and calyceal dilation associated with progressive renal atrophy of the kidney following outflow obstruction.* Causes include:

- Congenital anomalies (urethral valves or strictures, meatal stenosis, bladder neck obstruction, ureteropelvic junction obstruction, severe vesicoureteral reflux)
- Urinary calculi
- Prostatic hypertrophy
- Tumors of prostate, bladder, cervix, or uterus
- Inflammation (prostatitis, ureteritis, urethritis, retroperitoneal fibrosis)
- Sloughed papillae or blood clots
- Normal pregnancy
- Uterine prolapse and cystocele
- Functional disorders (neurogenic bladder)

Morphology (p. 961)

When obstruction is sudden and complete, GFR reduction leads to relatively modest pelvis and calyceal dilation, with only mild parenchymal atrophy. When the obstruction is subtotal or intermittent, GFR is not suppressed, and progressive dilation ensues. Obstruction also triggers interstial inflammatioin and fibrosis.

Clinical Features (p. 962)

Most early symptoms are the consequence of the underlying obstruction (e.g., renal colic from a stone). Unilateral obstruction can remain silent for long periods because the unaffected kidney can usually compensate. In bilateral partial obstruction, manifestations include polyuria, distal tubular acidosis, salt wasting, renal calculi, tubulointerstitial nephritis, atrophy, and hypertension. Complete bilateral obstruction results in oliguria or anuria; relief of such blockade is accompanied by a brisk post-obstructive diuresis.

Urolithiasis (Renal Calculi, Stones) (p. 962)

Calculi can arise at any level in the urinary tract, although most form in the kidney. In the United States, there is a 5% to 10% lifetime risk of urolithiasis, with men affected more commonly than women, and a peak incidence between ages 20 and 30 years. Hereditary associations are characterized by excessive production or secretion of stone-forming substances (e.g., gout, cystinuria, and primary hyperoxaluriua).

Pathogenesis (p. 962)

Increased concentrations of stone constituents, changes in urinary pH, decreased urine volume, and bacteria all play a role in stone formation. In addition, *loss of inhibitors* of crystal formation (e.g., citrate, pyrophosphate, glycosaminoglycans, osteopontin, and a glycoprotein called *nephrocalcin*) can also contribute.

There are four types of calculi; all also contain an organic matrix of mucoprotein (1% to 5% by weight):

- About 70% are *calcium-containing* stones composed of calcium oxalate and/or calcium phosphate. These are usually associated with hypercalcemia or hypercalciuria (i.e., 60%); hyperoxaluria and hyperuricosuria are contributory in others, and in 15% to 20%, there is no demonstrable metabolic abnormality.
- About 15% to 20% of calculi are *triple phosphate* or *struvite* stones composed of magnesium ammonium phosphate. Struvite stones precipitate in alkaline urine generated by bacterial infections that

convert urea to ammonia (e.g., *Proteus*). *Staghorn calculi*—occupying large parts of the renal pelvis—are struvite stones usually associated with infections.

- Roughly 5% to 10% are *uric acid stones*; more than half of such patients are neither hyperuricemic nor hyperuricosuric, instead they make exceptionally acidic urine (i.e., pH less than 5.5) that causes uric acid to precipitate.
- Between 1% and 2% of calculi are composed of *cysteine*, and are caused by genetic defects in renal amino acid resorption.

Clinical Features (p. 963)

Stones frequently cause clinical symptoms, including obstruction, ulceration, bleeding, and pain *(renal colic)*; they also predispose to renal infection.

Tumors of the Kidney (p. 963)

Benign Tumors (p. 963)

Renal Papillary Adenomas (p. 963)

Renal papillary adenomas are common (7% to 22% of autopsies), small (i.e., 0.5 cm), yellow cortical tumors. Histologically, most consist of vacuolated epithelial cells forming tubules and complex branching papillary structures. Adenomas are histologically indistinguishable from low-grade papillary renal cell carcinomas, and they share some of their cytogenetic features; 3 cm is the size cut-off separating those that metastasize from those that rarely do.

Angiomyolipoma (p. 963)

Angiomyolipoma is a hamartomatous lesion composed of vessels, smooth muscle, and fat; these are present in 25% to 50% of patients with tuberous sclerosis. They are clinically significant primarily for their susceptibility to spontaneous hemorrhage.

Oncocytoma (p. 964)

Oncocytoma is an epithelial tumor composed of eosinophilic cells arising from collecting duct intercalated cells; on electron microscopy, the cells are packed with mitochondria. They are common (5% to 15% of resected renal neoplasms) and can be large (up to 12 cm).

Malignant Tumors (p. 964)

Renal Cell Carcinoma (Adenocarcinoma of the Kidney) (p. 964)

Renal cell carcinoma represents 3% of all visceral cancers and 85% of renal cancers in adults; they usually occur in patients between the ages of 50 and 70 years and show a 2:1 male preponderance. Tobacco is the most significant risk factor, although obesity, hypertension, unopposed estrogens, and exposures to asbestos, petroleum products, and heavy metals are also implicated. Most renal cancer is sporadic, but autosomal dominant familial variants account for 4% of cases.

- *von Hippel-Lindau (VHL) syndrome:* 50% to 70% of patients with certain *VHL* mutations develop renal cysts, as well as bilateral, frequently multicentric renal cell carcinomas. A host of mutations in the *VHL* gene (see later discussion) are implicated in carcinogenesis of both familial and sporadic clear cell tumors; these do not necessarily induce the other manifestations of the syndrome.

- *Hereditary papillary carcinoma:* This is ascribed to mutations in the *MET* proto-oncogene; it is an autosomal dominant entity manifesting with multiple bilateral papillary tumors.

Classification and Pathogenesis (p. 964)

The classification of renal cell carcinoma is based on histology, cytogenetics, and genetics:

- *Clear cell (non-papillary) carcinoma* is the most common type (i.e., 70% to 80%); 95% are sporadic, and in 98% of these tumors—*whether familial, sporadic, or associated with VHL mutations*—there is a loss of sequences on chromosome 3p at a locus that harbors *VHL*. *VHL* is a tumor suppressor gene that encodes part of a ubiquitin ligase complex involved in targeting proteins for degradation. When *VHL* is mutated, hypoxia-inducible factor-1 levels remain high, and this constitutively active protein increases the production of growth and angiogenic factors that promote tumorigenesis.
- *Papillary carcinoma* accounts for 10% to 15% of renal cell cancers and occurs in both familial and sporadic forms. The familial form is associated with mutations of the *MET* proto-oncogene that serves as a tyrosine kinase receptor for *hepatocyte growth factor.*
- *Chromophobe renal carcinoma* constitutes 5% of renal cell cancers; they derive from collecting duct intercalated cells. Although they exhibit multiple chromosome losses and extreme hypodiploidy, they have an excellent prognosis.
- *Collecting duct (Bellini duct) carcinoma* makes up only 1% of renal cancers; this arises from medullary collecting duct cells.

Morphology (p. 965)

- *Clear cell carcinomas* are usually solitary, large (i.e., more than 3 cm) spherical bright yellow-gray masses that distort the renal outline. They exhibit large areas of ischemic opaque, gray-white necrosis, foci of hemorrhagic discoloration, and areas of softening. Tumors can bulge into the calyces and pelvis and invade the renal vein to grow as a solid column of cells within this vessel. Histologically, they can be solid, trabecular, or tubular growths; individual cells are polygonal with abundant clear cytoplasm, and there is a delicate arborizing vasculature.
- *Papillary carcinomas* can be multifocal and bilateral. These are typically hemorrhagic and cystic. Microscopically, these are composed of cuboidal cells arranged in papillary formations, often with interstitial foam cells and psammoma bodies (lamellated, calcified concretions).
- *Chromophobe renal carcinoma* is composed of pale, eosinophilic cells with perinuclear halos arranged in sheets around blood vessels.

Clinical Features (p. 966)

Patients classically (but only 10% of the time) present with flank pain, palpable mass, and hematuria. More commonly, tumors declare at a larger size (i.e., 10 cm) with fever, malaise, and weight loss. Renal cell carcinomas also produce a host of paraneoplastic syndromes attributable to hormone production: polycythemia, hypercalcemia, hypertension, feminization or masculinization, Cushing syndrome, eosinophilia, leukemoid reaction, and amyloidosis. *Prognosis* depends on tumor size and the extent of spread at diagnosis. Renal cell carcinoma tends to metastasize before symptoms are felt; in 25% of patients, there is radiographic evidence of metastases at presentation. On average, 45% of patients survive 5 years; without metastasis, the 5-year survival is 70%.

Urothelial Carcinomas of the Renal Pelvis (p. 967)

About 5% to 10% of renal tumors originate from renal pelvic urothelium; they tend to manifest relatively early due to hematuria or obstruction. Their histologic type is the same as for urothelial tumors in the bladder (Chapter 21), ranging from well-differentiated papillary lesions to anaplastic, invasive carcinomas. They are often multifocal, and in 50% of cases there is a concomitant bladder tumor. Five-year survival rate varies from 50% to 100% for low-grade superficial tumors to 10% with high-grade infiltrating tumors.

21

The Lower Urinary Tract and Male Genital System

THE LOWER URINARY TRACT (p. 972)

Ureters (p. 972)

Congenital Anomalies (p. 972)

Congenital ureteral anomalies are seen in 2% to 3% of autopsies; most have no clinical significance. However, congenital or acquired *ureteropelvic junction obstruction* can be an important cause of hydronephrosis, especially in children. The obstruction is secondary to disorganized junctional smooth muscle, excess stromal matrix, or rarely compression by renal vessels.

Tumors and Tumor-Like Lesions (p. 973)

Primary ureteral tumors are rare. *Benign ureteral neoplasms* are usually mesenchymal; *fibroepithelial polyps* present as small intraluminal projections, most commonly in children. *Malignant ureteral neoplasms* are primarily urothelial carcinomas comparable to similar tumors in the renal pelvis and bladder.

Obstructive Lesions (p. 973)

Ureteral obstruction can be secondary to calculi or clots, strictures (either extrinsic or due to congenital or post-inflammatory narrowing), tumors, or neurogenic bladder dysfunction. Ureteral dilation (hydroureter) is less important than the secondary renal hydrophrosis and/or pyelonephritis (Chapter 20).

Sclerosing *retroperitoneal fibrosis* (p. 973) is an uncommon cause of obstruction characterized by retroperitoneal inflammation and fibrosis that encases the ureters and leads to hydronephrosis; various drugs, inflammatory processes, and neoplasms can all contribute, but 70% have no obvious cause *(Ormond disease)*.

Urinary Bladder (p. 974)

Congenital Anomalies (p. 974)

- *Diverticula* (p. 974) are outpouchings of the bladder wall that can arise as congenital defects but more commonly are acquired in the setting of persistent urethral obstruction (e.g., with prostatic enlargement). Urinary stasis in the diverticuli predispose to infection and calculi formation, as well as vesicoureteric reflux; carcinomas arising within them tend to be more advanced due to thinning of the underlying wall.

- *Exstrophy* (p. 974) of the bladder is due to developmental failure of the anterior abdominal wall; the bladder communicates directly with the overlying skin or lies as an exposed sac. Complications include chronic infection and an increased incidence of adenocarcinoma; these can be surgically corrected.
- *Miscellaneous anomalies* (p. 974) include *vesicoureteral reflux* (most common; Chapter 20) and abnormal congenital connections between bladder and vagina, rectum, uterus, or umbilicus. The latter is often a remnant fistulous tract of the *urachus* that connected fetal bladder and allantois; occasionally only the central portion of the tract persists as a *urachal cyst*.

Inflammation (p. 974)

Acute and Chronic Cystitis (p. 974)

Urinary tract infections (UTIs) are extensively discussed in Chapter 20; they typically take the form of nonspecific acute and/or chronic inflammation. Besides the typical bacterial causes (mostly coliforms), infectious cystitis can be caused by *M. tuberculosis* (secondary to renal tuberculosis), fungi (mostly *Candida*), viruses, *Chlamydia,* and *Mycoplasma;* schistosomiasis cystitis is common in the Middle East. Radiation and chemotherapies can also precipitate bladder inflammation and/or hemorrhage. Classical cystitis symptoms are urinary frequency, lower abdominal pain, and *dysuria* (pain on urination).

Special Forms of Cystitis (p. 975)

- *Interstitial cystitis (chronic pelvic pain syndrome)* (p. 975) is a form of chronic cystitis, occurring usually in women. This causes pain and dysuria in the absence of infection. Punctate hemorrhages characterize early lesions, followed classically in late-stage disease by localized ulceration *(Hunner ulcer)* with inflammation and transmural fibrosis. Mast cells are characteristically seen but are of uncertain significance.
- *Malacoplakia* (p. 975) occurs in chronic bacterial cystitis (mostly due to *E. coli* or *Proteus* species) and is more common in immunosuppressed patients. Lesions are characterized by 3- to 4-cm soft, yellow, mucosal plaques, composed primarily of foamy macrophages stuffed with bacterial debris; the macrophages also display intra-lysosomal laminated calcified concretions called *Michaelis-Gutmann bodies*. The unusual appearance suggests defective macrophage phagocytic or degradative function.

Metaplasic Lesions (p. 975)

- *Cystitis glandularis and cystitis cystica* (p. 975) are common lesions in the setting of chronic cystitis, but they also occur in normal bladders. These are composed of nests of transitional epithelium *(Brunn nests)* that grow downward into the lamina propria and transform into cuboidal epithelium *(cystitis glandularis,* occasionally with intestinal metaplasia) or flattened cells lining fluid-filled cysts *(cystitis cystica).* They do not increase the risk of developing adenocarcinoma.
- *Squamous metaplasia* (p. 976) can occur as a response to injury.
- *Nephrogenic adenoma* (p. 976) results when shed tubular cells implant and proliferate at sites of injured urothelium. Although there can be extension into the superficial detrusor muscle, and lesions can be sizable, they are benign.

Neoplasms (p. 976)

In the United States, bladder cancer accounts for 7% of all malignancies and 3% of cancer deaths; 95% are of epithelial origin, the remainder being mesenchymal.

Urothelial Tumors (p. 976)

Urothelial tumors run the gamut from small benign lesions to aggressive cancers with a high mortality; these can occur anywhere from the renal pelvis to the distal urethra, and many are multifocal at presentation.

Precursor lesions to malignancy fall into two categories:

* *Non-invasive papillary tumors* are the most common, with lesions exhibiting a range of atypia that can reflect biologic behavior.
* *Carcinoma* in situ *(CIS)* represents a high-grade lesion of cytologically malignant cells present within a flat urothelium; the cells often lack cohesiveness and shed into the urine (detectable on urine cytology).

In half of patients, tumor has already invaded the bladder wall at the time of initial presentation. The absence of precursor lesions in such cases suggests obliteration by the high-grade invasive component. Although lamina propria invasion worsens prognosis, involvement of the muscularis propria (detrusor muscle) is the major determinant of outcome; at that stage there is a 50%, 5-year mortality.

Morphology (p. 977)

Urothelial malignancy ranges from papillary to nodular or flat.

* Most *papillary* lesions are low grade (i.e., less than 10% risk of invasion); they appear as red excrescences from 0.5 to 5 cm in size:

    Exophytic papillomas (urothelium over finger-like papillae with loose fibrovascular cores) have an extremely low incidence of progression or recurrence.

    Inverted papillomas (bland urothelium extending into the lamina propria) are uniformly benign.

    Papillary urothelial neoplasms of low malignant potential are slightly larger than papillomas with thicker urothelium and enlarged nuclei (but rare mitoses) and infrequent invasion.

    Low-grade papillary urothelial carcinomas characteristically have orderly cytology and architecture, with minimal atypia; they can invade but are rarely fatal lesions.

    High-grade papillary urothelial cancers contain discohesive cells with anaplastic features and architectural disarray; these have a high risk (i.e., 80%) for progression and metastases.

* CIS usually appears as an area of mucosal reddening, granularity, or thickening without producing an evident intraluminal mass. CIS is commonly multifocal; if untreated, 50% to 75% progress to invasive cancer.

Other Epithelial Tumors (p. 979)

* *Squamous cell carcinomas* are associated with chronic bladder infection and inflammation; these represent 3% to 7% of bladder cancers in the United States, but they occur much more frequently in countries endemic for urinary schistosomiasis.
* *Mixed urothelial carcinomas with areas of squamous carcinoma* are invasive, fungating, and/or ulcerating tumors; they are more common than purely squamous cell bladder cancers.
* *Adenocarcinomas* of the bladder are rare; they can arise from urachal remnants or in the setting of intestinal metaplasia.

Pathogenesis (p. 979)

Bladder cancer has a male to female ratio of 3:1 and is more common in industrialized nations, affecting urban populations more than rural dwellers; 80% of patients are between the ages of 50 and 80 years. Risk factors include:

- Cigarette smoking
- Industrial exposure to arylamines, particularly 2-naphthylamine
- *Schistosoma haematobium* infections (70% of such cases will be squamous)
- Chronic analgesic use
- Long-term cyclophosphamide exposure (causes hemorrhagic cystitis)
- Bladder radiation

The cytogenetic and molecular alterations are heterogeneous, but most tumors, even when multicentric, are clonal. Chromosome 9 deletions or monosomy are common (30% to 60% of tumors); 9p deletions involve the tumor-suppressor genes *p16* (*INK4a*) and *p15*. Many tumors also have 17p deletions (including *p53*) or *p53* mutations, suggesting a critical role in urothelial carcinoma progression.

Clinical Course of Bladder Cancer (p. 980)

Bladder tumors classically manifest with *painless hematuria*; frequency, urgency, and dysuria can also occur. At presentation, 60% of neoplasms are single and 70% are localized to the bladder.

Patients tend to develop new tumors (occasionally of higher grade) after primary excision; recurrences can reflect either new tumors or (because they share the same genetic changes as the initial tumor) represent shedding and implantation of the original tumor cells.

Prognosis depends upon the histologic grade and stage at diagnosis. Papillomas, papillary urothelial neoplasms of low malignant potential, and low-grade papillary urothelial cancer carry a 98%, 10-year survival rate regardless of the number of recurrences. In contrast, an initial high-grade cancer portends a 25% mortality rate.

Therapy depends on the grade and stage, as well as whether the lesion is flat or papillary. For small, low-grade papillary tumors, primary transurethral resection is sufficient (followed by life-long periodic cystoscopic and urine cytologic examinations). After primary resection, patients with higher-grade but still focal lesions can receive topical installation of an attenuated strain of tuberculous bacillus (BCG) that induces a therapeutic inflammatory response. Radical cystectomy is indicated for tumor invading the muscularis propria, CIS or high-grade papillary cancer refractory to immunotherapy, or CIS extending into the prostatic urethra and prostatic ducts. Metastatic bladder cancer requires chemotherapy.

Mesenchymal Tumors (p. 980)

Mesenchymal tumors are rare. *Benign tumors* resemble their counterparts elsewhere, with *leiomyomas* being most common. *Sarcomas* typically produce large (10 to 15 cm) exophytic masses; *embryonal rhabdomyosarcoma* is most common in children, and *leiomyosarcoma* is most common in adults.

Urethra (p. 981)

Inflammation (p. 981)

Urethritis is classically denoted as either *gonococcal* or *non-gonococcal* and is often accompanied by cystitis (women) or prostatitis (men). The most common non-gonococcal organisms are *E. coli* and other enterics; *Chlamydia* is responsible for 25% to 60% of non-gonococcal urethritis (NGU) in men and 20% in women, with *Mycoplasma* being a less frequent cause. Urethritis is also one component (along with arthritis and conjunctivitis) of the Reiter syndrome triad associated with NGU.

Tumors and Tumor-Like Lesions (p. 981)

- *Caruncles* are painful, small, red inflammatory lesions (essentially, polyps of inflamed granulation tissue) of the external urethral meatus in women; they are exquisitely friable and bleed easily. Excision is curative.
- *Peyronie disease* causes fibrosis of the penile corpus cavernosum, resulting in curvature and in pain during intercourse.
- *Urethral carcinoma* is uncommon; in the proximal urethra, these are analogous to bladder urothelial malignancy, whereas in the distal urethra, they are more commonly squamous cell carcinomas.

THE MALE GENITAL TRACT (p. 982)

Penis (p. 982)

Congenital Anomalies (p. 982)

Hypospadias and Epispadias (p. 982)

Malformations of the urethral canal can produce aberrant openings either on the *ventral* aspect of the penis *(hypospadias)* or the *dorsal* surface *(epispadias)*. These can be associated with other urogenital malformations, including *undescended testes*. Constriction can predispose to UTIs; severe displacement of the orifice can be a cause of sterility.

Phimosis (p. 982)

Phimosis is the designation for a prepuce (foreskin) orifice too small to permit normal retraction; it can be a primary developmental defect but is more often secondary to inflammation. Phimosis predisposes to secondary infections and carcinoma from chronic accumulation of secretions and other debris *(smegma)*.

Inflammation (p. 982)

Inflammations characteristically involve both the glans penis and the prepuce.

- The *sexually transmitted* causes of inflammation (e.g., syphilis, gonorrhea, chancroid, lymphopathia venereum, genital herpes, granuloma inguinale) are discussed in Chapter 8.
- *Balanoposthitis* refers to non-specific infection by other organisms (e.g., *Candida*, anaerobic or pyogenic bacteria and *Gardnerella*). Most are a consequence of poor local hygiene in uncircumcised males due to accumulated smegma and can lead to phimosis.

Tumors (p. 982)

Benign Tumors (p. 982)

- *Condyloma acuminatum* (p. 982) is a benign sexually-transmitted epithelial proliferation caused by *human papillomavirus (HPV)*, especially types 6 and 11. After excision it tends to recur, but it rarely transforms to malignancy.

Morphology (p. 983)

- *Grossly:* Single or multiple sessile or pedunculated red papillary excrescences 1 to 5 mm in size, often involving the coronal sulcus or inner prepuce.

- *Microscopically:* Branching papillae covered by hyperplastic (but orderly) stratified squamous epithelium, often with hyperkeratosis; epithelial cell vacuolation *(koilocytosis)* is common.

Malignant Tumors (p. 983)

- *Carcinoma* in situ *(CIS)* (p. 983): These lesions are strongly associated with HPV infection, especially type 16.

  Bowen disease can involve either male or female genitalia, generally in patients older than 35 years. Men typically present with solitary or multiple thickened, gray-white or red shiny plaques over the penile shaft. Histology reveals marked epithelial atypia with lack of orderly maturation but *no invasion.* Over the span of years transition to invasive squamous cell carcinoma occurs in approximately 10% of cases.

  Bowenoid papulosis presents as multiple, pigmented papular lesions on external genitalia in younger, sexually active patients. The lesions are histologically indistinguishable from Bowen disease, but evolution into invasive carcinoma is rare, and they frequently spontaneously regress.

- *Invasive carcinoma* (p. 984): Penile squamous cell carcinoma accounts for less than 1% of cancers in American men. The prevalence is higher in regions where circumcision is not routinely practiced. This prevalence is related to carcinogens within smegma accumulating under the foreskin, as well as HPV types 16 and 18. Most cases occur in men between ages 40 and 70 years.

Morphology (p. 984)

Squamous cell carcinoma typically presents as epithelial thickening on the glans or inner surface of the prepuce, progressing to ulceroinfiltrative or exophytic growth eroding the penile tip, shaft, or both. The histology is identical to squamous cell carcinomas elsewhere. *Verrucous carcinoma* is an uncommon well-differentiated variant with low malignant potential.

Clinical Features (p. 984)

The clinical course is characterized by slow growth; metastases can occur in regional (inguinal and iliac) lymph nodes, but distant metastases are uncommon. The 5-year survival rate is 66% for lesions confined to the penis and 27% with regional node involvement.

Testis and Epididymis (p. 984)

Congenital Anomalies (p. 984)

Cryptorchidism (p. 984)

Cryptochidism affects 1% of 1-year-old boys and represents *failure of descent;* it is usually unilateral and an isolated anomaly, but it is bilateral in 25% of patients and can occur with other genitourinary malformations. Although testes can be found anywhere along the normal abdomen-to-scrotal sac pathway, defects in transabdominal descent (under the control of *müllerian-inhibiting substance*) account for only 5% to 10% of cases; most cryptorchidism involves abnormalities in the descent through the inguinal canal into the scrotal sac (under the control of androgens) and, in most patients, the undescended testis is palpable in the inguinal canal.

Morphology (p. 985)

Histologic changes in maldescended testes can manifest as early as age 2 years; these include *decreased germ cell development, thickening* and *hyalinization* of seminiferous tubule basement membrane, and interstitial *fibrosis* along with relative sparing of Leydig cells. Histologic deterioration in the contralateral *descended* testis suggests an intrinsic defect in testicular development.

Beyond sterility, cryptorchidism is associated with *inguinal hernias* (10% to 20% of cases) and an increased incidence of *testicular malignancy.* Most cryptorchid testes spontaneously descend in the first year of life; for those that do not, surgical correction *(orchiopexy)* before the second birthday improves (but does not guarantee) fertility and reduces cancer risk.

Regressive Changes (p. 985)

Atrophy and Decreased Fertility (p. 985)

Atrophy and decreased fertility can be:

- Primary, due to a developmental abnormality (e.g., *Klinefelter syndrome*).
- Secondary to cryptorchidism, vascular disease (e.g., atherosclerosis), inflammatory disorders, hypopituitarism, malnutrition, persistently elevated levels of follicle-stimulating hormone, exogenous androgenic or anti-androgenic hormones, radiation, and chemotherapy.

The morphologic alterations are identical to those seen in cryptorchidism.

Inflammation (p. 986)

Inflammatory conditions are generally more common in the epididymis than in the testis; the exception is syphilis, which begins in the testis and secondarily progresses to involve the epididymis.

Nonspecific Epididymitis and Orchitis (p. 986)

Nonspecific epididymitis and orchitis typically result from a primary urinary tract infection that reaches the epididymis via the vas deferens or spermatic cord lymphatics. Causes vary with the age of the patient:

- *Childhood epididymitis* is usually associated with congenital genitourinary abnormalities and Gram-negative rod infections.
- In *sexually active men younger than 35 years, C. trachomatis* and *N. gonorrhoeae* are the common culprits.
- In men older than 35 years, common UTI agents (e.g., *E. coli* and *Pseudomonas*) are usually causal.

Morphology (p. 986)

This is characterized by non-specific epididymal congestion, edema, and neutrophilic infiltrates; severe cases can progress to generalized suppuration. Inflammation can extend to the testis via efferent ductules or local lymphatic channels, and resultant scarring can cause *infertility.* Leydig cells are less severely affected, so that testosterone levels are generally maintained.

Granulomatous (Autoimmune) Orchitis (p. 986)

Granulomatous (autoimmune) orchitis presents in middle age as a painless to moderately tender testicular mass of sudden onset; the histology reveals spermatic tubule granulomas. An autoimmune pathogenesis is suspected.

Specific Inflammations (p. 986)

- *Gonorrhea* (p. 986): Most cases represent *retrograde extension* of infection from the posterior urethra to the prostate, seminal vesicles, and epididymis; untreated, the infection can extend to the testis to produce suppurative orchitis.

- *Mumps* (p. 986): Mumps orchitis is uncommon in children, but it develops in 20% to 30% of postpubertal men infected with mumps. Acute interstitial orchitis typically develops about 1 week after onset of parotid inflammation.
- *Tuberculosis* (p. 986): Tuberculosis almost always begins in the *epididymis*, with secondary involvement of the testis; the histology of caseating granulomas is identical to that seen in other sites.
- *Syphilis* (p. 986): Syphilis can occur as both congenital and acquired forms and can present as isolated orchitis without involvement of adnexal structures. Histologically, there can be nodular *gummas* or *diffuse interstitial inflammation* with edema, lymphoplasmacytic inflammation, and obliterative endarteritis.

Vascular Disorders (p. 987)

Torsion (p. 987)

Twisting of the spermatic cord cuts off the testicular *venous drainage*; since the thick-walled arteries typically remain patent, there is intense vascular engorgement potentially followed by hemorrhagic infarction.

- *Neonatal torsion* occurs either *in utero* or shortly after birth; it lacks any associated anatomic defect.
- *Adult torsion* typically presents in adolescence as sudden dramatic testicular pain; it is associated with a *bilateral anatomic defect* giving the testis increased mobility *(bell-clapper abnormality)*.

Torsion often occurs without any inciting injury and can even occur during sleep. Torsion is a true urologic emergency; surgical untwisting within 6 hours of onset can preserve testicular viability. To prevent a recurrence or a similar fate in the contralateral testis, both testes are surgically fixed to the scrotum (orchiopexy).

Spermatic Cord and Paratesticular Tumors (p. 987)

- *Lipomas* commonly involve the proximal spermatic cord; in some cases, however, fat around the cord only represents retroperitoneal adipose tissue that has been pulled into the inguinal canal with a hernia sac.
- *Adenomatoid tumors* are the most common benign paratesticular neoplasms. These are small nodules of mesothelial cells usually near the upper epididymal pole.
- Of malignant tumors in this location, *rhabdomyosarcomas* are most common in children, and *liposarcomas* are most common in adults.

Testicular Tumors (p. 987)

Testicular tumors are generally divided into two major categories:

- *Germ cell tumors* (i.e., 95% of cases) are generally malignant; these are further divided into *seminomas* and *non-seminomas*.
- *Sex cord stromal tumors* are generally benign.

Germ Cell Tumors (p. 987)

Germ cell tumors have an incidence in the United States of 6 in 100,000 and involve whites five times more often than blacks; they constitute the most common malignancy in men between the ages of 15 and 34 years and account for 10% of cancer deaths in that group.

Pathogenesis (p. 988)

Several risk factors are implicated:

- *Cryptorchidism* is the most important; it is associated with 10% of cases.
- *Testicular dysgenesis syndrome (TDS)* includes cryptorchidism, hypospadias, and poor sperm quality; TDS has been related to pesticide and non-steroidal estrogen exposures *in utero.*
- *Genetic factors* are reflected by familial clustering and an increased incidence of testicular carcinoma among brothers and sons of affected individuals.

Most tumors arise from a focus of *intratubular germ cell neoplasia (ITGCN),* which occurs *in utero* but remains dormant until puberty. These cells retain expression of transcription factors OCT3/4 and NANOG associated with totipotentiality; they also share some of the genetic alterations found in many germ cell tumors (e.g., additional copies of chromosome 12p) and/or activating mutations of *c-KIT.* The neoplastic ITGCN cells then give rise to *seminomas* or transform into a *totipotential* neoplastic cell (e.g., *embryonal carcinoma*) capable of further differentiation.

SEMINOMA (p. 988)

Seminoma accounts for 50% of all testicular germ cell tumors; it has a peak incidence between ages 30 and 40 years.

Morphology (p. 988)

- *Grossly:* Seminomas are homogeneous, lobulated, gray-white masses, generally devoid of hemorrhage or necrosis; the tunica albuginea usually remains intact.
- *Microscopically:* This germ cell neoplasm is the one most likely to exhibit a single histologic pattern.

  The mass is composed of large polyhedral *seminoma cells* containing abundant clear cytoplasm (due to glycogen), large nuclei, and prominent nucleoli.

  A fibrous stroma of variable density divides the neoplastic cells into irregular *lobules,* and there is a lymphocytic (and occasionally granulomatous) infiltrate.

  Tumor cells are diffusely positive for c-KIT, OCT4, and placental alkaline phosphatase (PLAP).

  Roughly 15% contain syncytiotrophoblasts; human chorionic gonadotropin (hCG) is present in such cells.

SPERMATOCYTIC SEMINOMA (p. 989)

- Spermatocytic seminoma is an uncommon neoplasm (1% to 2% of all germ cell tumors), typically occurring in older patients (older than 65 years). These are usually indolent tumors with little tendency to metastasize; they are *not* associated with ITGCN.

Morphology (p. 989)

- *Grossly:* Soft, gray cut surfaces sometimes with mucoid cysts.
- *Microscopically:* Lesions composed of a *mixture* of three cell populations: small cells resembling secondary spermatocytes, medium-sized cells with a round nucleus and eosinophilic cytoplasm, and scattered giant cells.

EMBRYONAL CARCINOMA (p. 989)

- Embryonal carcinoma has a peak incidence between ages 20 and 30 years; these cancers are more *aggressive* than seminomas.

Morphology (p. 989)

- *Grossly:* Most are poorly demarcated, small, gray-white masses punctuated by hemorrhage and/or necrosis. Extension through the tunica albuginea into the epididymis or cord is common.
- *Microscopically:* Lesions are composed of primitive epithelial cells with indistinct cell borders, forming irregular sheets, tubules, alveoli, and papillary structures. Mitoses and giant cells are common; tumor cells are positive for OCT3/4, PLAP, cytokeratin, and CD30 but are negative for c-KIT.

YOLK SAC TUMOR (ENDODERMAL SINUS TUMOR) (p. 989)

Yolk sac tumor (endodermal sinus tumor) is the most common testicular neoplasm in patients younger than 3 years; the prognosis is very good. Most adult cases occur as a component of embryonal carcinoma.

Morphology (p. 990)

- *Grossly:* This is typically an infiltrative, homogeneous, yellow-white mucinous tumor.
- *Microscopically:* Lesions are composed of cuboidal neoplastic cells arrayed in a lacelike (reticular) network; solid areas and papillae may also be seen. Structures resembling primitive glomeruli *(Schiller-Duval bodies)* are seen in half. Eosinophilic hyaline globules containing immunoreactive *α-fetoprotein (AFP)* and *α1-antitrypsin* are associated with neoplastic cells.

CHORIOCARCINOMA (p. 990)

Choriocarcinoma is a highly malignant neoplasm composed of both cytotrophoblastic and syncytiotrophoblastic elements; it comprises less than 1% of all germ cell tumors.

Morphology (p. 990)

- *Grossly:* The neoplasm is often small, even in the presence of widespread systemic metastases; it ranges from a hemorrhagic mass to an inconspicuous lesion replaced by a fibrous scar.
- *Microscopically:* Lesions are composed of polygonal, comparatively uniform cytotrophoblastic cells growing in sheets and cords, admixed with multinucleated syncytiotrophoblastic cells; hCG is readily demonstrable.

TERATOMA (p. 990)

Teratoma is a neoplasm showing differentiation along endodermal, mesodermal, and ectodermal lines; these occur at any age. While pure teratomas are rare, the frequency of teratomas mixed with other germinal cell tumors approaches 50%. In children, mature teratomas behave as benign tumors, and patients have an excellent prognosis. In post-pubertal men, all teratomas are regarded as malignant regardless of the maturity or immaturity of the various elements.

Morphology (p. 991)

- *Grossly:* Tumors are usually large (5 to 10 cm), with a heterogeneous appearance; hemorrhage and necrosis suggest admixture with embryonal and/or choriocarcinoma.
- *Microscopically:* Teratomas are composed of a haphazard array of *differentiated* mesodermal (e.g., muscle, cartilage, adipose tissue), ectodermal (e.g., neural tissue, skin), and endodermal (e.g., gut, bronchial epithelium) elements. Tissues may be mature (resembling adult tissues) or immature (sharing histologic features with embryonic or fetal tissues).

Teratoma with malignant transformation signifies a non–germ cell malignancy developing within a teratoma. When the non–germ cell component spreads outside the testis it usually does not respond to chemotherapy; cure therefore depends on tumor resectability.

Clinical Consequences of Germ Cell Testicular Tumors (p. 991)

In 60% of cases, testicular germ cell tumors contain mixtures of multiple cell types; prognosis is a function of the most aggressive element. While most germ cell tumors are capable of rapid, wide dissemination, they usually respond to therapy.

- Most cases present with *painless enlargement of the testis;* clinical evaluation does not reliably distinguish between the various types.
- Since testicular biopsy could cause "tumor spillage" necessitating scrotal excision *in addition to* orchiectomy, standard management is radical orchiectomy based on a presumption of malignancy.
- Lymphatic metastases typically first involve *retroperitoneal para-aortic* nodes but can then spread more widely; *hematogenous* metastases predominantly involve the lung, followed by liver, brain, and bone. Because of the histologic mixtures present in many of these tumors, metastases need not be identical to the primary tumors, and they can contain other germ cell elements (e.g., teratomatous metastases from an "apparent" embryonal carcinoma primary).
- Non-seminomatous germ cell tumors (NSGCTs) are generally more aggressive than seminomas and do slightly worse.

  Seminomas are typically radiosensitive, and 70% present with localized (clinical stage I) disease. More than 95% of patients with stage I or stage II disease (extension to retroperitoneal nodes) are cured.

  NSGCTs are relatively radioresistant and 60% present with advanced disease (stage II, or stage III [metastases above the diaphragm]); 90% can achieve remission with chemotherapy.

  Pure choriocarcinomas are particularly aggressive, and extensive hematogenous metastases can be present even with small primary lesions. They have a poor prognosis.

- Germ cell neoplasms often produce hormones or enzymes that can be used for diagnosis and monitoring:

  AFP is markedly elevated in endodermal sinus tumors but present at lower levels in other germ cell tumors.

  High *hCG* is typical of choriocarcinomas but also present at lower levels in 15% of seminomas, as well as other NSGCT.

  Lactate dehydrogenase, while non-specific, can provide a rough measure of tumor burden.

Tumors of Sex Cord–Gonadal Stroma (p. 992)

Classification is based on Leydig versus Sertoli cell differentiation.

LEYDIG CELL TUMORS (p. 992)

Leydig cell tumors account for only 2% of all testicular tumors; most occur between the ages of 20 and 60 years. Tumors can produce androgens, estrogens, and/or corticosteroids; patients typically present with a *testicular mass* but can also exhibit changes referable to hormone elaboration (e.g., gynecomastia or sexual precocity). Most are benign, although 10% invade or metastasize.

Morphology (p. 992)

- *Grossly:* Tumors are grossly circumscribed nodules with a homogeneous, golden brown cut surface.
- *Microscopically:* Lesions are composed of polygonal cells with abundant granular, eosinophilic cytoplasm and indistinct cell borders. Lipochrome pigment, lipid droplets, and eosinophilic Reinke crystalloids are common.

SERTOLI CELL TUMORS (p. 992)

Sertoli cell tumors typically present only as a testicular mass and are hormonally silent; 10% pursue a malignant course.

Morphology (p. 992)

- *Grossly:* Tumors are homogeneous gray-white to yellow masses of variable size.
- *Microscopically:* Lesions exhibit tall, columnar cells in trabeculae, often forming cords or tubules.

Testicular Lymphoma (p. 993)

Testicular lymphomas account for 5% of all testicular neoplasms and are the most common testicular tumor in patients older than 60 years. Most are diffuse, large B-cell non-Hodgkin lymphomas and disseminate widely, with a high incidence of central nervous system (CNS) involvement.

Miscellaneous Lesions of Tunica Vaginalis (p. 993)

- *Hydrocele:* Accumulation of serous fluid within the mesothelial-lined tunica vaginalis, usually due to generalized edema
- *Hematocele:* Accumulation of blood secondary to trauma, torsion, or a generalized bleeding diathesis
- *Chylocele:* Accumulation of lymphatic fluid secondary to lymphatic obstruction (e.g., elephantiasis)
- *Spermatocele:* Local cystic accumulation of semen in dilated ductuli efferentes or rete testis
- *Varicocele:* Dilated vein in the spermatic cord; may be asymptomatic or contribute to infertility
- *Malignant mesothelioma* rarely arises in the tunica vaginalis

Prostate (p. 993)

Prostatic parenchyma can be divided into four biologically and anatomically distinct zones; the proliferative lesions are different for each region (Fig. 21-1).

Inflammation (p. 993)

- *Acute bacterial prostatitis* (p. 993): This is typically caused by organisms associated with UTI (e.g., E. coli, other Gram-negative rods, enterococci, and staphylococci).

  Prostatic infection occurs through urinary reflux or lymphohematogenous seeding from more distant sites; it can also follow catheterization or surgical manipulation.

  Patients present with fever, chills, dysuria, and a boggy, markedly tender prostate; diagnosis is based on clinical features and urine culture.

- *Chronic bacterial prostatitis* (p. 994): This is an insidious disorder that can be asymptomatic or associated with low back pain, suprapubic and perineal discomfort, and dysuria. It is frequently associated with a history of *recurrent UTI*, but without previous

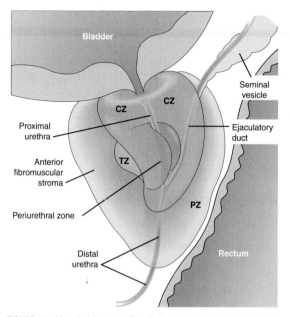

FIGURE 21-1 Normal adult prostate. Four distinct regions are appreciated: a central zone *(CZ)*, a peripheral zone *(PZ)*, a transitional zone *(TZ)*, and a periurethral zone. Most carcinomas arise in glands in the *PZ*, and can therefore be palpated during rectal digital examination. Nodular hyperplasia characteristically arises in the *TZ* and periurethral zone, typically leading to urinary obstruction earlier than does carcinoma.

acute prostatitis; the organisms are those typically involved in acute prostatitis.

Because antibiotics penetrate the prostate poorly, bacteria find safe haven and can recurrently seed the urinary tract.

Diagnosis is based on finding leukocytes and positive bacterial cultures in prostatic secretions.

- *Chronic abacterial prostatitis* (p. 994): This is the most common form of prostatitis.

  Manifestations are similar to chronic bacterial prostatitis but *without* recurrent urinary tract infections.

  Prostatic secretions contain more than 10 leukocytes per high-power field, but cultures are uniformly negative.

- *Granulomatous prostatitis* (p. 994): In the United States, the most common cause is related to installation of BCG to treat bladder cancer; in this setting, prostatic granulomas are of no clinical significance and require no treatment. Non-specific granulomatous prostatitis is relatively common and represents a reaction to secretions from ruptured prostatic ducts and acini.

Benign Enlargement (p. 994)

Benign Prostatic Hyperplasia or Nodular Hyperplasia (p. 994)

Benign prostatic hyperplasia (BPH) or nodular hyperplasia is an extremely common disorder caused by periurethral epithelial and stromal hyperplasia that compresses the urethra; symptoms are related to urinary flow obstruction. Histologic evidence of BPH is present in 20% of men by the age 40 years, 70% of men by age 60 years, and 90% by age 70 years; only half have clinically detectable prostate enlargement, and of those, only 50% develop clinical symptoms. Some 30% of white American men older than 50 years have moderate to severe symptoms.

Pathogenesis (p. 994)

The critical mediator in this process is dihydrotestosterone (DHT)—synthesized by the stromal cells of the prostate from circulating testosterone via the activity of 5α-reductase, type 2.

- DHT binds to the nuclear androgen receptor (AR) in stromal and epithelial cells, activating the transcription of androgen-dependent genes.
- DHT is not a direct mitogen, but it does increase the production of secondary growth factors and their receptors, particularly fibroblast growth factor-7 (FGF-7) by stromal cells.
- FGF-7 acts in a paracrine manner to stimulate stromal cell proliferation and inhibits epithelial apoptosis.
- Augmented FGF-1 and -2 and transforming growth factor-β (TGF-β) production also contribute by driving fibroblast proliferation.

Morphology (p. 995)

- *Grossly:* The gland is enlarged by nodules primarily in the transitional and periurethral zones (see Fig. 21-1); the cut surface demonstrates well-demarcated nodules that can vary from firm and pale gray (predominantly fibromuscular stromal) to yellow-pink and soft (mostly glands).
- *Microscopically:* Nodules are composed of variable mixtures of proliferating glands and fibromuscular stroma; glands are lined by two layers of cells—a basal layer of low cuboidal epithelium covered by a layer of columnar secretory cells. Other changes include *squamous metaplasia and infarcts.*

Clinical Features (p. 995)

The symptoms of lower urinary tract obstruction are due to the increased size of the prostate, the extrinsic compression of the urethra, and smooth muscle-mediated contraction of the prostate. In turn, the increased resistance to urinary outflow leads to bladder hypertrophy and distention, with urinary retention. Patients manifest with:

- Urinary frequency, nocturia, and difficulty starting and stopping the stream of urine
- Chronic urinary stasis with resultant bacterial overgrowth and UTIs
- Urinary bladder diverticula and hydronephrosis

Therapy can include α-blockers that inhibit the α_1-adrenergic receptors mediating prostate smooth muscle tone. In addition, 5-α-reductase inhibitors can reduce the underlying DHT-mediated stimulation, and for recalcitrant prostates, surgical (e.g., transurethral resection of the prostate [TURP]) and various other debulking approaches are available.

Tumors (p. 996)

Adenocarcinoma (p. 996)

Prostatic carcinoma is the *most common* form of cancer in men (29% of U.S. cancers) with a 1 in 6 lifetime risk; it is responsible for 9% of cancer deaths. Prostatic carcinoma occurs predominantly in men older than 50 years; the incidence increases from 20% for men in their fifties to 70% for men in their seventies. It is uncommon in Asians, and is more common in blacks than in whites. The clinical behavior ranges from aggressively lethal to indolent and incidental.

Pathogenesis (p. 996)

Clinical and epidemiologic data implicate advancing age, race, hormonal influences, genetic factors, and environmental factors (e.g., diet).

- *Androgens:* Prostate cancer cells depend on androgen interactions with AR to activate pro-growth and pro-survival genes.

  The X-linked AR gene contains a polymorphic sequence composed of CAG (glutamine) repeats. ARs with shorter glutamine repeats (common in African Americans) are more sensitive to androgens, whereas ARs with more numerous repeats (common in Asians) are less sensitive; Caucasians typically have intermediate-length repeats.

  Castration and anti-androgen therapies slow tumor progression, although most tumors eventually become resistant to androgen blockade (e.g., through mutations that allow activation by low-level androgens or non-androgen ligands or that bypass the need for AR).

- *Germline genes:* Risk increases with the number of first-degree relatives with prostate cancer (one relative = two-fold increased risk; two relatives = five-fold increased risk) and the onset of disease occurs at an earlier age.

  BRCA2 mutations increase risk 20-fold, but most familial prostate cancers are associated with loci that only modestly affect risk.

  Several risk loci are associated with innate immunity, suggesting that inflammation can underlie prostate cancer development.

- *Acquired mutations and epigenetic changes:*

  Chromosomal rearrangements that juxtapose an *ETS* family transcription factor gene next to the androgen-regulated *TMPRSS2* promoter lead to overexpression of the ETS transcription factors and make prostate epithelial cells more invasive.

  Hypermethylation of the glutathione *S*-transferase gene downregulates its expression and leads to increased susceptibility to a variety of carcinogens normally modified by the enzyme.

  Reduced expression of the adhesion molecule E-cadherin is associated with increased expression of the EZH-2 transcriptional repressor.

- *Diet:* Risk is associated with increased fat consumption; dietary products that appear to prevent or delay progression of prostate cancer include lycopenes (found in tomatoes), vitamin D, selenium, and soy products.

- *Precursor lesions:* Prostatic intraepithelial neoplasia (PIN) is now identified as a precursor on the spectrum to prostatic carcinoma; it contains many of the molecular changes seen in malignancy (e.g., *ETS* rearrangements)

Morphology (p. 998)

Most cases (i.e., 70%) arise in the peripheral zone of the prostate, usually in the posterior prostate.

- *Grossly:* Primary lesions characteristically are poorly demarcated, gritty, firm, and yellow. Locally advanced cases may infiltrate the seminal vesicles and urinary bladder; invasion of the rectum is uncommon.

- *Microscopically:* Most are well-differentiated *adenocarcinomas* with small, crowded glands lined by a single layer of epithelium *(lacking the outer basal layer of cells);* nuclei are large and often exhibit nucleoli. Perineural invasion is a sign of malignancy.

  High-grade PIN consisting of architecturally benign but cytologically atypical cells is associated with 80% of prostate carcinomas.

  The *Gleason system* stratifies prostate cancers into five grades based on their glandular patterns (i.e., 1 = closest to normal; 5 = no glandular differentiation), without regard to cytologic features. Low- to moderate-grade Gleason scores suggest treatable disease, whereas high-grade scores portend a grave prognosis.

Clinical Course (p. 1000)

- The treatment and prognosis of prostatic carcinoma are influenced primarily by the stage and Gleason grade of the disease. Localized (clinical stage T1 or T2) disease is treated primarily with *surgery or radiotherapy* with a 15-year survival rate of 90%.
- Many prostate cancers have a relatively indolent course; thus, it may take 10 years to see benefit from surgery or radiotherapy, and watchful waiting is an appropriate treatment for many older men (or those with significant co-morbidity).
- *Metastases* occur initially in obturator nodes, followed by spread to other nodal groups. *Hematogenous dissemination* occurs primarily to bone, most often in the form of *osteoblastic* metastases.
- External beam radiotherapy can be used to treat prostate cancer that is too locally advanced to be cured by surgery. Hormonal therapy for metastatic disease can include orchiectomy or the administration of synthetic analogues of luteinizing hormone–releasing hormone; tumors often eventually become refractory to anti-androgen therapies.

Prostate specific antigen (PSA) is the most important test used in the diagnosis and management of prostate cancer. PSA is a product of prostatic epithelium and is normally secreted in the semen; serum levels are elevated to a lesser extent in BPH than prostate cancer, although there is considerable overlap between the two entities. Important points:

- *PSA is organ-specific, yet not cancer-specific.* Other factors such as BPH, prostatitis, infarct, and instrumentation of the prostate can increase serum PSA levels. As men age, their prostates tend to enlarge with BPH, with corresponding higher serum PSA levels. Furthermore, 20% to 40% of patients with organ-confined prostate cancer have PSA below the thresholds usually set for screening for malignancy.
- *PSA velocity (rate of change of PSA)* may be a more useful measurement than just a single PSA value. This reflects the finding that PSA levels rise faster in prostate cancer than for age-related hyperplasia. Multiple measurements need to be made over a period of 1 to 2 years.
- In the setting of known prostatic carcinoma, PSA monitoring is useful in assessing response to therapy or progression of disease.

22

The Female Genital Tract

Development (p. 1006)
Anatomy (p. 1007)
Infections of the Female Genital Tract (p. 1008)

Most of the sexually transmitted infections are discussed in Chapter 8. The following are highlighted specifically for their role in female genital tract pathology.

Infections of the Lower Genital Tract (p. 1008)

- *Herpes simplex virus (HSV):* Although HSV-1 usually causes an oropharyngeal infection, and HSV-2 typically involves genital mucosa and skin, either virus can instigate lesions in either site. Infections present with red papules 3 to 7 days after contact; these progress to vesicles and painful, coalescent ulcers associated with fever, malaise, and tender lymphadenopathy. Although lesions spontaneously heal within 1 to 3 weeks, HSV establishes a latent infection in lumbosacral nerve ganglia and can be re-activated by stress, trauma, immunosuppression, or hormonal changes. Diagnosis is made on the basis of clinical findings and viral cultures. Antiviral agents can shorten the duration of symptomatic lesions, but they do not eliminate latent infections. The most important consequence of HSV infection is transmission to the neonate during birth.
- *Molluscum contagiosum:* This is a poxvirus infection of skin and mucous membranes. Of the four types, type I is most common; type II is most often sexually transmitted. After a 6-week incubation period, characteristic dimpled, dome-shaped lesions erupt; these contain cells with intracytoplasmic viral inclusions.
- *Fungal infections:* Fungal infections (especially *candidiasis*) are common; yeasts form part of the normal vaginal microflora and can expand to cause symptomatic infections when the characteristic host microbial ecosystem is disrupted (e.g., by diabetes, antibiotics, pregnancy, or immunosuppression).
- *Trichomonas vaginalis:* This is a flagellated protozoan transmitted by sexual contact; patients can be asymptomatic or present with yellow frothy vaginal discharge, vulvovaginal discomfort, dysuria, or dyspareunia.
- *Gardnerella vaginalis: Gardnerella vaginalis* is a Gram-negative bacillus and the major cause of bacterial vaginitis; patients present with a thin, green-gray, fishy-smelling discharge. Such infections can precipitate premature labor.

Infections Involving the Lower and Upper Genital Tract (p. 1009)

PELVIC INFLAMMATORY DISEASE (p. 1009)

Pelvic inflammatory disease (PID) results from infections that arise in the vulva or vagina and ascend to involve the other genital tract structures (e.g., cervix, uterus, fallopian tubes, and ovaries); symptoms include pelvic pain, adnexal tenderness, fever, and vaginal discharge. *Gonococcus* is the most common cause, followed by *Chlamydia* and postabortal or postpartum polymicrobial infections (e.g., staphylococci, streptococci, coliforms, and/or *Clostridium perfringens*). Ascending *gonococcal* infections tend to spread via the mucosal surfaces, eliciting an acute suppurative reaction; non-gonococcal infections—after abortion or other therapeutic procedures—are typically distributed through lymphatics and veins. Peritonitis and bacteremia (with systemic seeding) are acute complications; chronic sequelae include tubal scarring and obstruction, infertility, increased risk of ectopic pregnancy, pelvic pain, and gastrointestinal-pelvic adhesions that can cause intestinal obstruction.

VULVA (p. 1011)

Bartholin Cyst (p. 1011)

Bartholin gland cysts are common lesions resulting from occlusion of the draining ducts by inflammation; they are typically lined by flattened epithelium and can be large (i.e., 3 to 5 cm) and painful. Treatment involves excision or permanent opening *(marsupialization)*. Bartholin gland infections can also produce abscesses, requiring drainage.

Non-Neoplastic Epithelial Disorders (p. 1011)

A heterogeneous group of lesions—clinically designated *leukoplakia*—manifest as opaque, white, plaque-like thickenings and are often accompanied by pruritus and scaling. Pathologic evaluation is required to distinguish inflammatory etiologies from neoplastic causes (discussed later).

Lichen Sclerosus (p. 1011)

Lesions begin as papules or macules that eventually coalesce into smooth, white parchment-like areas. Microscopically, there is epidermal thinning, superficial hyperkeratosis, and dermal fibrosis with a scant mononuclear perivascular infiltrate. The labia can become atrophic and stiffened, with constriction of the vaginal orifice. An autoimmune response is implicated.

Squamous Cell Hyperplasia (p. 1012)

Also called *lichen simplex chronicus,* this is a non-specific response to recurrent rubbing or scratching to relieve pruritus; it is characterized by white plaques that histologically reveal thickened epithelium, hyperkeratosis, and dermal inflammation. Although lichen simplex chronicus does not exhibit epithelial atypia and there is no increased predisposition to malignancy, it is often present at the margins of vulvar carcinoma.

Benign Exophytic Lesions (p. 1012)

As opposed to *condyloma acuminatum* (due to human papillomavirus [HPV] infection, see later discussion) or *condyloma latum* (due to syphilis; Chapter 8), vulvar *fibroepithelial polyps* (skin tags) and *squamous papillomas* are not related to any infectious agent. Papillomas are benign exophytic proliferations lined by non-keratinizing squamous epithelium and can be single or numerous *(vulvar papillomatosis)*.

Condyloma Acuminatum (p. 1012)

These are verrucous lesions on the vulva, perineum, vagina, and (rarely) cervix that are sexually transmitted by HPV types 6 or 11. Histologically, they comprise sessile branching epithelial proliferations of stratified squamous epithelium; mature superficial cells exhibit characteristic perinuclear cytoplasmic clearing with nuclear atypia *(koilocytotic atypia)*. Condyloma acuminatum is not considered pre-cancerous.

Squamous Neoplastic Lesions (p. 1012)

Vulvar Intraepithelial Neoplasia and Vulvar Carcinoma (p. 1012)

Vulvar carcinoma is relatively uncommon, representing only 3% of female genital cancers; most occur in women older than 60 years. A third of cases are *basaloid* or *warty carcinomas* related to HPV infections; two thirds are keratinizing squamous cell carcinoma unrelated to HPV. Prognosis of vulvar carcinomas depends on size, depth of invasion, and lymph node status; regional lymph node metastasis portends a poor prognosis (less than 10% have 5-year survival). Uncommon variants (e.g., *verrucous carcinoma* and *basal cell carcinoma*) are locally aggressive but rarely metastasize.

- *Basaloid* and *warty carcinomas* arise from precancerous *in situ* lesions called *classic vulvular intraepithelial neoplasia (VIN)* (previously designated *carcinoma in situ* or *Bowen disease*); most are positive for HPV 16 and are often associated with vaginal and/or cervical HPV-related lesions. Cancer risk increases with age and with immunosuppression.

Morphology (p. 1013)

- *Classic VIN* lesions manifest as discrete, hyperkeratotic, flesh-colored or pigmented, slightly raised plaques. These are typically multicentric and demonstrate marked nuclear atypia with lack of cellular maturation.
- *Basaloid carcinoma* can be exophytic or indurated, often with ulceration; the tumors are characterized by nests and cords of small, tightly packed cells resembling immature basal cells.
- *Warty carcinoma* exhibits exophytic architecture with prominent koilocytic atypia.

Keratinizing squamous cell carcinomas typically arise in the setting of long-standing lichen sclerosus or squamous cell hyperplasia; the immediately pre-malignant lesions are called *differentiated VIN*, distinguished by basal atypia with apparently normal superficial epithelial maturation and differentiation. Risk of cancer development is a function of age, extent, and immune status.

Morphology (p. 1014)

These carcinomas typically develop as nodules in a background of vulvar inflammation. Histology reveals infiltrating nests and tongues of malignant squamous epithelium with prominent keratin pearls.

Glandular Neoplastic Lesions (p. 1015)

Papillary Hidradenoma (p. 1015)

This benign tumor arises from modified apocrine sweat glands. It presents as a sharply circumscribed nodule of tubular ducts lined by non-ciliated columnar cells atop a layer of flattened myoepithelial cells.

Extramammary Paget Disease (p. 1015)

This malignant lesion appears as a red, crusted, sharply demarcated, map-like area. Histologically there are large, anaplastic, mucin-containing tumor cells lying singly or in small clusters within the epidermis and its appendages; most lesions are confined to the epidermis and invasion is rare, but even with wide excision, there is a high recurrence rate.

Malignant Melanoma (p. 1015)

Vulvar melanomas constitute less than 5% of all vulvar malignancy and 2% of female melanomas; they have a peak incidence between ages 60 and 80 years. Histologic characteristics are comparable to melanomas at other sites, although 5-year survival is less than 32% due to delays in detection and rapid progression to a vertical growth phase.

VAGINA (p. 1016)

Developmental Anomalies (p. 1016)

- *Septate (i.e., double) vagina* accompanies a double uterus and arises from failure of complete fusion of the müllerian ducts. Causes include genetic syndromes, *in utero* exposure to diethyl-stilbestrol (DES), or abnormalities of epithelial-stromal signaling in fetal development.
- *Vaginal adenosis* is reflected by red, granular patches of remnant endocervical-type columnar epithelium that have not been replaced by the normal squamous epithelium characteristic of adult vaginal mucosa. It occurs at a low frequency in normal women, but is present in 35% to 90% of women exposed *in utero* to DES; in that latter setting, vaginal adenosis can be a substrate for the development of clear cell carcinoma.

Premalignant and Malignant Neoplasms (p. 1016)

Most *benign* vaginal tumors occur in reproductive-age women; these include stromal polyps, leiomyomas, and hemagiomas.

Vaginal Intraepithelial Neoplasia and Squamous Cell Carcinoma (p. 1016)

Primary vaginal carcinomas are rare; virtually all are *squamous cell carcinomas* associated with high-risk HPV infection. These arise from *vaginal intraepithelial neoplasia*, which is analogous to malignant precursor lesions in cervical carcinoma. The upper posterior vagina is the site most commonly affected.

Embryonal Rhabdomyosarcoma (p. 1017)

This is an uncommon, highly malignant vaginal tumor in infants and children consisting of embryonal rhabdomyoblasts. The tumors are polypoid, bulky masses composed of grapelike clusters (hence the alternative name, *sarcoma botryoides*) that can protrude from the vagina. Tumor cells are small, with oval nuclei and small eccentric cytoplasmic protrusions. Tumors tend to invade locally and cause death by penetration into the peritoneal cavity, or by obstructing the urinary tract.

CERVIX (p. 1017)

Inflammations (p. 1017)

Acute and Chronic Cervicitis (p. 1017)

Lactobacilli dominate the cervical and vaginal microbial ecosystem; their production of lactic acid (keeping the pH below 4.5) and hydrogen peroxide (H_2O_2) largely suppress the growth of other saprophytic and pathogenic species. However, higher pH (associated with douching, bleeding, or sexual intercourse) can reduce H_2O_2 levels, and antibiotic therapy can decimate the bacteria, potentially leading to overgrowth by pathogenic species (*acute cervicitis* or *vaginitis*).

Chronic cervicitis is found at a low level in virtually all women and is of little clinical significance. However, infections with *gonococci, chlamydiae, mycoplasmas,* and HSV can produce significant acute and/or chronic cervicitis, and can lead to upper genital tract disease and/or complications of pregnancy. Marked cervical inflammatiomn produces reactive and reparative epithelial changes that can lead to abnormal cytologic smears.

Endocervical Polyps (p. 1018)

Endocervical polyps are benign exophytic growths present in 2% to 5% of women; they can present with irregular vaginal "spotting." Most arise in the endocervical canal and are soft mucoid lesions composed of a loose connective tissue stroma harboring dilated glands and inflammation, covered by endocervical epithelium.

Premalignant and Malignant Neoplasms (p. 1018)

In the United States, 11,000 new cases of invasive cervical carcinoma are diagnosed annually. In comparison, almost 1 million precancerous lesions are discovered each year by cytology (*Pap smear*), indicating that wide-spread screening has allowed the detection and eradication of pre-invasive lesions that might have progressed to cancer if not treated.

Pathogenesis (p. 1018)

High oncogenic risk HPV types are the most important factor in cervical oncogenesis (low oncogenic risk types are associated with condyloma acuminatum); HPV 16 (60% of cases of cervical cancer) and 18 (10% of cases) are most important. Additional risk factors relate to likelihood of exposure (e.g., multiple sexual partners) and host immune responses. Most HPV infections are asymptomatic and do not cause any tissue changes; 50% are cleared within 8 months and 90% by 2 years. Persistent infection (as with high-risk types or immunocompromise) increases the risk of developing malignancy.

HPV are DNA viruses that infect only immature basal cells of the squamous epithelium (through a break in the epithelium) or metaplastic squamous cells at the cervical squamocolumnar junction. HSV *replicate*, however, in the maturing, normally non-proliferating squamous cells (such viral proliferation is reflected in koilocytotic change of the cells). In order for HSV to induce DNA replication in these cells, it must therefore reactivate the cellular mitotic cycle; HSV does so primarily by interfering with the function of the p53 and Rb tumor suppressors. Thus, viral E6 and E7 proteins:

- Increase cyclin E expression (through E7 induction of Rb degradation)
- Interrupt apoptotic pathways (through E6 induction of p53 degradation)
- Induce centrosome duplication and genomic instability (E6, E7)
- Increase telomerase expression (E6)

It is important to note that *all* HPV types increase the proliferation and life span of infected cells; the relative oncogenic risk of the different virus types may be related to whether the viral DNA is integrated (cancers) or is episomal (condylomas and pre-cancerous lesions), or whether the high-risk viruses induce additional genetic changes (e.g., 3p deletions). Definitive development of malignancy likely also depends on effects related to other co-infections, inflammatory responses, hormonal influences, and carcinogenic exposures.

Cervical Intraepithelial Neoplasia (p. 1019)

Precancerous cervical epithelial histologic changes are classified as *low-grade* or *high-grade squamous intraepithelial lesions* (LSIL and HSIL, respectively). More than 80% of LSIL and 100% of HSIL lesions are associated with high-risk HPV; HPV 16 is the most common type associated with both.

- *LSIL* show only mild dysplasia, involving the more basal layers of the epithelium. While associated with productive HPV infection, there is no significant alteration of the host cell cycle. Approximately 60% of LSIL spontaneously regress within 2 years, while another 30% persist over that period; only 10% progress to HSIL, and LSIL does not proceed directly to invasive carcinoma. It is therefore not treated like a premalignant lesion.
- *HSIL* exhibit moderate to severe dysplasia and involve progressively more of the epithelial thickness; this category also includes *carcinoma in situ.* There is further HPV-driven deregulation of the cell cycle, with increased proliferation, decreased epithelial maturation, and diminished viral replication. Approximately 30% of HSIL will regress over 2 years, 60% will persist, and 10% will progress to carcinoma within a 2- to 10-year period.

Morphology (p. 1020)

Lesions are classified according to distribution of cellular and nuclear atypia, including nuclear enlargement, hyperchromasia, chromatin granularity, size variation, and koilocytosis:

- In *LSIL,* the atypia is confined to the basal third of the epithelium.
- In *HSIL,* the atypia extends to two thirds (or more) of the epithelial thickness.

Cervical Carcinoma (p. 1021)

Squamous cell carcinoma constitutes 80% of cervical cancers, while adenocarcinoma comprises 15%, and adenosquamous and neuroendocrine carcinomas collectively amount to 5%; all are associated with high-risk HPV. Peak incidence of invasive cervical cancer is age 45 years; increasingly, cervical cancers are detected at subclinical stages by routine Pap smear screening.

Morphology (p. 1021)

- *Grossly:* Lesions can be exophytic or infiltrative.
- *Microscopically:* Squamous lesions can be keratinizing or non-keratinizing; adenocarcinomas tend to be glandular but relatively

mucin depleted; adenosquamous lesions are composed of inter-mixed malignant squamous and glandular elements; neuroendo-crine tumors resemble small cell malignancy of the lung.

- Staging is based on depth of invasion, involvement of adjacent structures, and/or metastatic spread.

Clinical Features (p. 1023)

Although early invasive cancers may be treated by cervical cone biopsy, most are managed by hysterectomy and lymph node dissec-tion, with irradiation for advanced disease. Prognosis and survival depends on stage more than grade; 5-year survival for micro-invasive carcinoma is 95% compared to less than 50% for the most advanced disease; neuroendocrine tumors have a particularly poor prognosis.

Cervical Cancer Screening and Prevention (p. 1023)

The false-negative error rate for Pap tests is between 10% and 20%, largely due to inadequate sampling. Adjunct HPV DNA testing can be added to the routine cytology screening; positivity for high-risk HPV types (even with normal cytology) mandates more frequent testing. An abnormal Pap smear is typically followed by a colposcopic examination with selected biopsies; LSIL lesions can be treated conservatively, while HSIL pathology is usually treated by cervical conization and life-long follow-up. Prophylactic vaccines directed against HPV types 6 and 11 (condylomas), and 16 and 18 (cervical cancer) can markedly reduce the incidence of HSIL but do not eliminate cancer risk from other HPV types.

BODY OF UTERUS AND ENDOMETRIUM (p. 1024)

Functional Endometrial Disorders (Dysfunctional Uterine Bleeding) (p. 1026)

The most common gynecologic problem during reproductive life is excessive bleeding during or between menstrual periods. The various causes differ depending on the age of the individual (Table 22-1). While bleeding can result from a well-defined organic lesion (e.g., submucosal leiomyoma, endometrial polyp, or chronic endo-metritis), the most common etiology is *dysfunctional uterine bleeding (DUB)*, defined as *abnormal bleeding in the absence of an organic lesion*.

Hyperestrogenic states are the most common basis for DUB, although other endocrine disorders (e.g., thyroid, adrenal, or pituitary) or generalized metabolic disturbances (e.g., obesity, malnutrition, or chronic systemic diseases) can be causal. Morphologically, hyper-estrogenic states produce cystic glandular changes associated with sporadic endometrial breakdown and bleeding.

- *Anovulatory cycle* (p. 1026): Lack of ovulation causes prolonged, excessive estrogen without the counteractive progestational phase; most anovulatory cycles have no obvious explanation and are attributed to subtle hormonal imbalances. DUB associated with menopause may be related to ovarian insufficiency and anovulatory cycles.
- *Inadequate luteal phase* (p. 1027): Inadequate corpus luteum function results in low progesterone output with early menses and is often associated with infertility.

Causes of Abnormal Uterine Bleeding by Age Group

Age Group	Causes
Prepuberty	Precocious puberty (hypothalamic, pituitary, or ovarian origin)
Adolescence	Anovulatory cycle, coagulation disorders
Reproductive age	Complications of pregnancy (abortion, trophoblastic disease, ectopic pregnancy) Organic lesions (leiomyoma, adenomyosis, polyps, endometrial hyperplasia, carcinoma) Anovulatory cycle Ovulatory dysfunctional bleeding (e.g., inadequate luteal phase)
Perimenopausal	Dysfunctional uterine bleeding Anovulatory cycle Irregular shedding Organic lesions (carcinoma, hyperplasia, polyps)
Postmenopausal	Organic lesions (carcinoma, hyperplasia, polyps) Endometrial atrophy

Inflammation (p. 1027)

Endometritis (p. 1027)

- *Acute endometritis* is uncommon. This condition is usually caused by bacterial infections occurring after delivery or miscarriage and is related to retained products of conception. Curettage and antibiotics are usually sufficient therapy.
- *Chronic endometritis* can present with abnormal bleeding, pain, discharge, and/or infertility; histologically, there is endometrial plasma cell and macrophage infiltration. It occurs in patients with:

  Chronic PID (*Chlamydia* is a common culprit.)
  Retained gestational tissue post-abortion or postpartum
  Intrauterine contraceptive devices
  Disseminated tuberculosis (rare)
  15% have no obvious cause

Endometriosis and Adenomyosis (p. 1028)

Endometriosis is the presence of endometrial tissue *outside* the uterus; it involves (in descending order) ovaries, uterine ligaments, rectovaginal septum, cul de sac, pelvic peritoneum, gastrointestinal tract, mucosa of the cervix, vagina, or fallopian tube, and laparotomy scars. These ectopic foci of endometrium are under the influence of ovarian hormones and therefore undergo cyclic menstrual changes with periodic bleeding, but they have no means of sloughing externally like normal endometrial lining.

The leading theory is that retrograde menstruation through the Fallopian tubes allows diffuse seeding of endometrial tissue; in rare cases, the endometrial foci may arise by coelomic epithelial metaplasia. Endometriotic tissue differs from normal endometrium by exhibiting marked activation of inflammatory cascades and increased stromal aromatase activity (and thus estrogen production). Overproduction of prostaglandins and estrogen (and relative progesterone resistance) enhances the survival and persistence of endometriotic foci.

Adenomyosis is a related disorder characterized by nests of endometrial tissues in the uterine myometrium. These are continuous with the endometrial lining, suggesting that they form by down-growth; 20% of women are affected. The symptomatology is similar to endometriosis.

Morphology (p. 1029)

- *Grossly:* Endometriosis manifests as red-blue to yellow-brown mucosal or serosal nodules. Extensive disease can be marked by organizing hemorrhage and fibrosis.
- *Microscopically:* Foci classically exhibit endometrial glands and stroma, with or without hemosiderin.

Clinical Features (p. 1029)

Endometriosis primarily affects women during their reproductive years (10% of all women are affected), and can present with severe dysmenorrheal (painful menses), pelvic pain, and/or infertility (30% to 40% of cases). Uncommonly, malignancy can develop from the ectopic foci.

Endometrial Polyps (p. 1029)

Endometrial polyps are exophytic masses of endometrial glands and stroma that project into the endometrial cavity; they may be associated with elevated estrogens or tamoxifen therapy. These polyps are usually benign and manifest primarily with abnormal bleeding, but they occasionally develop into adenocarcinoma.

Endometrial Hyperplasia (p. 1030)

Endometrial hyperplasia, defined as an increased proliferation of endometrial glands relative to the stroma, is an important cause of abnormal uterine bleeding; it is also clinically important as a precursor lesion in the continuum to endometrial carcinoma. This lesion is associated with prolonged estrogen stimulation of the endometrium; causes range from exogenous estrogen administration to anovulation, obesity, polycystic ovarian disease, and functioning estrogen-producing tumors. Endometrial hyperplasia is often associated with inactivation of the *PTEN* tumor suppressor gene (20% of cases), leading to enhanced AKT phosphorylation with increased proliferation and diminished apoptosis.

Morphology (p. 1030)

- *Simple hyperplasia without atypia (cystic or mild hyperplasia)* exhibits benign cystically dilated glands; these rarely progress to adenocarcinoma.
- *Simple hyperplasia with atypia* is uncommon; besides cystically-dliated glands, it exhibits cytologic atypia (e.g., loss of polarity, prominent nucleoli) and 8% progress to malignancy.
- *Complex hyperplasia without atypia* shows closely apposed glands of varying size crowded together into clusters; the epithelium remains cytologically normal and only 3% progress to cancer.
- *Complex hyperplasia with atypia* shows gland crowding and cytologic changes; there is substantial overlap with endometrial adenocarcinoma, and 23% to 48% of patients with such changes have concurrent malignancy.

Malignant Tumors of the Endometrium (p. 1031)

Carcinoma of the Endometrium (p. 1031)

Endometrial carcinoma accounts for 7% of all invasive cancers in women, with a peak incidence of 55 to 65 years; there are 39,000 new cases annually in the United States. Two epidemiologic and pathophysiologic categories are described:

Type I Carcinomas (p. 1031)

Type I carcinomas are the most common (80%); these are well-differentiated *(endometrioid carcinoma)* and typically arise in the setting of *endometrial hyperplasia* (with the same overall risk associations). *PTEN* mutations are seen in 30% to 80% of endometrioid carcinomas; in addition, tumors often exhibit micro-satellite instability, as well as mutations involving components of the PI3 kinase complex, and *KRAS* or β-catenin. *p53* mutations may be late events.

Morphology (p. 1032)

- *Grossly:* These can be localized polypoid tumors or diffuse spreading lesions.
- *Microscopically:* Most (85%) are endometrioid adenocarcinomas with epithelium resembling normal endometrium; grading depends on the mix of well-differentiated glands and more poorly differentiated solid tumor. Foci of squamous differentiation are seen in 20% of cases.

Type II Carcinomas (p. 1033)

Type II carcinomas typically arise a decade later than type I tumors and occur in the setting of *endometrial atrophy*; these are poorly differentiated tumors. The most common subtype is *serous carcinoma*, so-called due to biologic overlaps with similar ovarian lesions; *p53* mutations are present in at least 90% and appear to be early oncogenic events. Endometrial intraepithelial carcinoma (EIC) without invasion is a precursor to serous carcinoma.

Morphology (p. 1034)

- *Grossly:* Tumors are usually large and bulky and deeply invasive.
- *Microscopically:* Invasive lesions exhibit a papillary or glandular growth pattern with marked cellular atypia.

Clinical Course (p. 1034)

Patients typically present with uterine bleeding or an abnormal Pap smear. Prognosis depends largely on disease stage and grade; it is excellent (90% have 5-year survival) when cancer is confined to the uterine corpus and is well differentiated. However, serous tumors have a propensity for extensive for extrauterine spread even when apparently confined to the endometrium.

Malignant Mixed Müllerian Tumors (p. 1034)

Malignant mixed müllerian tumors (MMMT) are endometrial adenocarcinomas associated with concurrent malignant stroma changes attributable to a common neoplastic precursor for both lineages. The stromal component tends to differentiate into a variety of malignant mesodermal components. MMMT are highly malignant; 5-year survival rates are between 25% and 30%.

Morphology (p. 1035)

- *Grossly:* Tumors are bulky, fleshy, and polypoid.
- *Microscopically:* Lesions consist of malignant glandular and stromal elements; the stromal sarcomatous elements may show muscle, cartilage, and osteoid differentiation.

Tumors of the Endometrium with Stromal Differentiation (p. 1036)

These are relatively uncommon tumors, comprising less than 5% of endometrial cancers.

Adenosarcomas (p. 1036)

These estrogen-sensitive tumors exhibit *stromal neoplasia with benign glands*. Grossly, they are large polypoid growths, generally considered low-grade malignancies.

Stromal Tumors (p. 1036)

- *Benign stromal nodules* are discrete lumps of stromal neoplasia within the myometrium.
- *Endometrial stromal sarcomas* are lesions composed of malignant stroma interposed between myometrial bundles; they are distinguished by diffuse infiltration and/or lymphatic invasion. A recurrent t(7;17) translocation leads to the formation of a fusion transcript with anti-apoptotic features. Five-year survival rates approach 50%.

Tumors of the Myometrium (p. 1036)

Leiomyomas (p. 1036)

Commonly called *fibroids*, these are *benign masses of uterine smooth muscle cells*; they are the most common tumor in women. While most have a normal karyotype, some 40% have a balanced t(12;14) translocation, partial deletions of chromosome 7q, trisomy 12, or rearrangements of 6p, 3q, or 10q. Leiomyomas may be asymptomatic or can present with abnormal uterine bleeding, pain, urinary bladder disorders, and impaired fertility. Malignant transformation is extremely rare.

Morphology (p. 1037)

- *Grossly:* Tumors are sharply circumscribed, discrete, round, firm, gray-white nodules that occur within the myometrium (intramural), beneath the serosa (subserosal), or immediately beneath the endometrium (submucosal).
- *Microscopically:* Lesions show characteristically whorled bundles of relatively uniform smooth muscle cells with rare mitoses; variants can exhibit increased cellularity or atypical, bizarre cells.

Leiomyosarcomas (p. 1037)

Leiomyosarcomas are uncommon malignancies that form bulky, fleshy masses in the uterine wall or project into the lumen. Histologically, there is a wide range of atypia; features that distinguish these from benign leiomyomas include increased numbers of mitoses (5 to 10 per 10 high-power fields), particularly when accompanied by cellular atypia and/or necrosis.

These tumors disseminate throughout the abdominal cavity and aggressively metastasize. The overall 5-year survival rate is 40%, although anaplastic tumors have 5-year survivals of only 10% to 15%.

FALLOPIAN TUBES (p. 1038)

Inflammations (p. 1038)

Suppurative salpingitis is typically a component of PID; gonococcal infections account for 60% of cases, although any of the pyogenic organisms can be involved; *Chlamydia* is less often a factor.

Tuberculous salpingitis is rare in the United States but is an important cause of infertility worldwide.

Tumors and Cysts (p. 1038)

- The most common primary lesions are benign *paratubal cysts* (1 to 2 mm translucent cysts filled with serous fluid); larger versions near the fimbria are called *hydatids of Morgagni.*
- Benign neoplasms include *adenomatoid tumors,* comprising small nodules of mesothelial cells.
- Primary tubal *adenocarcinoma* is rare and can be associated with germline *BRCA* mutations. Even early stage tumors have a 40%, 5-year mortality; prognosis worsens with higher stages.

OVARIES (p. 1039)

Non-Neoplastic and Functional Cysts (p. 1039)

Follicle and Luteal Cysts (p. 1039)

Extremely common findings, these are typically multiple and usually less than 2 cm; they are lined by follicular or luteinized cells with a clear, serous fluid. Cysts derive from unruptured Graafian follicles, or follicles that have resealed after rupture. While typically asymptomatic, they can rupture with ensuing peritoneal inflammation and pain.

Polycystic Ovarian Disease and Stromal Hyperthecosis (p. 1039)

Polycystic ovarian disease (PCOD) (*Stein-Leventhal syndrome*) affects 3% to 6% of reproductive-age women; it presents with numerous cystic follicles, often with associated oligomenorrhea, persistent anovulation, obesity, hirsuitism, and insulin resistance. Disturbances in androgen biosynthesis are causally implicated. The ovaries are enlarged with cortical fibrosis; innumerable subcortical cysts (i.e., up to 1 cm) exhibit theca interna hyperplasia.

Stromal hyperthecosis is a disorder of ovarian stroma typically in postmenopausal women; it is reflected by stromal hypercellularity and luteinization visible as discrete nests of cells with vacuolated cytoplasm. The clinical manifestations are similar to PCOD, although virilization can be profound.

Ovarian Tumors (p. 1040)

Ovarian tumors can arise from the epithelium, germ cells, or sex cord stroma; overall, 80% are benign, and most occur in women aged 20 to 45 years (Table 22-2; Fig. 22-1). Malignant tumors typically occur in older women (45 to 65 years) and represent 3% of all female cancers; because most are detected only after spreading beyond the ovary, they account for a disproportionate number of cancer deaths.

Tumors of Surface (Müllerian) Epithelium (p. 1041)

Most primary ovarian neoplasms fall in this category. Classification is based on the proliferation and differentiation of the epithelium; greater proliferation generally connotes greater malignant potential. Most of these tumors ultimately derive from transformed

TABLE 22-2 Frequency of Major Ovarian Tumors

Type	Percentage of Malignant Ovarian Tumors	Percentage that Are Bilateral
Serous		
Benign (60%)		25
Borderline (15%)		30
Malignant (25%)	45	65
Mucinous		
Benign (80%)		5
Borderline (10%)		10
Malignant (10%)	5	<5
Endometrial carcinoma	20	40
Undifferentiated carcinoma	10	–
Clear cell carcinoma	6	40
Granulosa cell tumor	5	5
Teratoma		15
Benign (96%)		
Malignant (4%)	1	Rare
Metastatic	5	>50
Others	3	–

coelomic epithelium; the serous, mucinous, or endometrioid varieties speak to the plasticity of the original cells.

Serous Tumors (p. 1042)

Serous tumors account for 30% of all ovarian tumors; 70% are benign or borderline. Serous carcinomas are the most common ovarian malignancy (40% of the total). Prognosis is linked to stage and tumor grade; even with extensive extra-ovarian spread, low-grade tumors can progress relatively slowly. Five-year survivals for borderline and malignant tumors confined to the ovary are 100% and 70%, respectively; 5-year survival for similar tumors involving the peritoneum is 90% for borderline tumors and 25% for malignant tumors.

Pathogenesis (p. 1042)

Nulliparity, gonadal dysgenesis, family history, and hereditable mutations are important risk factors. *BRCA1* and *-2* mutations incur a risk of ovarian cancer developing by age 70 years in 20% to 60% of patients; most are high-grade. Low-grade tumors tend to arise in serous borderline tumors and have *KRAS* and *BRAF* mutations; conversely, high-grade tumors have a high frequency of *p53* mutations. Many of these tumors appear to arise from the fimbriated end of the fallopian tube.

Morphology (p. 1043)

- *Grossly:* These are typically large cystic masses filled with serous fluid; intracystic loculations can occur. Benign cystadenomas have a smooth and glistening inner lining. The *cystadeno-carcinomas* can have small mural nodularities or papillary projections. Bilaterality is common.

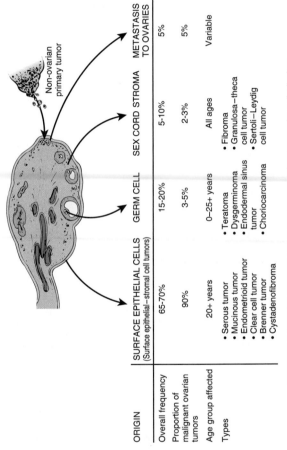

ORIGIN	SURFACE EPITHELIAL CELLS (Surface epithelial–stromal cell tumors)	GERM CELL	SEX CORD STROMA	METASTASIS TO OVARIES
Overall frequency	65–70%	15–20%	5–10%	5%
Proportion of malignant ovarian tumors	90%	3–5%	2–3%	5%
Age group affected	20+ years	0–25+ years	All ages	Variable
Types	• Serous tumor • Mucinous tumor • Endometrioid tumor • Clear cell tumor • Brenner tumor • Cystadenofibroma	• Teratoma • Dysgerminoma • Endodermal sinus tumor • Choriocarcinoma	• Fibroma • Granulosa–theca cell tumor • Sertoli–Leydig cell tumor	

Non-ovarian primary tumor

FIGURE 22-1 Derivation of various ovarian neoplasms with frequency and age distributions.

- *Microscopically:*

  Benign lesions are lined by a single layer of tall, columnar, ciliated epithelial cells, occasionally forming microscopic papillae.

  Frankly malignant cystadenocarcinomas have multilayered epithelium with many papillary areas and large, solid epithelial masses focally invading the stroma.

  Borderline tumors demonstrate mild atypia with complex micropapillary epithelial architecture without invasion.

Mucinous Tumors (p. 1044)

Mucinous tumors account for roughly 30% of all ovarian neoplasms; 80% are benign or borderline. Primary mucinous carcinomas amount to less than 5% of all ovarian malignancies. Smoking is a risk factor, and *KRAS* mutations are a common feature. These tumors can seed the peritoneum with numerous implants that produce extensive mucinous ascites, called *pseudomyxoma peritonei* (although this condition is more commonly due to primary appendiceal tumors). Five-year survival rates for stage I disease are more than 90%.

Morphology (p. 1044)

- *Grossly:* Tumors tend to produce large multiloculated cystic masses filled with sticky, gelatinous fluid. Less than 10% are bilateral.
- *Microscopically:*

  Benign lesions are lined by tall, columnar non-ciliated epithelium with apical mucin akin to benign cervical or intestinal epithelium; *Müllerian mucinous tumors* are associated with endometriosis and have cells resembling cervical or endometrial epithelium.

  Cystadenocarcinomas usually exhibit intestinal-type epithelium and display solid tumor growth, necrosis, and stroma invasion.

  Borderline mucinous tumors exhibit complex growth analogous to serous tumors but lack solid growth or stromal infiltration.

Endometrioid Tumors (p. 1045)

Endometrioid carcinomas account for 20% of all ovarian cancers; they exhibit epithelium resembling benign or malignant endometrium. About 15% to 20% of cases occur in the setting of concurrent endometriosis, although direct origin from the ovarian surface is also possible. In 15% to 30% of cases, independent endometrial carcinomas also occur. *PTEN, KRAS,* and β-catenin mutations occur frequently, as well as microsatellite instability; *p53* mutations are common in poorly differentiated tumors. Five-year survival for stage I disease is 75%.

Morphology (p. 1046)

- *Grossly:* Lesions are a combination of solid and cystic masses; 40% are bilateral.
- *Microscopically:* The glandular patterns bear a strong resemblance to endometrial adenocarcinoma.

Clear Cell Adenocarcinoma (p. 1046)

Clear cell adenocarcinoma is uncommon; it is considered a variant of endometrioid adenocarcinoma. Tumors can be cystic or solid; the large epithelial cells contain abundant clear cytoplasm. Patients with cancer confined to the ovary have 5-year survivals of 65%; with extra-ovarian spread, 5-year survival is unusual.

Brenner Tumor (p. 1046)

Brenner tumor is a variably sized (1 to 30 cm), solid tumor (*adenofibroma*) characterized by dense fibrous stroma and nests of epithelium resembling urinary transitional or rarely columnar epithelium. They are usually unilateral; the vast majority of these tumors are benign.

Clinical Course, Detection, and Prevention of Surface Epithelial Tumors (p. 1047)

- These tumors tend to have similar manifestations: lower abdominal pain and enlargement, with symptoms secondary to bowel or bladder compression. Benign lesions are readily resected; malignant lesions are associated with progressive cachexia, and dissemination beyond the capsule can cause massive ascites and/or diffuse peritoneal studding. Most patients are diagnosed only after the tumor has become large or disseminated, leading to poor overall survival statistics.
- CA-125 (a high-molecular-weight glycoprotein marker of ovarian cancer) is present in the serum of more than 80% of patients with serous or endometrioid carcinomas. However, it is more useful as a tool in monitoring disease progression than in primary diagnosis since non-specific peritoneal inflammation also increases the serum levels. Elevated osteopontin levels may allow earlier ovarian cancer detection.
- Fallopian tubal ligation and oral contraceptive use reduce risk of developing ovarian malignancy.

Germ Cell Tumors (p. 1047)

Germ cell tumors represent 15% to 20% of all ovarian tumors; most are *benign cystic teratomas*. They are similar to male germ cell tumors and arise from neoplastic transformation of totipotential germ cells capable of differentiating into the three germ cell layers.

Teratomas (p. 1047)

- *Mature (benign) teratomas* (*dermoid cysts*; p. 1047) typically arise in young women during their active reproductive years. The karyotype of virtually all benign teratomas is 46XX, and they likely arise from an ovum after the first meiotic division. Mature teratomas are characteristically cystic masses lined by squamous epithelium with adnexal structures including hair shafts and sebaceous glands; tooth structures and tissues from other germ cell layers can often also be identified (e.g., cartilage, bone, thyroid, and neural tissues). Tumors are bilateral in 10% to 15% of cases. The vast majority of such tumors are cured by excision; 1% undergo malignant transformation, most commonly as squamous cell carcinoma.
- *Monodermal or specialized teratomas* (p. 1048) differentiate along the line of a single abnormal tissue. The most common is *struma ovarii*, composed entirely of mature thyroid tissue; ovarian carcinoid is another variant.
- *Immature (malignant) teratomas* (p. 1048) are rare tumors composed of embryonic (rather than adult) elements resembling immature fetal tissues. These occur chiefly in adolescents and young women. Although they grow rapidly and frequently penetrate the capsule, low-grade tumors have an excellent prognosis, and even high-grade malignancies can respond well to chemotherapy.

Dysgerminoma (p. 1048)

Dysgerminoma is the ovarian counterpart of testicular seminoma. These account for 2% of all ovarian cancers but about half of the malignant germ cell tumors. Most occur between ages 20 and

40 years, and most have no endocrine function. Oct3, Oct4, and Nanog transcription factor expression by dygerminomas maintain pluripotency; the tumors also express the c-KIT receptor tyrosine kinase. All dysgerminomas are malignant, but only about one third are highly aggressive; because they are chemosensitive, overall survival exceeds 80%.

Morphology (p. 1049)

- *Grossly:* Tumors are solid, yellow-white to gray-pink, and fleshy; 80% to 90% are unilateral.
- *Microscopically:* Lesions consist of sheets and cords of large vesicular cells separated by scant fibrous stroma.

Endodermal Sinus (Yolk Sac) Tumor (p. 1049)

Endodermal sinus (yolk sac) tumor is a rare malignancy resulting from differentiation of germ cells toward yolk sac structures. Histologically, there are glomerulus-like structures with a central vessel enveloped by germ cells within a cystic space lined by additional germ cells *(Schiller-Duvall body)*. Intracellular and extracellular hyaline droplets are conspicuous and can contain α-fetoprotein (AFP). The tumors occur in children and young women and grow aggressively, although they are chemoresponsive.

Choriocarcinoma (p. 1049)

Choriocarcinoma is another example of extra-embryonic differentiation of malignant germ cells; most such tumors exist in combination with other germ cell tumors. Histologically, they are identical to placental malignancies and elaborate chorionic gonadotropins. Ovarian choriocarcinomas are highly malignant, metastasize widely, and are much more resistant to chemotherapy than their placental counterparts.

Sex Cord–Stromal Tumors (p. 1050)

These tumors originate from ovarian stroma, which, in turn, derives from the sex cords of the embryonic gonad. The tumors frequently produce estrogens or androgens.

Granulosa–Theca Cell Tumors (p. 1050)

Granulosa–theca cell tumors constitute 5% of all ovarian tumors; they are composed of various combinations of theca and granulosa cells. Two thirds occur in postmenopausal women. *Inhibin* produced by granulosa cells can be a useful biomarker to diagnose and monitor tumors.

- These tumors can elaborate large amounts of estrogen and thus produce precocious sexual development and endometrial hyperplasia; they predispose to endometrial carcinoma. Occasionally, granulosa cell tumors produce masculinizing androgens.
- While 5% to 25% of granulosa cell tumors are malignant, most have an indolent course, with 10-year survival rates of 85%. Pure thecomas are virtually always benign.

Morphology (p. 1050)

- *Grossly:* Tumors are usually unilateral, solid, and white-yellow.
- *Microscopically:* The granulosa cell component consists of small cuboidal-to-polygonal cells growing in cords, sheets, or strands; there can be occasional gland-like structures with acidophilic material *(Call-Exner body)*. The thecal cell components are composed of sheets of plump spindle cells often containing lipid droplets.

Fibromas, Thecomas, and Fibrothecomas (p. 1051)

Fibromas, thecomas, and fibrothecomas account for 4% of all ovarian neoplasms; the vast majority of these are benign. They are usually unilateral, solid, hard, gray-white masses. The fibroma component is composed of well-differentiated fibroblasts and scant collagenous connective tissue; the thecoma portion contains plump spindle cells with lipid droplets.

Curiously, 40% of tumors are associated with ascites and occasionally right-sided hydrothorax *(Meigs syndrome)*. They can also be associated with basal cell nevus syndrome (Chapter 25).

Sertoli–Leydig Cell Tumors (Androblastomas) (p. 1051)

Sertoli–Leydig cell tumors (androblastomas) recapitulate the cells of the testes and commonly produce masculinization or defeminization. They are usually unilateral and consist of tubules composed of Sertoli cells and/or Leydig cells interspersed with stroma.

Metastatic Tumors (p. 1052)

Metastatic tumors of the ovary most commonly derive from tumors of müllerian origin (e.g., uterus, fallopian tube, contralateral ovary, or pelvic peritoneum); the sources of the most common extra-müllerian metastases are carcinomas of the breast and gastrointestinal tract. *Krukenberg tumors* are ovarian cancers (often bilateral) caused by metastatic mucin-producing signet cells, usually originating from the stomach.

GESTATIONAL AND PLACENTAL DISORDERS (p. 1052)

Disorders of Early Pregnancy (p. 1053)

Spontaneous Abortion (p. 1053)

Spontaneous abortion ("miscarriage") is defined as pregnancy loss before 20 weeks' gestation; 10% to 15% of clinically recognized pregnancies (and a significant number of unrecognized pregnancies) terminate spontaneously. Causes are:

- Maternal (e.g., diabetes, luteal-phase defects, and other endocrine disorders)
- Fetal, with 50% having chromosomal abnormalities, and additional numbers with more subtle genetic defects
- Uterine defects (e.g., leiomyomas, polyps, or malformations)
- Systemic disorders affecting the maternal vasculature (e.g., antiphospholipid antibody syndrome, coagulopathies, or hypertension)
- Infections (e.g., *Toxoplasmosis*, *Mycoplasma*, *Listeria*, and several viruses)
- Idiopathic

Ectopic Pregnancy (p. 1053)

Ectopic pregnancy denotes embryo implantation at a site other than the uterus, often in the fallopian tubes (90%) but also in the ovary or abdominal cavity; it occurs in 1 of 150 pregnancies. Predisposing factors include PID with scarring, intrauterine devices (2.5-fold increased risk), and peritubal adhesions related to endometriosis or prior surgery; 50% occur in apparently normal tubes.

Clinical Features (p. 1054)

Tubal pregnancy has one of four outcomes:

- Intratubal hemorrhage with the formation of *hematosalpinx*
- Tubal rupture with intraperitoneal hemorrhage
- Spontaneous regression with resorption of the products of conception
- Extrusion into the abdominal cavity (tubal abortion)

Tubal rupture is a medical emergency characterized by acute abdomen and shock; diagnosis is suggested by high human chorionic gonadotropin (hCG) levels, ultrasonographic findings, and an endometrial biopsy showing decidual changes and absent chorionic villi.

Disorders of Late Pregnancy (p. 1054)

A multitude of disorders can arise as a consequence of various placental pathologies; outcomes range from mild intrauterine growth retardation to fetal demise, and they can also precipitate maternal preeclampsia.

Twin Placentas (p. 1054)

Twin pregnancies arise from fertilization of two ova (i.e., dizygotic) or division of one fertilized ovum (i.e., monozygotic). The resulting placentas can be mono- or dichorionic; a single chorion indicates monozygotic twins, and depending on the time of splitting these can be mono- or diamnionic. Dichorionic placentas are always diamniotic and can occur with either mono- or dizygotic twins.

In monochorionic twin pregnancies, vascular anastomoses can allow sharing of the fetal circulations. *Twin-twin transfusion syndrome* occurs if imbalanced flow occurs through an arteriovenous shunt; subsequent disparities in blood volume can lead to death of one or both fetuses.

Abnormalities of Placental Implantation (p. 1055)

- *Placenta previa* denotes placental implantation in the lower uterine segment or cervix and is associated with severe third-trimester bleeding. Complete coverage of the cervical os requires a cesarean delivery to avert the placental rupture and maternal exsanguination of a vaginal delivery.
- *Placenta accreta* occurs when there is absence of decidua and the placenta adheres directly to the myometrium; at delivery, the placenta fails to separate, and there is potentially life-threatening hemorrhage.

Placental Infections (p. 1055)

- Ascending (usually bacterial) infections via the birth canal are most common; these can cause infection of the chorionic membranes (*acute chorioamnionitis*) that then produces premature membrane rupture and preterm delivery. Inflammation involves the chorion-amnion and fetal umbilical and chorionic plate vessels.
- Hematogenous infections can result from a maternal septicemia, including listerial, streptococcal, and TORCH (i.e., toxoplasma, rubella, syphilis, cytomegalovirus, herpes) organisms. These are characterized by villous chronic inflammation (*villitis*).

Preeclampsia and Eclampsia (p. 1055)

Preeclampsia is a syndrome characterized by hypertension, proteinuria, and edema; it occurs in 3% to 5% of pregnancies, usually in the third trimester. *Eclampsia* is a more severe form associated with seizures and coma. Patients can also present with hypercoagulability, renal failure, and pulmonary edema; 10% develop HELLP syndrome (Chapter 18), that is, *h*emolysis, *e*levated *l*iver enzymes, and *l*ow *p*latelets.

Pathogenesis (p. 1056)

The syndromes are associated with systemic endothelial dysfunction, vasoconstriction, and increased vascular permeability driven by placental-derived factors.

- *Abnormal placental vasculature* is an underlying precursor lesion. In normal pregnancy, fetal trophoblast cells convert the maternal high-resistance decidual spiral arteries into high capacitance uteroplacental vessels lacking a smooth muscle coat. In preeclampsia, the remodeling does not occur, and the placenta cannot meet the perfusion demands of late pregnancy. Placental vessel thrombosis or fibrinoid necrosis can have a similar outcome.
- In response to hypoxia, the ischemic placenta releases copious amounts of anti-angiogenic factors (i.e., sFlt-1 and endoglin) that reduce placental vascular development.
- Placental sFlt-1 and endoglin in the circulation also lead to widespread maternal endothelial dysfunction by inhibiting vascular endothelial growth factor (VEGF)-and transforming growth factor-β (TGF-β)-dependent nitric oxide and prostacyclin production. The consequences include systemic hypertension; the ensuing endothelial dysfunction leads to proteinuria, edema, and hypercoagulability.

Morphology (p. 1057)

The placenta exhibits numerous small, peripheral infarcts (with accelerated villous maturation indicative of chronic ischemia), and retroplacental hematomas.

Clinical Features (p. 1057)

Preeclampsia usually occurs after 34 weeks' gestation; onset is typically insidious. Delivery is the only definitive treatment, but mild pre-term disease can be managed conservatively with monitoring and bedrest. In severe disease, anti-hypertensive therapy does not affect the course or outcome.

Gestational Trophoblatic Disease (p. 1057)

Gestational trophoblastic disease is a spectrum of tumors and tumor-like conditions, characterized by proliferation of trophoblastic tissue.

Hydatidiform Mole (p. 1057)

Hydatidiform moles are characterized by cystic swelling of chorionic villi, accompanied by variable trophoblastic proliferation; these can be precursors of choriocarcinoma. Risk of a mole is highest at either extreme of the reproductive years; the incidence in the United States is 1 per every 1000 to 2000 pregnancies. Benign noninvasive moles are classified as *complete* and *partial,* based by histologic, cytogenetic, and flow cytometric studies (Table 22-3).

- *Complete mole* (p. 1058) occurs when an egg that has lost its chromosomes is fertilized by 1 or 2 sperm; all genetic material is therefore paternally derived. About 90% of complete moles derive from the duplicated genetic material of one sperm and are 46,XX; the remainder derive from two sperm and are 46, XX or 46,XY. There is a 2.5% risk of choriocarcinoma.

TABLE 22-3   Features of Complete Versus Partial Hydatidiform Mole

Feature	Complete Mole	Partial Mole
Karyotype	46,XX (46,XY)	Triploid
Villous edema	All villi	Some villi
Trophoblast proliferation	Diffuse, circumferential	Focal; slight
Atypia	Often present	Absent
Serum hCG	Elevated	Less elevated
hCG in tissue	++++	+
Behavior	2% choriocarcinoma	Rare choriocarcinoma

hCG, Human chorionic gonadotropin.

- *Partial mole* (p. 1058) occurs when an egg with normal chromosomal content is fertilized by two sperm to get a triploid complement of genetic material; the karyotype is 69,XXX or 69,XXY. There is no increased risk of choriocarcinoma.

Morphology (p. 1058)

- *Grossly:* Moles consist of masses of thin-walled, translucent, cystic, grapelike structures. Fetal parts are rarely seen in complete moles and are more common in partial moles.
- *Microscopically:* Complete moles show hydropic swelling of villi, inadequate vascularization of villi, and significant trophoblastic proliferation. Partial moles show only focal edema and focal and slight trophoblastic proliferation.

Clinical Features (p. 1059)

Moles can be diagnosed by ultrasound examination and by serum hCG, revealing levels exceeding those produced by a normal pregnancy of similar age. Thorough curettage is adequate therapy for most moles, although 10% develop into invasive moles (see later discussion), and 2.5% develop into choriocarcinoma; follow-up hCG determinations can identify those at risk.

Invasive Mole (p. 1059)

An invasive mole penetrates and may even perforate the uterine wall, associated with proliferating cytotrophoblasts and syncytiotrophoblasts; villi can embolize to distant sites but do not grow. Invasive moles are associated with persistently elevated hCG. The tumor responds well to chemotherapy but can result in uterine rupture.

Choriocarcinoma (p. 1059)

Choriocarcinoma is a malignant tumor arising in 1:20,000 to 1:30,000 pregnancies in the United States. Half arise in hydatidiform moles, 25% in previous abortions, 22% in normal pregnancies, and the rest in ectopic pregnancies.

Morphology (p. 1060)

- *Grossly:* Tumors are large, soft, yellow-white, fleshy masses with areas of necrosis and hemorrhage.
- *Microscopically:* Lesions consist of mixed cytotrophoblast and syncytiotrophoblast proliferations. The tumor invades the underlying

endometrium, penetrates blood vessels and lymphatics, and can metastasize widely.

Clinical Features (p. 1060)

Choriocarcinomas manifest with vaginal bleeding and discharge that can appear in the course of an apparently normal pregnancy, after a miscarriage, or after curettage; hCG titers are elevated to levels above those seen in hydatidiform mole. Commonly, widespread metastases are already present at the time of initial discovery. Gestational choriocarcinomas are highly sensitive to chemotherapy, with 100% remission rates and high cure rates.

Placental-Site Trophoblastic Tumor (p. 1061)

Placental-site trophoblastic tumor (PSTT) comprises less than 2% of gestational trophoblastic tumors; it represents neoplastic prolife-ration of extravillous (intermediate) trophoblasts. The lesion differs from choriocarcinoma because syncytio- and cytotrophoblastic elements are absent and the tumors make lower levels of hCG. Most are only locally invasive, but 10% to 15% result in metastases and death.

23

The Breast

Breast pathology is best understood in the context of its normal anatomy (Fig. 23-1). Breasts are composed of specialized epithelium and stroma, either of which can develop benign or malignant lesions. It is worth noting that two cell types (derived from the same precursor stem cells) line the ducts and lobules: *myoepithelial cells* on the basement membrane and overlying luminal *epithelial cells*. The stroma also takes two forms: (1) *interlobular stroma* composed of intermixed adipose and dense fibrous connective tissue and (2) *intralobular stroma* around acini composed of hormone-responsive breast-specific fibroblast-like cells. Stroma and epithelial interactions promote normal breast structure and function.

THE FEMALE BREAST (p. 1066)

Disorders of Development (p. 1067)

- *Milkline remnants* (p. 1067): These can produce hormone-responsive supernumerary nipples or breast tissue from the axilla to the perineum. These mainly come to attention secondary to painful pre-menstrual enlargement.
- *Accessory axillary breast tissue* (p. 1067): Occasionally, normal ductal tissue extends into subcutaneous tissue of the axilla or chest wall. This can present as a lump in the setting of lactational hyperplasia, or it can give rise to carcinoma outside the breast proper.
- *Congenital nipple inversion* (p. 1067): This is common and usually spontaneously corrects during pregnancy or with traction; *acquired nipple inversion* is concerning for carcinoma or inflammatory conditions.

Clinical Presentations of Breast Disease (p. 1067)

- *Pain* is a common breast symptom. Diffuse cyclic pain has no pathologic correlate; therapy targets hormone levels. Non-cyclic pain is usually localized and can occur secondary to infection, trauma, or ruptured cysts. Roughly 95% of painful masses are benign, although 10% of breast cancer presents with pain.
- *Discrete palpable masses* are also common, but they need to be differentiated from normal breast "lumpiness"; a breast mass typically becomes palpable when larger than 2 cm. The most common lesions are cysts, fibroadenomas, and carcinoma, with the likelihood of malignancy increasing with age. Thus, 10% of dominant masses in women younger than age 40 years are cancer; whereas in women older than age 50 years, 60% of dominant masses are malignant.

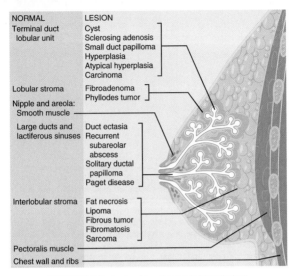

NORMAL	LESION
Terminal duct lobular unit	Cyst Sclerosing adenosis Small duct papilloma Hyperplasia Atypical hyperplasia Carcinoma
Lobular stroma	Fibroadenoma Phyllodes tumor
Nipple and areola: Smooth muscle	
Large ducts and lactiferous sinuses	Duct ectasia Recurrent subareolar abscess Solitary ductal papilloma Paget disease
Interlobular stroma	Fat necrosis Lipoma Fibrous tumor Fibromatosis Sarcoma
Pectoralis muscle	
Chest wall and ribs	

FIGURE 23-1 Anatomic origins of common breast lesions.

- *Nipple discharge* is a less common symptom but is worrisome for cancer when unilateral and spontaneous; cancer-associated discharge occurs in 7% of malignancies in women younger than 60 years and in 30% of cancers in women older than 60 years. Bloody or serous discharges are most commonly due to cysts or intraductal papillomas, and benign bloody discharge can also occur during pregnancy. Milky discharge (galactorrhea) outside of pregnancy can be related to prolactin-producing pituitary adenomas, hypothyroidism, anovulatory cycles, or certain medications.
- The principal *mammographic signs* associated with carcinoma are *densities* and *calcifications*. Most neoplasms (benign and malignant) are radiologically denser than normal breast tissue; the value of mammography is the ability to detect lesions as small as 1 cm. Calcifications form on secretions, necrotic debris, or hyalinized stroma and are associated with both benign and malignant lesions.
- The sensitivity and specificity of mammography increases with age, due to the progressive replacement of radiodense fibrous youthful breast tissue with fatty, radiolucent stroma. At age 40 years, mammographic lesions reflect carcinoma in only 10% of cases; this increases to 25% in patients older than 50 years.

Inflammatory Disorders (p. 1069)

Inflammatory conditions *(mastitis)* are rare except during lactation. "Inflammatory carcinoma" mimics inflammation by obstructing dermal lymphatics; it should be suspected in a non-lactating woman with the clinical appearance of mastitis.

Acute Mastitis (p. 1069)

Almost all cases occur during the first month of lactation when the breast is vulnerable to bacterial infections *(Staphylococcus* and *Streptococcus)* through nipple cracks and fissures. Acute mastitis usually resolves with antibiotic treatment and continued breastfeeding.

Periductal Mastitis (p. 1069)

Squamous metaplasia of the nipple ducts results in keratin shedding and subsequent ductal plugging; duct dilation and rupture then leads to intense chronic and granulomatous inflammation that presents as a painful subareolar mass in both sexes. Synonymous terms include *recurrent subareolar abscess, squamous metaplasia of lactiferous ducts,* and *Zuska disease.* Smoking is associated with 90% of cases. Secondary bacterial infections can occur, and recurrent cases may be complicated by periareolar fistulous tracts and/or nipple inversion. Treatment includes surgical excision of the involved ducts.

Mammary Duct Ectasia (p. 1070)

Mammary duct ectasia usually presents as an ill-defined, usually painless periareolar mass with viscous white nipple secretions. It tends to occur in multiparous women between ages 50 and 70 years old; there is no association with smoking. The lesion is characterized by inspissation of secretions, duct dilation without squamous metaplasia, and periductal inflammation that can lead to fibrosis and skin retraction.

Fat Necrosis (p. 1070)

Fat necrosis presents as a painless palpable mass, skin thickening or retraction, or mammographic density and/or calcifications. It is associated with prior trauma or surgery. Histologically, lesions progress from hemorrhage with acute inflammation and liquefactive fat necrosis to chronic inflammation with giant cells and hemosiderin to scar tissue.

Lymphocytic Mastopathy (Sclerosing Lymphocytic Lobulitis) (p. 1070)

Lesions present as single or multiple, rock-hard, palpable masses; histology reveals collagenized stroma around atrophic ducts with a prominent lymphocytic infiltrate. An association with type 1 diabetes and autoimmune thyroid disease suggests an autoimmune etiology.

Granulomatous Mastitis (p. 1070)

This can be associated with systemic diseases (e.g., sarcoidosis, Wegener granulomatosis), foreign bodies (e.g., piercings), or granulomatous infections (e.g., mycobacteria or fungi). *Granulomatous lobular mastitis* is a rare entity occurring in parous women, attributed to hypersensitivity responses to lactational epithelium.

Benign Epithelial Lesions (p. 1070)

These lesions are categorized according to the risk of developing breast malignancy (Table 23-1); in the vast majority of cases, *breast cancer does not develop.*

Nonproliferative Breast Changes (Fibrocystic Changes) (p. 1071)

These lesions have essentially no malignant potential; they represent the common findings seen in "lumpy bumpy" breasts.

Morphology (p. 1071)

- *Cysts* form by lobular dilation and unfolding, and they can coalesce to form larger lesions; they are lined by flattened atrophic epithelium or metaplastic apocrine cells and frequently exhibit calcifications.

TABLE 23-1 **Epithelial Breast Lesions and the Risk of Developing Invasive Carcinoma**

Pathologic Lesion	Relative Risk (Absolute Lifetime Risk)*
Nonproliferative Breast Changes (Fibrocystic changes)	1.0 (3%)
Duct ectasia	
Cysts	
Apocrine change	
Mild hyperplasia	
Adenosis	
Fibroadenoma w/o complex features	
Proliferative Disease without Atypia	1.5 to 2.0 (5% to 7%)
Moderate or florid hyperplasia	
Sclerosing adenosis	
Papilloma	
Complex sclerosing lesion (radial scar)	
Fibroadenoma with complex features	
Proliferative Disease with Atypia	4.0 to 5.0 (13% to 17%)
Atypical ductal hyperplasia (ADH)	
Atypical lobular hyperplasia (ALH)	
Carcinoma *In Situ*	8.0 to 10.0 (25% to 30%)
Lobular carcinoma *in situ* (LCIS)	
Ductal carcinoma *in situ* (DCIS)	

*Relative risk is the risk compared to women without any risk factors. Absolute lifetime risk is the percentage of patients expected to develop invasive carcinoma if untreated.

- *Fibrosis* occurs secondary to cyst rupture and inflammation.
- *Adenosis* is defined as increased numbers of acini per lobule; it occurs normally during pregnancy and can be a focal finding in non-pregnant breasts. Acini are often enlarged but are not distorted and are lined by columnar epithelium that can exhibit atypia; calcification is occasionally present.

Proliferative Breast Disease without Atypia (p. 1071)

These lesions are characterized by epithelial or stromal proliferation, but without cytologic or architectural atypia.

Morphology (p. 1071)

- *Epithelial hyperplasia* is defined by more than two cell layers around ducts and lobules.
- *Sclerosing adenosis* is reflected by increased numbers of acini per lobule with central distortion and compression and peripheral dilation.
- *Complex sclerosing lesions* have components of sclerosing adenosis, papillomas and epithelial hyperplasia.
- *Papillomas* reflect epithelial growth and associated fibrovascular cores within dilated ducts; more than 80% of large duct papillomas produce a nipple discharge.

Proliferative Breast Disease with Atypia (p. 1073)

Lesions include atypical ductal and atypical lobular hyperplasia, occasionally associated with radiologic calcifications.

Morphology (p. 1073)

Atypical hyperplasia lacks sufficient features to diagnose carcinoma; however, these epithelia have many of the same acquired genetic changes present in *carcinoma in situ*.

- *Atypical ductal hyperplasia* shares some morphologic features with ductal carcinoma *in situ* (DCIS) but is limited in extent.
- *Atypical lobular hyperplasia* shares features with lobular carcinoma *in situ* (LCIS), but cells do not distend more than 50% of acini within a lobule.

Carcinoma of the Breast (p. 1073)

Breast carcinoma is the most common non-skin malignancy in women; a female living to age 90 years has a one in eight chance of developing breast cancer. However, less than 20% of women with invasive breast cancer die of it.

Incidence and Epidemiology (p. 1074)

Due to mammographic screening, breast cancer incidence increased in the 1980s; this was accompanied, however, by a downward trend in the clinical stage at presentation—now predominantly DCIS or stage I disease without nodal metastases—and declining mortality rates.

Major risk factors:

- *Gender:* Only 1% of breast cancers occur in men.
- *Age:* Breast cancer is rare before age 25 years. The incidence increases with age with the average age at diagnosis being 61 years old for Caucasian women, 56 years old for Hispanic women, and 46 years old for African-American women. Carcinoma in young women is associated with the loss of estrogen receptors (ERs) or increased human epidermal growth factor receptor 2 (HER2/neu) expression.
- *Age at menarche:* Early menarche (i.e., younger than 11 years) and late menopause increase risk.
- *Age at first live birth:* Earlier full-term pregnancy (i.e., younger than 20 years) halves the risk relative to nulliparous women or women with a first birth after age 35 years; this is attributed to lactation-induced terminal differentiation of luminal cells that removes them from the potential pool of cancer precursors.
- *First-degree relatives with breast cancer:* Risk increases with the number of affected first-degree relatives, although 87% with such a history will not develop malignancy. Most family risk is probably due to the interaction of low-risk susceptibility genes and non-genetic factors.
- *Atypical hyperplasia:* This increases risk (see Table 23-1).
- *Race/Ethnicity:* The risk that a 50-year-old woman will develop invasive carcinoma within 20 years is roughly 7% for Caucasian women, 5% for African-American women, and less than 4% for Hispanic women and Asian/Pacific Islanders. However, African-American and Hispanic women tend to present with more advanced malignancy and have higher mortality rates, in part related to variation in cancer risk genes.
- *Estrogen exposure:* Postmenopausal hormone replacement therapy increases risk 1.2- to 1.7-fold, although oral contraceptives do not increase risk. Reducing endogenous estrogens through oophorectomy or hormonal blockade decreases breast cancer risk.
- *Breast density, radiation exposure,* and *carcinoma of the endometrium or contralateral breast* (likely reflecting prolonged estrogen exposures): All of these increase risk.

- *Geographic influence:* Four- to seven-fold higher incidences of breast cancer in the United States and Europe are attributed to cultural differences in reproductive number and timing, breastfeeding, diet, obesity, and physical activity.
- *Diet:* Heavy alcohol consumption increases risk, while caffeine intake appears to decrease incidence.
- *Obesity:* Obesity in people younger than age 40 years reduces risk by increasing anovulatory cycling, while postmenopausal obesity increases risk through augmented estrogen synthesis.
- *Breastfeeding:* The greater the duration of breastfeeding, the greater the reduction in overall risk.

Pathogenesis (p. 1077)

The major risk factors for breast cancer are genetic and hormonal; tumors can therefore be divided into hereditary cases associated with germline mutations and sporadic cases related to hormonal exposures with *de novo* mutations.

Hereditary Breast Cancer (p. 1077)

Germ-line mutations underlie approximately 12% of breast cancers; hereditary etiology is suggested in the setting of multiple affected first-degree relatives, premenopausal cancers, or family members with specific malignancies (see later discussion) (Table 23-2). The major susceptibility genes are tumor suppressors with roles in DNA repair, cell cycle control, and regulation of apoptosis. However, the known high-risk breast cancer genes only account for 25% of all familial breast cancers. Thus the remaining cases are likely caused through the interaction of multiple genes with individually weak effects.

BRCA1 and -2 mutations account for the majority of breast malignancies that can be attributed to single-gene mutations and about 3% of all breast cancers. Penetrance varies from 30% to 90% depending on the specific mutation (only 0.1% to 0.2% of mutations in the general population actually increase breast cancer risk), and these tumors tend to be poorly differentiated. BRCA mutations also increase the risk of ovarian, prostatic, and pancreatic cancers. Mutations in *CHEK2*, *p53*, *PTEN*, and *LKB1/STK11* collectively account for less than 10% of hereditary breast carcinomas.

Sporadic Breast Cancer (p. 1079)

Hormone exposure is the major risk factor for sporadic cancers; moreover, most of these tumors are ER positive and occur in post-menopausal women. Hormone exposure increases the number of target cells by stimulating breast growth; by driving proliferation, hormones also place cells at risk for stabilizing DNA mutations. Metabolites of estrogen can also directly cause mutations or generate DNA-damaging free radicals.

Overview of Carcinogenesis and Tumor Progression (p. 1079)

Since the majority of breast cancers are ER-positive, the most likely cell of origin is an ER-expressing luminal cell; ER-negative carcinomas may arise from ER-negative myoepithelial cells (or by de-differentiation of an ER-expressing precursor). Initial lesions are typically marked by proliferative changes; atypical ductal and lobular hyperplasia show increased hormone receptor expression and abnormal proliferative capacity (due to increased pro-growth signals, diminished apoptosis, or loss of growth-inhibitory signals). At some point the tumor becomes immortalized and develops angiogenic capabilities. The final step—progressing from *in situ*

TABLE 23-2 Most Common "Single Gene" Mutations Associated with Hereditary Susceptibility to Breast Cancer

GENE (location) Syndrome (Incidence)*	% of "Single Gene" Hereditary Cancers[†]	Breast Cancer Risk by Age 70[‡]	Changes in Sporadic Breast Cancer	Other Associated Cancers	Functions	Comments
BRCA1 (17q21) Familial breast and ovarian cancer (1 in 860)	52% (~2% of all breast cancers)	40% to 90%	Mutations rare; inactivated in 50% of some subtypes (e.g. medullary and metaplastic) by methylation	Ovarian, male breast cancer (but lower than BRCA2), prostate, pancreas, fallopian tube	Tumor suppressor, transcriptional regulation, repair of double-stranded DNA breaks	Breast carcinomas are commonly poorly differentiated and triple negative (basal-like), and have p53 mutations.
BRCA2 (13q12-13) Familial breast and ovarian cancer (1 in 740)	32% (~1% of all breast cancers)	30% to 90%	Mutations and loss of expression rare	Ovarian, male breast cancer, prostate, pancreas, stomach, melanoma, gallbladder, bile duct, pharynx	Tumor suppressor, transcriptional regulation, repair of double-stranded DNA breaks	Biallelic germline mutations cause a rare form of Fanconi anemia (Chapter 7)
p53 (17p13.1) Li-Fraumeni (1 in 5000)	3% (<1% of all breast cancers)	>90%	Mutations in 20%, LOH in 30% to 42%; most frequent in triple negative cancers	Sarcoma, leukemia, brain tumors, adrenocortical carcinoma, others	Tumor suppressor with critical roles in cell cycle control, DNA replication, DNA repair, and apoptosis	p53 is the most commonly mutated gene in sporadic breast cancers
CHEK2 (22q12.1) Li-Fraumeni variant (1 in 100)	5% (~1% of all breast cancers)	10% to 20%	Mutations rare (<5%); loss of protein expression in at least one third by unknown mechanism(s)	Prostate, thyroid, kidney, colon	Cell cycle checkpoint kinase, recognition and repair of DNA damage, activates BRCA1 and p53 by phosphorylation	May increase risk for breast cancer after radiation exposure

*Frequency of heterozygotes in the U.S. population; the incidence of gene mutations is higher in some ethnic populations (e.g., BRCA1 and BRCA2 mutations occur at high frequencies in Askenazi Jews).
[†]Defined as familial breast cancers showing a pattern of inheritance consistent with a major effect of a single gene.
[‡]Risk varies with specific mutations and is likely modified by other genes.
LOH, Loss of heterozygosity.

to invasive carcinoma—is poorly understood and may involve inflammation and/or wound healing–like tissue reactions.

Classification of Breast Carcinoma (p. 1079)

More than 95% are adenocarcinomas; these may be *in situ* (i.e., proliferation limited to ducts and lobules by the basement membrane) or invasive (i.e., penetrating the basement membrane with metastatic capacity). Different histologic types have characteristic clinical, biologic, and prognostic implications (Table 23-3).

DUCTAL CARCINOMA IN SITU (P. 1080)

- DCIS now constitutes 15% to 30% of all breast cancers in well-screened populations; most are detected mammographically, presenting with calcifications more often than periductal fibrosis. It is bilateral in 10% to 20% of cases. Left untreated, low-grade DCIS will progress to invasive cancer at a rate of 1% per year. Mastectomy is curative in more than 95% of patients; excision followed by radiation has slightly higher rates of recurrence relating to grade, size, and margins. Regardless of treatment, less than 2% of women with DCIS will die of breast cancer.

Morphology (p. 1080)

- *Comedocarcinoma* is characterized by ducts and lobules dilated by sheets of high-grade pleomorphic cells with zones of central necrosis.
- *Noncomedo DCIS* consists of a monomorphic population of cells of varying nuclear grades; patterns include cribriform, solid, papillary, and micropapillary.
- *Paget disease* of the nipple occurs rarely (1% to 4% of cases); malignant cells extend from ductal DCIS into nipple skin without crossing the basement membrane. These cells disrupt the epithelial barrier and allow extracellular fluid to seep out, creating an erythematous eruption with a scaly crust.
- *Microinvasion* is defined by stromal invasion less than 0.1 cm; if only a few foci are present, the prognosis is similar to DCIS.

TABLE 23-3   Distribution of Histologic Types of Breast Cancer

Total Cancers	Percent
Carcinoma *In Situ**	15-30
Ductal carcinoma *in situ* (DCIS)	80
Lobular carcinoma *in situ* (LCIS)	20
Invasive Carcinoma	70-85
No special type of carcinoma ("ductal")	79
Lobular carcinoma	10
Tubular/cribriform carcinoma	6
Mucinous (colloid) carcinoma	2
Medullary carcinoma	2
Papillary carcinoma	1
Metaplastic carcinoma	<1

*The proportion of *in situ* carcinomas detected depends on the number of women undergoing mammographic screening and ranges from less than 5% in unscreened populations to almost 50% in patients with screen-detected cancers. Current observed numbers are between these two extremes.

The data on invasive carcinomas are modified from Dixon JM, et al: Long-term survivors after breast cancer, *Br J Surg* 72:445, 1985.

LOBULAR CARCINOMA IN SITU (p. 1082)

LCIS comprises 1% to 6% of all breast cancers and is always an incidental biopsy finding since it does not induce calcifications or stromal responses; it is bilateral in 20% to 40% of cases, with the vast majority occurring in premenopausal women. Left untreated, LCIS progresses to invasive cancer at a rate of about 1% per year. Therapy can entail mastectomy or tamoxifen but typically now involves close follow-up with mammographic screening.

Morphology (p. 1082)

Lesions consist of discohesive cells (in some cases due to loss of E-cadherin expression), often with intracellular mucin forming signet ring cells. Most express ER and PR.

Invasive (Infiltrating) Carcinomas (p. 1083)

Invasive (infiltrating) carcinomas can present as palpable masses or radiodense mammographic lesions (see Table 23-2). Mammography-identified tumors are typically half the size of palpable masses and only 20% have nodal metastases; conversely, palpable tumors are associated with nodal metastases in more than 50% of patients. Larger tumors can be fixed to the chest wall, can cause skin dimpling or nipple retraction, or can invade dermal lymphatics (blocking outflow) with the resulting lymphedema leading to a *peau d'orange* appearance. *Inflammatory carcinoma* refers to tumors that present with a swollen, erythematous breast due to extensive lymphatic invasion and destruction; the overall prognosis is poor.

Invasive Carcinoma, No Special Type (NST; Invasive Ductal Carcinoma) (p. 1083)

Invasive carcinoma comprises 70% to 80% of breast cancers. Newer *molecular classifications* are based on gene expression profiling and correlate with prognosis and therapeutic responses:

- "Luminal A" (40% to 55% of no special type cancers): Tumors are ER positive and HER2/neu negative; the genetic signature is dominated by estrogen-responsive genes. Most are well differentiated and occur in postmenopausal women. They are slow-growing and respond to hormone therapy, but are less sensitive to traditional chemotherapy.
- "Luminal B" (15% to 20%): Tumors are also ER positive but tend to be higher grade, with greater proliferation, and HER2/neu over-expression (i.e., "triple-positive tumors"). They often present with nodal metastases and may respond to chemotherapy.
- "Normal breast-like" (6% to 10%): Well-differentiated, ER-positive, HER2/neu-negative tumors with gene signatures and most like normal breast tissue.
- "Basal-like" (13% to 25%): These tumors lack ER, PR, or HER2/neu ("triple negative carcinomas"); instead they express myoepithelial cell markers; many arise in the context of *BRCA1* mutations. Many are high grade and proliferative and pursue an aggressive course; a subset (15% to 20%) may exhibit complete response to chemotherapy.
- "HER2 positive" (7% to 12%): These are ER-negative tumors that over-express HER2/neu, often due to 17q21 chromosomal amplification; this amplicon dominates the gene signature. These cancers are usually poorly differentiated and aggressively metastatic.

ER-positive tumors respond to hormone blockade, whereas HER2/neu over-expressing cancers respond to a combination of chemotherapy and monoclonal antibodies (trastuzumab) directed against HER2/neu.

Morphology (p. 1083)

- *Grossly:* Most tumors are firm to hard, with an irregular border and a gritty sensation on cutting.
- *Microscopically:* Lesions range from well differentiated with tubule formation, small round nuclei, and rare mitoses to poorly differentiated with sheets and nests of cells with enlarged irregular nuclei, multiple mitoses, and focal necrosis.

Invasive Lobular Carcinoma (p. 1085)

Invasive lobular carcinoma usually presents as a palpable mass or mammographic density; however, in 25% of cases, the tumor invades with little desmoplasia, making detection by any modality difficult. Well-differentiated and moderately differentiated invasive lobular carcinoma are usually diploid, ER-positive, associated with LCIS, and have a gene expression profile akin to luminal A cancers. Poorly differentiated tumors are usually aneuploid and lack hormone receptors, and they can over-express HER2/neu. Lobular carcinomas tend to metastasize to peritoneum and retroperitoneum, gastrointestinal tract, leptomeninges, ovaries, and uterus.

Morphology (p. 1087)

The histologic hallmark is discohesive infiltrating tumor cells, often arranged in single-file or loose clusters; these often have a signet ring appearance, and desmoplasia is typically minimal.

Medullary Carcinomas (p. 1087)

Medullary carcinomas typically present after age 60 years as rapidly-growing, well-circumscribed masses. These tumors have a "basal-like" gene expression pattern, and two thirds exhibit hypermethylation of the *BRCA1* promoter. Their prognosis is slightly better than NST carcinomas; over-expression of intercellular adhesion molecules and E-cadherin may limit metastatic spread.

Morphology (p. 1087)

- *Grossly:* Tumors are characteristically soft and fleshy with a pushing border and little desmoplastic response.
- *Microscopically:* Lesions exhibit solid sheets of large cells with vesicular pleomorphic nuclei and prominent nucleoli, multiple mitoses, and a lymphoplasmacytic infiltrate.

Mucinous (Colloid) Carcinomas (p. 1087)

Mucinous (colloid) carcinomas are slow-growing well-differentiated ER-positive tumors that occur at a median age of 71 years; nodal metastases are uncommon.

Morphology (p. 1087)

- *Grossly:* Tumors are soft to rubbery with a gel-like consistency.
- *Microscopically:* Malignant cells grow in clusters within large mucin lakes.

Tubular Carcinoma (p. 1087)

Tubular carcinomas are typically detected as small irregular mammographic densities in women in their forties; they may be multifocal and/or bilateral. Tubular carcinomas are associated with atypical lobular hyperplasia, LCIS, or low-grade DCIS; 95% are well-differentiated, diploid, ER-positive, and HER2/neu-negative. They have an excellent prognosis.

Prognostic and Predictive Factors (p. 1089)

The following major prognostic factors are incorporated into the breast cancer staging system (five stages [0 to IV] that correlate with survival):

- *Invasive carcinoma versus* in situ *disease:* By definition, carcinoma *in situ* cannot metastasize; thus, adequate DCIS treatment is usually curative. Deaths associated with DCIS are attributed to subsequent invasive carcinoma or occult areas of invasion. In contrast, half of invasive cancers have metastasized at the time of diagnosis.
- *Distant metastases:* Once distant metastases are present, cure is unlikely, although long-term remissions and palliation can be achieved.
- *Lymph node metastases:* In the absence of distant metastases, lymph node status is the most important prognostic factor. If nodes are cancer-free, 10-year disease-free survival rate is 70% to 80%; that falls to 35% to 40% with 1 to 3 positive nodes and 10% to 15% with more than 10 positive nodes. Most breast cancers drain into 1 to 2 "sentinel nodes" in the ipsilateral axilla identifiable by colored dye or radioactive tracer injected prior to surgical excision. Women with negative sentinel nodes can be spared the morbidity of a full axillary dissection.
- *Tumor size:* Tumor size is an independent prognostic factor and also predicts the likelihood of metastasis. Women with node-negative carcinomas less than 1 cm in size have a 10-year survival rate more than 90%; survival drops to 77% for cancers more than 2 cm.
- *Locally advanced disease:* Carcinomas invading into skin or skeletal muscle are usually large and have a worse prognosis.
- *Inflammatory carcinoma:* Dermal lymphatic involvement portends a very poor prognosis with 3% to 10% 3-year survivals.

Minor Prognostic and Predictive Factors (p. 1089)

Histologic subtype: In general, carcinomas classified as a special type (e.g., tubular, mucinous, or medullary) have a better prognosis than NST carcinomas.

Histologic grade: Patients with low-grade, well-differentiated tumors have almost two-fold better survival on average than individuals with poorly differentiated carcinomas.

ERs and progesterone receptors (PRs): Hormone receptor expression predicts hormone responsiveness but also lack of sensitivity to conventional chemotherapy. Conversely, tumors lacking hormone receptors do not usually respond to hormones but are more susceptible to chemotherapy.

HER2/neu: Over-expression of HER2/neu connotes a worse prognosis but predicts response to trastuzumab.

Lymphovascular invasion (LVI): This is a poor prognostic factor in women without lymph node metastases and is a risk factor for local recurrence.

Proliferative rate: A high proliferative rate is a poor prognostic factor.

DNA content: Aneuploidy (DNA content greater than diploid) connotes a slightly worse prognosis.

Response to neoadjuvant therapy: Such therapy prior to surgery strongly predicts long-term outcome; good responses are more common in ER-negative, poorly differentiated tumors with focal areas of necrosis.

Gene expression profiling: This can predict outcomes, but it does not correlate with tumor size or node status, suggesting that it is identifying other independent factors.

Current therapeutic approaches include combinations of surgery (mastectomy or breast-conserving surgery) and postoperative radiation, with systemic hormonal treatment, chemotherapy, or both. Newer therapeutic strategies include inhibitors of membrane-bound growth factor receptors (e.g., HER2/neu), stromal proteases, and angiogenesis.

Stromal Tumors (p. 1091)

Breast-specific intralobular stroma gives rise to biphasic (i.e., stroma and epithelium) breast tumors, fibroadenomas, and phyllodes tumors; interlobular stroma gives rise to the same benign and malignant tumors that occur in other stroma (e.g., lipomas and sarcomas).

Fibroadenomas (p. 1091)

Fibroadenomas are the most common benign tumor of the female breast, occurring most often during the reproductive years, and regressing and calcifying after menopause; no consistent cytogenetic changes have been demonstrated. Fibroadenomas present clinically as rubbery, well-circumscribed palpable masses; ovoid mammographic densities; or mammographic calcifications. Fibroadenoma epithelium is hormone responsive; tumors can grow during pregnancy. Some fibroadenomas are polyclonal hyperplasias of lobular stroma, responding to specific stimuli (e.g., cyclosporine).

Phyllodes Tumor (p. 1092)

Phyllodes tumors occur most commonly after age 60 years, typically presenting as palpable masses. The stroma frequently overgrows the epithelial component, forming clefts and slits and creating bulbous protrusions; increased cellularity, mitotic activity, stromal overgrowth, and infiltrative borders differentiate them from fibroadenomas. The frequency of chromosomal changes increases with grade; high-grade lesions also have epidermal growth factor (EGF) receptor amplification. Most phyllodes tumors can be cured by wide local excision; nodal or distant metastases are rare.

Benign Stromal Lesions (p. 1092)

Tumors of interlobular stroma are composed of stromal cells without an epithelial component. These include *pseudoangiomatous stromal hyperplasia* and *fibromatosis* (fibroblasts and myofibroblasts), *myofibroblastoma* (myofibroblasts), and lipomas.

Malignant Stromal Tumors (p. 1092)

Malignant stromal tumors are rare; the most common is angiosarcoma, arising as a primary tumor in young women, after radiation therapy for breast cancer, or in the skin of a chronically edematous arm after mastectomy (Stewart-Treves syndrome). Primary angiosarcomas are usually high grade and carry a poor prognosis.

Other Malignant Tumors of the Breast (p. 1093)

Malignant tumors (identical to their counterparts elsewhere) can arise from breast skin or adnexal structures. Breast can be a primary site of lymphomas or can be involved by a systemic lymphoma; most are diffuse large B-cell type. Metastases to the breast are rare and typically arise from a contralateral breast carcinoma; non-mammary metastases are most commonly melanomas and lung cancers.

THE MALE BREAST (p. 1093)

Gynecomastia (p. 1093)

Gynecomastia can be uni- or bilateral and presents as a button-like subareolar enlargement; it is significant primarily as an indicator of estrogen and androgen imbalance. Gynecomastia can occur during puberty, in Klinefelter syndrome, due to hormone-producing tumors, in men with cirrhosis, or as a side effect of drugs. Histologically, there is ductal epithelial and stromal hyperplasia; lobule formation is rare.

Carcinoma (p. 1093)

Carcinoma of the male breast is rare (1% of all breast cancers). Risk factors and prognostic factors are similar to those for women (e.g., first-degree relatives, increased estrogen exposures, etc.). Male breast cancer is strongly associated with BRCA2 (BRCA2 mutations will be present in 60% to 76% of families with a male having breast cancer); BRCA1 mutations are less frequently associated. The same histologic types of breast cancer are found in men and women. Because of the scant amount of male breast tissue, carcinomas tend to invade skin and chest wall earlier and present at higher stages. Matched by stage, however, prognosis is similar in men and women.

24

The Endocrine System

Endocrine signaling occurs through secreted hormones acting on target cells distant from the site of synthesis; target tissue responses also typically include feedback regulation of the original hormone production. Hormones are broadly classified as:

* Peptide or amino acid–derived hormones that interact with *cell surface receptors*
* Steroid hormones that diffuse across plasma membranes and interact with *intracellular receptors*

Endocrine disorders result from either:

* Hormone underproduction or overproduction
* Mass lesions that can be nonfunctional or can be associated with abnormal hormone levels

PITUITARY GLAND (p. 1098)

The pituitary gland, along with the hypothalamus, plays a critical role in the regulation of most other endocrine glands. It is composed of two morphologically and functionally distinct components:

* Anterior lobe (adenohypophysis; 80% of the pituitary). Hypo-thalamic factors carried to the anterior pituitary by a portal circulation influence hormone production by the five basic ante-rior lobe cell types:

  Somatotrophs: Growth hormone (GH)
  Lactotrophs: Prolactin (Prl)
  Corticotrophs: Adrenocorticotropic hormone (ACTH), pro-opiomelanocortin (POMC), melanocyte-stimulating hormone (MSH), endorphins, and lipotropin
  Thyrotrophs: Thyroid-stimulating hormone (TSH)
  Gonadotrophs: Follicle-stimulating hormone (FSH) and luteinizing hormone (LH)

* *Posterior lobe (neurohypophysis)* comprises modified glial cells *(pituicytes)* and axonal processes extending from the hypothala-mus; oxytocin and vasopressin (antidiuretic hormone [ADH]) synthesized by the hypothalamus are stored in the axon terminals. Oxytocin stimulates smooth muscle cell contraction in the gravid uterus and around mammary lactiferous ducts; ADH participates in water regulation.

Clinical Manifestations of Pituitary Disease (p. 1100)

- *Hyperpituitarism* (increased hormone production) results from anterior pituitary adenomas (most common), hyperplasia, or malignancy, hormone secretion by non-pituitary tumors, or hypothalamic disorders.
- *Hypopituitarism* (decreased hormone production) can be caused by ischemic injury, surgery, radiation, inflammation, or non-functional (but compressive) pituitary adenomas.
- *Local mass effects* include optic nerve compression, diplopia, visual field abnormalities (classically *bitemporal hemianopsia*), and increased intracranial pressure with headache, nausea, and vomiting. Mass effects can arise gradually or abruptly; the latter occurs with enlargement due to acute hemorrhage into an adenoma *(pituitary apoplexy)*.
- *Posterior pituitary lesions* typically manifest due to elevated or depressed ADH.

Pituitary Adenomas and Hyperpituitarism (p. 1100)

Functional pituitary adenomas are usually composed of a single cell type, producing one predominant hormone (Table 24-1); GH and Prl is the most common dual combination. Conversely, pituitary adenomas can be non-functional and cause hypopituitarism by destroying normal parenchyma. *Microadenomas* are defined as less than 1 cm; *macroadenomas* are defined as more than 1 cm. Non-functional tumors are usually macroadenomas since they come to attention primarily due to mass effects. Overall, the population prevalence of pituitary adenomas is 14%; the peak

TABLE 24-1	Classification of Pituitary Adenomas	
Pituitary Cell Type	**Hormone**	**Associated Syndrome***
Corticotroph	ACTH and other POMC-derived peptides	Cushing syndrome Nelson syndrome
Somatotroph	GH	Gigantism (children) Acromegaly (adults)
Lactotroph	Prolactin	Galactorrhea and amenorrhea (in females) Sexual dysfunction, infertility
Mammosomatotroph	Prolactin, GH	Combined features of GH and prolactin excess
Thyrotroph	TSH	Hyperthyroidism
Gonadotroph	FSH, LH	Hypogoandism, mass effects, and hypopituitarism

ACTH, Adrenocorticotropic hormone; *FSH,* follicle-stimulating hormone; *GH,* growth hormone; *LH,* luteinizing hormone; *POMC,* pro-opiomelanocortin; *TSH,* thyroid-stimulating hormone.
*Note that the non-functional adenomas in each category typically present with *mass effects* accompanied by *hypopituitarism* due to destruction of normal parenchyma.
Adapted from Ezzat S, Asa L: Mechanisms of disease: the pathogenesis of pituitary tumors, *Nat Clin Prac Endocrinol Metab* 2:200-230, 2006.

incidence is between the ages of 35 and 60 years. The majority of adenomas are sporadic, although 5% have a hereditable cause.

Pathogenesis (p. 1101)

- Spontaneous mutations of the α-subunit of the G_S stimulatory G protein (encoded by the *GNAS* gene on chromosome 20q13) that interfere with the intrinsic GTPase activity occur in 40% of somatotroph adenomas (and a smaller fraction of corticotroph adenomas); such mutations result in persistent cAMP generation and unchecked proliferation.
- A number of germline mutations are associated with familial adenomas but occur infrequently in sporadic adenomas:

  MEN1 mutations (affecting the tumor suppressor protein *menin*) underlie the multiple endocrine neoplasia-1 (MEN-1) syndrome; see later).

  CDKN1B encodes the cell-cycle checkpoint regulator p27; mutations give rise to an "MEN-1–like syndrome."

  Protein kinase A regulatory subunit 1α (PRKAR1A) encodes a tumor suppressor that regulates protein kinase A activity, downstream of cAMP-mediated signaling. It is mutated in *Carney syndrome,* an autosomal dominant disorder associated with pituitary and other endocrine tumors.

  AIP codes for the tumor suppressor *aryl hydrocarbon receptor–interacting protein;* mutations often lead GH-producing adenomas and acromegaly.

Morphology (p. 1102)

- *Grossly:* Tumors are usually solitary, forming discrete soft masses within the sella turcica. Larger adenomas can compress or infiltrate adjacent structures *(invasive adenomas).*
- *Microscopically:* Adenomas are generally composed of uniform, monomorphous cell populations arrayed in sheets, cords, or nests with scant extracellular matrix. Immunohistochemistry can be used to identify the hormone product. Nuclear atypia, necrosis, and hemorrhage can occur but do not imply malignancy; however, a subset of adenomas with increased mitotic activity (more than 3% of nuclei) are associated with *p53* mutations and have a greater propensity for aggressive behavior.

Prolactinomas (p. 1103)

Prolactinomas are the most common functional pituitary tumor (30%). Even microadenomas can secrete sufficient Prl to cause hyperprolactinemia although serum Prl concentrations tend to correlate with adenoma size. Hyperprolactinemia can produce amenorrhea (25% of cases), galactorrhea, loss of libido, and infertility.

Hyperprolactinemia is physiologic in pregnancy. Besides adenomas, pathologic hyperprolactinemia can be caused by *lactotroph hyperplasia,* occurring when the normal dopamine inhibition of Prl secretion is blocked. This can result from damage to the hypothalamic dopaminergic neurons, pituitary stalk transsection (e.g., head trauma), or drugs that block dopamine receptors; any suprasellar mass can potentially disturb the normal hypothalamic inhibitory pathways. Consequently, mild Prl elevations (even in the presence of a pituitary adenoma) does not necessarily indicate a Prl-secreting tumor.

Growth Hormone Cell (Somatotroph) Adenomas (p. 1104)

GH-secreting tumors are the second most common functioning adenoma. Hypersecretion of GH stimulates hepatic production of insulin-like growth factor-1 (IGF-1, somatomedin C), which causes many of the clinical manifestations; the effects depend on the age of onset. If somatotroph adenomas appear *before* epiphyseal closure, elevated GH results in *gigantism* characterized by a generalized increase in body size and disproportionately long arms and legs. If increased GH appears *after* epiphyseal closure, patients develop *acromegaly* with enlargement of head, hands, feet, jaw, tongue, and soft tissues. GH excess is also associated with gonadal dysfunction, diabetes mellitus, muscle weakness, hypertension, arthritis, congestive heart failure, and increased risk of gastrointestinal cancers.

Diagnosis relies on documenting elevated serum GH and IGF-1 levels; failure to suppress GH production by an oral glucose load is the most sensitive assay. Tumors can be surgically removed, or GH secretion can be reduced by drug therapy with somatostatin analogues or GH receptor antagonists. Effective control of GH levels leads to gradual recession of the tissue overgrowth and resolution of the metabolic abnormalities.

ACTH Cell (Corticotroph) Adenomas (p. 1104)

Corticotroph cell adenomas are typically microadenomas at the time of diagnosis, because ACTH production leads to early symptoms related to adrenal hypercortisolism *(Cushing disease)*. Besides adenomas, a wide variety of conditions can also cause elevated cortisol levels *(Cushing syndrome*, discussed under *Adrenal Pathology)*. Surgical removal of the adrenals results in loss of inhibitory feedback to the pituitary corticotrophs and can induce the formation of large, destructive adenomas *(Nelson syndrome)*; these can also cause hyperpigmentation through effects on melanocytes of other products of the ACTH precursor.

Other Anterior Pituitary Adenomas (p. 1104)

- *Gonadotroph adenomas* (10% to 15% of pituitary adenomas) typically occur in middle-aged men and women. Because they produce hormones somewhat variably and the secretory products do not cause recognizable symptoms, most tumors are detected only when they become large enough to cause neurologic symptoms. Impaired LH production is the most common gonadotroph deficiency; in men, the resulting low serum testosterone manifests as decreased energy and libido, whereas in premenopausal women, the outcome is amenorrhea.
- *Thyrotroph adenomas* (1% of pituitary adenomas) are rare causes of hyperthyroidism.
- *Nonfunctioning pituitary adenomas* (25% to 30% of pituitary adenomas) include non-secretory ("silent") variants of functioning adenomas, as well as true hormone-negative adenomas; the latter are unusual. Patients with nonfunctioning adenomas typically present with mass effects.
- *Pituitary carcinomas* are quite rare (less than 1%); most are functional (secreting Prl or ACTH most commonly). Diagnosis of carcinoma requires the demonstration of metastases.

Hypopituitarism (p. 1105)

Hypopituitarism can result from diseases of the hypothalamus and/or pituitary. Hypofunction occurs when 75% of the parenchyma is lost. Manifestations depend on which hormone(s) are lacking. Causes include the following:

- *Tumors and other mass lesions* in the sella (adenomas, metastases, or cysts) can cause damage by compression of adjacent normal pituitary.

- *Traumatic brain injury* and/or *subarachnoid hemorrhage.*
- *Pituitary surgery or radiation.* Surgical excision of a pituitary adenoma may inadvertently remove sufficient normal tissue to cause hypopituitarism; radiation to prevent regrowth of residual tumor can damage nonadenomatous tissue.
- *Pituitary apoplexy* can present dramatically with sudden onset of excruciating headache, diplopia, and hypopituitarism; it is a neurosurgical emergency because in severe cases it can precipitate cardiovascular collapse and sudden death.
- *Sheehan syndrome* results from sudden infarction of the anterior lobe occurring in the setting of obstetric hemorrhage or shock. This occurs because the pituitary enlarges to almost twice its normal size during pregnancy, but it does so without accompanying increases in vascular perfusion; it can then become frankly ischemic with any substantial blood loss or diminished perfusion pressure. Ischemic pituitary necrosis can also be encountered in other conditions, such as disseminated intravascular coagulation (DIC), sickle cell anemia, elevated intracranial pressure, traumatic injury, or shock.
- *Rathke cleft cysts* can accumulate proteinaceous fluid and expand.
- *Empty sella syndrome* can occur with any condition that destroys part or all of the pituitary gland:

   In *primary empty sella*, defects in the diaphragma sellae allow arachnoid matter and cerebrospinal fluid to herniate into the sella, causing pituitary compression. Classically, affected individuals are obese multigravidas. Besides hypopituitarism, patients can present with visual field defects and hyperprolactinemia due to loss of inhibitory hypothalamic tracts.

   In *secondary empty sella*, surgery or radiation leaves behind a vacant space; hypopituitarism results from the treatment or spontaneous infarction.

- *Genetic defects* are rare; the best-described are mutations in the pituitary-specific homeobox gene *POU1F1*, causing deficiencies in GH, Prl, and TSH.
- *Hypothalamic lesions* (e.g., tumors, trauma, etc.) interfere with the delivery of pituitary hormone–releasing factors.
- *Inflammatory disorders and infections.*

Posterior Pituitary Syndromes (p. 1106)

- Inappropriate *oxytocin* secretion has not been associated with clinical abnormalities.
- *ADH deficiency (diabetes insipidus)* results in *hypernatremia* due to ineffective renal water resorption; patients present clinically with polyuria and polydipsia. It can result from head trauma, tumors, inflammatory disorders, or surgery involving the hypothalamus or pituitary.
- *Syndrome of inappropriate ADH secretion (SIADH)* results in *hyponatremia* due to excessive renal water resorption; patients present clinically with cerebral edema and resultant neurologic dysfunction. The most frequent causes include ectopic ADH secretion by malignancies (especially lung small cell carcinoma), non-neoplastic pulmonary diseases (e.g., tuberculosis, pneumonia), and hypothalamus and/or posterior pituitary injury.

Hypothalamic Suprasellar Tumors (p. 1106)

Such tumors can induce anterior pituitary hypofunction or hyperfunction and/or diabetes insipidus; the most common lesions are gliomas (Chapter 28) and craniopharyngiomas. *Craniopharyngiomas* derive from Rathke pouch remnants, are slow-growing, and account for 1% to 5% of intracranial tumors. There is a bimodal age distribution with one peak between ages 5 and 15 years and the second peak after age 65 years. Children usually present with endocrine deficiencies (e.g., growth retardation) while adults present with visual disturbances and headaches. Even with local invasion, these tumors have an excellent prognosis; malignant transformation is rare.

Morphology (p. 1106)

- *Grossly:* Tumors average 3 to 4 cm in diameter and are characteristically cystic or multi-loculated.
- *Microscopically:* Lesions are composed of a mixture of squamous epithelial elements and stroma; two variants are recognized:

  Adamantinomatous craniopharyngioma is more common in children. These lesions commonly calcify. There is a "spongy" reticulum with peripheral palisading of the epithelium and compact, lamellar keratin ("wet keratin"). Cysts in these tumors contain cholesterol-rich, thick brownish-yellow fluid likened to "machinery oil."

  Papillary craniopharyngioma is more common in adults. These lesions rarely calcify; they are composed of sheets and papillae of well-differentiated squamous epithelium lacking keratin or cysts.

THYROID GLAND (p. 1107)

TSH binding to thyroid epithelial receptors leads to activation of a coupled G_S protein and increased intracellular cAMP; this, in turn, promotes epithelial proliferation, thyroglobulin synthesis and systemic thyroxine (T_4) release (with lesser amounts of triiodothyronine [T_3]). T_4 and T_3 circulate bound to thyroxine-binding globulin (TBG); in the periphery, most free T_4 is deiodinated to T_3, which binds to nuclear thyroid receptors (TR) in target cells with 10-fold greater affinity than T_4 and has proportionately greater activity. Thyroid hormone–TR complexes regulate target gene transcription by binding to thyroid hormone response elements (TREs); the result is a globally augmented basal metabolic rate with broadly increased protein synthesis, as well as carbohydrate and lipid catabolism. *Goitrogens* diminish T_4/T_3 synthesis, which increases TSH release, and in turn, causes hyperplastic thyroid enlargement *(goiter)*; propylthiouracil blocks iodide oxidation (blocking thyroid hormone production) and inhibits T_4 de-iodination to T_3, while high-dose iodide inhibits thyroglobulin proteolysis.

Thyroid *parafollicular (C) cells* secrete *calcitonin*; this blocks calcium resorption by osteoclasts and augments skeletal calcium deposition.

Hyperthyroidism (p. 1108)

Thyrotoxicosis is a hypermetabolic state caused by elevated circulating levels of free T_3 and T_4; it is most commonly due to primary hyperactivity of the thyroid *(hyperthyroidism)*. Causes include:

- Thyroid hyperplasia (Graves disease; 85% of cases)
- Hyperfunctional multinodular goiter
- Hyperfunctional thyroid adenoma

Secondary causes include pituitary thyrotroph adenomas, excess exogenous thyroid hormone (e.g., as treatment for hypothyroidism), and thyroid inflammatory diseases.

Clinical Course (p. 1108)

The symptoms and signs of hyperthyroidism relate to the resulting hypermetabolic state, as well as to overactivity of the sympathetic nervous system:

- *Cardiac:* Increased cardiac contractility and increased peripheral oxygen requirements can cause cardiomegaly, tachycardia, palpitations, and arrhythmias (particularly atrial fibrillation); congestive failure may supervene, particularly with pre-existing cardiac disease.
- *Ocular:* Wide, staring gaze and lid lag are due to sympathetic overstimulation of the levator palpebrae superioris; patients with Graves disease can also have a deposition ophthalmopathy (see later).
- *Neuromuscular:* Sympathetic nervous system overactivity (with increased β-adrenergic tone) causes tremor, hyperactivity, emotional lability, anxiety, inability to concentrate, and insomnia. Proximal muscle weakness and diminished mass are also common.
- *Cutaneous:* Increased blood flow and peripheral vasodilation leads to warm, moist, and flushed skin; Graves patients can also develop an infiltrative dermopathy.
- *Gastrointestinal:* Hypermotility, malabsorption, and diarrhea are due to sympathetic hyperstimulation.
- *Skeletal:* Enhanced bone resorption leads to osteoporosis and increased risk of fractures.
- *Thyroid storm:* This designates abrupt onset of severe hyperthyroidism; it usually occurs in Graves patients due to acute elevation in circulating catecholamines (e.g., secondary to injury, surgery, infection, or any exogenous stress) and is a medical emergency due to the risk of fatal arrhythmia.
- Thyrotoxicosis in the elderly may be blunted by various comorbidities, leading to so-called *apathetic hyperthyroidism;* diagnosis is made during laboratory evaluation for unexplained weight loss or cardiovascular deterioration.

Serum TSH levels are the most useful single screening test for hyperthyroidism; TSH is decreased even at the earliest stages and is usually associated with increased free serum T_4. Treatments include β-blockade to reduce adrenergic tone, propylthiouracil or similar agents to block hormone synthesis and peripheral T_4 to T_3 conversion, and iodine to block thyroglogulin proteolysis; radioiodine can ablate thyroid epithelium over a period of 6 to 18 weeks.

Hypothyroidism (p. 1109)

Hypothyroidism is caused by any structural or functional derangement that interferes with adequate thyroid hormone production; overt hypothyroidism affects 0.3% of the population, and subclinical disease occurs in more than 4%.

- *Primary hypothyroidism* (vast majority of cases) can be accompanied by thyroid enlargement (goiter). In iodine-sufficient areas of the world, the most common cause of hypothyroidism is *autoimmune thyroiditis* (most frequently, *Hashimoto thyroiditis*); patients typically have circulating anti-microsomal, anti-thyroid peroxidase, and anti-thyroglobulin autoantibodies. Other causes of primary hypothyroidism include dietary iodine deficiency–associated endemic goiter, inborn errors of metabolism, and goitrogens. Genetic causes include 1) *Pendred syndrome* (hypothyroidism and sensorineural hearing loss) due to *SLC26A4* mutations encoding the pendrin anion transporter on thyroid and inner ear epithelium, and 2) inactivating mutations of the TSH receptor. Hypothyroidism can also follow thyroid surgery or radiation and can be due to infiltrative disorders.

- *Secondary hypothyroidism* is caused by TSH deficiency (or, more rarely, by thyrotropin-releasing hormone [TRH] deficiency).

An elevated TSH level is the most sensitive screening test for primary hypothyroidism owing to a loss of feedback inhibition of TRH and TSH production; T_4 levels are reduced in any cause of hypothyroidism. Clinical manifestations are *cretinism* if thyroid deficiency develops *in utero* through early childhood, and *myxedema* in older children and adults.

Cretinism (p. 1110)

Cretinism is associated with dietary iodine deficiency and goiter (endemic form), as well as rarely with defects in hormone synthesis (sporadic form). Manifestations include impaired development of the skeletal and central nervous system (CNS), with mental retardation, short stature, umbilical hernia, and coarse facial features including wide-set eyes and an enlarged, protruding tongue. The severity of mental impairment depends on the timing of any *in utero* deficiency. Maternal thyroid hormones cross the placenta and are critical for normal fetal brain development in the period prior to fetal thyroid development; maternal thyroid hormone deficiency occurring later in pregnancy may therefore allow normal brain development.

Myxedema (p. 1111)

Older children with hypothyroidism exhibit signs and symptoms intermediate between those of the cretin and those of the hypothyroid adult. Adult hypothyroidism is associated with insidious slowing of physical and mental activity, associated with fatigue, cold intolerance, and apathy; decreased sympathetic activity reduces sweating and causes constipation. Signs include periorbital edema, coarsening of skin and facial features, cardiomegaly with congestive failure, and lipid profiles that promote atherogenesis, pericardial effusion, hair loss, and accumulation of mucopolysaccharide-rich ground substance within the dermis *(myxedema)* and other tissues.

Thyroiditis (p. 1111)

Thyroid inflammation *(thyroiditis)* can have diverse manifestations ranging from acute illness with severe pain (e.g., infectious thyroiditis) to thyroid dysfunction with little inflammation (subacute lymphocytic thyroiditis).

Acute infectious thyroiditis can occur via hematogenous spread or through direct seeding (e.g., via a laryngeal fistula). *Chronic infectious thyroiditis* typically occurs in immunocompromised hosts, and causes include mycobacterial, fungal, and *Pneumocystis* infections. Inflammation can cause sudden thyroid-localized neck pain, accompanied by fever and rigors.

Hashimoto Thyroiditis (p. 1111)

Hashimoto thyroiditis is the most common cause of hypothyroidism in locations where iodine levels are sufficient; it is a major cause of nonendemic goiter in children. It is characterized by insidious thyroid failure, and it is most prevalent between ages 45 and 65 years with a 10:1 to 20:1 female predominance. There is a 40% concordance of disease in monozygotic twins; half of asymptomatic siblings of Hashioto thyroiditis patients have circulating anti-thyroid antibodies.

Pathogenesis (p. 1111)

Hashimoto thyroiditis is an autoimmune disease directed against thyroid antigens. Autoimmune injury is mediated by circulating antibodies to thyroglobulin and thyroid peroxidase, CD8+ cytotoxic T cells, and/or T_H1 cytokine activation of macrophages. The inciting events leading to Hashimoto thyroiditis are unknown, but the disease is linked to genetic polymorphisms in proteins that negatively regulate T-cell responses (cytotoxic T lymphocyte–associated antigen-4 [CTLA-4] and protein tyrosine phosphatase-22 [PTPN22]). Thyroid autoimmunity is accompanied by progressive thyroid epithelium depletion, mononuclear cell infiltration, and fibrosis.

Morphology (p. 1112)

- *Grossly:* The thyroid is typically diffusely enlarged with pale parenchyma and an intact capsule.
- *Microscopically:* Lesions exhibit an exuberant infiltrate of lymphocytes, plasma cells, and macrophages; occasional germinal centers; atrophic follicles with eosinophilic granular cytoplasm in residual follicular cells *(Hürthle cells)*; and delicate fibrosis.

Clinical Course (p. 1113)

Hashimoto thyroiditis presents with painless thyroid enlargement usually associated with some degree of hypothyroidism. Hyperthyroidism *(hashitoxicosis)* can be seen early but is transient. Patients have an increased risk of developing other autoimmune diseases (e.g., type 1 diabetes, autoimmune adrenalitis, systemic lupus erythematosus, and Sjögren syndrome). There is a small risk of subsequent B-cell non-Hodgkin lymphoma.

Subacute (Granulomatous) Thyroiditis (p. 1113)

Also called *de Quervain thyroiditis*, this occurs much less frequently than Hashimoto thyroiditis. It most commonly affects women (i.e., 4:1) between the ages of 40 and 50.

Pathogenesis (p. 1113)

Subacute thyroiditis is attributed to a viral infection or postviral inflammatory process, resulting in cytotoxic T-cell–mediated follicular epithelial damage. Because the immune response is virus initiated, it is self-limited.

Morphology (p. 1113)

- *Grossly:* There is variable symmetric or irregular glandular enlargement.
- *Microscopically:* Early lesions include thyroid follicular disruption with a neutrophilic infiltrate. Later features include lymphocyte, macrophage, and plasma cell infiltrates around damaged thyroid follicles, with fibrosis and occasional multinucleated giant cells.

Clinical Course (p. 1113)

Subacute thyroiditis is the most common cause of thyroid pain. Any hyperthyroidism is transient and fades in 2 to 6 weeks; normal thyroid function usually recovers after 6 to 8 weeks.

Subacute Lymphocytic (Painless) Thyroiditis (p. 1113)

This is an uncommon cause of hyperthyroidism, occurring most commonly in middle-aged women; a similar process occurs in up to 5% of postpartum women. Both entities have anti-thyroid antibodies and are likely variants of Hashimoto thyroiditis.

Morphology (p. 1114)

The thyroid appears grossly normal. Histology demonstrates lymphocyte infiltrates with germinal centers and follicular disruption, but no fibrosis or Hürthle cell metaplasia.

Clinical Course (p. 1114)

Patients present with painless goiter and/or hyperthyroidism; a third can progress to overt hypothyroidism, although 80% of postpartum thyroiditis patients are euthyroid within a year.

Riedel thyroiditis is an uncommon fibrosing process of unknown etiology associated with replacement of thyroid parenchyma by dense fibrous tissue penetrating the capsule and extending into contiguous neck structures. There are circulating anti-thyroid autoantibodies, and patients are hypothyroid; the entity may be associated with fibrosis in other sites (e.g., retroperitoneum).

Graves Disease (p. 1114)

This is the most common cause of endogenous hyperthyroidism; a clinical triad includes:

- Hyperthyroidism due hyperfunctional, diffuse thyroid enlargement
- Infiltrative ophthalmopathy with resultant exophthalmos
- Localized infiltrative dermopathy present in a minority of patients

Women are affected seven times more frequently than men; peak incidence is between ages 20 and 40 years with the disease affecting up to 2% of American women. There is a 30% to 40% concordance rate among identical twins, and genetic susceptibility is linked to CTLA-4 and PTPN22 polymorphisms; patients are at risk of developing other autoimmune disorders.

Pathogenesis (p. 1114)

Graves disease is an autoimmune disorder caused predominantly by autoantibodies directed against the TSH receptor (TSHR):

- *Thyroid-stimulating immunoglobulin* binds to the TSHR and mimics the action of TSH, leading to T_3 and T_4 release. It is relatively specific for Graves disease.
- *Thyroid growth-stimulating immunoglobulin* is also directed against TSHR, but these autoantibodies induce thyroid follicular epithelium proliferation.
- *TSH-binding inhibitor immunoglobulin* binds to TSHR and prevents TSH from interacting with the receptor. Such antibodies can mimic TSH (stimulating thyroid epithelial activity) or can inhibit thyroid cell function.

Autoimmunity also contributes to the characteristic *infiltrative ophthalmopathy*; orbital preadipocyte fibroblasts express TSHR, thereby becoming another target of the autoimmune attack. The volume of retro-orbital connective tissues and extraocular muscles increases due to:

- Marked infiltration by mononuclear cells, predominantly T cells
- Inflammatory edema and swelling of extraocular muscles
- Accumulation of extracellular matrix components such as hyaluronic acid and chondroitin sulfate
- Increased fatty infiltration

Morphology (p. 1115)

- *Grossly:* The thyroid gland is mildly and symmetrically enlarged with an intact capsule and soft parenchyma.

- *Microscopically:* Lesions show diffuse hypertrophy and hyperplasia of follicular epithelium, manifested by crowding into irregular papillary folds. Colloid is substantially decreased. Interfollicular parenchyma contains hyperplastic lymphoid tissue and increased numbers of blood vessels.

Changes in extrathyroidal tissue include generalized lymphoid hyperplasia. Both ophthalmopathy and dermopathy (most common over the shins; called *pretibial myxedema*) are characterized by lymphocyte infiltration and accumulation of hydrophilic glycosaminoglycans.

Clinical Course (p. 1115)

T_4 and T_3 levels are elevated and TSH is depressed. Clinical manifestations are referable to thyrotoxicosis, diffuse thyroid hyperplasia, ophthalmopathy, and dermopathy. Ophthalmopathy may be self-limited or can progress to severe proptosis despite control of the hyperthyroidism. Patients are treated with β-blockade and measures to diminish thyroid hormone synthesis as discussed previously.

Diffuse and Multinodular Goiters (p. 1116)

Thyroid enlargement *(goiter)* is the most common manifestation of thyroid disease; it reflects impaired synthesis of thyroid hormone with resultant TSH production and follicular hyperplasia to restore a euthyroid state. If the compensatory hyperplasia cannot overcome the impairment in hormone synthesis, then *goitrous hypothyroidism* results.

Diffuse Nontoxic (Simple) Goiter (p. 1116)

This form diffusely involves the entire gland without producing nodularity; enlarged follicles are filled with colloid, hence the alternative term *colloid goiter.*

- *Endemic goiters* occur in geographic areas with low iodine levels (e.g., Alps, Andes, and Himalayas). With dietary iodine supplementation, the frequency and severity have declined significantly; nevertheless, subsistence on diets with high goitrogen content (e.g., cruciferous vegetables like cassava and cabbage) can also precipitate simple goiters.
- *Sporadic goiters* occur less frequently; there is a striking preponderance of young females. Causes include goitrogen ingestion or hereditary defects in thyroid hormone synthesis.

Morphology (p. 1116)

Two stages can be identified in the evolution of diffuse goiter:

- *Hyperplastic stage:*

  Grossly: The thyroid gland is diffuse and symmetrically enlarged.
  Microscopically: There is follicular epithelium hypertrophy and hyperplasia; some follicles are hugely distended while others remain small.

- *Colloid involution stage* (as thyroid hormone demand is met):

  Grossly: The cut surface is glassy, brown, and translucent.
  Microscopically: There is variable involution of follicular epithelium to form an enlarged, colloid-rich gland.

Clinical Course (p. 1116)

Most patients with simple goiters are clinically euthyroid; thus, clinical manifestations are primarily related to mass effects. TSH levels are elevated.

Multinodular Goiter (p. 1116)

Recurrent episodes of stimulation and involution of diffuse goiters result in irregularly enlarged *multinodular goiters* and can produce extreme thyroid enlargements. Multinodular goiters occur due to variations in follicular cell responses to hormonal stimulation; acquired mutations in the TSH signaling pathway (leading to constitutive activation) can also eventually result in formation of nodules with autonomous growth.

Morphology (p. 1117)

- *Grossly:* Multinodular goiters are multilobulated, asymmetrically enlarged glands and can be massively enlarged (i.e., more than 2000 g). Irregular expansion can produce lateral pressure on the trachea and esophagus, or can present as a single dominant mass. Cut section reveals variable amounts of brown gelatinous colloid, focal hemorrhage, fibrosis, calcification, and cystic change.
- *Microscopically:* There is variable degree of colloid accumulation, inactive flattened epithelium interspersed with follicular epithelial hyperplasia, and focal intervening areas of scarring and hemorrhage.

Clinical Course (p. 1117)

- Mass effects (occasionally complicated by acute expansion by hemorrhage) dominate the clinical picture: cosmetic deformity, esophageal compression with dysphagia, tracheal compression, and superior vena cava obstruction can occur.
- Most patients are euthyroid or subclinically hyperthyroid (evidenced by reduced TSH). However, in 10% of patients, a hyperfunctioning nodule can develop and cause hyperthyroidism (toxic multinodular goiter, or *Plummer syndrome*); this is not accompanied by the infiltrative ophthalmopathy and dermopathy of Graves disease.

Neoplasms of the Thyroid (p. 1118)

Solitary thyroid nodules occur in 1% to 10% of the U.S. population (with significantly higher rates in endemic goitrous regions); female to male ratio is 4:1, and the incidence increases throughout life. Although less than 1% of solitary thyroid nodules are malignant, this represents 15,000 new U.S. cases of thyroid carcinoma annually; most are indolent with 90% survival at 20 years. Risk of malignancy increases with:

- Solitary nodules more than multiple nodules
- Nodules in younger patients (i.e., younger than 40 years)
- Nodules in men more than women
- A history of head or neck radiation treatment
- Nodules that do not take up radioactive iodine in imaging studies *(cold nodules)*

Adenomas (p. 1118)

Thyroid adenomas are discrete, solitary masses derived from follicular epithelium *(follicular adenomas).* Most are non-functional, and they are rarely precursors to malignancy.

Pathogenesis (p. 1118)

Gain-of-function somatic mutations of components of the TSH receptor signaling pathway (commonly TSHR or GNAS) lead to autonomous proliferation and underlie roughly 50% of toxic adenomas; these changes are rare in thyroid malignancy. *RAS* or phoshphatidylinositol-3-kinase subunit *(PIK3CA)* mutations occur in 20% of non-functioning adenomas (these are also common in follicular carcinomas).

Morphology (p. 1118)

- *Grossly:* Most adenomas are gray-white to red-brown (depending on cellularity and colloid content) well-demarcated, solitary encapsulated lesions, occasionally with fibrosis, hemorrhage, or calcification.
- *Microscopically:* Constituent cells typically form uniform-appearing follicles containing colloid; the epithelium shows little nuclear variability or mitotic activity, and the follicular growth pattern is usually distinct from adjacent non-neoplastic thyroid. *Hürthle cell adenomas,* exhibiting granular, eosinophilic cells, behave like conventional adenomas. Follicular adenomas are distinguished by an intact well-formed capsule; follicular carcinomas demonstrate capsular and/or vascular invasion.

Clinical Features (p. 1119)

Most lesions present as dominant painless masses. Non-functioning adenomas take up less radioactive iodine than adjacent normal thyroid ("cold nodule"), but less than 10% of cold nodules eventually prove to be malignant. Because capsular integrity is a critical distinguishing feature, definitive diagnosis can be made only after careful histologic examination of the resected specimen.

Carcinomas (p. 1119)

Thyroid carcinoma accounts for 1.5% of all malignancies in the United States. Most occur in adults, with a slight female predominance; the vast majority of cases are well-differentiated lesions derived from thyroid follicular epithelium.

- Papillary carcinoma (more than 85%)
- Follicular carcinoma (5% to 15%)
- Anaplastic (undifferentiated) carcinomas (less than 5%)
- Medullary carcinoma (5%; not derived from follicular epithelium)

Pathogenesis (p. 1120)

- *Genetic factors:* The epithelial-derived thyroid malignancies are associated with gain-of-function mutations in the mitogen-activated protein (MAP) kinase and the PI3 kinase/AKT pathways; these lead to constitutive cell activation in the absence of TSH ligand binding.
- *Papillary carcinomas:* These are associated with MAP kinase pathway mutations:

  Rearrangements of *RET* or *NTRK1* (neurotrophic tyrosine kinase receptor 1) tyrosine kinase receptors place the kinase domain of these receptors under the transcriptional control of genes that are constitutively active in thyroid epithelium. *RET* has more than 15 potential fusion partners; novel *RET/PTC* (RET/papillary thyroid cancer) fusion proteins are present in 20% to 40% of papillary thyroid cancers, while similar *NTRK1* fusion proteins occur in 5% to 10%. Constitutive expression of these proteins leads to ongoing MAP kinase activation.

  Gain-of-function *BRAF* mutations occur in 33% to 50% of papillary thyroid cancers and also result in constitutive MAP kinase activation.

- *Follicular carcinomas* are associated with:

  Gain-of-function mutations in *RAS* or *PIK3CA*, amplification of *PIK3CA*, or loss-of-function mutations in the *PTEN* tumor suppressor gene (PTEN negatively regulates the pathway). These lead to constitutive activation of the *PI-3kinase*/AKT pathway and are associated with up to 50% of follicular carcinomas.

A t(2;3)(q13;p25) translocation fuses *PAX8* (a thyroid homeobox gene) with a peroxisome proliferator–activated receptor gene *(PPARG)* coding for a nuclear hormone receptor implicated cellular differentiation cells. These are associated with up to 50% of follicular carcinomas.

- *Anaplastic (undifferentiated) carcinomas* exhibit *RAS* or *PIK3CA* mutations, as well as mutations in *p53* or β-catenin that may underlie their aggressive behavior.
- *Medullary thyroid carcinomas* arise from thyroid parafollicular C cells. Familial versions occur in multiple endocrine neoplasia type 2 (see later), associated with germline activating mutations of the *RET* proto-oncogene mutations; similar *RET* mutations occur in half of sporadic medullary thyroid cancers.

Environmental Factors

The major risk factor is *ionizing radiation exposure*, particularly in the first two decades of life. *Iodine deficiency* is linked to a higher frequency of follicular carcinomas.

Papillary Carcinoma (p. 1121)

Papillary carcinoma occurs most commonly between ages 25 and 50 years; these account for the vast majority of thyroid carcinomas associated with previous radiation exposure.

Morphology (p. 1121)

- *Grossly:* Tumors are solitary or multifocal lesions; they may be circumscribed or infiltrate adjacent parenchyma. Calcification, fibrosis, and cystic changes are common. Conventional papillary carcinomas less than 1 cm and confined to the thyroid are called *papillary microcarcinomas;* these are often incidental findings in surgical resections.
- *Microscopically:* There are more than a dozen histologic variants often associated with particular mutations; lesions vary from papillary (with dense fibrovascular cores) to follicular (*follicular variant* of papillary carcinoma) to sclerosing, and lesions may have different clinical behaviors. *Psammoma bodies* (concentric calcifications) and foci of lymphatic invasion variably occur. Definitive diagnosis is based on nuclear features even in the absence of papillary architecture:

  Hypochromatic empty nuclei ("Orphan Annie eyes") and nuclear grooves
  Eosinophilic intranuclear inclusions (cytoplasmic invaginations)

Clinical Course (p. 1122)

Most papillary carcinomas present as isolated, asymptomatic, "cold" thyroid nodules, although the first manifestation may be cervical node metastasis. Thyroid lesions move freely during swallowing and are grossly indistinguishable from benign nodules; hoarseness, dysphagia, cough, or dyspnea suggests advanced disease. Ten-year survivals exceed 95%; unfavorable factors include age older than 40 years, extrathyroidal extension, and distant metastases.

Follicular Carcinoma (p. 1123)

Follicular carcinoma accounts for 5% to 15% of thyroid cancers; they are three-fold more common in women, with a peak incidence between 40 and 60 years, and there is an increased prevalence in areas of dietary iodine deficiency.

Morphology (p. 1123)

- *Grossly:* Tumors are single nodules that may be well-circumscribed or infiltrative. Distinguishing minimally invasive follicular carcinomas from follicular adenomas requires extensive sampling of the thyroid-tumor interface.
- *Microscopically:* The nuclear features noted in papillary carcinomas are absent. Most tumors exhibit a microfollicular pattern, with relatively uniform, colloid-filled follicles reminiscent of normal thyroid. Other patterns include a trabecular or sheetlike architecture, and histologic variants contain large numbers of Hürthle cells.

Clinical Course (p. 1123)

Most present as slowly-growing, painless, "cold" nodules. Lymphatic invasion is rare, but hematogenous metastasis to bone, lungs, and liver is common. Prognosis depends on the stage and extent of invasion: minimally invasive follicular carcinoma has a 10-year survival rate more than 90%, while invasive carcinoma with metastases has a 50%, 10-year mortality. Therapy involves resection, radioactive iodine to ablate metastatic lesions, and thyroid hormone administration to reduce TSH that could be potentially stimulatory for malignant epithelium.

Anaplastic (Undifferentiated) Carcinoma (p. 1124)

Anaplastic (undifferentiated) carcinoma is an aggressive variant most common in elderly patients (i.e., older than 65 years) and associated with prior or concurrent well-differentiated thyroid cancer.

Morphology (p. 1124)

- *Microscopically:* These neoplasms are composed of highly anaplastic cells, including large, pleomorphic giant cells and spindle cells with a sarcomatous appearance.

Clinical Course (p. 1124)

Tumors usually present as rapidly enlarging bulky masses that have already invaded neck structures or metastasized to lung at the time of original diagnosis. These are almost uniformly fatal; death is usually secondary to aggressive local growth.

Medullary Carcinoma (p. 1124)

Medullary carcinoma is a neuroendocrine neoplasm; like normal C cells, these secrete *calcitonin* (and can also produce serotonin, ACTH, and vasoactive intestinal peptide [VIP]). Some 70% of cases are sporadic with the remainder occurring in the setting of MEN-2 syndromes or familial medullary thyroid carcinoma (FMTC). *RET* protooncogene mutations are involved in both sporadic and familial cases.

Morphology (p. 1124)

- *Grossly:* Sporadic tumors are usually solitary; bilaterality and multicentricity are typical of familial cases. Tumors are firm, gray-tan, and infiltrative, occasionally with hemorrhage and focal necrosis.
- *Microscopically:* Cells are polygonal to spindle-shaped and are arrayed in nests, trabeculae, and, occasionally, follicles. Stromal *amyloid deposits* (from altered calcitonin) are often present. Multifocal C-cell hyperplasia is often present in familial cases but is typically absent in sporadic cases.

Clinical Course (p. 1125)

- Sporadic cases usually present as a thyroid mass, sometimes associated with dysphagia, or hoarseness. Initial manifestations may be paraneoplastic related to hormone secretion (e.g., diarrhea due to VIP, or Cushing syndrome due to ACTH); hypocalcemia is uncommon despite elevated calcitonin levels.
- Familial cases can present with thyroid or extra-thyroid neoplasms, or may be identified through screening of asymptomatic relatives of affected patients.
- Medullary carcinomas arising in the context of MEN-2B are more aggressive and metastasize more often than those arising sporadically or with other familial syndromes.

Congenital Anomalies (p. 1126)

Thyroglossal duct cysts are developmental remnants of thyroid migration from the tongue foramen cecum. They are the most common clinically significant congenital thyroid anomaly and can present at any age, primarily as a mid-line masses anterior to the trachea. Cysts high in the neck are lined by stratified squamous epithelium; those more inferior are lined by thyroidal acinar epithelium. Lymphocytic infiltrates are often conspicuous. Superimposed infections can generate abscess cavities; rarely, they can give rise to carcinoma.

PARATHYROID GLANDS (p. 1126)

Parathyroid activity is controlled by the level of free (ionized) circulating calcium; elevated calcium levels inhibit parathyroid hormone (PTH) synthesis and secretion, whereas hypocalcemia stimulates PTH production. PTH increases calcium levels by:

- Driving osteoclast differentiation (and thereby bone resorption) by increasing osteoblast expression of receptor activator for nuclear factor-κB ligand (RANKL), which binds to RANK on osteoclast precursors
- Increasing renal tubular reabsorption of calcium
- Increasing renal vitamin D conversion to the active 1,25 dihydroxylated form
- Increasing urinary phosphate excretion
- Augmenting gastrointestinal calcium absorption

Malignancy, secondary to paraneoplastic production of PTH-related protein (PTHrP), is the most common cause of clinically apparent hypercalcemia; primary hyperparathyroidism is a more common cause of asymptomatic hypercalcemia. Besides increasing osteoblast RANKL expression, PTHrP also inhibits the expression of osteoprotegerin a "decoy receptor" that normally binds to RANKL and blocks its interactions with RANK.

Hyperparathyroidism (p. 1126)

Primary Hyperparathyroidism (p. 1127)

This is a common endocrine disorder (25 cases per 100,000 population in the United States) and an important etiology of hypercalcemia; most cases are sporadic, occurring in patients older than 50 years with a 3:1 female predominance. Causes include:

- Adenoma (85% to 95%)
- Primary hyperplasia (5% to 10%)

- Parathyroid carcinoma (1%)
- *Sporadic hyperparathyroidism:* Most cases of sporadic parathyroid hyperplasia and the vast majority of parathyroid adenomas are monoclonal. In sporadic adenomas, two acquired defects have pathogenic import:

  Cyclin D1 overexpression is associated with 40% of sporadic parathyroid adenomas; approximately half of these occur through relocation of the *cyclin D1* gene adjacent to the 5′ flanking region of the *PTH* gene.

  MEN1 mutations leading to homozygous inactivation occur in 20% to 30% of sporadic adenomas.

- *Familial hyperparathyroidism:*

  MEN-1 syndrome: parathyroid adenomas and hyperplasia can be associated with germline *MEN1* mutations.

  MEN-2 syndrome is due to activating mutations of the *RET* tyrosine kinase receptor.

  Familial hypocalciuric hypercalcemia (FHH) is an autosomal dominant disorder resulting from decreased sensitivity to extracellular calcium caused by inactivating mutations of the parathyroid calcium-sensing receptor gene *(CASR).*

Morphology (p. 1127)

Morphologic changes involve the parathyroid glands as well as all other organs affected by hypercalcemia.

- Parathyroid adenomas:

  Grossly: Tumors are almost all solitary, well-circumscribed, tan-brown nodules that average 0.5 to 5 g; they are surrounded by a delicate capsule; remaining glands are usually normal size or smaller secondary to hypercalcemic feedback inhibition.

  Microscopically: Lesions are composed predominantly of chief cells arrayed in uniform sheets, trabeculae, or follicles; foci of oxyphil cells may be present, and bizarre atypia is not uncommon. Adipose tissue is inconspicuous.

- Primary hyperplasia:

  Grossly: All glands are typically involved although not necessarily uniformly; combined weights rarely exceed 1 g.

  Microscopically: Chief cell hyperplasia typically involves glands in a diffuse or multinodular pattern. Adipose tissue is inconspicuous.

- Parathyroid carcinoma may be grossly and microscopically difficult to distinguish from an adenoma:

  Grossly: Typically, one gland is enlarged by a gray-white, irregular mass sometimes exceeding 10 g.

  Microscopically: Lesional cells are usually uniform and not too dissimilar from normal parathyroid cells; diagnosis of malignancy is based on the presence of local invasion and/or metastases.

- Other organs:

  Skeletal changes include osteoclast activation with bone resorption. In severe cases, affected bones show thinned cortices with increased marrow fibrous tissue accompanied by foci of hemorrhage and cyst formation *(osteitis fibrosa cystica).*

  Hypercalcemia promotes *nephrolithiasis,* renal interstitial and tubular calcification *(nephrocalcinosis),* and *metastatic calcifications* elsewhere.

Clinical Course (p. 1128)

- *Asymptomatic hyperparathyroidism* is caused most commonly by primary hyperparathyroidism and is typically discovered by routine serum calcium measurements; serum PTH levels are inappropriately elevated for the level of serum calcium (conversely, PTH levels are low in the hypercalcemia, resulting from non-parathyroid diseases). Malignancy is a much less common etiology but merits exclusion in patients with hypercalcemia.
- *Symptomatic primary hyperparathyroidism* is traditionally associated with a constellation of symptoms: painful bones, renal stones, abdominal groans, and psychic moans:

  Bone disease and pain with fractures occur secondary to osteoporosis and osteitis fibrosa cystica.

  Nephrolithiasis (renal stones) occurs in 20% of patients; pain is secondary to obstructive uropathy. Chronic renal insufficiency can cause polyuria and polydipsia.

  Gastrointestinal disturbances include constipation, nausea, peptic ulcers, pancreatitis, and gallstones.

  CNS alterations include depression, lethargy, and eventually seizures.

  Other findings include weakness, fatigue, and cardiac valve calcifications.

Secondary Hyperparathyroidism (p. 1129)

Secondary hyperparathyroidism results from any condition associated with chronic hypocalcemia that leads to compensatory parathyroid overactivity; *renal failure is the most common etiology.* Renal failure triggers phosphate retention and hyperphosphatemia; elevated phosphate levels directly depress serum calcium, causing a compensatory PTH hypersecretion. Renal disease also leads to reduced 1-hydroxylation of vitamin D, which impairs gastrointestinal calcium absorption; reduced vitamin D also removes normal feedback inhibitory mechanisms on PTH secretion. Parathyroid glands and bones exhibit the same morphologic features (albeit usually less severe) as for other causes of hyperparathyroidism. Metastatic calcifications in vessels can lead to significant ischemic damage to skin and other organs *(calciphylaxis).* Secondary hyperparathyroidism responds to correction of the underlying renal disease or to vitamin D supplementation with phosphate binders to reduce the hyperphosphatemia. Occasionally, an autonomous adenoma develops *(tertiary hyperparathyroidism),* which requires surgical resection.

Hypoparathyroidism (p. 1129)

Hypoparathyroidism is much less common than hyperparathyroidism; causes include:

- Surgical (e.g., thyroidectomy or treatment of hyperparathyroidism)
- Autoimmune hypoparathyroidism associated with autoimmune polyendocrine syndrome, type I (see later)
- Autosomal dominant hypoparathyroidism due to gain-of-function mutations in the *CASR* gene (causing increased sensitivity of the calcium receptor)
- Familial isolated hypoparathyroidism, due either to primary PTH mutations that affect its precursor processing (autosomal dominant) or loss-of function mutations in the *GCM2 gene responsible for parathyroid development (autosomal recessive)*
- Congenital absence of all glands (e.g., DiGeorge syndrome)

Manifestations are related to the chronicity and severity of the hypocalcemia:

- *Tetany* (characterized by neuromuscular irritability) is the hypocalcemic hallmark: symptoms range from muscle cramps and carpopedal spasms to laryngeal stridor and convulsions
- *Mental status changes* (e.g., anxiety, depression, or psychosis)
- *Intracranial manifestations*, including basal ganglia calcifications, parkinsonian-like movement disorders, and elevated intracranial pressure
- *Ocular changes* with lens calcification and cataract formation
- *Cardiac conduction defects*, producing a characteristic prolongation of the QT interval
- *Dental developmental defects* (when hypoparathyroidism is present early in development), including hypoplasia, and defective enamel and root formation

Pseudohypoparathyroidism (p. 1130)

Pathogenesis is related to *GNAS1* mutations that code for a defective G-protein normally responsible for mediating PTH activity. Target tissues are relatively resistant to PTH, resulting in hypocalcemia, compensatory parathyroid hyperfunction, and a variety of skeletal and developmental abnormalities. Since the same G-protein mediates the action of TSH and LH/FSH, hypothyroidism and hypogonadism can also occur.

THE ENDOCRINE PANCREAS (p. 1130)

Diabetes Mellitus (p. 1131)

Diabetes mellitus is a group of metabolic disorders sharing the *common underlying feature of hyperglycemia*. The net effect is a chronic disorder of carbohydrate, fat, and protein metabolism with long-term complications affecting blood vessels, kidneys, eyes, and nerves; it is the leading cause of end-stage renal disease, adult-onset blindness, and non-traumatic lower extremity amputation. In the United States, 20 million people (7% of the population) are diabetic, with 1.5 million new cases diagnosed annually; worldwide, more than 150 million people are affected.

Diagnosis (p. 1131)

Blood glucose is normally maintained between 70 and 120 mg/dL. Diabetes mellitus is diagnosed by demonstrating blood glucose elevations by any one of three criteria:

- Random glucose level 200 mg/dL or more, with classic signs and symptoms (see later)
- Fasting glucose level 126 mg/dL or more on more than one occasion
- Abnormal oral glucose tolerance test (OGTT), that is, glucose 200 mg/dL or more 2 hours after a standard carbohydrate load

Individuals with fasting glucose between 100 and 126 mg/dL or OGTT values between 140 and 200 mg/dL are have impaired glucose tolerance and are considered to be "pre-diabetic." Such patients have a 5% to 10% risk per year of progressing to full-blown diabetes.

In patients with long-standing diabetes, glycemic control is monitored by measuring the circulating levels hemoglobin A1c (Hb$_{A1c}$). Hb$_{A1c}$ is a glycated modification of hemoglobin that occurs nonenzymatically in the presence of glucose metabolites; normal level in nondiabetics is 4% to 6% of the total hemoglobin content. Unlike blood glucose levels, Hb_{A1c} allows the integration of glucose levels over the 120-day life span of an erythrocyte; in diabetics with good glycemic control, it should constitute less than 7%.

Classification (p. 1132)

The causes of diabetes mellitus vary widely (Table 24-2), although the vast majority of cases fall into one of two broad types (Table 24-3):

- *Type 1 diabetes* is an autoimmune disease characterized by pancreatic β-cell destruction and an absolute insulin deficiency. It accounts for 5% to 10% of all cases and is the most common cause in patients younger than 20 years.
- *Type 2 diabetes* is caused by a combination of peripheral insulin resistance and inadequate compensatory responses by pancreatic β-cells ("relative insulin deficiency"). It accounts for 90% to 95% of cases; the vast majority of patients are overweight.

Glucose Homeostasis (p. 1132)

Normal glucose homeostasis is tightly regulated by three interrelated processes: hepatic glucose production, glucose uptake by peripheral tissues (chiefly skeletal muscle), and the actions of insulin and counter-regulatory hormones (e.g., glucagon). During fasting, low insulin and high glucagon maintain peripheral glucose levels by facilitating hepatic gluconeogenesis and glycogenolysis, as well as by decreasing glycogen synthesis. After feeding, rising insulin and diminished glucagon lead to glucose uptake and utilization (primarily in skeletal muscle), as well as hepatic glycogen synthesis.

Regulation of Insulin Release (p. 1133)

A rise in glucose leads to increased uptake into β cells through the GLUT-2 insulin-independent glucose transporter (Fig. 24-1); as glucose is metabolized, intracellular ATP increases. This inhibits the activity of an ATP-sensitive K^+ channel, leading in turn to membrane depolarization, influx of extracellular Ca^{+2}, and insulin release from pre-formed stores. Persistent stimulus also results in increased insulin synthesis.

Insulin Action and Insulin Signaling Pathways (p. 1133)

The principal metabolic function of insulin is to increase glucose transport into target cells—primarily skeletal muscle and adipocytes; glucose uptake into most other cell types is insulin independent. Once internalized, glucose either is stored as glycogen (skeletal muscle) or lipid (adipose tissue) or is oxidized to generate ATP. Insulin inhibits lipid catabolism by adipocytes, inhibits glycogen breakdown, and promotes amino acid uptake and protein synthesis while diminishing protein degradation; it is also mitogenic for several cell types. Insulin acts through a heterodimeric insulin receptor; binding stimulates receptor kinase activity and induces phosphorylation of several insulin receptor substrate (IRS) proteins with activation of downstream cascades including the PI3 and MAP kinase pathways. These lead eventually to AKT pathway activation, culminating in movement of the GLUT-4 glucose transporter protein to the plasma membrane; the outcome is increased glucose transport. A variety of phosphatases (e.g., protein tyrosine phosphatase 1B and PTEN) can negatively regulate this activation cascade.

TABLE 24-2 Classification of Diabetes Mellitus

1. **Type 1 diabetes** (β-cell destruction, usually leading to absolute insulin deficiency)
   Immune-mediated
   Idiopathic
2. **Type 2 diabetes** (combination of insulin resistance and β-cell dysfunction)
3. **Genetic defects of β-cell function**
   Maturity-onset diabetes of the young (MODY), caused by mutations in:
      Hepatocyte nuclear factor 4α (*HNF4A*), MODY1
      Glucokinase (*GCK*), MODY2
      Hepatocyte nuclear factor 1α (*HNF1A*), MODY3
      Pancreatic and duodenal homeobox 1 (*PDX1*), MODY4
      Hepatocyte nuclear factor 1β (*HNF1B*), MODY5
      Neurogenic differentiation factor 1 (*NEUROD1*), MODY6
   Neonatal diabetes (activating mutations in *KCNJ11* and *ABCC8*, encoding Kir6.2 and SUR1, respectively)
   Maternally inherited diabetes and deafness (MIDD) due to mitochondrial DNA mutations (m.3243A→G)
   Defects in proinsulin conversion
   Insulin gene mutations
4. **Genetic defects in insulin action**
   Type A insulin resistance
   Lipoatrophic diabetes, including mutations in *PPARG*
5. **Exocrine pancreatic defects**
   Chronic pancreatitis
   Pancreatectomy/trauma
   Neoplasia
   Cystic fibrosis
   Hemochromatosis
   Fibrocalculous pancreatopathy
6. **Endocrinopathies**
   Acromegaly
   Cushing syndrome
   Hyperthyroidism
   Pheochromocytoma
   Glucagonoma
7. **Infections**
   Cytomegalovirus
   Coxsackie B virus
   Congenital rubella
8. **Drugs**
   Glucocorticoids
   Thyroid hormone
   Interferon-α
   Protease inhibitors
   β-adrenergic agonists
   Thiazides
   Nicotinic acid
   Phenytoin (Dilantin)
   Vacor
9. **Genetic syndromes associated with diabetes**
   Down syndrome
   Kleinfelter syndrome
   Turner syndrome
   Prader-Willi syndrome
10. **Gestational diabetes mellitus**

American Diabetes Association: Position statement from the American Diabetes Association on the diagnosis and classification of diabetes mellitus, *Diabetes Care* 31 (Suppl. 1):S55–S60, 2008.

TABLE 24-3	Type 1 versus Type 2 Diabetes Mellitus	
Feature	**Type 1 Diabetes Mellitus**	**Type 2 Diabetes Mellitus**
Clinical	Onset: usually childhood and adolescence	Onset: usually adult; increasing incidence in childhood and adolescence
	Normal weight or weight loss preceding diagnosis	Vast majority are obese (80%)
	Progressive decrease in insulin levels	Increased blood insulin (early); normal or moderate decrease in insulin (late)
	Circulating islet auto-antibodies (anti-insulin, anti-GAD, anti-ICA512)	No islet auto-antibodies
	Diabetic ketoacidosis in absence of insulin therapy	Nonketotic hyperosmolar coma more common
Genetics	Major linkage to MHC class I and II genes; also linked to polymorphisms in CTLA4 and PTPN22, and insulin gene VNTRs	No HLA linkage; linkage to candidate diabetogenic and obesity-related genes (*TCF7L2, PPARG, FTO,* etc.)
Pathogenesis	Dysfunction in regulatory T cells (Tregs) leading to breakdown in self-tolerance to islet auto-antigens	Insulin resistance in peripheral tissues, failure of compensation by β-cells
		Multiple obesity-associated factors (circulating nonesterified fatty acids, inflammatory mediators, adipocytokines) linked to pathogenesis of insulin resistance
Pathology	Insulitis (inflammatory infiltrate of T cells and macrophages)	No insulitis; amyloid deposition in islets
	β-cell depletion, islet atrophy	Mild β-cell depletion

HLA, Human leukocyte antigen; *MHC,* major histocompatibility complex; *VNTRs,* variable number of tandem repeats.

Pathogenesis of Type 1 Diabetes
Mellitus (p. 1134)

This form of diabetes results from autoimmune β-islet cell destruction. Although the clinical onset is typically abrupt (occurring after more than 90% of β-cells have been destroyed), the autoimmune process starts many years before the disease becomes evident. Pathogenesis involves a combination of genetic susceptibility and environmental insults.

- *Genetic susceptibility:* By far the most important genetic association (50% of susceptibility) is attributable to the class II major histocompatibility complex (MHC) HLA locus. Approximately 90% to 95% of whites with type 1 diabetes have HLA-DR3 or

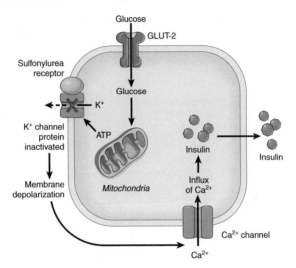

FIGURE 24-1 Insulin secretion and synthesis. Glucose enters β-islet cells via the GLUT-2 insulin-independnet glucose transporter. Resulting ATP production leads to inhibition of a K+ channel receptor (a heterodimer of the sulfonylurea receptor [SUR1] and the Kir6.2 K+-channel protein) and membrane depolarization with Ca²⁺ influx. Increased intracellular calcium leads to release of stored insulin. The sulfonylurea class of oral hypoglycemic agents binds to the SUR1 receptor protein and mediates mebrane depolarization and subsequent insulin release.

DR4 haplotypes (compared to 40% of normal subjects), and an associated DQ8 haplotype incurs the greatest inherited risk. Non-MHC polymorphisms associated with disease susceptibility include the insulin gene itself, CTLA-4, and PTPN22.

- *Environmental factors:* Several viral agents have been implicated as potential triggers for an autoimmune attack, including coxsackieviruses, mumps, cytomegalovirus, and rubella. Postulated mechanisms:

  Viral infection causes islet injury and inflammation, leading to release of cryptic β-cell antigens and autoreactive T-cell activation ("bystander damage")

  Viruses produce proteins that mimic β-cell antigens, and host immune responses to the infection cross-reacts with self tissues ("molecular mimicry")

  Viral infection early in life persists in the tissue of interest; subsequent infection with a related virus bearing similar epitopes leads to immune responses against the latently-infected β-cells.

- *Mechanisms of β-cell destruction* (p. 1135): The fundamental immune abnormality is failure of T-cell self-tolerance:

  CD4+ T$_H$1 cells cause tissue injury by releasing cytokines (e.g., interferon-γ [IFN-γ] and tumor necrosis factor [TNF]) that activate macrophages.

  CD8+ cytotoxic T lymphocytes directly kill β cells.

  Autoantibodies against islet cells and insulin may also participate; β-cell antigens include the enzyme glutamic acid decarboxylase (GAD) and islet cell auto-antigen 512. In susceptible children who have not developed diabetes, islet cells autoantibodies can be predictive of diabetes development.

Pathogenesis of Type 2 Diabetes
Mellitus (p. 1136)

This form of diabetes is a complex multifactorial disease; it results from a collection of multiple genetic defects (there is 35% to 60% disease concordance in monozygotic twins), each contributing its own predisposing risk and modified by environmental factors. There is no evidence to suggest an autoimmune etiology. Rather, polymorphisms in genes associated with β-cell function and insulin secretion confer the greatest genetic risk; *transcription factor 7-like-2 (TCF7L2)* encoding a *WNT* signaling pathway transcription factor has the most reproducible association. Type 2 diabetes is characterized by:

- Decreased responses of peripheral tissues to insulin *(insulin resistance)*
- β-cell dysfunction (i.e., inadequate insulin secretion in the setting of hyperglycemia)

Insulin Resistance (p. 1136)

Insulin resistance is reflected by diminished skeletal muscle glucose uptake, reduced hepatic glycolysis and fatty acid oxidation, and the inability to suppress hepatic gluconeogenesis. Obesity plays a dominant role.

- *Obesity and insulin resistance* (p. 1136): Diabetes risk increases as the body mass index increases; central obesity (abdominal fat) is more closely linked to insulin resistance than is peripheral obesity (gluteal and subcutaneous fat).

  Nonesterified fatty acids (NEFA): These acids are correlated with insulin resistance. Intracellular NEFA are markedly increased in muscle and liver of obese individuals and can overwhelm the fatty acid oxidation pathways. This leads to accumulation of potentially "toxic" intermediates such as ceramide and diacylglycerol; these can drive aberrant serine/threonine *(not tyrosine)* phosphorylation of the insulin receptor and IRS proteins that *attenuate* insulin signaling responses. NEFA can also compete with glucose for substrate oxidation, leading to feedback inhibition of glycolysis.

  Adipokines: Fat is a source of cytokines, including those that are pro-glycemic (e.g., resistin and retinol binding protein 4) and anti-glycemic (e.g., leptin and adiponectin). The latter improve tissue insulin sensitivity by enhancing AMP-activated protein kinase (AMPK) activity, thus promoting fatty acid oxidation (notably, AMPK is the target of the oral hypoglycemic agent metformin). Adiponectin levels are reduced in obesity.

  Inflammation: Adipose tissue production of pro-inflammatory cytokines (e.g., IL-6, TNF) can also reduce insulin sensitivity by driving systemic inflammation

  Peroxisome proliferator-activated receptor γ (PPARγ): This is a nuclear receptor critical for adipocyte differentiation. PPARγ activation promotes adiponectin production and shifts NEFA away from muscle and liver and into fat depots. The thiazolidinedione class of hypoglycemic medications improves insulin sensitivity by acting as PPARγ agonist ligands.

β-Cell Dysfunction (p. 1137)

In states of insulin resistance, β-islet cells attempt to maintain normoglycemia by increased insulin output; unfortunately, in most patients this compensatory mechanism ultimately fails and hyperglycemia supervenes. Such eventual β-cell dysfunction is linked to *TCF7L2* and other genes; it is probably also driven by the same mechanisms that underlie insulin resistance. *Amyloid replacement* of the islet is a characteristic finding in patients with long-standing type 2 diabetes, and it may be directly cytotoxic.

Monogenic Forms of Diabetes (p. 1137)

These are uncommon, and they result from either a primary defect in β-cell function or insulin-receptor signaling (see Table 24-2).

Genetic Defects in β-Cell Function (p. 1137)

Genetic defects in β-cell function affect β-cell mass and/or insulin production (without β-cell loss) and are responsible for 1% to 2% of diabetes cases. The causes are heterogeneous but are typified by:

- Autosomal-dominant inheritance with high penetrance
- Early onset, usually before age 25 years and even in the neonatal period
- Absence of obesity
- Absence of β-cell autoantibodies

Maturity-onset diabetes of the young (MODY) is the largest subgroup in this category. Six distinct loss-of-function genetic defects have been identified (see Table 24-2), including glucokinase mutations that block glucose entry into the glycolytic cycle and thus raise the glucose threshold necessary to trigger insulin release.

Permanent neonatal diabetes results from gain-of-function mutations of the subunits of the β-cell ATP-sensitive K^+ channel (see Fig. 24-1); these cause constitutive channel activation and membrane hyperpolarization and thus prevent insulin release, leading to hypoinsulinemic diabetes.

Maternally inherited diabetes and deafness results from mitochondrial DNA mutations; impaired ATP synthesis in β-cells results in diminished insulin release. Patients also have bilateral sensorineural deafness.

Genetic Defects in Insulin Action (p. 1138)

Rarely, mutations affecting receptor synthesis, insulin binding, or intracellular signaling can result in severe insulin resistance and diabetes. Such patients may also exhibit *acanthosis nigricans* (velvety hyperpigmented cutaneous macules), and (in women) polycystic ovaries and elevated androgens. *Lipoatrophic diabetes* is hyperglycemia accompanied by loss of subcutaneous adipose tissue; one form is caused by dominant-negative mutations of PPARγ that interfere with its normal nuclear transcription activity.

Pathogenesis of the Complications of Diabetes (p. 1138)

The morbidity associated with long-standing diabetes of any cause is attributable to *macrovascular disease* (accelerated atherosclerosis) precipitating myocardial infarction, stroke, or extremity gangrene, and *microvascular disease* (capillary dysfunction) causing nephropathy, retinopathy, and neuropathy. Hyperglycemia is the major factor, although insulin resistance and dyslipidemia can contribute.

Formation of Advanced Glycation End Products (p. 1138)

Formation of advanced glycation end products (AGEs) occurs through nonenzymatic interactions between protein amino groups and glucose-derived metabolites; a natural baseline rate of AGE formation is markedly accelerated by hyperglycemia. AGEs bind to a specific receptor (RAGE) expressed on vascular wall and inflammatory cells; this leads to pro-inflammatory cytokine release, generation of reactive oxygen species, increased procoagulant activity, and enhanced vascular smooth muscle proliferation and matrix synthesis. AGEs can also directly cross-link matrix proteins, leading to protein deposition, loss of vascular wall elasticity, poor endothelial adhesion, leaky basement membranes, and persistence of poorly degradable, cross-linked adducts.

Activation of Protein Kinase C (p. 1139)

Intracellular hyperglycemia stimulates the *de novo* synthesis of diacylgylcerol, which in turn activates protein kinase C (PKC); PKC activation leads to:

- Production of vascular endothelial growth factor (VEGF)
- Increased endothelin-1 and diminished nitric oxide (increased vascular tone)
- Increased fibrosis due to TGF-β production
- Production of plasminogen activator inhibitor-1 (PAI-1), reducing fibrinolysis and promoting thrombosis
- Production of pro-inflammatory cytokines by endothelium

Intracellular Hyperglycemia and Disturbances in Polyol Pathways (p. 1139)

In tissues that do not require insulin for glucose transport (e.g., nerves, lens, kidney, blood vessels), hyperglycemia leads to increased intracellular glucose. This glucose is metabolized to sorbitol and then fructose (using NADPH reducing equivalents), so that an equilibrium with extracellular solute is not achieved. The accompanying osmotic load leads to water influx and osmotic cell injury. Reductions in NADPH also lead to reduced glutathione regeneration and increased cellular susceptibility to oxidative stress.

Morphology of Diabetes and Its Late Complications (p. 1139)

Morphology (p. 1139)

- *Pancreas:* Findings are variable.

  Type 1: Islet number and size are reduced and a lymphocytic infiltrate *(insulitis)* may be present.
  Type 2: Subtle reduction in islet cell mass may be accompanied by amyloid deposition, occasionally effacing the islets.

- *Diabetic macrovascular disease* is manifested as accelerated/exacerbated atherosclerosis in the aorta and large and medium-sized arteries; hyaline arteriolosclerosis is more prevalent and severe.
- *Diabetic microangiopathy* is reflected by diffuse basement membrane thickening, most evident in the capillaries of the skin, skeletal muscle, retina, renal glomeruli, and renal medulla. Such capillaries are more leaky than normal to plasma proteins. Basement membrane thickening can also affect nonvascular structures (e.g., renal tubules, Bowman capsule, peripheral nerves, and placenta).
- *Diabetic nephropathy:*

  Glomerular involvement includes diffuse basement membrane thickening, mesangial sclerosis, nodular glomerulosclerosis *(Kimmelstiel-Wilson lesion)*, and/or exudative lesions.
  Vascular effects include renal artery atherosclerosis and arteriolosclerosis with hypertension.
  There is increased incidence of infections, including pyelonephritis and sometimes necrotizing papillitis.

- *Diabetic ocular complications* take the form of retinopathy, cataracts, or glaucoma (Chapter 29).
- *Diabetic neuropathy* is a combination of direct neural injury as well as microvascular ischemia (Chapter 27).

Clinical Features of Diabetes (p. 1143)
(see Table 24-3)

- *Type 1 diabetes* can occur at any age. Its manifestations are due to altered metabolism; glycosuria induces osmotic diuresis and polyuria, with profound loss of water and electrolytes. Intense thirst (polydipsia) develops, with increased appetite (polyphagia), completing the classic clinical triad. There is also unopposed glucagon and growth hormone production, and despite an increased appetite, catabolic effects prevail, resulting in weight loss and muscle weakness.

  Diabetic ketoacidosis occurs as a result of severe insulin deficiency and absolute or relative increases in glucagon: excessive release of free fatty acids from adipose tissue and hepatic oxidation generates ketone bodies (β-hydroxy-butyric acid and acetoacetic acid). Ketonemia and ketonuria, with dehydration, can cause life-threatening systemic metabolic ketoacidosis.

  Metabolic derangement and insulin need are directly related to physiologic stress, including deviations from normal dietary intake, increased physical activity, infections, and surgery. In the initial 1 to 2 years after initial presentation, exogenous insulin requirements may be minimal due to residual low-level endogenous insulin production ("honeymoon period"); however, any residual reserve is eventually exhausted and insulin requirements increase dramatically.

- *Type 2 diabetics* are usually older than 40 years and typically obese; they can also present with polyuria and polydipsia but are most often discovered by routine blood glucose screening. Ketoacidosis is uncommon due to persistent insulin production that minimizes ketone body production. *Non-ketotic hyperosmolar coma* can occur in compromised individuals who become dehydrated secondary to osmotic diuresis and inadequate water intake.
- Complications of long-standing diabetes:

  Cardiovascular events (e.g., myocardial infarction, renal vascular insufficiency, and stroke) are the most common causes of death. Diabetics have a four-fold greater risk of dying of cardiovascular causes compared to the non-diabetic population. In most instances, these occur 15 to 20 years after hyperglycemic onset; diabetes-associated hypertension, dyslipidemia, and hypercoagulability are frequent associated conditions.

  Diabetic nephropathy is a leading cause in the United States of end-stage renal disease; 30% to 40% of all diabetics develop some degree of nephropathy, with the frequency influenced by ethnic make-up (i.e., African Americans and Native Americans have greater risk than Caucasian Americans). Microalbuminuria is the earliest manifestation (between 30 and 300 mg/day); without intervention, 80% of type 1 diabetics and 20% to 40% of type 2 diabetics develop overt nephropathy with macroalbuminuria (more than 300 mg/day), and 75% and 20%, respectively, progress to end-stage renal disease within 20 years.

  Diabetic retinopathy develops in 60% to 80% of patients within 15 to 20 years of diagnosis. The fundamental lesion is neovascularization attributable to hypoxia-induced over-expression of VEGF in the retina.

Diabetic neuropathy typically presents with extremity *distal symmetric polyneuropathy,* affecting both sensory and motor function. *Autonomic neuropathy* can produce bladder, bowel, or sexual dysfunction, and *diabetic mononeuropathy* can manifest with sudden cranial nerve palsy or foot or hand drop.

Enhanced susceptibility to infections is attributable to compromised tissue perfusion, diminished neutrophil function, and impaired macrophage cytokine production.

Pancreatic Endocrine Neoplasms (p. 1146)

Also known as *islet cell tumors,* these constitute only 2% of all pancreatic neoplasms; they may be single or multiple, benign or malignant, and can secrete hormones or be nonfunctional. Insulinomas are the most common islet cell tumor, and 90% are benign; 60% to 90% of other pancreatic endocrine neoplasms are malignant. Unequivocal criteria for malignancy include metastases, vascular invasion, and/or local infiltration.

Hyperinsulinism (Insulinoma) (p. 1146)

β-cell tumors can elaborate sufficient insulin to cause hypoglycemia; symptoms (e.g., confusion, stupor, or loss of consciousness) occur with serum glucose below 50 mg/dL.

Morphology (p. 1146)

Most are solitary lesions, less than 2 cm and well encapsulated, composed of cords and nests of well-differentiated β-cells; carcinomas (about 10% of cases) are diagnosed based on metastasis or invasion.

Clinical Features (p. 1147)

Hypoglycemic symptoms are mild in all but 20% of cases; surgical resection yields prompt normalization of glycemia. Hyperinsulinism can also be caused by diffuse islet hyperplasia (in neonates and infants in the setting of maternal diabetes, Beckwith-Wiedemann syndrome, and rare metabolic disorders).

Zollinger-Ellison Syndrome (Gastrinomas) (p. 1147)

Gastrin hypersecretion is usually due to gastrin-producing *gastrinomas;* these can occur in the pancreas, duodenum, or peripancreatic soft tissue. The classic "Z-E" syndrome comprises a triad of severe peptic ulcer disease, gastric hypersecretion, and pancreatic islet lesions.

Clinical Features (p. 1147)

The majority of patients present with diarrhea; duodenal and gastric ulcers are often multiple. Although the ulcers are identical to those found in the general population, they are often intractable to therapy; they may also occur in unusual locations such as the jejunum. More than half of the gastrinomas have metastasized or are locally invasive at the time of diagnosis; approximately 25% arise in conjunction with other endocrine tumors as part of the MEN-1 syndrome.

Other Rare Pancreatic Endocrine Neoplasms (p. 1147)

- *α-Cell tumors (glucagonomas)* are associated with elevated glucagon and a syndrome that includes mild diabetes, necrolytic migratory erythema (a skin rash), and anemia.

- δ-*cell tumors (somatostatinomas)* exhibit high somatostatin levels and a syndrome comprising diabetes mellitus, cholelithiasis, steatorrhea, and hypochlorhydria.
- *VIPoma* causes a w*atery* d*iarrhea,* h*ypokalemia,* and a*chlorhydria (WDHA) syndrome;* neural crest tumors (e.g., neuroblastomas) can present with the same syndrome.
- *Pancreatic carcinoid tumors* produce serotonin.
- *Pancreatic polypeptide-secreting endocrine tumors* are rare and usually asymptomatic.

ADRENAL GLANDS (p. 1148)

Adrenal Cortex (p. 1148)

Adrenocortical Hyperfunction (Hyperadrenalism) (p. 1148)

Adrenal hyperfunction syndromes are related to overproduction of one or more of the three basic adrenal cortical steroids:

- Cushing syndrome (excess glucocorticoids)
- Hyperaldosteronism (excess mineralocorticoids)
- Adrenogenital syndromes (excess androgens)

Hypercortisolism (Cushing Syndrome) (p. 1148)

Hypercortisolism (Cushing syndrome) occurs with:

- Administration of *exogenous* glucocorticoids (most common cause)
- Primary hypothalamic-pituitary disorders associated with ACTH hypersecretion
- Cortisol hypersecretion by adrenal adenoma, carcinoma, or nodular hyperplasia
- Ectopic ACTH production by a non-endocrine neoplasm

Pituitary ACTH hypersecretion (Cushing disease) typically occurs in women (4:1 ratio), and accounts for 70% of cases of *endogenous* hypercortisolism. Most cases are associated with an ACTH-producing pituitary adenoma. Serum ACTH is elevated and is not suppressed by low-dose dexamethasone challenge but is reduced by high-dose challenge.

Ectopic ACTH secretion by non-pituitary tumors accounts for 10% of cases of endogenous *Cushing syndrome.* It occurs most commonly in men between the ages of 40 and 60 years and is associated with lung small cell carcinoma, although carcinoid tumors, thyroid medullary carcinoma, and islet cell tumors can also be ACTH sources. Serum ACTH is elevated and its secretion is completely insensitive to either low-dose or high-dose dexamethasone. Rarely, Cushing syndrome can be associated with ectopic secretion of corticotropin-releasing factor (CRF), with resultant ACTH overproduction and hypercortisolism.

Primary adrenal neoplasms, for example, adenoma (10% of cases) or carcinoma (5% of cases) are the most common causes for *ACTH-independent* Cushing syndrome. ACTH levels are quite low (feedback inhibition), and dexamethasone challenge has no effect on cortisol levels.

ACTH-independent primary cortical hyperplasia is uncommon; it is often reflected by adrenal cortical *macronodular hyperplasia.* Although macronodular hyperplasia is ACTH-autonomous, cortisol production can instead be driven by *non-ACTH hormones* (e.g., LH, ADH, or serotonin) for which the epithelium has overexpressed the corresponding receptors. Macronodular hyperplasia also occurs in the setting of the *McCune-Albright syndrome* (due to activating mutations in *GNAS*), and when genes controlling intracellular cAMP are mutated.

Morphology (p. 1149)

- *Pituitary:* Regardless of etiology, elevated glucocorticoid levels induce *Crooke hyaline change*—the normal granular, basophilic cytoplasm of ACTH-producing cells becomes pale and homogeneous due to keratin filament deposition.
- *Adrenals:* Morphology depends on the cause of hypercortisolism.

  Exogenous glucocorticoids suppress endogenous ACTH and result in cortical atrophy; the zona glomerulosa is of normal thickness since it functions independently of ACTH.

  Endogenous elevations of ACTH cause bilateral cortical hyperplasia.

  Macronodular hyperplasia exhibits almost complete replacement of the cortex by nodules 3 cm or smaller that contain an admixture of lipid-poor and lipid-rich cells.

  Primary neoplasms resemble non-functional cortical neoplasms (see later); adenomas are generally small (less than 30 g), yellow, and well-circumscribed, while carcinomas tend to be larger and unencapsulated. There is atrophy of the adjacent residual cortex and the contralateral gland.

Clinical Course (p. 1150)

Cushing syndrome develops slowly, and early manifestations (hypertension and weight gain) are non-specific. The full-blown syndrome complex, however, has a number of characteristic features, including:

- Adipose tissue redistribution with central obesity, moon facies, and fat accumulation on the posterior neck and back (so-called "buffalo hump")
- Atrophy of type 2 fast-twitch myofibers with decreased muscle mass and proximal muscle weakness
- Hyperglycemia, glucosuria, and polydipsia *(secondary diabetes)* due to cortisol-induced gluconeogenesis and inhibition of glucose uptake
- Poor wound healing and abdominal striae due to catabolic effects on collagen
- Bone resorption and osteoporosis with increased risk of fractures
- Increased risk of infection due to immunosuppression
- Hirsuitism and menstrual abnormalities
- Mental disturbances including depression and frank psychosis

Primary Hyperaldosteronism (p. 1151)

Primary hyperaldosteronism is characterized by autonomous aldosterone secretion; this leads to sodium retention and potassium excretion, with resultant hypertension and hypokalemia. The renin-angiotensin system is suppressed, and thus plasma renin activity is low. Causes include the following:

- *Primary idiopathic hyperaldosteronism* accounts for 60% of cases; the etiology is unknown.
- *Adrenocortical neoplasm* (35% of cases); these are usually solitary aldosterone-secreting adenomas *(Conn syndrome),* typically arising in middle age with a female to male ratio of 2:1. Adrenocortical carcinoma is a rarer cause, except in children.
- *Glucocorticoid-remediable hyperaldosteronism* is a rare hereditable form caused by fusion between *CYP11B1* (the 11β-hydroxylase

gene) and *CYP11B2* (the aldosterone synthase gene); aldosterone secretion is regulated by ACTH and is thus suppressible by exogenous glucocorticoids.

In *secondary hyperaldosteronism,* aldosterone release occurs through activation of the renin-angiotensin system; it is encountered in conditions such as congestive heart failure, decreased renal perfusion, and pregnancy (due to increased angiotensinogen synthesis).

Morphology (p. 1152)

- *Grossly: Aldosterone-producing adenomas* are usually solitary, small, yellow encapsulated lesions; they occur more commonly on the left side. Adjacent normal cortex is not atrophic.
- *Microscopically:* Cells in adenomas are lipid-laden and usually resemble zona fasciculata cells; they frequently exhibit *PAS*-reactive, eosinophilic, laminated cytoplasmic inclusions (*spironolactone bodies*).

  Primary idiopathic hyperplasia is characterized by hyperplasia of cells resembling normal zona glomerulosa

Clinical Course (p. 1152)

Hypertension is the major feature; sodium retention increases the total body sodium and expands the extracellular fluid volume. Aldosterone also contributes to endothelial dysfunction, leading to reduced nitric oxide synthesis and increased oxidative stress. Hypokalemia, when present, results from renal potassium wasting and can cause a variety of neuromuscular manifestations, including weakness, paresthesias, visual disturbances, and occasionally tetany. Therapy involves resection of adenomas, aldosterone antagonists (e.g., spironolactone) for primary idiopathic aldosteronism, and correction of the underlying cause in cases of secondary hyperaldosteronism.

Adrenogenital Syndromes (p. 1152)

Disorders of sexual differentiation (e.g., female virilization or male precocious puberty) can be caused by primary gonadal (Chapter 22) or adrenal disorders. Unlike gonadal androgens, ACTH regulates adrenal androgen formation; thus over-secretion can be primary or a component of Cushing disease (Fig. 24-2).

- *Androgen-secreting adrenal cortical neoplasms* are more likely to be carcinomas than adenomas.
- *Congenital adrenal hyperplasia (CAH)* is a group of autosomal recessive metabolic disorders affecting enzymes involved in adrenal steroid synthesis; cortisol production is mainly affected, although certain defects are also associated with salt wasting due to impaired aldosterone synthesis. Steroidogenesis is then channeled into other pathways (see Fig. 24-2) leading to increased production of androgens; in all cases, adrenals exhibit bilateral cortical hyperplasia.

21-Hydroxylase Deficiency (p. 1152)

21-Hydroxylase deficiency is caused by mutations in *CYP21A* and results in defective conversion of progesterone to 11-deoxycorticosterone; it accounts for more than 90% of CAH and, depending on the nature of the mutation, can manifest as three different syndromes:

- *Salt-wasting syndrome* is associated with a complete deficiency of 21-hydroxylase activity and thus absent aldosterone or cortisol

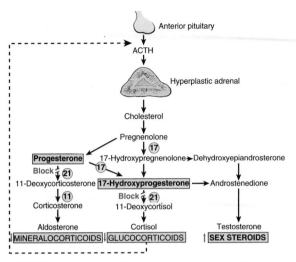

FIGURE 24-2 Consequences of 21-hydroxylase deficiency. Absence of the enzyme impairs both cortisol and aldosterone synthesis. Subsequent loss of feedback inhibition *(dashed line)* leads to increased ACTH production with cortical hyperplasia and steroidogenesis being funneled into testosterone synthesis. The sites of action of 11-, 17-, and 21-hydroxylase are shown by the circled numbers.

production. It is recognized shortly after birth, by salt wasting, hyponatremia, and hyperkalemia—leading to acidosis, hypotension, and cardiovascular collapse; females exhibit virilization.

- *Simple virilizing adrenogenital syndrome without salt wasting* is associated with incomplete loss of hydroxylase activity (about one third of patients). Patients have sufficient aldosterone to avoid a salt-wasting crisis, but reduced cortisol production still drives ACTH secretion and ultimately increased testosterone synthesis.
- *Non-classic (late onset) adrenal virilism* is more common than the other syndromes; partial 21-hydroxylase deficiency in this case results in either no symptoms or only subtle features of androgenic excess later in life (e.g., hirsuitism, acne, or menstrual irregularities).

Clinical Course (p. 1154)

Clinical consequences are determined by the specific enzyme deficiency; effects are related to androgen excess and/or aldosterone and glucocorticoid deficiency. CAH should be suspected in any neonate with ambiguous genitalia; severe enzyme deficiency in infancy can be a life-threatening. CAH patients are treated with exogenous glucocorticoids and/or mineralocorticoid supplementation for salt-wasting variants.

Adrenocortical Insufficiency (p. 1154)

Insufficiency can occur through either acute or chronic primary loss of adrenal function or through secondary to diminished ACTH production.

Primary Acute Adrenocortical Insufficiency (p. 1154)

Primary acute adrenocortical insufficiency can occur due to:

- A sudden increase in glucocorticoid requirements in patients with chronic insufficiency *(adrenal crisis)*

- Rapid withdrawal of steroids, or failure to increase steroid doses in periods of stress, in patients with adrenal suppression secondary to long-term glucocorticoid therapy
- Massive adrenal hemorrhage (e.g., neonatal adrenal hemorrhage, postsurgical disseminated intravascular coagulation, Waterhouse-Friderichsen syndrome)

Waterhouse-Friderichsen Syndrome *(p. 1155)*

Waterhouse-Friderichsen syndrome is an uncommon but catastrophic event characterized by:

- Overwhelming septicemic infection, classically due to meningococcus (although other virulent bacterial infections can also be responsible)
- Rapidly progressive hypotension and shock
- DIC with purpura
- Massive adrenal hemorrhage with adrenal insufficiency; the clinical course can be devastatingly abrupt unless recognition is prompt and appropriate antibiotic therapy is provided.

Primary Chronic Adrenocortical Insufficiency (Addison Disease) *(p. 1155)*

Primary chronic adrenocortical insufficiency (Addison disease) is an uncommon condition associated with the destruction of at least 90% of the adrenal cortex. Causes include:

- *Autoimmune adrenalitis* (60% to 70% of cases):

  Autoimmune polyendocrinopathy syndrome type 1 (APS1) is caused by mutations in the autoimmune regulator *(AIRE)* gene. *AIRE* codes for a thymic transcription factor that drives the expression of many peripheral tissue antigens; thymic expression of these antigens allows self-reactive T cells to undergo clonal deletion. In the absence of normal AIRE function, central tolerance is compromised and autoimmunity develops. APS1 is characterized by chronic mucocutaneous candidiasis and abnormalities of skin, dental enamel, and nails (ectodermal dystrophy), occurring in association with a combination of organ-specific autoimmune disorders (e.g., autoimmune adrenalitis, autoimmune hypoparathyroidism, idiopathic hypogonadism, pernicious anemia).
  Autoimmune polyendocrinopathy syndrome type 2 (APS2) usually presents in early adulthood as a combination of adrenal insufficiency and autoimmune thyroiditis or type 1 diabetes; mucocutaneous candidiasis and ectodermal dysplasia do not occur.

- *Infectious processes,* particularly tuberculosis and those caused by fungi such as *Histoplasma capsulatum* and *Coccidioides immitis.* Patients with AIDS are at risk for developing adrenal insufficiency from complications of their disease (e.g., cytomegalovirus, *Mycobacterium avium-intracellulare,* Kaposi sarcoma).
- *Metastatic neoplasms,* most commonly lung and breast carcinomas.
- Rare genetic disorders including *adrenal hypoplasia congenita* (an X-linked disorder caused by mutations in a transcription factor involved in adrenal development) and *adrenoleukodystrophy* (Chapter 28).

Clinical Course *(p. 1156)*

Features of Addison disease include insidious onset of weakness, fatigue, and anorexia; patients also develop hyperkalemia, hyponatremia, and hypotension due to mineralocorticoid insufficiency. Cutaneous hyperpigmentation can result from elevation of POMC (due to loss of cortisol feedback on the pituitary), which is the precursor peptide to both ACTH and melanocyte-stimulating hormone. Acute stresses (e.g., trauma or infection) can precipitate acute adrenal crisis, with rapid progression to death unless corticosteroid therapy is promptly initiated.

Secondary Adrenocortical Insufficiency (p. 1157)

Secondary adrenocortical insufficiency occurs with any hypothalamic or pituitary disorder leading to diminished ACTH production (e.g., tumor, infection, infarction); it can be an isolated deficiency or associated with decreased levels of other pituitary hormones *(panhypopituitarism)*. It is distinguished from primary hypoadrenalism by:

- Absence of hyperpigmentation
- Near-normal aldosterone levels since production is largely independent of ACTH; thus, hyponatremia and hyperkalemia are not features of secondary adrenocortical insufficiency.

Adrenocortical Neoplasms (p. 1157)

Most adrenal cortical neoplasms are sporadic, although *Li-Fraumeni syndrome* (associated with germline *p53* mutations) and *Beckwith-Wiedemann syndrome* (an imprinting disorder) are associated with a predilection for adrenal cortical carcinomas. Adrenal cortical carcinomas are highly malignant neoplasms (mean survival is 2 years) and are usually large infiltrative lesions at the time of primary diagnosis; they tend to invade the adrenal vein, inferior vena cava, and lymphatics. Functional adenomas are commonly associated with hyperaldosteronism and Cushing syndrome; functional carcinomas tend to be virilizing. Functioning and non-functioning tumors cannot be distinguished morphologically; differentiation requires laboratory measurement of hormones or relevant metabolites.

Morphology (p. 1157)

- Adenomas

    Grossly: Tumors are typically well-circumscribed, yellow-brown lesions up to 2.5 cm. In nonfunctioning adenomas, the adjacent cortex is normal thickness; in functioning neoplasms, the adjacent cortex is typically atrophic.

    Microscopically: Lesions resemble the normal cortical cells, although nuclear atypia is not uncommon.

- Adrenal cortical carcinomas

    Grossly: Tumors are typically variegated with areas of hemorrhage, cystic change, and necrosis.

    Microscopically: Cells range from well-differentiated to markedly anaplastic.

Other Lesions of the Adrenal (p. 1159)

The prevalence of "adrenal incidentalomas" discovered by computed tomography (CT) scans is approximately 4%, with an age-dependent increase in prevalence; the vast majority are non-secreting cortical adenomas. Other lesions include adrenal cysts and *adrenal myelolipomas;* the latter are benign lesions composed of mature fat and hematopoietic elements.

Adrenal Medulla (p. 1159)

Most adrenal medullary disorders are neoplasms; neuroblastomas and other neuroblastic tumors are discussed in Chapter 10.

Pheochromocytoma (p. 1159)

Pheochromocytomas are relatively uncommon tumors of chromaffin cells. The tumors produce catecholamines and typically present with hypertension; they are therefore significant as surgically correctable causes of high blood pressure. They are memorable for obeying a "rule of 10s":

- 10% are extra-adrenal (e.g., organ of Zuckerkandl or carotid body), in which they are designated *paragangliomas*.
- 10% of sporadic adrenal pheochromocytomas are bilateral (in comparison, 50% of cases associated with familial syndromes are bilateral).
- 10% are biologically malignant (i.e., associated with metastasis); malignancy occurs in 20% to 40% in familial syndromes or in extra-adrenal pheochromocytomas.
- 10% are *not* associated with hypertension.
- As many as 25% (not 10%, unfortunately) of pheochromocytomas arise in familial syndromes associated with germline mutations in at least one of six different genes, including MEN-2A and -2B syndromes (*RET* mutations, described later), type I neurofibromatosis (*NF1* mutations, Chapter 7), von Hippel-Lindau (VHL) syndrome (Chapter 28), and familial paraganglioma syndromes (mutations in the subunits of the succinate dehydrogenase complex).

Morphology (p. 1159)

- *Grossly:* Tumors range from 1 g to 4 kg. Tumors are highly vascular; the cut surface is usually yellow-tan and associated with hemorrhage, necrosis, or cystic change. Incubation of fresh tissue with potassium dichromate turns the tumor dark black due to catecholamine oxidation (hence the term *chromaffin*).
- *Microscopically:* Tumors are composed of clusters ("zellballen") of polygonal to spindle-shaped chief cells (exhibiting neuroendocrine markers) admixed with sustentacular cells (expressing S-100), all delimited by a rich vascular network. Cellular and nuclear pleomorphism is common. Metastasis is the sole criterion of malignancy.

Clinical Course (p. 1161)

The dominant clinical consequence in patients with pheochromocytoma is hypertension; this is typically paroxysmal (due to sudden catechol release) with abrupt blood pressure elevations, tachycardia, palpitations, headache, sweating, tremor, and a sense of foreboding. The acute hypertension can precipitate congestive heart failure, myocardial infarcts, cardiac arrhythmia, and/or cerebral hemorrhage. Cardiac complications are also attributed to ischemic myocardial damage secondary to catecholamine-induced vasoconstriction. Laboratory diagnosis is based on increased urinary catecholamines and their metabolites (e.g., vanillylmandelic acid). Surgical excision requires on-board adrenergic blockade to prevent hypertensive crisis; therapy for metastatic disease requires long-term blood pressure control.

MULTIPLE ENDOCRINE NEOPLASIA SYNDROMES (p. 1161)

Multiple endocrine neoplasia (MEN) is a group of heritable diseases resulting in proliferative lesions (e.g., hyperplasia, adenomas, and carcinomas) of multiple endocrine organs (Table 24-4). Relative to sporadic tumors, those associated with MEN:

TABLE 24-4 Multiple Endocrine Neoplasia (MEN) Syndromes

	MEN-1	MEN-2A	MEN-2B
Pituitary	Adenomas		
Parathyroid	Hyperplasia +++ Adenomas +	Hyperplasia +	
Pancreatic islets	Hyperplasia ++ Adenomas ++ Carcinomas +++		
Adrenal	Cortical hyperplasia	Pheochromocytoma ++	Pheochromocytoma +++
Thyroid		C-cell hyperplasia +++ Medullary carcinoma +++	C-cell hyperplasia +++ Medullary carcinoma +++
Extraendocrine changes			Mucocutaneous ganglioneuromas Marfanoid habitus
Mutant gene locus	MEN1	RET	RET

Relative frequency: +, uncommon; +++, common.

- Occur at a younger age than their sporadic counterparts
- Arise in multiple organs, either synchronously (at the same time) or sequentially
- Are often multifocal
- Are usually preceded by asymptomatic endocrine hyperplasia
- Are usually preceded by an asymptomatic stage of endocrine hyperplasia involving the cell of origin (e.g., C-cell hyperplasia adjacent to medullary thyroid cancers)
- Are usually more aggressive and recur in a higher proportion of cases

Multiple Endocrine Neoplasia, Type 1 (p. 1162)

Multiple endocrine neoplasia type 1 (MEN-1) (Wermer syndrome) is classically characterized by 3 "Ps":

- *Parathyroid:* Primary hyperparathyroidism, due to hyperplasia or adenomas, occurs in 80% to 95% of cases, and is often the initial manifestation.
- *Pancreas:* Endocrine tumors are typically aggressive (presenting with metastases) and are often functional. Pancreatic peptide is the most common hormone produced so that there is not necessarily an accompanying hypersecretory syndrome; insulinomas and gastrinomas are next in frequency.
- *Pituitary:* Anterior adenomas are most commonly prolactinomas.

Notably, the duodenum (*not* a "P") is the most common source of gastrinomas in MEN-1; these patients can also develop carcinoid tumors, thyroid and adrenocortical adenomas, and lipomas. MEN-1 is caused by germline mutations in the *MEN1* tumor suppressor gene, encoding the protein *menin*—a component of several different transcription factor complexes. Peptide hormone over-production dominates the clinical picture, with malignant behavior by one of the tumors often being the cause of death.

Multiple Endocrine Neoplasia, Type 2 (p. 1162)

MEN-2 is divided into three distinct syndromes:

- *MEN-2A (Sipple syndrome)* is characterized by thyroid medullary carcinoma (almost 100% of cases), pheochromocytoma (40% to 50%), and parathyroid hyperplasia with hypercalcemia (10% to 20%). It is caused by germline gain-of-function *RET* protooncogene mutations (Chapter 7).
- *MEN-2B* is characterized by thyroid medullary carcinoma and pheochromocytomas, but hyperparathyroidism does not develop; instead patients develop neuromas or ganglioneuromas of multiple sites and exhibit a marfanoid habitus, with long axial skeletal features and hyperextensible joints. The sydrome is caused by a unique, single amino acid substitution in RET, leading to constitutive activation of its tyrosine kinase activity.
- *Familial medullary thyroid cancer* is a variant of MEN-2A, with a strong predisposition to thyroid malignancy but without the other clinical manifestations.

Although MEN-1 genetic screening has questionable long-term value, screening of at-risk family members in the MEN-2 syndromes can be life-saving since early thyroidectomy can potentially mitigate the fatal complications of medullary thyroid carcinoma.

PINEAL GLAND (p. 1163)

The principal pineal secretory product is melatonin, involved in control of circadian rhythms, including sleep-wake cycles.

Pineal tumors are exceptionally rare; most (50% to 70%) arise from sequestered embryonic germ cells (Chapter 28), and they commonly take the form of *germinomas* resembling testicular seminomas.

Pinealomas (p. 1163)

Pinealomas are true tumors of pineocytes (as opposed to germ-cell tumors). They are classified based on their degree of differentiation (i.e., pineoblastomas vs. pineocytomas); less differentiated tumors (pineoblastomas) are typically more aggressive.

25

The Skin

The Skin: More Than a Mechanical Barrier (p. 1166)

- *Squamous epithelial cells (keratinocytes)* constitute the majority of epidermal cells and synthesize the keratin mechanical barrier; they also produce cytokines that regulate the cutaneous environment.
- *Melanocytes* produce *melanin* pigment to screen ultraviolet (UV) light.
- *Dendritic cells* (called *Langerhans cells* in the epidermis) process and present antigen to activate the immune system; a subset of T lymphocytes specifically home to the skin through the expression of cutaneous lymphocyte-associated antigen (CLA).
- *Neural end organs* detect pain and temperature; neuroendocrine Merkel cells also reside in the epidermal basal layer.
- *Sweat glands* permit cooling.
- *Hair follicles* elaborate hair shafts and are repositories for epithelial stem cells.

DEFINITIONS

Macroscopic Terms (p. 1167):

Bulla Elevated fluid-filled lesion more than 5 mm

Excoriation Linear, traumatic epidermal disruption (i.e., a deep scratch)

Lichenification Thick, rough skin with prominent skin markings, usually due to repeated rubbing

Macule Flat, circumscribed area 5 mm or more distinguished by coloration

Onycholysis Separation of a nail from the underlying skin

Nodule Elevated dome-shaped lesion more than 5 mm

Papule Elevated lesion 5 mm or more

Plaque Elevated flat-topped lesion more than 5 mm

Pustule Discrete, pus-filled raised lesion

Scale Dry, plate-like excrescence due to aberrant cornification

Vesicle Elevated fluid-filled lesion 5 mm or more

Wheal Pruritic, elevated, erythematous lesion secondary to dermal edema

Microscopic Terms (p. 1168):

Acantholysis Loss of intercellular keratinocyte connections

Acanthosis Epidermal hyperplasia

Dyskeratosis Abnormal keratinization below the stratum granulosum

Erosion Focal incomplete epidermal loss

Exocytosis Epidermal inflammatory cells

Hydropic swelling (ballooning) Intracellular keratinocyte edema

Hypergranulosis Stratum granulosum hyperplasia, usually due to rubbing

Hyperkeratosis Stratum corneum thickening, often with aberrant keratinization

Lentiginous Linear (non-nested) melanocyte proliferation within the epidermal basal cell layer

Papillomatosis Surface elevation due to dermal papillae hyperplasia

Parakeratosis Stratum corneum keratinization with retained nuclei

Spongiosis Epidermal intercellular edema

Ulceration Focal, complete epidermal loss

Vacuolization Vacuoles within or adjacent to keratinocytes

Disorders of Pigmentation And Melanocytes (p. 1168)

Freckles (Ephelis) (p. 1168)

Freckles are common pigmented lesions of childhood: they are 1 to 10 mm, tan-red to brown macules, fading and recurring depending on the amount of sun exposure.

Morphology (p. 1168)

Melanocyte density is normal so that hyperpigmentation is a result of focal melanin over-production and/or enhanced pigment donation to basal keratinocytes.

Lentigo (p. 1168)

Lentigo (plural, *lentigines*) is a benign, hyperpigmented macule (5 to 10 mm) common in infancy and childhood; lentigines do not darken with sun exposure.

Morphology (p. 1169)

Lesions characteristically exhibit hyperpigmented linear basal melanocyte hyperplasia, often with rete ridge elongation and thinning.

Melanocytic Nevus (Pigmented Nevus, Mole) (p. 1169)

Melanocytic nevi are congenital or acquired *melanocyte neoplasms*; common acquired moles are well-demarcated, uniformly tan-brown papules 6 mm or less, but there are several variants (Table 25-1).

Morphology (p. 1169)

- Moles arise from basal melanocytes—rounded cells exhibiting uniform nuclei and inconspicuous nucleoli (Fig. 25-1); nevi mature through characteristic stages:

  Junctional nevi (i.e., nests of nevus cells at the dermoepidermal junction) are the earliest lesions.

  Compound nevi develop as nests or cords of melanocytes extending into the underlying dermis.

  In *dermal nevi*, the epidermal component is lost.

  As nevus cells enter the dermis they undergo maturation, becoming smaller and nonpigmented, resembling neural tissue *(neurotization)*.

- In comparison, melanomas exhibit little to no maturation.

Pathogenesis (p. 1170)

Many nevi have acquired mutations in *BRAF* or *NRAS*, genes involved in *RAS* signaling (see later). These changes cause a limited

TABLE 25-1 Variant Forms of Nevocellular Nevi

Nevus Variant	Diagnostic Architectural Features	Diagnostic Cytologic Features	Clinical Significance
Congenital nevus	Deep dermal and sometimes subcutaneous growth around adnexa, neurovascular bundles, and blood vessel walls	Identical to ordinary acquired nevi	Present at birth; large variants have increased melanoma risk
Blue nevus	Non-nested dermal infiltration, often with associated fibrosis	Highly dendritic, heavily pigmented nevus cells	Black-blue nodule; often confused with melanoma clinically
Spindle and epithelioid cell nevus (Spitz nevus)	Fascicular growth	Large, plump cells with pink-blue cytoplasm; fusiform cells	Common in children; red-pink nodule; often confused with hemangioma clinically
Halo nevus	Lymphocytic infiltration surrounding nevus cells	Identical to ordinary acquired nevi	Host immune response against nevus cells and surrounding normal melanocytes
Dysplastic nevus	Large, coalescent intraepidermal nests	Cytologic atypia	Potential precursor of malignant melanoma

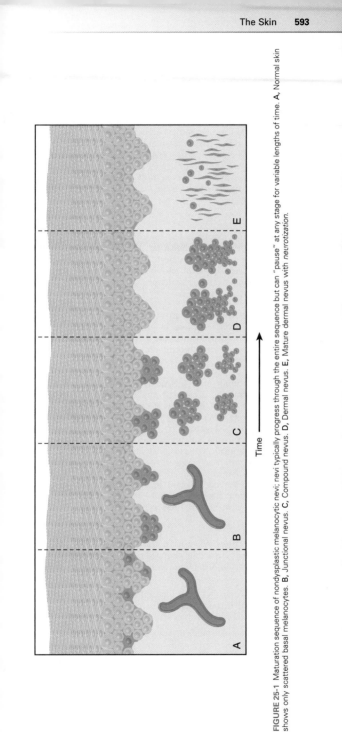

FIGURE 25-1 Maturation sequence of nondysplastic melanocytic nevi; nevi typically progress through the entire sequence but can "pause" at any stage for variable lengths of time. A, Normal skin shows only scattered basal melanocytes. B, Junctional nevus. C, Compound nevus. D, Dermal nevus. E, Mature dermal nevus with *neurotization*.

period of proliferation, followed—in most cases—by permanent growth arrest due to accumulation of p16/INK4a (an inhibitor of cyclin-dependent kinases).

Dysplastic Nevi (p. 1170)

Dysplastic nevi are larger (more than 5 mm) than most acquired nevi; they are flat macules to slightly raised plaques with variegated pigmentation and irregular borders occurring in both sun-exposed and protected skin. They can number in the hundreds in individuals with the *dysplastic nevus syndrome*—half of such patients develop melanomas by age 60 years, some of which arise within a dysplastic nevus. However, most dysplastic nevi are clinically stable, and sporadic isolated lesions have a low risk of malignant transformation.

Morphology (p. 1171)

Histologically, most dysplastic nevi are compound nevi exhibiting cytologic and architectural atypia; i.e., enlarged and fused nests of nevus cells, lentiginous melanocyte hyperplasia, linear papillary dermal fibrosis, and pigment incontinence (release of melanin from dead melanocytes into the dermis).

Pathogenesis (p. 1171)

Dysplastic nevus syndrome is an autosomal dominant disorder often associated with mutations in proteins associated with cell cycling (e.g., cyclin-dependent kinase 4 [CDK4]); acquired *NRAS* and *BRAF* mutations are also common.

Melanoma (p. 1171)

This malignant tumor most commonly arises in skin, but it can also occur in oral and anogenital mucosal surfaces, esophagus, meninges, and eye. The incidence of cutaneous malignant melanoma is increasing, with roughly 60,000 cases and 8000 deaths annually in the United States.

Cutaneous melanoma can present with pain or pruritus, but most are asymptomatic. The majority are more than 10 mm at diagnosis and are usually associated with color variegations (including black, brown, blue, red, and gray); the most consistent clinical signs are recent changes in size, shape, or color. The borders are often irregular and/or notched, with zones of hypopigmentation due to focal regression.

Morphology (p. 1172)

Melanomas are composed of large cells with expanded, irregular nuclei containing peripherally clumped chromatin and prominent eosinophilic nucleoli. Melanomas progress from *radial* to *vertical growth* patterns:

- *Radial growth* describes horizontal spread within the epidermis and superficial dermis; tumor cells typically lack the capacity to metastasize. Lesions include:

  Lentigo maligna: An indolent lesion on the face that may not progress for decades
  Superficial spreading: The most common form of melanoma, usually involving sun-exposed skin
  Acral/mucosal lentiginous: Melanoma unrelated to sun exposure

- *Vertical growth* occurs unpredictably and is characterized by dermal invasion of an expanding clonal mass of cells, lacking cellular maturation. These cells often have the capacity to metastasize, with the probability of distal spread correlating with the depth of invasion; the distance (called the *Breslow thickness*) is measured from the epidermal granular layer to the deepest intra-dermal tumor cells.

Prognostic Factors (p. 1173)

Prognostic factors predict the risk of metastatic spread; these include the following (more favorable determinants are in parentheses):

- Breslow thickness (less than 1.7 mm)
- Number of mitoses (few)
- Evidence of regression (absent)
- Presence of tumor-infiltrating lymphocytes (many)
- Gender (female)
- Location (extremity)
- Sentinel node micrometastasis (absent)

Pathogenesis (p. 1174)

Sun exposure and inherited genes are most important.

- Most melanomas arise in sun-exposed areas, with lightly pigmented individuals at greater peril; severe sunburns early in life are the most important risk factor.
- 10% to 15% of melanomas are familial and often occur in the setting of dysplastic nevus syndrome.
- Polymorphisms linked to melanin production modestly increase risk in light-skinned individuals.
- Mutations that increase RAS and PI3K/AKT proliferation pathways are strongly associated with sporadic melanomas; activating *BRAF* mutations (encoding a serine/threonine kinase downstream of *RAS*) occur in 60% to 70% of melanomas.
- Mutations that reduce RB protein activity or affect genes encoding CDK inhibitors (e.g., p16/INK4a) are strongly associated with both familial and sporadic melanomas and are probably important in the loss of cellular senescence in melanomas.

Benign Epithelial Tumors (p. 1175)

Seborrheic Keratoses (p. 1175)

Seborrheic keratoses typically arise in middle-aged and older individuals, most commonly on the trunk; similar smaller facial lesions in non-whites are called *dermatosis papulosa nigra*. When seborrheic keratoses occur explosively in large numbers, they may represent a paraneoplastic syndrome *(sign of Leser-Trélat)*, due to tumor elaboration of transforming growth factor-α (TGF-α). Activating mutations in fibroblast growth factor receptor-3 (FGFR-3) likely drive the growth of many sporadic lesions.

Morphology (p. 1175)

- *Grossly:* Lesions are uniform, tan-brown, velvety or granular round plaques millimeters to several centimeters in diameter; keratin-filled plugs may be evident.
- *Microscopically:* Lesions are sharply demarcated and exophytic, with hyperplasia of variably pigmented basaloid cells and *hyperkeratosis;* keratin-filled *horn cysts* are common features. When irritated and inflamed, the basaloid cells undergo squamous differentiation.

Acanthosis Nigricans (p. 1175)

Lesions are thickened, velvety hyperpigmented plaques typically occurring in flexural areas (e.g., axilla, groin, neck, anogenital region); they can be a marker of benign or malignant conditions:

- The *benign* type makes up 80% of all cases; it develops gradually, usually arising in childhood through puberty, and can be an autosomal dominant trait with variable penetrance (related to activating *FGFR-3* mutations), associated with obesity or endocrine disorders (especially diabetes), or a component of several rare congenital disorders.
- The *malignant* type arises in middle-aged and older individuals, often in association with an occult adenocarcinoma (possibly due to tumor elaboration of epidermal growth factors).

Morphology (p. 1176)

Lesions exhibit hyperkeratosis, with prominent rete ridges and basal hyperpigmentation (without melanocyte hyperplasia).

Fibroepithelial Polyp (p. 1176)

Also called *acrochordon, squamous papilloma,* or *skin tag,* fibroepithelial polyps are found on the neck, trunk, face, or intertriginous zones and are exceptionally common benign lesions in middle-aged and older individuals. These are soft, flesh-colored tumors attached by a slender fibrovascular stalk covered by benign epidermis. The vast majority are sporadic, but they may be associated with pregnancy, diabetes, or intestinal polyposis.

Epithelial Cyst (Wen) (p. 1176)

Epithelial cysts are common lesions presenting as well-circumscribed, firm subcutaneous nodules formed by downgrowth and cystic expansion of epidermal or follicular epithelium.

Morphology (p. 1176)

Lesions are filled with keratin and variable amounts of lipid and debris from sebaceous secretions; they are subclassified based on the cyst wall characteristics:

- *Epidermal inclusion cyst:* Wall is almost identical to normal epidermis.
- *Pilar (trichilemmal) cyst:* Wall resembles follicular epithelium (i.e., without a granular cell layer).
- *Dermoid cyst:* Wall is similar to epidermis but has multiple skin appendages, especially hair follicles.
- *Steatocystoma multiplex:* Wall resembles sebaceous gland ductal epithelium with numerous compressed sebaceous lobules (frequently occurs as a dominantly inherited lesion).

Adnexal (Appendage) Tumors (p. 1176)

These are typically nondescript, flesh-colored benign papules or nodules; some have a predilction for specific body surfaces (e.g., *eccrine poromas* on palms and soles). Although most are localized and not aggressive, a subset can be malignant (e.g., *sebaceous carcinoma* arising in eyelid meibomian glands); others have a mendelian pattern of inheritance and occur as multiple disfiguring lesions. Some can serve as markers for visceral malignancies; for example, multiple trichilemmomas in *Cowden syndrome* (due to germline mutations in the tumor suppressor gene *PTEN*) are associated with increased risk of breast cancer.

- *Cylindromas* usually occur on the scalp and forehead; lesions are composed of islands of basaloid cells with apocrine or eccrine differentiation that may coalesce to form hat-like growths *(turban tumor)*. Lesions can be dominantly inherited, associated with inactivating mutations of the *CYLD* tumor suppressor gene.

- *Syringomas* usually occur as multiple, small, tan papules near the lower eyelids and are composed of basaloid epithelium with eccrine differentiation.
- *Sebaceous adenomas* exhibit lobular proliferations of sebocytes with frothy, lipid-filled cytoplasm. They can be associated with internal malignancy in the Muir-Torre syndrome (a subset of the HNPCC syndrome; Chapter 17), linked to germline deficits in DNA mismatch repair proteins.
- *Trichoepitheliomas* are proliferations of basaloid cells that form hair follicle–like structures.
- *Pilomatrixomas* are proliferations of basaloid cells that show hair-like differentiation; they are associated with activating mutations of the *CTNNB1* gene encoding β-catenin.
- *Apocrine carcinomas* occur in the axilla and scalp and exhibit ductal differentiation showing prominent apocrine secretion.

Premalignant and Malignant Epidermal Tumors (p. 1178)

Much has been learned about the molecular underpinnings of skin cancers from otherwise rare hereditary cancer syndromes that also happen to have frequent skin manifestations (Table 25-2).

Actinic Keratosis (p. 1178)

This is a premalignant dysplastic lesion associated with chronic sun exposure, especially in light-skinned individuals; ionizing radiation, hydrocarbons, and arsenicals can induce similar lesions. Because many undergo malignant transformation, local eradication is indicated. Imiquimod can be used to eradicate the abnormal cells through activation of innate immunity via toll-like receptor (TLR) stimulation.

Morphology (p. 1178)

- *Grossly:* Lesions are usually less than 1 cm, tan-brown, red, or flesh-colored with a rough consistency; exuberant keratin production can form "cutaneous horns."
- *Microscopically:* Lesions exhibit cytologic atypia in the lower epidermis, frequently with basal cell hyperplasia and dyskeratosis; intercellular bridges are present. *Hyperkeratosis* and *parakeratosis* are common, although epidermal atrophy can occur. The dermis exhibits thickened, blue-gray elastic fibers *(elastosis)* due to aberrant synthesis by sun-damaged fibroblasts.

Squamous Cell Carcinoma (p. 1178)

Squamous cell carcinoma is the second most common tumor of sun-exposed skin of older individuals (basal cell carcinoma holds the dubious distinction of being first); it occurs more frequently in men than in women, with the exception of lower leg lesions; less than 5% of lesions metastasize to regional nodes.

Morphology (p. 1179)

- *Grossly: In situ* squamous cell carcinomas are well-demarcated, red, scaling plaques; invasive lesions are nodular, variably hyperkeratotic, and prone to ulceration.
- *Microscopically: In situ carcinoma* has full-thickness epidermal atypia; invasive tumors vary from well differentiated (with prominent keratinization) to highly anaplastic with necrosis.

Keratoacanthoma is a self-limited, often *spontaneously resolving,* rapid-growing lesion; it is controversial whether it represents a

TABLE 25-2 A Survey of Familial Cancer Syndromes with Cutaneous Manifestations

Disease	Inheritance	Chromosomal Location	Gene/Protein	Function/Manifestation
Ataxia-telangiectasia	AR	11q22.3	ATM/ATM*	DNA repair after radiation injury; p53 signaling/neurologic and vascular lesions
Nevoid basal cell carcinoma syndrome	AD	9q22.3	PTCH/PTCH	Developmental gene/multiple basal cell carcinomas; jaw cysts, etc.
Cowden syndrome	AD	10q23	PTEN, MMAC1/PTEN, TEP1, MMAC1	Lipid phosphatase/benign follicular appendage tumors (trichilemmomas); internal adenocarcinoma (often breast)
Familial melanoma syndrome	AD	9p21	CDKN2/p16INK4 CDKN2/p14ARF	Inhibits CDKs from phosphorylating Rb, thus arresting cell cycle/melanoma Binds MDM2 and thus, preserves p53/melanoma
Muir-Torre syndrome	AD	2p22	hMSH2/hMSH2	Involved in DNA mismatch repair/benign and malignant sebaceous tumors; internal adenocarcinoma
Neurofibromatosis I	AD	17q11.2	NF1/neurofibromin	Negatively regulates Ras family of signal molecules/neurofibromas
Neurofibromatosis II	AD	22q12.2	NF2/merlin	Integrates cytoskeletal signaling/neurofibromas and acoustic neuromas
Tuberous sclerosis	AD	9q34 16p13.3	TSC1/hamartin TSC2/tuberin	Interacts with tuberin; function unkown Interacts with hamartin; may regulate Ras proteins/angiofibromas, mental retardation
Xeroderma pigmentosum	AR	9q22 and others	XPA/XPA and others	Nucleotide excision repair/melanoma and nonmelanoma skin cancers

AD, Autosomal dominant; AR, autosomal recessive; CDK, cyclin-dependent kinase.
*By convention, genes are italicized and proteins are not italicized.

variant of *squamous cell carcinoma* that regresses because of host-tumor interactions or is a distinct entity. *Grossly,* lesions are symmetric, cup-shaped nodules with central keratin-filled craters. *Histologically,* lobules of glass squamous cells keratinize without progressing through a granular layer. As lesions mature, they elicit a brisk lymphocytic and eosinophilic inflammatory response.

Pathogenesis (p. 1180)

UV radiation is the greatest predisposing factor, primarily by inducing DNA damage but also by dampening the immune functioning of Langerhans cells; immunosuppression (e.g., by chemotherapy) also reduces host surveillance and increases keratinocyte susceptibility to infection and transformation by oncogenic viruses (especially human papillomavirus [HPV] subtypes 5 and 8). Other risks include industrial carcinogens (tars), chronic skin ulcers, old burn scars, draining osteomyelitis, ionizing radiation, and (for oral mucosa) tobacco or betel nut chewing. Acquired or germline (e.g., xeroderma pigmentosum) *p53* mutations may allow cell-cycle progression despite low-fidelity DNA repair of UV-induced damage; this leads to rapid accumulation of mutations and eventual carcinogenesis.

Basal Cell Carcinoma (p. 1180)

Basal cell carcinoma (BCC) is the most common invasive human cancer (1 million cases in the United States annually); they are slow growing and rarely metastasize. Immunosuppression and defects in DNA repair (e.g., xeroderma pigmentosum) increase the incidence.

Morphology (p. 1180)

- *Grossly:* Tumors typically present as pearly papules, often with prominent telangiectatic vessels; some are melanin-pigmented. Advanced lesions ulcerate and can show extensive local invasion, hence the term *rodent ulcer.*
- *Microscopically:* lesions exhibit monotonous basal cell proliferation, either as *multifocal superficial growths* over a large area (several centimeters) of skin or as *nodules* extending deeply into the dermis.

Pathogenesis (p. 1181)

Nevoid basal cell carcinoma syndrome (NBCCS or Gorlin syndrome) is a rare autosomal dominant disorder characterized by multiple basal cell carcinomas usually manifesting before age 20 years; patients also develop medulloblastomas, ovarian fibromas, odontogenic keratocysts, and pits of the palms and soles and can have multiple developmental abnormalities.

The responsible *PTCH* gene on chromosome 9q22.3 is the human homologue for the *Drosophila* developmental gene *patched;* it encodes the receptor for the *sonic hedgehog gene (SHH)* gene product. In the absence of SHH, PTCH binds to another transmembrane protein (SMO, for "smoothened") and blocks its activation of downstream signals. When SHH and PTCH interact, SMO is released and can trigger a signal cascade that involves the GLI1 transcription factor.

Absence of *PTCH* (as in NBCSS) or acquired *PTCH* or *SMO* mutations (sporadic tumors) lead to constitutive SMO activation and the development of BCC; 30% of sporadic BCC have *PTCH* mutations. Additional *p53* mutations are present in 40% to 60% of BCC.

Tumors of the Dermis (p. 1182)

Benign Fibrous Histiocytoma (Dermatofibroma) (p. 1182)

Benign fibrous histiocytomas are a heterogeneous group of indolent neoplasms of dermal fibroblasts and histiocytes usually occurring in adults; they frequently occur on the legs of young women. Antecedent trauma and aberrant healing are often causally implicated.

Morphology (p. 1182)

- *Grossly:* Lesions are firm tan-brown, occasionally tender papules, occasionally as large as several centimeters; lateral compression causes inward dimpling.
- *Microscopically: Dermatofibromas* are most common; these exhibit spindle-shaped fibroblasts in a well-defined, mid-dermal nonencapsulated mass, occasionally extending into subcutaneous fat. Many cases have overlying epidermal hyperplasia.

Dermatofibrosarcoma Protuberans (p. 1183)

This well-differentiated, slow-growing fibrosarcoma is locally aggressive but rarely metastasizes.

Morphology (p. 1183)

- *Grossly:* Tumors are firm nodules arising as protuberant, occasionally ulcerated aggregates within an indurated plaque, typically on the trunk.
- *Microscopically:* Lesions are cellular and composed of radially oriented fibroblasts; mitoses are rare. The overlying epidermis is thinned, and there often is microscopic extension into subcutaneous fat.

Pathogenesis (p. 1183)

The molecular hallmark is a balanced translocation between the collagen 1A1 and platelet-derived growth factor-β (PDGFβ) genes; this juxtaposes the COL1A1 promoter and the coding region of PDGFβ, leading to PDGFβ over-expression and tumor cell proliferation. Treatment involves inhibition of the PDGF receptor tyrosine kinase.

Tumors of Cellular Migrants to the Skin (p. 1183)

These are proliferative disorders of cells that arise elsewhere but home to skin (e.g., Langerhans cells, T lymphocytes, and mast cells).

Mycosis Fungoides (Cutaneous T-Cell Lymphoma) (p. 1184)

Cutaneous T-cell lymphoma (CTCL) represents a spectrum of T-cell lymphoproliferative disorders of the skin; *mycosis fungoides* is a chronic process, while *mycosis fungoides d'emblee* is a more aggressive nodular variant.

Mycosis fungoides is a CTCL that can evolve into a generalized lymphoma; most cases afflict individuals older than 40 years and remain localized to skin for many years. *Sézary syndrome* occurs with seeding of the blood by malignant T cells, accompanied by diffuse erythema and scaling *(erythroderma)*. The proliferating cells in CTCL are CD4+, with clonal T-cell receptor gene rearrangements; CLA expression is responsible for the cutaneous homing behavior.

Morphology (p. 1185)

- *Grossly:* Early lesions resemble eczema and typically arise on the trunk; these progress to scaly, red-brown patches, scaling plaques (similar to psoriasis), or fungating nodules (up to 10 cm) on various body surfaces, correlating with systemic spread.
- *Microscopically: The hallmark* of mycosis fungoides is the *Sézary-Lutzner cell*, a malignant CD4+ (T-helper) cell with a hyperconvoluted or *cerebriform* nucleus; these form band-like dermal infiltrates with single cell invasion into the epidermis *(Pautrier microabscesses).*

Mastocytosis (p. 1185)

Mastocytosis is a spectrum of rare disorders characterized by increased numbers of cutaneous mast cells. Symptoms reflect the consequences of mast cell degranulation; histamine release causes pruritus, flushing, rhinorrhea, or dermal edema and erythema. *Wheal* formation when lesional skin is rubbed is termed the *Darier sign; dermatographism* indicates wheal formation evoked by rubbing normal skin. Rarely, mast cell heparin release can cause epistaxis or gastrointestinal bleeding; bone pain can occur secondary to osteoclastic and osteoblastic involvement.

Urticaria pigmentosa (50% of all cases) is an exclusively cutaneous form of mastocytosis occurring mainly in children, with a generally favorable prognosis. Systemic mastocytosis occurs in 10% of patients, usually adults, and carries a much poorer prognosis. Many cases are caused by point mutations of the c-KIT receptor tyrosine kinase, leading to mast cell proliferation and survival.

Morphology (p. 1185)

- *Grossly:* Skin lesions are multiple, round-oval, nonscaling, red-brown papules and plaques.
- *Microscopically:* Lesions exhibit variable dermal fibrosis, edema, eosinophils, and numerous mast cells.

Disorders of Epidermal Maturation (p. 1186)

Ichthyosis (p. 1186)

Ichthyosis is a spectrum of disorders of epidermal maturation leading to chronic excessive keratin accumulation *(hyperkeratosis)* resembling fish scales (hence the name). There are X-linked, autosomal recessive, and autosomal dominant forms; acquired variants (e.g., *ichthyosis vulgaris*) can be associated with various malignancies. The primary defect in most forms is increased cell-cell adhesion resulting in abnormal desquamation.

Morphology (p. 1186)

Microscopically: Lesions exhibit compacted stratum corneum with minimal inflammation; thickness of the epidermis or stratum granulosum is used to subclassify the disorders.

Acute Inflammatory Dermatoses (p. 1187)

This is an enormous family of conditions, characterized by short-lived (i.e., days to weeks), mononuclear inflammatory infiltrates associated with edema and variable tissue damage.

Urticaria (p. 1187)

Urticaria ("hives") is characterized by focal mast cell degranulation, with histamine-mediated dermal edema and pruritus (*wheal* formation). Individual lesions develop and regress within hours, but sequential lesions can occur for months. *Angioedema* is distinguished by the presence of both *dermal* and *subcutaneous fat* edema.

Morphology (p. 1187)

- *Grossly:* Lesions vary from small, pruritic papules to large edematous plaques. Areas exposed to pressure (e.g., trunk, distal extremities, and ears) are more prone to urticaria.
- *Microscopically:* Sparse mononuclear perivascular infiltrates are associated with edema and occasional dermal eosinophils.

Pathogenesis (p. 1187)

Most lesions are driven by antigen-specific cross-linking of IgE bound to mast cells (Chapter 6). *Immunoglobulin E (IgE)-independent urticaria* can occur through chemical-induced mast cell degranulation (e.g., opiates, certain antibiotics, curare, or radiocontrast materials) or by suppression of prostaglandin synthesis (i.e., with aspirin). Persistent urticaria may reflect an inability to clear the inciting antigen or can reflect cryptic collagen vascular disorders or Hodgkin lymphoma. *Hereditary angioneurotic edema* is caused by deficient C1 esterase inhibitor and subsequent unregulated activation of the early complement components.

Acute Eczematous Dermatitis (p. 1187)

These are a family of disorders of differing etiology, but common immune-driven morphology. Eczematous dermatitis is subdivided based on the initiating factors:

- Allergic contact dermatitis (e.g., poison ivy)
- Atopic dermatitis
- Drug-related eczematous dermatitis
- Photoeczematous dermatitis
- Primary irritant dermatitis

Morphology (p. 1188)

- *Grossly:* Lesions range from pruritic, red, and papulovesicular to blistered, oozing, and crusted. With chronic exposure, these can evolve into psoriasis-like scaling plaques. Bacterial superinfection produces a yellow crust *(impetiginization)*.
- *Microscopically:* Early *spongiosis* progresses to frank fluid accumulation, splaying keratinocytes apart and forming intraepidermal vesicles. Dermal perivascular lymphocytic infiltrates are associated with mast cell degranulation and papillary dermal edema. Drug hypersensitivity lesions may have eosinophils. In chronic lesions, the vesicular phase is replaced with progressive *acanthosis* and *hyperkeratosis*.

Pathogenesis (p. 1188)

Many forms of *eczema* constitute a cutaneous, delayed-type hypersensitivity response driven by Langerhans cell presentation of antigens acquired at the epidermal surface. The subsequent pathogenesis is attributed to cytokine release by recruited memory cells, and nonspecific accumulation of additional inflammatory cells. UV exposures and neuropeptides released near the epidermis can affect Langerhans cell function.

Erythema Multiforme (p. 1189)

Erythema multiforme is an uncommon, self-limited hypersensitivity response; triggers can be certain drugs, infections, malignancy, or collagen vascular disorders. Patients present with an array of "multiform" lesions including the characteristic targetoid lesion.

- *Stevens-Johnson syndrome* is a severe, febrile form typically occurring in children; there are erosions and hemorrhagic crusting of the lips, oral mucosa, conjunctiva, urethra, and anogenital regions. Bacterial superinfection may be life threatening.
- *Toxic epidermal necrolysis* is another variant, characterized by diffuse mucocutaneous epithelial necrosis and sloughing; it is clinically analogous to extensive third-degree burns.

Morphology (p. 1189)

- *Grossly: Multiform* lesions include macules, papules, vesicles, and bullae; *targets* are red maculopapular lesions with central pallor. Symmetric involvement of the extremities is common.
- *Microscopically:* Early lesions show dermal-epidermal and perivascular lymphocytic infiltrates with dermal edema and focal basal keratinocyte degeneration and necrosis. Exocytosis is associated with epidermal necrosis, blistering, and shallow erosions. *Target lesions* show central necrosis with associated perivenular inflammation.

Pathogenesis (p. 1189)

The etiology shares similarities to other immunologic cutaneous disorders (e.g., graft-versus-host disease and skin allograft rejection). Epithelial cells are injured by skin-homing (CLA+) CD8+ cytotoxic T lymphocytes (CTL); these are prominent in the central portion of lesions, while CD4+ T cells localize to the raised erythematous periphery.

Chronic Inflammatory Dermatoses (p. 1189)

These are persistent inflammatory disorders (months to years in duration) characterized by excessive scaling and desquamation.

Psoriasis (p. 1190)

Psoriasis affects 1% to 2% of the U.S. population and can be associated with other disorders (e.g., arthritis, myopathy, enteropathy, spondylitic joint disease, or AIDS). It most commonly affects the elbows, knees, scalp, lumbosacral area, intergluteal cleft, and glans penis; occasionally the entire body can be affected *(erythroderma).* Nail changes (30% of cases) consist of yellow-brown discoloration with onycholysis, thickening, and crumbling. Rarely, small pustules form on erythematous plaques *(pustular psoriasis);* when localized to hands and feet, this is benign, but systemic involvement can be life threatening.

Morphology (p. 1190)

- *Grossly:* Classic lesions are well-demarcated, salmon-pink plaques with silvery scaling. *Annular, linear, gyrate,* or *serpiginous* variations occur.
- *Microscopically:* Lesions exhibit marked acanthosis with downward rete elongation and with mitoses well above the basal layer. The stratum granulosum is thinned or absent, with extensive overlying parakeratosis. The epidermis adjacent to the acanthotic rete is markedly thinned; dilated vessels in the underlying dermal papillae yield pinpoint bleeds when the overlying scale is removed *(Auspitz sign).* Aggregates of epidermal neutrophils occur within small spongiotic foci in the stratum spinosum *(spongiform pustules)* or within the parakeratotic stratum corneum *(Munro microabscesses).* Larger, abscess-like accumulations may also occur in pustular psoriasis.

Pathogenesis (p. 1191)

An association with certain human leukocyte antigen (HLA) types suggests a genetic component; the genesis of new lesions at sites of trauma *(Koebner phenomenon)* suggests a role for exogenous stimuli. Sensitized CD4+ T_H1 and T_H17 cells and activated CTL accumulate in the epidermis and may drive keratinocyte proliferation by elaborating cytokines, for example, interleukin-12 (IL-12), interferon-γ (INF-γ), and IL-17; tumor necrosis factor (TNF), in particular, is a major pathogenic mediator.

Seborrheic Dermatitis (p. 1191)

Seborrhea affects 1% to 3% of the general population; although it typically involves skin with high densities of sebaceous glands (e.g., scalp, forehead, nasolabial folds, and presternum), it is *not* a disease of sebaceous glands. In infants, seborrheic dermatitis can present as "cradle cap," but it can also be a component of *Leiner disease* with generalized seborrhea, diarrhea, and failure to thrive. An especially severe form of seborrheic dermatitis occurs in the setting of acquired immunodeficiency syndrome (AIDS).

Morphology (p. 1191)

- *Grossly:* Lesions are macules or papules on a greasy, yellow erythematous base, often with scaling and crusting. Dandruff is the common expression of scalp lesions.
- *Microscopically:* Early lesions resemble spongiotic dermatitis, while later lesions are more reminiscent of acanthotic psoriasis. Mounds of parakeratosis admixed with acute inflammatory cells accumulate around hair follicles; there is also a superficial perivascular infiltrate of neutrophils and lymphocytes.

Pathogenesis (p. 1191)

The etiology is unknown, although the efficacy of antifungal agents suggests that lipophilic yeasts (e.g., *Malassezia furfur*) may be involved; sebum production can also be correlated to disease severity.

Lichen Planus (p. 1191)

Lichen planus is usually a self-limited disease that resolves after 1 to 2 years, leaving only postinflammatory hyperpigmentation; oral lesions may persist longer and occasionally become malignant.

Morphology (p. 1192)

- *Grossly:* Lesions are *pruritic, purple, polygonal planar papules* that may coalesce into *plaques;* lesions are often highlighted by white dots or lines (areas of hypergranulosis) called *Wickham striae.* Lesions are typically multiple and symmetrically distributed, often on the wrists and elbows and on the glans penis; oral mucosal lesions are generally white and netlike. A form with preferential involvement of hair follicle epithelium is called *lichen planopilaris.*
- *Microscopically:* There is a dense, bandlike dermal-epidermal junction lymphocytic infiltrate with basal cell degeneration and necrosis, and jagged rete sawtoothing. Necrotic basal cells may be sloughed into inflamed papillary dermis, forming *colloid* or *Civatte bodies.* Chronic changes include acanthosis, hyperkeratosis, and thickening of the granular cell layer.

Pathogenesis (p. 1192)

The etiology is unknown, but T-cell infiltrates with Langerhans cell hyperplasia suggest cell-mediated immune injury to altered antigens in basal cells; notably, the Koebner phenomenon also occurs in lichen planus.

Blistering (Bullous) Diseases (p. 1192)

These are *primary* blistering disorders, as opposed to vesicles and bullae that occur as a *secondary* phenomenon in a variety of unrelated conditions. The level within the skin where the blister occurs is important for diagnosis and is understandable based on knowledge of intercellular and cell-matrix attachments (Fig. 25-2).

Inflammatory Blistering Disorders (p. 1192)

Pemphigus (p. 1192)

Pemphigus is an uncommon and potentially life-threatening autoimmune disorder typically affecting patients 30 to 60 years old; treatment involves immunosuppression to reduce the titers of the pathogenic autoantibodies. There are multiple variants, depending on the level of the blister and the clinical manifestations:

- *Pemphigus vulgaris* accounts for 80% of cases; it involves oral mucosa, scalp, face, intertriginous zones, trunk, and pressure points. Lesions are superficial, easily ruptured blisters that leave shallow, crusted erosions. If untreated, it is almost uniformly fatal.
- *Pemphigus vegetans* is a rare form presenting with large, moist verrucous plaques studded with pustules, typically in flexural and intertriginous zones.
- *Pemphigus foliaceus* is a more benign form occurring epidemically in South America and sporadically elsewhere. Lesions occur mainly on the face, scalp, and upper trunk. Bullae are extremely superficial, leaving only slight erythema and crusting after rupture.
- *Pemphigus erythematosus* is a localized, milder variant of pemphigus foliaceus, typically involving only a malar distribution.
- *Paraneoplastic pemphigus* occurs in association with various malignancies, most commonly non-Hodgkin lymphoma.

Morphology (p. 1193)

Microscopically: All variants are characterized by *acantholysis* with intercellular clefting and *intraepithelial* blisters, with a variable dermal inflammatory infiltrate. For pemphigus vulgaris and vegetans, the separation occurs immediately above the basal layer *(suprabasal blister)*, leaving an intact layer of tombstone-like basal cells; in the vegetans variant, there is also overlying epidermal hyperplasia. In the foliaceus variant, only the stratum granulosum is involved. With anti-immunoglobulin or anti-complement immunofluorescence, netlike *(reticular)* staining may be seen in the epidermis, outlining each keratinocyte.

Pathogenesis (p. 1194)

Patients have circulating IgG directed against desmoglein components (see Fig. 25-2). Binding of these autoantibodies directly disrupts intercellular adhesion and also activates intercellular proteases.

Bullous Pemphigoid (p. 1195)

Bullous pemphigoid is an autoimmune blistering disease of skin and mucosa typically affecting elderly individuals. Bullae do not rupture as easily as in pemphigus and, if uninfected, heal without scarring.

Morphology (p. 1195)

- *Grossly:* Lesions are 2 to 8 cm tense bullae containing clear fluid; inner thigh, forearm flexor surfaces, lower abdomen, and intertriginous zones are common sites, and oral mucosa is involved in 10% to 15% of patients.

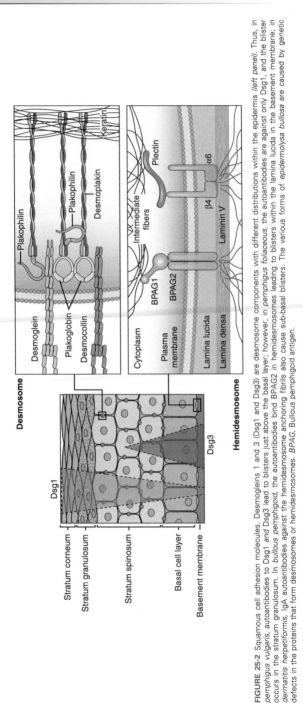

FIGURE 25-2 Squamous cell adhesion molecules. Desmogleins 1 and 3 (Dsg1 and Dsg3) are desmosome components with different distributions within the epidermis (*left panel*). Thus, in *pemphigus vulgaris*, autoantibodies to Dsg1 and Dsg3 lead to blisters just above the basal layer; however, in *pemphigus foliaceous*, the autoantibodies are against only Dsg1, and the blister occurs in the stratum granulosum. In *bullous pemphigoid*, the autoantibodies bind BPAG2 in hemidesmosomes leading to blisters within the lamina lucida in the basement membrane; in *dermatitis herpetiformis*, IgA autoantibodies against the hemidesmosome anchoring fibrils also cause sub-basal blisters. The various forms of *epidermolysa bullosa* are caused by genetic defects in the proteins that form desmosomes or hemidesmosomes. *BPAG*, Bullous pemphigoid antigen.

- *Microscopically:* Subepidermal, non-acantholytic blister with *linear* dermoepidermal junction staining for immunoglobulin and complement. There is a variable, superficial, perivascular dermal inflammatory cell infiltrate, and degranulated eosinophils are typically seen directly beneath the basal epithelial cells.

Pathogenesis (p. 1195)

Bullous pemphigoid is caused by autoantibodies against hemi-desmosome proteins (bullous pemphigoid antigen [BPAG]) that attach epidermal cells to the basal membrane; only antibodies against BPAG2 cause blistering. Bound autoantibodies cause injury via complement activation and granulocyte recruitment.

Dermatitis Herpetiformis (p. 1196)

Dermatitis herpetiformis is an uncommon disorder, characterized by intensely pruritic urticaria and grouped vesicles; typically occurring in young men, it is associated with celiac disease (Chapter 17) and responds to a gluten-free diet.

Pathogenesis (p. 1196)

Dermatitis herpetiformis is presumably mediated either by immune complex deposition in the skin or by gliadin (a gluten protein) antibodies cross-reacting with junction-anchoring components (e.g., reticulin).

Morphology (p. 1196)

- *Grossly:* Plaques and grouped vesicles are typically bilateral and symmetric, involving the extensor surfaces, upper back, and buttocks.
- *Microscopically:* Neutrophils and fibrin accumulate in the tips of dermal papillae *(microabscesses)* with overlying basal vacuolization coalescing to large subepidermal blisters. Immunofluorescence shows granular IgA deposits at the dermal papillae tips.

Noninflammatory Blistering Disorders (p. 1196)

Epidermolysis Bullosa (p. 1196)

Epidermolysis bullosa is a large group of non-inflammatory disorders (10 or so) that have in common blistering at pressure sites or trauma due to defects in the structural proteins forming the dermoepidermal junction.

- *Simplex type* results from mutations in keratins 5 or 14, leading to structural defects in the epidermal basal cell layer.
- *Junctional type* shows blistering at the lamina lucida in otherwise histologically normal skin.
- *Dystrophic type* shows blistering beneath the lamina densa due to type VII collagen mutations; this form typically leads to cutaneous scarring.

Porphyria (p. 1196)

Porphyria is a group of inborn or acquired disturbances of porphyrin metabolism (there are five major types based on biochemical and clinical features); porphyrins are the ring structures that bind metal ions in hemoglobin, myoglobin, and cytochromes. The cutaneous lesions consist of urticaria and vesicles that are exacerbated by sun exposure and heal without scarring. Histologically, there are subepidermal vesicles with marked thickening of the walls of superficial dermal vessels. The pathogenesis is unknown.

Disorders of Epidermal Appendages (p. 1197)

Acne Vulgaris (p. 1197)

Acne vulgaris is a common chronic lesion of hair follicles (particularly the sebaceous glands), typically occurring in middle to late adolescence and in males more often than in females. It is associated with hormonal changes and alterations in hair follicle maturation and can be induced by sex hormones, corticosteroids, occupational exposure (e.g., coal tars), or occlusive conditions (e.g., heavy clothes). There may be a heritable component.

Morphology (p. 1197)

- *Grossly:*

  Noninflammatory acne is characterized by *open comedones*—follicular papules with central black keratin plugs (the color is due to oxidized melanin), and *closed comedones*—follicular papules with central plugs trapped beneath the epidermis. The latter can rupture and cause inflammation.

  Inflammatory acne presents with erythematous papules, nodules, and pustules.

- *Microscopically:* Comedones are composed of expanding masses of lipid and keratin at the midportion of hair follicles, with follicular dilation, and epithelial and sebaceous gland atrophy. There is a variable lymphohistiocytic infiltrate, but with rupture there is extensive acute and chronic inflammation, occasionally with ensuing scar formation.

Pathogenesis (p. 1198)

Speculatively, acne involves bacterial *(Propionibacterium acnes)* lipase degradation of sebaceous oils to form highly irritating fatty acids and incite the early inflammatory lesions. Antibiotics (e.g., tetracyclines) may be effective by inhibiting the lipase activity, and vitamin A derivatives (13-*cis*-retinoic acid) have efficacy through their anti-sebaceous action.

Rosacea (p. 1198)

Rosacea affects up to 3% of the U.S. population, with a predilection for middle-aged women.

Morphology (p. 1198)

- *Grossly:* The disorder has four characteristic stages: (1) flushing; (2) persistent erythema and telangiectasia; (3) pustules and papules; and (4) *rhinophyma* (i.e., permanent thickening of the nasal skin by confluent papules and follicles).
- *Microscopically:* Lesions exhibit a nonspecific perifollicular lymphocyte infiltrate with dermal edema and telangiectasia. In the pustular phase, neutrophilic infiltrates and follicular rupture can elicit a dermal granulomatous response. Rhinophyma is associated with sebaceous hyperplasia and follicular plugging by keratotic debris

Pathogenesis (p. 1199)

Inappropriate activation of the innate immune system (characterized by increased cathelicidin production) is implicated.

Panniculitis (p. 1199)

Panniculitis is inflammation of subcutaneous fat; it may be acute or chronic, and it commonly involves the lower extremities.

Erythema Nodosum (p. 1199)

Erythema nodosum is the most common form; it typically has an acute onset and may be idiopathic or can occur in association with specific drugs, infections, sarcoidosis, inflammatory bowel disease, or visceral malignancy. It presents with ill-defined, exquisitely tender erythematous nodules, occasionally with fever and malaise. With time, old lesions flatten and become ecchymotic without scarring, while new lesions develop. Deep wedge biopsy shows distinctive early septal widening (i.e., edema, fibrin deposition, and neutrophil infiltration) and lymphohistiocytic infiltration (occasionally with giant cells and eosinophils) without vasculitis.

Erythema Induratum (p. 1199)

Erythema induratum is an uncommon form of panniculitis, typically affecting adolescents and menopausal women. It may represent a primary vasculitis of subcutaneous fat with subsequent inflammation and necrosis of adipose tissue. It presents as an erythematous, slightly tender nodule that eventually ulcerates and scars. Early lesions show necrotizing vasculitis in small- to medium-sized vessels in deep dermis and subcutis. Eventually the fat lobules develop granulomatous inflammation and necrosis.

Weber-Christian disease (relapsing febrile nodular panniculitis) is a rare, lobular form of panniculitis; it presents as crops of erythematous plaques or nodules, mainly on the legs, associated with deep lymphohistiocytic infiltrates and occasional giant cells. *Factitial panniculitis* (from self-administered foreign substances), deep mycotic infections in immunocompromised hosts, and occasionally disorders such as SLE can mimic the clinical and histologic appearance of primary panniculitis.

Infection (p. 1199)

Verrucae (Warts) (p. 1200)

Verrucae are common, spontaneously regressing (i.e., 6 months to 2 years) lesions, typically seen in children and adolescents. They are caused by human papillomaviruses (HPV), transmitted by direct contact.

Verrucae are classified by appearance and anatomic location:

- *Verruca vulgaris* is most common, typically found on the hand dorsum; lesions are gray-white to tan, flat to convex, less than 1 cm papules with a rough surface.
- *Verruca plana (flat wart)* usually present on the face or hand dorsum as flat, smooth, tan papules smaller than verruca vulgaris.
- *Verruca plantaris (soles) or palmaris (palms)* are rough, scaly 1 to 2 cm lesions; these can coalesce and be confused with calluses.
- *Condyloma acuminatum (anogenital and venereal warts)* are soft, tan, cauliflower-like masses measuring up to many centimeters in diameter.

Morphology (p. 1200)

Microscopically: All variants have undulant *(verrucous)* epidermal hyperplasia and superficial keratinocyte perinuclear vacuolization *(koilocytosis)*. Electron microscopy reveals numerous intranuclear viral particles.

Pathogenesis (p. 1201)

More than 150 types of HPV have been identified, many capable of causing lesions; the clinical variants of warts are often associated with specific HPV subtypes. Thus anogenital warts are caused predominantly by HPV 6 and 11, and type 16 is associated with dysplasia and *in situ* squamous cell carcinoma.

Molluscum Contagiosum (p. 1201)

This is a common, self-limited poxvirus infection transmitted by direct contact.

Morphology (p. 1201)

* *Grossly:* Firm, pruritic, pink to skin-colored, umbilicated papules 0.2 to 2 cm are seen on the trunk or anogenital regions; cheesy material containing diagnostic molluscum bodies can be expressed from the central umbilications.
* *Microscopically:* Lesions exhibit cuplike verrucous epidermal hyperplasia with pathognomonic *molluscum bodies*—eosinophilic cytoplasmic inclusions in the stratum granulosum or stratum corneum containing numerous virions.

Impetigo (p. 1201)

Impetigo is a common superficial bacterial infection; *Staphylococcus aureus* is the most common agent although β-hemolytic streptocci can also cause lesions. It is highly contagious; infection typically involves exposed skin, particularly the face and hands. A bullous form occurs mainly in children.

Morphology (p. 1201)

* *Grossly:* Lesions begin as erythematous macules that progress to small pustules and eventually to shallow erosions with a honey-colored crust.
* *Microscopically:* Characteristically, these are subcorneal pustules filled with neutrophils and Gram-positive cocci accompanied by non-specific dermal inflammation. The crust is formed by superficial layering of serum, neutrophils, and cellular debris.

Pathogenesis (p. 1201)

Epidermal bacterial infections provoke a destructive innate immune response with a serous exudate. Blister formation is driven by bacterial production of a toxin that cleaves Dsg1.

Superficial Fungal Infections (p. 1202)

Superficial fungal infections are confined to the nonviable stratum corneum; they are caused by dermatophytes derived from soil or animal contacts.

* *Tinea capitis* typically occurs in children. It causes asymptomatic hairless patches on the scalp, associated with mild erythema, crusting, and scale.
* *Tinea barbae* affects the beard area in men.
* *Tinea corporis* is a common superficial dermatophytosis of the body, especially in children. Predisposing factors are excessive heat or humidity, exposure to infected animals, and chronic foot or nail dermatophytosis. It typically presents with an expanding erythematous plaque with an elevated scaling border.
* *Tinea cruris* is typically found in the inguinal areas; obesity, heat, friction, and maceration are pre-disposing factors. It presents as moist red patches with raised scaling borders.
* *Tinea pedis (athlete's foot)* affects 30% to 40% of the population at some point; it is characterized by erythema and scaling, beginning in the webbed spaces between the digits. Most of the inflammation is due to secondary bacterial superinfection.

- *Tinea versicolor* (due to the yeast *Malassezia furfur*) typically presents on the upper trunk as groups of various-sized hyperpigmented or hypopigmented macules with a peripheral scale.
- *Onychomycosis* is a nail dermatophytosis characterized by discoloration, thickening, and deformity of the nail plate.

Morphology (p. 1202)

There is histologic variability depending on the organism, the host response, and the extent of bacterial superinfection; nevertheless, lesions characteristically exhibit reactive epidermal changes similar to mild eczematous dermatitis. Fungal organisms in the stratum corneum are revealed by special stains and can be cultured from scrapings of affected areas.

26

Bones, Joints, and Soft-Tissue Tumors

BONES (p. 1206)

- *Osteoblasts* are responsible for bone matrix synthesis and initiating mineralization; they derive from *osteoprogenitor cells*—pluripotent mesenchymal stem cells—through activation of the RUNX2/CBFA1 transcription factor network and WNT/β-catenin signaling pathway.
- *Osteocytes* are long-lived cells responsible for local bone calcium and phosphate homeostasis and for translating mechanical forces into biologic activity *(mechanotransduction);* they derive from osteoblasts.
- *Osteoclasts* are short-lived (2 weeks) multinucleated cells responsible for bone resorption; macrophage colony-stimulating factor (M-CSF), interleukin-1 (IL-1), and tumor necrosis factor (TNF) derive their differentiation from the same hematopoietic precursors as monocytes and macrophages.
- *Bone homeostasis* involves a balance of bone deposition by osteoblasts and resorption by osteoclasts; stromal cells and osteoblasts also critically regulate the differentiation and activation of osteoclasts (Fig. 26-1).

Developmental Abnormalities in Bone Cells, Matrix, and Structure (p. 1210)

While acquired bone disorders usually present in adulthood, most developmental anomalies are caused by genetic mutations and typically manifest during early stages of bone formation (Table 26-1).

- *Dysostoses:* Developmental anomalies due to abnormal mesenchymal cell migration or differentiation; these often result from mutations in homeobox transcription factor genes.

  Synpolydactyly is caused by mutation of the homeobox HOXD-13 transcription factor and manifests as an extra digit (polydactyly) and/or finger fusion (syndactyly).

- *Dysplasias:* mutations in signal molecules or matrix constituents (see later discussion) leading to more global skeletal disorders.

  Achondroplasia is the most common form of dwarfism; some cases are familial, but 80% involve new mutations, most arising in the paternal allele. All cases are caused by mutations in the fibroblast growth factor receptor-3 (FGFR-3), leading to constitutive

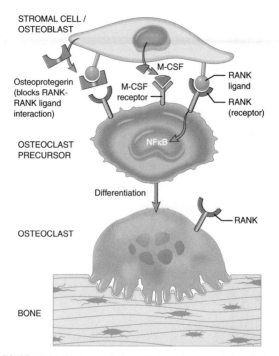

FIGURE 26-1 Molecular mechanisms that regulate osteoclast activation. Osteoblast or stromal cell RANKL binds to RANK on osteoclast precursors; in the presence of M-CSF, RANK-RANKL interactions induce osteoclast differentiation. Stromal cells also secrete osteoprotegerin (OPG), a "decoy" receptor for RANKL that blocks its ability to stimulate osteoclast precursors—thus inhibiting osteoclast differentiation and subsequent bone resorption. Not shown is a pathway involving stromal cell WNT binding to LRP5 and LRP6 receptors on osteoblasts (LRP = low-density lipoprotein receptor-related protein); this interaction activates β-catenin and induces OPG production. RANKL and OPG expression are also regulated by various hormones (e.g., parathyroid horme, estrogen, testosterone, and glucocorticoids), vitamin D, inflammatory cytokines (e.g., IL-1), and selected growth factors (e.g., bone morphogenic proteins). *M-CSF,* Macrophage colony-stimulating factor; *RANK,* receptor activator for nuclear factor-κB; *RANKL,* receptor activator for nuclear factor-κB ligand.

activation. Anatomically, the growth plates are shortened and disordered, resulting in abnormally short extremity bones; because appositional growth is not affected, bones are of normal width and the skull appears comparatively enlarged.

- *Increased bone mass* (causing diseases such as endosteal hyperostosis and osteopetrosis type I) can result from low-density lipoprotein receptor-related protein-5 (LRP5) gain-of-function mutations that drive constitutive osteoblast activation via the WNT/β-catenin pathway. Conversely, inactivating LRP5 mutations causes severe osteoporosis and multiple fractures.

Diseases Associated with Defects in Extracellular Structural Proteins *(p. 1210)*

Type 1 Collagen Diseases (Osteogenesis Imperfecta, Brittle Bone Disease) *(p. 1211)*

Type 1 collagen diseases represent a group of related genetic disorders caused by qualitatively or quantitatively abnormal type I collagen synthesis (constituting about 90% of bone organic matrix).

TABLE 26-1 Molecular Genetics of Diseases of the Skeleton

Human Disorder	Gene Mutation	Affected Molecule	Phenotype
Defects in Transcription Factors Producing Abnormalities in Mesenchymal Condensation and Related Cell Differentiation			
Synpolydactyly	HOXD-13	Transcription factor	Extra digit with fusion
Waardenburg syndrome	PAX-3	Transcription factor	Hearing loss, abnormal pigmentation, craniofacial abnormalities
Greig syndrome	GLI3	Transcription factor	Synpolydactyly, craniofacial abnormalities
Campomelic dysplasia	SOX9	Transcription factor	Sex reversal, abnormal skeletal development
Oligodontia	PAX9	Transcription factor	Congenital absence of teeth
Nail-patella syndrome	LMX1B	Transcription factor	Hypoplastic nails, hypoplastic or aplastic patellae, dislocated radial head, progressive nephropathy
Holt-Oram syndrome	TBX5	Transcription factor	Congenital abnormalities, forelimb anomalies
Ulnar-mammary syndrome	TBX3	Transcription factor	Hypoplasia or absent ulna, 3rd–5th digits, breast, and teeth, delayed puberty
Cleidocranial dysplasia	CBFA1	Transcription factor	Abnormal clavicles, wormian bones, supernumerary teeth
Defects in Extracellular Structural Proteins			
Osteogenesis imperfecta types 1-4	COL1A1, COL1A2	Type 1 collagen	Bone fragility, hearing loss, blue sclerae, dentinogenesis imperfecta
Achondrogenesis II	COL2A1	Type 2 collagen	Short trunk, severely shortened extremities, relatively enlarged cranium, flattened face
Hypochondrogenesis	COL2A1	Type 2 collagen	Short trunk, shortened extremities, relatively enlarged cranium, flattened face
Stickler syndrome	COL2A1	Type 2 collagen	Myopia, retinal detachment, hearing loss, flattened face, premature osteoarthritis
Multiple epiphyseal dysplasia	COL9A2	Type 9 collagen	Short or normal stature, small epiphyses, early-onset osteoarthritis
Schmid metaphyseal chondrodysplasia	COL10A1	Type 10 collagen	Mild short stature, bowing of lower extremities, coxa vara, metaphyseal flaring

TABLE 26-1 Molecular Genetics of Diseases of the Skeleton—cont'd

Human Disorder	Gene Mutation	Affected Molecule	Phenotype
Defects in Hormones and Signal Transduction Mechanisms Producing Abnormal Proliferation or Maturation of Chondrocytes and Osteoblasts			
Brachydactyly type C	CDMP1	Signaling molecule	Shortened metacarpals and phalanges
Jansen metaphyseal chondroplasia	PTHrp receptor	Receptor	Short bowed limbs, clinodactyly, facial abnormalities, hypercalcemia, hypophosphatemia
Achondroplasia	FGFR-3	Receptor	Short stature, rhizomelic shortening of limbs, frontal bossing, midface deficiency
Hypochondroplasia	FGFR-3	Receptor	Disproportionate short stature, micromelia, relative macrocephaly
Thanatophoric dwarfism	FGFR-3	Receptor	Severe limb shortening and bowing, frontal bossing, depressed nasal bridge
Crouzon syndrome	FGFR-2	Receptor	Craniosynostosis
Osteoporosis-pseudoglioma syndrome	LRP5	Receptor	Congenital or infant-onset loss of vision, skeletal fragility

Data from Mundlos S, Olsen BR: Heritable diseases of the skeleton. Part I: Molecular insights into skeletal development—transcription factors and signaling pathways, *FASEB J* 11:125-132, 1997; Mundlos S, Olsen BR: Heritable diseases of the skeleton. Part II: Molecular insights into skeletal development—matrix components and their homeostasis, *FASEB J* 11:227-233, 1997; Superti-Furga A, et al: Molecular-pathogenetic classification of genetic disorders of the skeleton, *Am J Med Genet* 106:262-293, 2001.

- Classically, these involve autosomal dominant mutations in the genes coding the collagen α1 and α2 chains; in most cases, other amino acids are substituted in place of glycines in the primary sequence.
- Mutations leading to decreased synthesis of qualitatively normal collagen usually exhibit mild skeletal abnormalities; severe—and even lethal—phenotypes are associated with mutations that cause abnormal polypeptides that cannot be assembled into triple helices.
- Morphologically, there is *osteopenia* (too little bone), with marked cortical thinning and trabecular rarefaction, leading to increased fracture susceptibility. The classic "blue sclera" is due to decreased collagen content, causing translucent sclera that permits visualization of the underlying choroid; hearing loss is related in part to impeded conduction due to abnormalities of bones of the middle and inner ear; dental imperfections are due to dentin deficiency.
- There are four major subtypes based on the specific biosynthetic abnormality and the clinical manifestations. Syndromes range from *type II* that is uniformly fatal in the perinatal period (from multiple bone fractures) to other variants with increased risk of fractures but compatible with survival.

Diseases Associated with Mutations of Types 2, 9, 10, and 11 Collagen (p. 1212)

Diseases associated with mutations of types 2, 9, 10, and 11 collagen are related to abnormal hyaline cartilage synthesis (see Table 26-1); in severe disorders, absence of type 2 collagen synthesis leads to insufficient bone formation, whereas milder forms are associated with reduced synthesis of normal type 2 collagen.

Diseases Associated with Defects in Folding and Degradation of Macromolecules (p. 1212)

Mucopolysaccharidoses (p. 1212)

Mucopolysaccharidoses are a group of lysosomal storage diseases caused by deficiencies in enzymes that degrade mucopolysaccharides (e.g., dermatan sulfate, heparan sulfate, and keratan sulfate). Since chondrocytes are responsible for mucopolysaccharide metabolism, hyaline cartilage (e.g., growth plates, costal cartilages, and articular surfaces) is typically most affected; patients are frequently short and have malformed bones and chest abnormalities.

Diseases Associated with Defects in Metabolic Pathways (Enzymes, Ion Channels, and Transporters) (p. 1212)

Osteopetrosis (p. 1212)

Osteopetrosis (marble bone disease, Albers-Schönberg disease) is a group of genetic disorders characterized by reduced osteoclastic activity; although there is increased mass, the bone is abnormally brittle and fractures like chalk. Diffuse skeletal sclerosis also impinges on the medullary cavity and impairs hematopoiesis.

Pathogenesis (p. 1213)

Most mutations interfere with osteoclast acidification of the resorptive pit, a step required to dissolve matrix calcium hydroxyapatite prior to bone resorption. Thus, mutations in carbonic anhydrase II reduce the formation of protons from carbon dioxide (CO_2) and water (they also block renal tubular acidification of urine). Other mutations in the chloride channel gene *CLCN7* or in the *TCIRG1* gene (encodes part of the proton pump) interfere with the function of the osteoclast H^+-ATPase proton pump. Yet other mutations in the genes encoding RANK, RANKL, M-CSF, or OPG can lead to reduced numbers of osteoclasts.

Clinical Features (p. 1214)

Fractures and anemia are frequently early heralds of osteopetrosis; patients can also have hydrocephaly and cranial nerve defects (e.g., optic atrophy, deafness, and facial paralysis) due to abnormal skull bone remodeling. Recurrent infections (inadequate white cell production) and hepatosplenomegaly (due to extramedullary hematopoiesis) are also features. The disease can be treated with bone marrow transplantation, since osteoclasts derive from monocyte precursors.

Diseases Associated with Decreased Bone Mass (p. 1214)

Osteoporosis (p. 1214)

Osteoporosis is characterized by porous bones and reduced bone mass, predisposing to fracture; it can be localized to a specific site (e.g., disuse osteoporosis of a limb) or can be a generalized disorder of primary (senile) or secondary causes (due to endocrine abnormalities, malabsorption, or neoplasia). Osteoporosis occurs most commonly in aged individuals and is most pronounced in postmenopausal women.

Pathogenesis (p. 1214)

Senile and postmenopausal osteoporosis are multifactorial disorders (Fig. 26-2).

- Genetic factors influence 60% to 80% of peak bone density; polymorphisms in RANKL, RANK, OPG, LRP5, and the estrogen and vitamin D receptors have all been implicated. Physical activity, muscle strength, diet (e.g., calcium and vitamin D), and hormonal status also influence bone deposition. After achieving

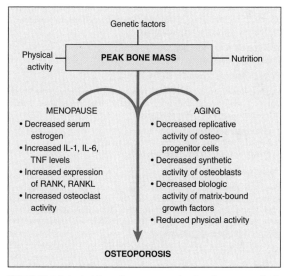

FIGURE 26-2 Pathophysiology of postmenopausal and senile osteoporosis. *IL,* Interleukin; *RANK,* receptor activator for nuclear factor κB; *RANKL,* RANK ligand; *TNF,* tumor necrosis factor.

peak bone mass in young adulthood, each cycle of bone turnover accrues a predictable shortfall in bone formation relative to absorption, averaging a 0.7% deficit each year regardless of gender.

- Age-related changes diminish osteoblast proliferation and biosynthetic potential; osteogenic growth factors bound to the extracellular matrix also show diminished activity with increasing age.
- Decreased physical activity accelerates bone loss because mechanical forces stimulate normal bone remodeling; the magnitude of bone loading influences bone density more than the number of load cycles.
- In postmenopausal women, decreased estrogen levels promote increased osteoclastic activity by increasing monocyte production of IL-1, IL-6, and TNF; these cytokines recruit and activate osteoclasts by increasing RANKL expression while reducing OPG synthesis. Compensatory osteoblastic activity occurs, but it does not keep pace with the bone loss.

Morphology (p. 1215)

Although the entire skeleton is involved in postmenopausal and senile osteoporosis, increased osteoclast activity mainly affects bone with increased surface area (e.g., the cancellous compartment of vertebral bodies). Progressive thinning of trabeculae leads to progressive microfractures and eventual bony collapse. Cortical bone is thinned by subperiosteal and endosteal resorption, and haversian systems are widened.

Clinical Course (p. 1216)

Microfractures cause pain and loss in height and stability of the vertebral column. Osteoporosis also predisposes to fractures of pelvis, femoral neck, and spine; complications (including pulmonary embolism and pneumonia) are responsible for 50,000 deaths per year. Osteoporosis cannot be reliably identified on standard radiographs until 30% to 40% of bone mass has been lost; early detection requires bone densitometry measurements. Therapy involves exercise, calcium and vitamin D supplementation, and osteoclast inhibition with bisphosphonates.

Diseases Caused by Osteoclast Dysfunction (p. 1216)

Paget Disease (Osteitis Deformans) (p. 1216)

Paget disease results in a focal increase in bone mass; the excess bone is disordered and architecturally unsound. Paget disease progresses through three stages:

- Osteolytic bone resorption
- Mixed osteolytic and osteoblastic activity
- Burnt-out, quiescent osteosclerosis

Pathogenesis (p. 1216)

Both environmental and genetic factors are implicated; mutations in the *SQSTM1* gene (enhancing RANK signaling) increase susceptibility and are present in 40% to 50% of familial cases and 5% to 10% of sporadic cases. A contributory role for paramyxovirus infection remains unproved.

Morphology (p. 1217)

- The *osteolytic phase* is marked by resorption by numerous, large osteoclasts (some containing more than 100 nuclei).
- The *mixed phase* exhibits osteoclasts and osteoblasts lining bone surfaces with disordered woven and lamellar bone formation;

adjacent marrow spaces are replaced by loose connective tissue. The lamellar bone assumes a pathognomonic *mosaic* pattern.

- The *burnt-out phase* is marked by bone sclerosis composed of coarsely thickened trabeculae and cortices; the bone is soft and porous and lacks structural stability.

Clinical Course (p. 1217)

Paget disease has an average age of onset of 70 years; the prevalence is high in the United States (1%) and Europe but low in China, Japan, and Africa. It is monostotic in 15% of cases, and the axial skeleton or proximal femur is involved in 80% of patients.

- Pain is a common feature, associated with fractures, nerve compression, osteoarthritis, and skeletal deformities (e.g., tibial bowing, skull enlargement).
- Facial bone coarsening may produce *leontiasis ossea* (lion-like facies). Less commonly, the vascularity of polyostotic lesions can cause high-output heart failure. In 1% of patients, secondary sarcoma develops.
- Most affected individuals have mild symptoms suppressible by calcitonin and bisphosphonates.

Diseases Associated with Abnormal Mineral Homeostasis (p. 1218)

Rickets and Osteomalacia *(p. 1218)*

Rickets (children) and osteomalacia (adults) are disorders characterized by defective matrix mineralization; these are most often secondary to vitamin D deficiency or other calcium metabolic disturbance (Chapter 9).

Hyperparathyroidism *(p. 1218)*

Hyperparathyroidism, either primary or secondary (e.g., in renal failure), is characterized by increased parathyroid hormone (PTH) with unabated osteoclastic bone resorption.

Morphology (p. 1218)

- The entire skeleton is affected, although some sites more than others; cortical bone is affected more than cancellous bone.
- Increased bone resorption is also associated with increased osteoblast activity; fibrovascular tissues replace the surrounding marrow spaces.
- Microfractures and associated hemorrhages elicit an influx of macrophages with reparative fibrous tissue, called *brown tumors;* this is designated *osteitis fibrosa cystica* (also known as *von Recklinghausen disease of bone*).

Renal Osteodystrophy *(p. 1218)*

Renal osteodystrophy refers to the various bone changes associated with chronic renal failure: increased osteoclastic activity, delayed matrix mineralization *(osteomalacia)*, osteosclerosis, growth retardation, and osteoporosis. Patients exhibit some combination of *high-turnover osteodystrophy* (characterized by increased bone resorption and formation) and *low-turnover disease* (manifested by largely quiescent bone).

Pathogenesis (p. 1219)

- Chronic renal failure results in phosphate retention (hyperphosphatemia), leading to increased PTH production *(secondary hyperparathyroidism)* and increased osteoclast activity.
- Hypocalcemia develops due to diminished 25-hydroxylation of vitamin D by damaged kidneys and reduced intestinal absorption of calcium.

- Reduced 1,25-$(OH)_2D_3$ leads to increased PTH production, and renal failure leads to diminished excretion of PTH.
- Metabolic acidosis associated with renal failure stimulates bone resorption and calcium hydroxyapatite release.
- Aluminum—from dialysis solutions and aluminum-containing oral phosphate binders—is deposited in bone and interferes with calcium hydroxyapatite deposition (causing osteomalacia).
- Hemodialysis patients have elevated levels of β_2-microglobulin (not removed by dialysis) leading to formation of amyloid in bone and periarticular structures.

Fractures (p. 1219)

Fractures are classified as:

- *Complete* or *incomplete*
- *Closed (simple)* when the overlying tissue is intact; *compound* when the fracture communicates with the skin
- *Comminuted* when the bone is splintered
- *Displaced* when the ends of the fractured bone are not aligned
- *Pathologic fractures* are breaks in bones altered by a disease process
- *Stress fractures* are slowly developing breaks associated with repetitive physical loading

Fracture healing—regulated by cytokines and growth factors—involves reactivating bone formation pathways that normally occur during embryogenesis:

- *Procallus formation:* Within a week of breaking, fracture site hematomas are organized by an influx of inflammatory cells, fibroblasts, and new vessels; platelets and inflammatory cells release platelet-derived growth factor (PDGF), transforming growth factor-β (TGF-β), fibroblast growth factor (FGF), and interleukins that trigger osteoprogenitor cells and stimulate osteoclast and osteoblast activity.
- The procallus is converted to a *fibrocartilaginous callus* composed of reactive mesenchymal cells; the new cartilage along the fracture line undergoes enchondral ossification (analogous to bone formation at a growth plate), eventually forming a *bony callus*. Progressive mineralization increases callus stiffness and strength.
- The osseous callus is eventually remodeled along lines of weight bearing to complete the repair.

If fractures are well aligned and the original weight-bearing strains are restored, virtually perfect repair is accomplished. Imperfect results are seen with malalignment, comminution, inadequate immobilization, infection, and superimposed systemic abnormality (e.g., dietary deficiency, osteoporosis). Nonunion with excessive motion along the fracture gap can cause callus cystic degeneration; the luminal surface can then become synovium-lined to create a false joint *(pseudoarthrosis)*.

Osteonecrosis (Avascular Necrosis) (p. 1220)

Bone and marrow infarction is relatively common; traumatic fracture, which causes vascular interruption, is the most common cause, with most other osteonecrosis being either idiopathic or associated with corticosteroid administration. Other, less frequent causes include infection, radiation therapy, vasculitis, sickle cell and other anemias, Gaucher disease, and air embolism *(caisson disease)*.

Morphology (p. 1220)

Medullary infarcts are geographic and involve cancellous bone and marrow. Cortical bone is usually not affected because of collateral blood flow; articular cartilage over subchondral infarcts remains viable by virtue of nutrient diffusion from synovial fluid. Necrotic bone shows empty lacunae; ruptured adipocytes can have associated fat saponification. *Creeping substitution* with new bone occurs from the margin of the infarct. In subchondral infarcts, the articular cartilage may collapse into the necrotic bone.

Clinical Course (p. 1221)

Patients may be asymptomatic, but subchondral lesions often cause joint pain and predispose to subsequent osteoarthritis. More than 10% of the half million joint replacements in the United States annually are for complications of osteonecrosis.

Infections—Osteomyelitis (p. 1221)

Pyogenic Osteomyelitis (p. 1221)

Pyogenic osteomyelitis is almost always bacterial; seeding occurs by:

- Hematogenous spread (most common in children, typically involving long bones)
- Extension from a contiguous infection (e.g., diabetic foot ulcer)
- Open fracture or surgical procedure

In half of cases, no organism can be identified. *S. aureus* is responsible for 80% to 90% of the remainder, largely related to receptors that enhance adherence to bone matrix; patients with sickle cell anemia are prone to *Salmonella* infections.

Morphology (p. 1222)

Morphologic changes are dependent on the chronicity and location of the infection. Once in bone, bacteria proliferate and engender an acute inflammatory response.

- Entrapped bone undergoes necrosis within the first 48 hours, and bacteria and inflammation can then percolate within the shaft and along haversian systems to involve the periosteum.
- Lifting of the periosteum further compromises vascular supply to the area and leads to a zone of bone necrosis; rupture of the periosteum can lead to a soft-tissue abscess and a *draining sinus*.
- A dead piece of bone is called a *sequestrum*.
- After the first week, chronic inflammatory infiltrates stimulate osteoclastic bone resorption, ingrowth of fibrous connective tissue, and deposition of reactive bone. The subperiosteal new bone encasing the inflammatory focus is called an *involucrum*. A small, walled-off intracortical abscess is called a *Brodie abscess*.

Clinical Course (p. 1222)

Pyogenic osteomyelitis is classically an acute febrile illness associated with local pain; subtle lesions can present in infants as unexplained fever or in adults as focal pain without fever. Antibiotics and surgical drainage are usually curative, although 5% to 25% of cases persist as chronic infections (usually due to extensive bone necrosis, inadequate therapy, or immunocompromise). Complications include pathologic fracture, amyloidosis, endocarditis, and development of squamous cell carcinoma in the sinus tract or sarcoma in the infected bone.

Tuberculous Osteomyelitis (p. 1222)

Tuberculous osteomyelitis occurs in 1% to 3% of patients with pulmonary or extrapulmonary tuberculosis. Organisms are typically blood-borne, although direct extension or lymphatic seeding can occur; bony infection is usually solitary unless the patient is immunocompromised. The spine is involved in 40% of cases *(Pott disease)* with frequent invasion into soft tissues and abscess formation; knees and hips are other common sites. Lesions exhibit typical granulomatous reaction with caseous necrosis.

Bone Tumors and Tumor-Like Lesions (p. 1223)

Most bone tumors are asymptomatic and are detected as incidental findings; others present with pain or as a slow-growing mass, and a small number announce as pathologic fractures. In diagnosing bone tumors, patient age, neoplasm location, and radiologic appearance are important (Table 26-2); biopsy and histologic evaluation are necessary. Benign tumors greatly outnumber their malignant counterparts, although in the elderly, a bone tumor is more likely to be malignant. While bone sarcomas occur in the setting of *p53* and *RB* mutations, the cause of most bone malignancies is unknown; secondary causes (e.g., Paget disease, chronic osteomyelitis, radiation, etc.) account for only a small fraction.

Bone-Forming Tumors (p. 1224)

Bone production by the neoplastic cells is the common feature of these tumors; most of the bone is deposited as woven trabeculae (except osteomas) and is variably mineralized.

TABLE 26-2	Classification of Major Primary Tumors Involving Bones	
Histologic Type	**Benign**	**Malignant**
Hematopoietic (40%)		Myeloma Malignant lymphoma
Chondrogenic (22%)	Osteochondroma Chondroma Chondroblastoma Chondromyxoid fibroma	Chondrosarcoma Dedifferentiated chondrosarcoma Mesenchymal chondrosarcoma
Osteogenic (19%)	Osteoid osteoma Osteoblastoma	Osteosarcoma
Fibrogenic	Fibrous cortical defect (fibroma) Non-ossifying fibroma Fibrous histiocytoma Desmoplastic fibroma	Fibrosarcoma
Unknown origin (10%)	Giant-cell tumor Unicameral cyst Aneurysmal bone cyst	
Neuroectodermal		Ewing sarcoma
Notochordal	Benign notochordal cell tumor	Chordoma

Data on percentage of each type from Unni KK: *Dahlin's bone tumors,* ed 5, Philadelphia, 1996, Lippincott-Raven, p 4.

Osteoma (p. 1224)

Osteomas are bosselated, sessile tumors projecting from the subperiosteal surface of the cortex; skull and facial bones are most commonly affected. Most are solitary; multiple lesions occur in the setting of *Gardner syndrome* (Chapter 17). Osteomas are typically composed of well-formed cortical bone. Unless their location (e.g., nasal sinus, inner skull) compromises local organ function or produces cosmetic deformities, they are of little clinical significance.

Osteoid Osteoma and Osteoblastoma (p. 1224)

Osteoid osteoma and osteoblastoma are benign neoplasms with identical histologic features but differing size, location, and symptoms.

- *Osteoid osteomas* are small (less than 2 cm) and usually occur between ages 10 and 30 years; men outnumber women 2:1. There is a predilection for extremities and spine, with half arising in the femur or tibia. They classically manifest with nocturnal pain (due to prostaglandin E2 production) relieved by aspirin. Treatment often involves radioablation.
- *Osteoblastomas* are longer than 2 cm, and more frequently involve the spine; the pain is dull, achy, and unresponsive to salicylates. Tumors are usually curetted on excised *en bloc*; malignant transformation is rare except following radiation treatment.

Morphology (p. 1224)

- *Grossly:* Lesions are round-oval masses of hemorrhagic gritty tan tissue.
- *Microscopically:* Tumors are well-circumscribed nodules of radiologically translucent woven bone (nidus) rimmed by osteoblasts; this is surrounded by highly vascular loose connective tissue enclosed by radiologically dense reactive sclerotic bone.

Osteosarcoma (p. 1225)

Osteosarcoma is a malignant mesenchymal tumor where neoplastic cells produce bone matrix; 75% occur before age 20 years, with most of the remainder developing in geriatric patients with known risk factors (e.g., Paget disease, radiation). Most are solitary, arising in the medullary cavity of the metaphyses of extremity long bones; roughly half occur around the knee.

Pathogenesis (p. 1225)

Osteosarcomas tend to occur at sites of bone growth (presumably because proliferation makes cells prone to acquiring mutations), and they frequently exhibit *p53* or *RB* mutations; genetic abnormalities of p16 (cell cycle regulator) and p14 (aids p53 function) are also associated.

Morphology (p. 1225)

- *Grossly:* Tumors are large, destructive, tan-white, gritty, and sometimes bloody and cystic masses.
- *Microscopically:* Osteosarcomas are composed of large, hyperchromatic, pleomorphic, mitotically active tumor cells. They can exhibit osteoblastic, chondroblastic, or fibroblastic differentiation; *all form neoplastic bone that frequently has a coarse lace-like pattern.* Vascular invasion is usually conspicuous, and more than half of any given tumor may be necrotic.

Clinical Course (p. 1226)

Osteosarcomas typically present as painful, progressively enlarging masses. Radiographs show destructive and infiltrative lesions with mixed blastic and lytic features; when the tumor breaks through the cortex and lifts the periosteum, it forms a characteristic (but not diagnostic) *Codman triangle*. Osteosarcomas are aggressive malignancies with 10% to 20% having demonstrable pulmonary metastases at the time of first diagnosis; many more have likely occult metastatic disease. Surgery and adjuvant chemotherapy yields a 60% to 70%, 5-year survival in the absence of detectable metastases; with overt distal disease, the 5-year survival falls to 20%.

Cartilage-Forming Tumors (p. 1227)

Cartilage-forming tumors constitute the majority of primary bone neoplasms; most form hyaline or myxoid cartilage. Benign tumors are considerably more common than malignant ones.

Osteochondroma (p. 1227)

Osteochondroma is the most common benign bone tumor; the male to female ratio is 3:1. Also called *exostosis*, these can be solitary sporadic lesions (85% of cases) or occur as multiple tumors in the autosomal-dominant *multiple hereditary exostosis syndrome*. Hereditary lesions are associated with loss-of-function mutations in *EXT1* or *EXT2* genes (encoding proteins that participate in the synthesis of heparan sulfate proteoglycans); sporadic lesions are associated with only *EXT1* inactivation. Reduced EXT activity leads to defective enchondral ossification, setting the stage for abnormal growth.

Osteochondromas commonly develop in the metaphyseal region (near the growth plate) of long bones, especially near the knee. They present as slow-growing lesions that can be painful if they impinge on nerves or the stalk is fractured. In multiple hereditary exostosis, the underlying bone may be bowed and shortened, reflecting abnormal epiphyseal growth. They infrequently give rise to chondrosarcomas.

Morphology (p. 1227)

- *Grossly:* Lesions are mushroom-shaped surface protrusions 1 to 20 cm in size, covered by perichondrium overlying a hyaline cartilage cap.
- *Microscopically:* The cartilage cap has the appearance of disorganized growth plate and undergoes enchondral ossification. The outer stalk cortex and medullary cavities of the cap are in continuity with the cortex and marrow cavity of the underlying bone.

Chondromas (p. 1227)

Chondromas are benign tumors composed of hyaline cartilage; *enchondromas* arise within the medullary cavity, while *juxtacortical chondromas* arise on the bone surface. They are usually solitary metaphyseal lesions of tubular bones, commonly occurring between ages 20 and 40 years. A syndrome with multiple enchondromas is called *Ollier disease;* similar enchondromatosis associated with hemangiomas is designated *Maffucci syndrome.*

Morphology (p. 1227)

- *Grossly:* Enchondromas are usually less than 3 cm and translucent gray-blue.
- *Microscopically:* Lesions are composed of well-circumscribed nodules of benign hyaline cartilage; there can be peripheral enchondral ossification and central calcification and necrosis.

Clinical Features (p. 1228)

Chondromas are usually asymptomatic but may cause bone deformity (especially in enchondromatosis), pain, and fracture. Radiologic imaging reveals characteristic circumscribed oval lucencies with a thin rim of radio-dense bone; matrix calcification is detected as irregular opacification. Most tumors are stable, and treatment involves only curettage. Solitary lesion rarely undergo malignant transformation; evolution to sarcomas occurs more frequently with enchondromatosis. Patients with Maffucci syndrome are at increased risk of ovarian carcinoma and central nervous system (CNS) gliomas.

Chondroblastoma (p. 1228)

Chondroblastoma is a rare benign tumor, typically occurring in young men (2:1 male to female ratio); it has a predilection for the epiphyses of bones around the knees. Lesions are usually painful; radiologically, there is a well-defined lucency with spotty calcifications. Tumors often recur after curettage, and pulmonary metastases can also rarely occur.

Morphology (p. 1228)

Tumor cells are polygonal, arranged in sheets, and sometimes surrounded by a lacelike pattern of focally hyaline cartilage. Their nuclei are often deeply indented or longitudinally grooved. Multinucleated, osteoclast-like giant cells may be present, as well as hemorrhagic cystic degeneration.

Chondromyxoid Fibroma (p. 1229)

Chondromyxoid fibroma is the rarest of the cartilage-forming tumors; it typically affects males between the ages of 10 and 30 years, and most commonly involves the metaphyses of long tubular bones. Patients typically present with dull, achy pain; radiographs exhibit an area of lucency with a rim of sclerotic bone. Treatment involves curettage; even when fibromas recur, metastasis or malignant transformation do not occur.

Morphology (p. 1229)

- *Grossly:* Tumors are 3 to 8 cm, well-circumscribed, solid, glistening, and tan-gray.
- *Microscopically:* Lesions exhibit nodules of poorly-formed hyaline cartilage and myxoid tissue delineated by fibrous septae. There is variable cellularity and cytologic atypia, with focal calcification and scattered non-neoplastic, osteoclast-type giant cells.

Chondrosarcoma (p. 1229)

Chondrosarcoma is the second most common malignant matrix-producing bone tumor; it is roughly half as common as osteosarcoma. Most patients are older than 40 years, and the male to female ratio is 2:1. Most cases (85%) arise *de novo* with the remainder occurring in a preexisting enchondroma or osteochondroma. The majority occur in the central portion of the skeleton (i.e., pelvis, shoulders, ribs), and distal extremities are rarely involved. Tumors typically present as painful, progressively enlarging masses. Radiologically, there is endosteal scalloping and flocculent-appearing matrix calcification; slow-growing tumors cause reactive cortical thickening, whereas high-grade neoplasms destroy the cortex and form a soft-tissue mass. Treatment involves wide surgical excision and often chemotherapy. Lung and skeleton are favored metastatic sites.

Morphology (p. 1229)

- *Grossly:* Tumors are lobulated, gray, glistening and semitranslucent; necrosis and spotty calcification are frequently present.
- *Microscopically:* Lesions are classified by histologic type and as *intramedullary* or *juxtacortical*; 90% are intramedullary *conventional* (hyaline or myxoid) chondrosarcomas. The histologic

grade (based on cellularity, cytologic atypia, and mitotic activity) correlates with biologic behavior; most tumors are low-grade. Grade 1 or 2 lesions have 5-year survivals of 90% and 81%, respectively, and grade 3 lesions have a 43%, 5-year survival.

Fibrous and Fibro-Osseous Tumors (p. 1230)

Fibrous Cortical Defect And Non-Ossifying Fibroma (p. 1230)

Fibrous cortical defect and non-ossifying fibroma are closely related benign tumors. Radiologically, they are elongated, sharply demarcated radiolucencies surrounded by a thin rim of sclerosis.

- *Fibrous cortical defects* are small (0.5 cm) developmental defects (rather than neoplasms) occurring in 30% to 50% of children older than 2 years. Most arise in the metaphysis of the distal femur or proximal tibia and are asymptomatic; the majority of these defects are eventually replaced by normal cortical bone.
- *Nonossifying fibomas* are 5 to 6 cm in size and develop from enlargement of fibrous cortical defects. These can present with a pathologic fracture; curettage and histologic evaluation are necessary to exclude other tumors.

Morphology (p. 1230)

These are gray-yellow cellular lesions containing cytologically bland fibroblasts and macrophages; the latter may be foamy or multi-nucleated.

Fibrous Dysplasia (p. 1230)

Fibrous dysplasia is a benign lesion akin to a localized developmental arrest; all the elements of normal bone are present but do not differentiate into mature structures.

- In 70% of patients, only one bone is involved *(monostotic disease)*. Lesions typically arise in early adolescence and stop growing at the point of epiphyseal fusion; boys and girls are equally affected. Most lesions are asymptomatic, but pain, fracture, discrepancies in limb length, or distortion of craniofacial bones can occur.
- *Polyostotic disease without endocrine dysfunction* accounts for 27% of cases; it manifests at a slightly earlier age than monostotic disease. Craniofacial, shoulder, and pelvic girdle involvement are extremely common and can cause crippling deformities (e.g., shepherd-crook deformity of the proximal femur).
- *Polyostotic disease associated with café-au-lait skin pigmentation and endocrinopathies (McCune-Albright syndrome)* accounts for 3% of cases. This is associated with gain-of-function mutations of the *GNAS* gene leading to constitutive activation of the $G_S\alpha$ G-protein subunit and elevated intracellular cAMP. Such mutations can cause pituitary adenomas (Chapter 24), as well as sexual precocity, hyperthyroidism, and primary adrenal hyperplasia (hence the various associated endocrinopathies).

Morphology (p. 1231)

- *Grossly:* Lesions are well-circumscribed, intramedullary masses that are tan-white, gritty, and variable in size.
- *Microscopically:* Lesions are composed of curvilinear trabeculae of woven bone (likened to Chinese ideographs). Cystic degeneration, hemorrhage, foamy macrophages, and nodules of hyaline cartilage (resembling disorganized growth plates) can also be present.

Clinical Course (p. 1231)

The natural history depends on the extent and location of skeletal involvement. Isolated lesions can be cured by conservative surgery, whereas polyostotic involvement is often progressive and may require multiple procedures. Bisphosphonates can reduce bone pain. Rarely, there is malignant transformation.

Fibrosarcoma Variants (p. 1232)

Fibrosarcoma variants are collagen-producing sarcomas with a fibroblast phenotype; they are most common in middle age and beyond, with equal gender distribution. Fibrosarcoma typically presents as an enlarging painful mass in the metaphysis of long bones or pelvis; pathologic fractures are common. Large, high-grade tumors that are difficult to resect have a poor prognosis.

Morphology (p. 1232)

- *Grossly:* Tumors are large, hemorrhagic tan-white masses that destroy the underlying bone and invade into adjacent soft tissues.
- *Microscopically:* Lesions are composed of cytologically malignant cells arranged in a herringbone storiform pattern. Variants with pleomorphic cells resembling histiocytes were previously called *malignant fibrous histiocytomas.*

Miscellaneous Tumors (p. 1232)

Ewing Sarcoma and Primitive Neuroectodermal Tumor (p. 1232)

These are malignant, small, round-cell tumors of bone and soft tissue (Chapter 10), accounting for 6% to 10% of all primary malignant bone tumors. They share a t(11;22) translocation and differ only in their degree of neural differentiation. Ewing sarcomas are undifferentiated, whereas primitive neuroectodermal tumors (PNET) exhibit neural differentiation; the distinction has no clinical significance. The translocation juxtaposes the *EWS* gene on chromosome 22 with an *ETS* family transcription factor (usually *FLI1*), producing chimeric transcription factors that drive aberrant cell proliferation and survival. Most tumors present before age 20 years, with a slight male preponderance and a striking predilection for Caucasians.

Morphology (p. 1232)

- *Grossly:* Tumors usually invade cortex and penetrate the periosteum to produce a tan-white soft-tissue mass, often with focal hemorrhage and necrosis.
- *Microscopically:* Lesions are composed of sheets of uniform small, round cells with scant clear cytoplasm, rich in glycogen. *Homer-Wright pseudorosettes*—tumor cells arrayed in a circle about a central fibrillary space—indicate neural differentiation.

Clinical Features (p. 1232)

Ewing sarcoma and PNET typically present as painful, enlarging, warm masses in the diaphysis of long tubular bones; fever, elevated sedimentation rate, and leukocytosis can mimic infection. Radiographs reveal an invasive lytic lesion; a characteristic periosteal reaction produces layers of reactive bone deposited in an onion-skin fashion. With combined radiation, chemotherapy, and surgery, there is a 75%, 5-year survival rate.

Giant-Cell Tumor (p. 1233)

These are benign but locally aggressive neoplasms of epiphyses and metaphyses occurring most commonly between the ages of 20 and 50 years.

Morphology (p. 1233)

- *Grossly:* Tumors are large and red-brown with frequent cystic degeneration.
- *Microscopically:* Plump, uniform mononuclear cells constitute the proliferating component of the tumor. In the background are scattered osteoclast-like, multinucleated giant cells. The mononuclear cells in the lesions express RANKL, and characteristic osteoclast-like giant cells are formed through RANK-RANKL signaling pathways. Focal necrosis, hemorrhage, hemosiderin deposition, and reactive bone can also occur.

Clinical Course (p. 1233)

More than half these tumors arise near the knees, but virtually any bone can be involved; location near joints frequently manifests as arthritis-like symptoms, but patients can also present with pathologic fractures. Most are solitary; radiology shows erosion into subchondral bone with a soft tissue mass delineated by a thin rim of reactive bone. Conservative surgery with curettage has a 40% to 60% recurrence rate, with up to 4% exhibiting lung metastasis.

Aneurysmal Bone Cyst (p. 1234)

This benign tumor often presents as a rapidly growing expansile mass; it is associated with 17p13 translocations that cause increased expression of a USP6 deubiquitinating enzyme.

Morphology (p. 1234)

- *Grossly:* Lesions consist of multiple, blood-filled cystic spaces separated by thin, tan-white septa.
- *Microscopically:* The walls are composed of plump uniform fibroblasts, multinucleated osteoclast-like giant cells, and reactive woven bone; a third of cases exhibit an unusual cartilage-like matrix called *blue bone*.

Clinical Course (p. 1234)

Lesions generally present as pain and swelling, typically in the first two decades of life; long bone metaphyses or posterior elements of vertebral bodies are most often affected. Radiology shows expansile lytic lesions with a thin shell of reactive bone. Conservative surgical curettage is usually sufficient; the recurrence rate is low.

Metastatic Disease (p. 1235)

In adults, more than 75% of skeletal metastases originate from cancers of the prostate, breast, kidney, and lung. In children, metastatic disease derives most commonly from neuroblastoma, Wilms tumor, osteosarcoma, Ewing sarcoma/PNET, and rhabdomyosarcoma. Osteolytic lesions are due to tumor cell elaboration of prostaglandins, interleukins, and PTH-related protein that stimulate osteoclastic bone resorption. In turn, lysis of bone tissue rich in growth factors (e.g., TGF-β, IGF-1, FGF, PDGF, and bone morphogenic proteins) helps drive tumor growth. Osteosclerotic responses (most often induced by prostate cancer) occur through tumor elaboration of WNT proteins that stimulate osteoblastic activity.

JOINTS (p. 1235)

Hyaline cartilage is an elastic shock absorber and a wear-resistant surface situated at the end of apposed bones in synovial joints. Chondrocytes synthesize the type 2 collagen and proteoglycan matrix elements of hyaline cartilage and secrete the degradative enzymes responsible for matrix turnover. Degradative enzymes are secreted as inactive precursors, and chondrocytes also enrich the matrix with enzyme inhibitors. Thus, diseases that destroy articular cartilage do so by activating catabolic enzymes and by decreasing inhibitor synthesis. Cytokines such as TNF and IL-1—derived from chondrocytes, synoviocytes, fibroblasts, and inflammatory cells—can trigger the degradative process.

Arthritis (p. 1235)

Osteoarthritis (Degenerative Joint Disease) (p. 1235)

Degenerative joint disease (DJD) is characterized by progressive erosion of articular cartilage:

- *Primary DJD* appears insidiously, largely as an aging phenomenon and only in a few joints; knees and hands are affected more in women, and hips are affected more in men.
- *Secondary DJD* appears at any age in a previously damaged or congenitally abnormal joint or in patients with systemic disorders such as diabetes, ochronosis, or hemochromatosis.

Pathogenesis (p. 1236)

Osteoarthritis (OA) has both genetic and environmental components. Genome-wide association studies implicate polymorphisms in prostaglandin synthesis and WNT signaling (among others), and epidemiology studies incriminate variables such as aging, obesity, muscle strength, and joint architecture. Phases of OA include:

- Chondrocyte injury due to aging, biochemical and genetic effects, and trauma
- Chrondrocyte proliferation and secretion of matrix and inflammatory mediators, resulting in cartilage remodeling and secondary changes in synovium and subchondral bone
- Chondrocyte drop-out and cartilage loss due to repetitive injury and chronic inflammation

Morphology (p. 1236)

- *Grossly:* The articular surface is soft with dislodged fragments of cartilage and subchondral bone forming loose bodies *(joint mice)*. Exposed subchondral bone is burnished by the opposing degenerated articular surface *(bone eburnation)*, and the underlying cancellous bone becomes sclerotic. Small fractures allow synovial fluid to be expressed into the subchondral bone to form cystic spaces. Bony overgrowths *(osteophytes)* capped by cartilage also develop at the edges of the articular cartilage; Heberden nodes are osteophytes of the distal interphalangeal joints (common in women)
- *Microscopically:* In early OA, there is chrondrocyte proliferation, with increased matrix water and decreased proteoglycan content; this is followed by *fibrillation* and cracking of the matrix as superficial layers are degraded. The synovium is mildly congested with scattered chronic inflammation.

Clinical Course (p. 1236)

DJD is an insidious and slowly progressive disease; patients characteristically develop deep achy joint pain that worsens with use, morning stiffness, crepitus, and limited range of motion. Osteophyte compression on spinal foramina can cause radicular pain, muscle spasm or atrophy, and neurologic deficits. There is no known way of preventing or arresting DJD.

Rheumatoid Arthritis (p. 1237)

Rheumatoid arthritis (RA) is a chronic systemic inflammatory disease that principally attacks joints, producing a non-suppurative proliferative synovitis that progresses to joint destruction and ankylosis; blood vessels, skin, heart, lungs, and muscles can also be impacted. About 1% of the world's population is affected; women are affected three- to five-fold more commonly than men; peak ages are between 40 and 70 years.

Morphology (p. 1237)

- *Joints:*

  Grossly: In early stages, the synovium is edematous and hyperplastic, exhibiting delicate and bulbous fronds. At later stages, a *pannus* of proliferative synovium, inflammatory cells, and fibroblasts encroaches on the hyaline cartilage, leading to its destruction; the pannus can bridge apposing bones to form a *fibrous ankylosis* that will eventually ossify.

  Microscopically: Lesions show a dense, perivascular mononuclear inflammatory cell infiltrate with focal lymphoid aggregates; neutrophils accumulate on the synovial surface and in the synovial fluid. Vasodilation and increased vascular permeability is reflected by hemosiderin deposits and aggregates of organizing fibrin. There is osteoclast activation with bone erosion, osteoporosis, and subchondral cysts.

- *Skin:*

  Grossly: Rheumatoid *nodules* are firm, non-tender nodules arising in subcutaneous tissues in a quarter of patients, typically in regions subjected to recurrent pressure (e.g., elbows); they can also occur in lungs, spleen, heart valves, aorta, and other viscera.

  Microscopically: Lesions exhibit a central zone of fibrinoid necrosis, surrounded by a palisade of activated macrophages.

- *Blood vessels:*

  Patients with severe disease and high titers of rheumatoid factor are at increased risk of developing small- to medium-sized vessel vasculitis comparable to polyarteritis nodosa (Chapter 11).

Pathogenesis (p. 1237)

RA is triggered by exposure of a genetically susceptible host to an arthritogenic antigen, resulting in loss of self-tolerance and a chronic autoimmune response (Fig. 26-3).

- *Genetic susceptibility:* RA is linked to specific HLA-DRB1 alleles; these have the same β chain sequences involved in antigen binding and thus disease association may be related to presentation of the putative arthritogenic peptide(s). RA is also associated with PTPN22, a tyrosine phosphatase that regulates T cell activation.
- *Environmental arthritogen:* Microbial triggers (e.g., Epstein-Barr virus [EBV], retroviruses, mycobacteria, *Borrelia*, and *Mycoplasma*) are implicated but not proved. Host proteins modified by conversion of arginine to citrulline (e.g., by smoking) can induce robust autoresponses in some patients.
- *Autoimmunity:* Once an inflammatory synovitis is initiated, the ensuing CD4+ autoimmune response may be propagated by autoimmunity to type 2 collagen and glyocsaminoglycans, with continued activation of CD4+ T_H1 and T_H17 cells. Antibodies against citrulline-modified peptides are present in many RA

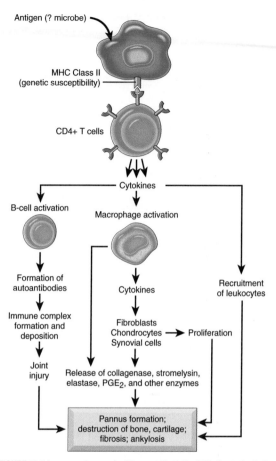

FIGURE 26-3 Immunopathogenesis of rheumatoid arthritis. *PGE₂,* Prostaglandin E₂.

patients and may contribute to disease chronicity. Autoantibodies to the Fc portion of autologous IgG *(rheumatoid factor)* also occur in 80% of RA patients and, while not causal, are good markers of disease activity.

Tissue damage occurs through cytokines produced by CD4+ T cells that coordinate an ongoing response. These include interferon-γ and IL-17, which act on macrophages and synoviocytes, inducing those cells to produce a host of mediators (e.g., IL-1, IL-6, IL-23, PGE₂, TGF-β) and *especially TNF* that can drive RANKL expression and osteoclastogenesis, as well as mediate synoviocyte hyperplasia. Local production of matrix metalloproteinases and immune complex activation of complement and neutrophils further contribute to cartilage destruction.

Clinical Course (p. 1239)

Although the clinical course is variable, non-specific malaise, fatigue, and generalized musculoskeletal pain progresses insidiously to localized joint involvement. RA generally involves small joints first (digits before wrist, ankles, elbows, and knees) in a bilaterally symmetric pattern; affected joints are swollen, warm, and painful, particularly following inactivity. There is typically progressive joint involvement over months to years, with some fluctuation in tempo; the greatest damage occurs in the first 4 to 5 years. Destruction of tendons, ligaments, and joint capsules leads to classic lesions including radial deviation of the wrist, ulnar deviation of the fingers, and flexion-hyperextension abnormalities of the digits. Ultimately, the deformed joints lose stability and have minimal range of motion. Radiologically, there are joint effusions, with juxta-articular osteopenia and narrowing of the joint space as articular cartilage is lost. Therapies include corticosteroids, methotrexate, and TNF antagonists.

Juvenile Idiopathic Arthritis (p. 1240)

Previously called *juvenile rheumatoid arthritis, juvenile idiopathic arthritis (JIA)* encompasses at least seven (!!) different clinical subsets of arthritis that occur before age 16 years, each persisting for at least 6 weeks; 30,000 to 50,000 children are affected annually in the United States. Like RA, JIA is associated with both environmental factors and genetic susceptibility; the CD4+ dysregulation and the inflammatory synovitis are also similar. JIA *differs from* RA because in JIA:

- Oligoarthritis is more common.
- Systemic disease is more frequent.
- Large joints are affected more often than small joints.
- Rheumatoid nodules and rheumatoid factor are usually absent.
- Antinuclear antibody (ANA) seropositivity is common.

The long-term prognosis of JIA is variable; while some individuals will have sustained disease activity, only 10% develop serious functional disability.

Seronegative Spondyloarthropathies (p. 1241)

These represent a group of putatively autoimmune diseases initiated by environmental factors (especially infections) in genetically predisposed individuals; the manifestations are immune mediated. All have similar synovial inflammation but are distinguished by various overlapping patterns of extra-articular involvement (e.g., skin, cardiovascular system, and eyes). Many are associated with the human leukocyte antigen (HLA)-B27 allele, but without specific autoantibodies (hence "seronegative").

Ankylosing Spondyloarthritis (p. 1241)

Ankylosing spondyloarthritis *(Marie-Strümpell disease)* is a chronic ankylosing synovitis of vertebrae and sacroiliac joints; the male to female ratio is 2:1 to 3:1 with onset in the twenties to thirties. It follows a progressive course that involves hips, knees, and shoulders in one third of patients; uveitis, aortitis, and amyloidosis are complications. While 90% of patients are HLA-B27 positive, there is also association with the IL23 receptor, and *ARTS1*, a gene encoding a peptidase that trims peptides for HLA class I presentation.

Reiter Syndrome (p. 1241)

Reiter syndrome comprises the triad of arthritis, nongonococcal urethritis or cervicitis, and conjunctivitis. The typical patient is a 20- to 30-year-old man; 80% of patients express HLA-B27. Prior gastrointestinal or genitourinary infections are implicated as triggers since symptoms begin several weeks after urethritis or diarrheal illness. Ankles, knees, and feet in an asymmetric distribution are affected most often, but chronic disease progresses to spine involvement reminiscent of ankylosing spondylitis. Extra-articular manifestations include conjunctivitis, cardiac conduction abnormalities, and aortic regurgitation. Although symptoms in half of patients resolve over a period of months, the remainder have recurrent arthritis, tendinitis, and fasciitis with significant functional impairment.

Enteritis-Associated Arthritis (p. 1241)

Enteritis-associated arthritis is caused by gastrointestinal infections with *Yersinia, Salmonella, Shigella,* or *Campylobacter.* The arthritis appears abruptly and tends to involve knees and ankles; it typically remits after a year, without anklyosing spondylitis.

Psoriatic Arthritis (p. 1241)

Psoriatic arthritis develops in 10% of patients with psoriasis. The arthritis usually affects small hand and foot joints but can extend to ankles, knees, hips, and wrists; spinal disease occurs in 20% to 40%. Psoriatic arthritis is not as severe as RA, and there is less joint destruction.

Infectious Arthritis (p. 1241)

Joints can be seeded hematogenously or by direct extension from a soft-tissue abscess or osteomyelitis; infectious arthritis can rapidly destroy a joint and produce permanent deformities.

Bacterial Arthritis (p. 1242)

Bacterial arthritis is most commonly caused by gonococcus, staphylococcus, streptococcus, *Haemophilus influenzae* (especially children younger than 2 years), and Gram-negative bacilli; individuals with sickle cell disease are prone to infection with *Salmonella.* In most instances, a single joint is affected, with the knee being most common. Predisposing conditions include immune deficiency, debilitating illness, joint trauma, chronic arthritis, and intravenous drug use.

Tuberculous Arthritis (p. 1242)

Tuberculous arthritis is an insidious chronic arthritis involving hematogenous spread or nearby tuberculous osteomyelitis; hips, knees, and ankles are commonly involved. Chronic disease results in severe destruction with fibrous ankylosis.

Lyme Arthritis (p. 1242)

Lyme arthritis occurs in 60% to 80% of untreated individuals several weeks to 2 years after the initial skin infection by *Borrelia burgdorferi.* The arthritis is oligoarticular, remitting, and migratory and primarily involves large joints (i.e., knees, shoulders, elbows, and ankles). The articular involvement histologically resembles RA; in most cases, it clears spontaneously or with antibiotic therapy, but in about 10%, a presumed autoimmune arthritis supervenes, resulting in permanent deformities.

Viral Arthritis (p. 1242)

Viral arthritis can occur with a wide variety of viral infections, but it is unclear whether the joint symptoms result from direct infection or secondary to an autoimmune response; arthritic syndromes associated with human immunodeficiency virus (HIV) infections are presumed autoimmune.

Crystal-Induced Arthritis (p. 1242)

Both endogenous (urate, hydroxyapatite) and exogenous (talc, prosthetic biomaterials) crystals can trigger cytokine-mediated cartilage destruction.

Gout (p. 1243)

Gout is characterized by transient attacks of *acute arthritis* initiated by crystallization of urates around joints, leading eventually to *chronic gouty arthritis* and *tophi* (large aggregates of urate crystals and associated inflammation). Hyperuricemia (more than 6.8 mg/dL) occurs in 10% of the U.S. population and is necessary for gout, but only 0.5% of these hyperuricemic individuals actually develop disease.

Pathogenesis (p. 1243)

- *Hyperuricemia* can be due to overproduction or reduced renal excretion (notably, humans are one of few mammals that lack uricase to degrade uric acid). Alcohol and obesity increase the risk of gout; certain drugs (e.g., thiazides) reduce urate excretion, and lead toxicity can also precipitate disease.

  Overproduction (10% of cases): Most cases are associated with increased nucleic acid turnover (e.g., cancer, psoriasis, tumor lysis). Others can be related to deficiency of hypoxanthine guanine phosphoribosyl transferase (HGPRT), an enzyme involved in the purine salvage pathway; lack of HGPRT (e.g., Lesch-Nyhan syndrome) leads to decreased recycling of precursors into purine metabolic pathways and increased uric acid accumulation.

  Reduced renal excretion (90% of cases): Decreased filtration and under-excretion of uric acid underlie most cases; the urate transporter gene *URAT1* has an important role in the reabsorption process.

- *Inflammation:* Deposition of monosodium urate (MSU) in joints is affected by temperature and by the intra-articular concentrations of urates and cations. Once accumulated, MSU is phagocytosed by macrophages, culminating in inflammasome activation and release of activated IL-1β. IL-1β induces chemokine and adhesion molecule production to recruit and activate neutrophils, which are responsible for the acute arthritis. Recurrent rounds of acute arthritis eventually result in chronic arthritis and tophus formation, with cartilage damage and functional joint compromise.

Morphology (p. 1244)

- *Acute arthritis:* Lesions exhibit a dense neutrophilic infiltrate within the synovium and synovial fluid; slender, birefringent MSU crystals are present in the edematous and congested synovium and within neutrophils; there is scattered chronic inflammation.
- *Chronic tophaceous arthritis:* Urates can encrust the articular surfaces and form grossly visible synovial deposits. The synovium becomes hyperplastic and fibrotic with increased inflammatory infiltrates; a synovial pannus extends from the cartilage into juxta-articular bone, causing erosions and fibrosis and eventually producing a bony ankylosis.
- *Tophi are pathognomonic lesions:* These are masses of urates, crystalline or amorphous, surrounded by intense mononuclear inflammation with foreign body giant cells. Tophi tend to occur on the ear, in the olecranon and patellar bursae, and in periarticular ligaments and connective tissue.
- *Gouty nephropathy* (Chapter 20) is associated with renal medullary MSU deposition (including tophi) and uric acid stones; obstruction can cause a secondary pyelonephritis.

Clinical Course (p. 1244)

After years of asymptomatic hyperuricemia, acute gouty arthritis is classically announced by excruciating joint pain accompanied by localized hyperemia and warmth; most first presentations are monoarticular, and half of the initial attacks involve the great toe (followed by insteps, ankles, or heels and knees). Typically, the acute episode resolves, followed by an *asymptomatic intercritical period.* Although some patients never have another flare, in the majority, attacks tend to recur with greater frequency and become polyarticular. Eventually (12 years, on average) chronic tophaceous gout develops with joint effacement. Cardiovascular disease (atherosclerosis and hypertension) is a common accompanying pathology, and 20% of patients die of renal failure secondary to gouty nephropathy.

Calcium Pyrophosphate Crystal Deposition Disease (Pseudo-Gout) *(p. 1246)*

Calcium pyrophosphate crystal deposition disease (CPPD) is also called *chondrocalcinosis.* CPPD typically occurs after age 50 years with a 30% to 60% prevalence by age 85 years; the hereditary variant presents somewhat earlier and the phenotype is more severe. An autosomal dominant form of the disease is due to mutations in the *ANKH* gene encoding a pyrophosphate transport channel. The most common *secondary* form is associated with a variety of etiologies, including trauma, hyperparathyroidism, hemochromatosis, and diabetes; altered matrix synthesis and degradation of pyrophosophates is implicated.

The *clinicopathologic features are similar to gout.* The crystals initially form in cartilage; as deposits enlarge they rupture and seed the joint where macrophages engulf them and activate their inflammasomes to generate IL-1β. Subsequent neutrophil recruitment and recurrent bouts of inflammation result in joint damage in more than 50% of patients. Knees, wrists, elbows, shoulders, and ankles are affected (in decreasing order).

Morphology *(p. 1246)*

- *Grossly:* Crystals form chalky white, friable deposits; they rarely deposit in masses reminiscent of tophi.
- *Microscopically:* Crystals stain as oval, blue-purple aggregates; they are weakly birefringent and have geometric shapes. Chronic lesions exhibit mononuclear cell infiltrates with fibrosis.

Tumors and Tumor-Like Lesions *(p. 1246)*

Ganglion and Synovial Cysts *(p. 1247)*

- *Ganglions* are small (1 to 1.5 cm), multiloculated, cystic lesions of connective tissues near joint capsules or tendon sheaths (the wrist is a common site). They arise through myxoid degeneration and softening of connective tissues; they are not lined by epithelium and do not communicate with joint spaces.
- *Synovial cysts* are herniations of synovium through joint capsules (e.g., a *Baker cyst* arising in the popliteal fossa). The synovial lining may be hyperplastic and contain scattered inflammation.

Tenosynovial Giant-Cell Tumor (Localized and Diffuse) *(p. 1247)*

This is the term for a group of closely related benign neoplasms involving synovial membranes, tendon sheaths, and bursae. They all share a t(1;2) chromosomal translocation that fuses the gene for colony-stimulating factor 1 *(CSF1)* to the promoter for the α3 chain of collagen type VI. As a result, the lesions overexpress CSF1, leading to the accumulation of swarms of macrophages. Variants include:

- *Diffuse type* (previously called *pigmented villonodular tenosynovitis*), typically presenting in the knee (80%) with pain, "locking", and swelling; range of motion is decreased and aggressive lesions erode into the bone and adjacent soft tissue.

- *Localized type (giant cell tumor of the tendon sheath),* commonly manifesting as a solitary painless mass involving the tendon sheaths of the wrist and fingers; cortical bone erosion affects 15%.

Morphology (p. 1247)

- *Grossly:* Lesions are red-brown to mottled orange-yellow. In diffuse disease, the synovium is a tangled mat of red-brown folds, nodules, and finger-like projections that spread along the articular surface and infiltrate the subsynovial tissue. In the localized form, tumors are well-circumscribed and nodular, and they may be attached to the synovium by a pedicle.
- *Microscopically:* Neoplastic cells (2% to 16% of the total cellularity) are polyhedral and resemble synoviocytes. Both types of lesions are heavily infiltrated by macrophages, often contain hemosiderin, and form multinucleated giant cells.

SOFT-TISSUE TUMORS AND TUMOR-LIKE LESIONS (p. 1248)

Soft tissue tumors are mesenchymal proliferations of extra-skeletal non-epithelial tissues, excluding viscera, meninges, and lymphatics. These are typically classified according to the tissue they recapitulate, although some have no apparent normal tissue counterpart. Benign lesions outnumber malignant 100:1; only 8000 sarcomas are diagnosed annually in the United States, but these tend to be highly lethal, commonly with hematogenous metastasis to bone and lung.

Pathogenesis and General Features (p. 1248)

The cause in most cases is unknown, although individual soft-tissue tumors can be associated with radiation, prior trauma or chemical injury, chemical exposures, and infection (e.g., human herpesvirus 8 and Kaposi sarcoma). Most are sporadic, and a minority are associated with hereditable syndromes (e.g., neurofibromatosis type 1 and Gardner syndrome). In several cases, specific translocations give rise to aberrant transcription factor expression that drive neoplastic transformation (Table 26-3). Males are affected 1.4 times more frequently than females, and 15% of soft-tissue tumors arise in children.

Prognosis is influenced by:

- Histologic classification and grade, the latter based on cytologic atypia, mitotic activity, and necrosis
- Staging—size and spread
- Location—the more superficial, the better the prognosis

Fatty Tumors (p. 1249)

Lipomas (p. 1249)

Lipomas are the most common benign soft tissue tumor of adults; they are subclassified according to morphologic features (e.g., fibrolipoma, angiolipoma, spindle cell lipoma), and some have characteristic genetic rearrangements. They are usually soft, mobile, and painless (except angiolipomas) and are cured by simple excision.

TABLE 26-3   Chromosomal and Genetic Abnormalities in Soft Tissue Sarcomas

Tumor	Cytogenetic Abnormality	Genetic Abnormality
Extraosseous Ewing sarcoma and primitive neuroectodermal tumor	t(11:22)(q24;q12)	FLI1-EWS fusion gene
	t(21:22)(q22;q12)	ERG-EWS fusion gene
	t(7;22)(q22;q12)	ETV1-EWS fusion gene
Liposarcoma—myxoid and round cell type	t(12:16)(q13;p11)	CHOP/TLS fusion gene
Synovial sarcoma	t(x;18)(p11;q11)	SYT-SSX fusion gene
Rhabdomyosarcoma— alveolar type	t(2;13)(q35;q14)	PAX3-FKHR fusion gene
	t(1;13)(p36;q14)	PAX7-FKHR fusion gene
Extraskeletal myxoid chondrosarcoma	t(9;22)(q22;q12)	CHN-EWS fusion gene
Desmoplastic small round cell tumor	t(11;22)(p13;q12)	EWS-WT1 fusion gene
Clear cell sarcoma	t(12;22)(q13;q12)	EWS-ATF1 fusion gene
Dermatofibrosarcoma protuberans	t(17:22)(q22;q15)	COLA1-PDGFB fusion gene
Alveolar soft part sarcoma	t(X;17)(p11.2;q25)	TFE3-ASPL fusion gene
Congenital fibrosarcoma	t(12;15)(p13;q23)	ETV6-NTRK3 fusion gene

Morphology (p. 1249)

Lipomas are well-encapsulated tumors (of variable size) of mature adipocytes. Infrequently, they can be large, intramuscular, and poorly circumscribed.

Liposarcoma (p. 1250)

Liposarcomas are some of the more common adult sarcomas; they typically appear between ages 40 and 70 years, presenting as large masses in deep soft tissues of the proximal extremities and retroperitoneum. Well-differentiated forms are relatively indolent, while the pleomorphic variant is highly aggressive, and the myxoid/round cell type (with a characteristic t[12;16] translocation) is intermediate in its behavior.

Morphology (p. 1250)

In well-differentiated liposarcomas, the tumor cells are readily recognized as lipocytes. In other variants, adipogenic differentiation may not be obvious. Nevertheless, cells showing fatty differentiation are almost always present; such *lipoblasts* mimic fetal fat cells with clear cytoplasmic lipid droplets that scallop the nucleus.

Fibrous Tumors and Tumor-Like Lesions (p. 1250)

Reactive Pseudosarcomatous Proliferations (p. 1250)

These are non-neoplastic lesions that either are idiopathic or develop in response to trauma; they can grow rapidly and can be alarming due to hypercellularity, high mitotic activity, and reactive mesenchymal cells.

Nodular Fasciitis (p. 1250)

Nodular fascilitis is also called *pseudosarcomatous fasciitis;* patients typically present with a several-week history of a solitary, rapidly growing, and sometimes painful mass, usually on the volar forearm, chest, or back. Preceding trauma is reported in 10% to 15% of cases. Lesions rarely recur after excision.

Morphology (p. 1250)

- *Grossly:* Neoplasms are typically large and nodular, with ill-defined margins.
- *Microscopically:* Lesions are cellular and highly mitotic, with plump, reactive, immature-appearing fibroblasts and myofibroblasts arranged randomly or in intersecting fascicles. Lesions often exhibit myxoid stroma and scattered lymphocytes.

Myositis Ossificans (p. 1251)

Myositis ossificans is distinguished from other reactive fibroblastic proliferations by the presence of *metaplastic bone*. It usually occurs following trauma in the proximal extremity musculature in adolescents and young adults. Although initially painful, the lesion evolves into a painless, hard, well-demarcated mass. Simple excision is usually curative.

Morphology (p. 1251)

Initial lesions resemble nodular fasciitis (see preceding discussion). Thereafter, a surrounding zone of osteoblasts deposits ill-defined trabeculae of woven bone; this mineralizes from the periphery into well-formed cancellous bone. Eventually the entire lesion ossifies, and the intertrabecular areas accrue marrow elements.

Fibromatoses (p. 1251)

Superficial Fibromatosis (Palmar, Plantar, and Penile Fibromatoses) (p. 1251)

Superficial fibromatosis encompass a group of benign fibroproliferative lesions with abundant dense collagen. Males are affected more frequently than females.

- *Palmar fibromatosis (Dupuytren contracture)* presents with irregular thickening of the palmar fascia; it is bilateral in 50% of affected individuals. Attachment to the overlying skin leads to skin puckering, and patients develop a slowly progressive flexion contracture of the fourth and fifth fingers.
- *Plantar fibromatosis* is essentially the same process occurring on the foot; however, bilaterality and contractures are uncommon.
- *Penile fibromatosis (Peyronie disease)* usually occurs on the dorsolateral penis, leading to abnormal curvature and/or urethral constriction.

Deep-Seated Fibromatosis (Desmoid Tumor) (p. 1251)

These neoplasms have no metastatic potential but are nevertheless locally aggressive and frequently recur after incomplete excision. *APC* or *β-catenin* gene mutations are typically present. Besides surgery, tumors can be treated with tamoxifen, chemotherapy, or radiation. Three clinical types are recognized, all with similar gross and microscopic features:

- *Extra-abdominal fibromatosis* occurs equally in men and women, principally in the musculature of the shoulder, chest wall, back, and thigh.
- *Abdominal fibromatosis* arises in the anterior abdominal wall in women during or after pregnancy.
- *Intra-abdominal fibromatosis* occurs in the mesentery or pelvic walls, usually in patients with Gardner syndrome.

Morphology (p. 1252)

- *Grossly:* Tumors are 1 to 15 cm, gray-white, rubbery, poorly demarcated masses.
- *Microscopically:* Lesions are composed of banal fibroblasts arrayed in broad sweeping fascicles that infiltrate neighboring tissues.

Fibrosarcoma (p. 1252)

Fibrosarcomas arise in deep soft tissue, often in the extremities. More than half recur after excision, and more than 25% metastasize.

Morphology (p. 1252)

- *Grossly:* Tumors are unencapsulated, infiltrative, soft (fish-flesh consistency) masses often with focal hemorrhage and necrosis.
- *Microscopically:* All degrees of differentiation can be seen, from that resembling cellular fibromatosis to highly cellular anaplastic appearance.

Fibrohistiocytic Tumors (p. 1252)

Benign Fibrous Histiocytoma (Dermatofibroma) (p. 1253)

These are common painless and slow-growing lesions of the dermis and subcutis (Chapter 25).

Malignant Fibrous Histiocytoma (p. 1253)

Although previously a designation for soft tissue tumors characterized by extensive pleomorphism and a storiform architecture, this term is no longer used; such tumors are now mainly classified as fibrosarcoma variants.

Tumors of Skeletal Muscle (p. 1253)

Most skeletal muscle tumors are malignant. The benign counterpart, rhabdomyoma, is rare; cardiac rhabdomyomas occur in association with tuberous sclerosis (Chapter 12).

Rhabdomyosarcoma (p. 1253)

Rhabdomyosarcoma is the most common soft-tissue sarcoma of children; most occur in the head and neck or in the genitourinary tract. These are aggressive neoplasms, treated with surgery, radiation, and chemotherapy. Lesions are histologically subclassified into three major types that have slightly different clinical features:

- *Embryonal rhabdomyosarcoma* is the most common (60% of cases); it typically occurs in children younger than 10 years and involves the nasal cavity, orbit, middle ear, prostate, and paratesticular region. Tumors often have parental isodisomy of chromosome 11p15 leading to over-expression of the imprinted *IGFII* gene. The *botryoides* subtype develops in the walls of hollow, mucosa-lined structures (e.g., nasopharynx, common bile duct, bladder, and vagina) and overall has the best prognosis.
- *Alveolar rhabdomyosarcoma* (20%) tends to arise in middle adolescence in the deep musculature of extremities. This type is associated with translocations that fuse either *PAX3* or *PAX7* to *FOXO1a* (t[2,13] or t[1,13] translocations, respectively) (see Table 26-3).
- *Pleomorphic rhabdomyosarcoma* is rare, occurring in the deep soft tissue of adults.

Morphology (p. 1253)

The rhabdomyoblast is the diagnostic cell; although they can be round or elongate, all contain sarcomeres (sometimes only apparent by electron microscopy) and express myogenic markers (e.g., desmin, MYOD1, and myogenin).

- *Embryonal rhabdomyosarcomas* present as soft, gray infiltrative masses; the botryoid variant resembles a cluster of grapes. Tumor cells form sheets of round and spindled cells in a myxoid stroma.
- *Alveolar rhabdomyosarcomas* exhibit a network of fibrous septae that divide the tumor cells into clusters or aggregates resembling alveoli; tumor cells are moderate-sized but may have little cytoplasm.
- *Pleomorphic rhabdomyosarcomas* resemble other pleomorphic sarcomas.

Tumors of Smooth Muscle (p. 1254)

Leiomyomas (p. 1254)

Benign smooth muscle tumors occur predominantly in the uterus (Chapter 22), but can occur at other body sites where smooth muscle is well represented. Lesions are usually smaller than 1 to 2 cm and composed of fascicles of bland-appearing smooth muscle cells with few mitoses. A syndrome of multiple cutaneous leiomyomas arising from arrector pili muscles, in association with uterine leiomyomas and renal cell carcinomas, can be transmitted as an autosomal dominant disorder; it is linked to a loss-of-function mutation in the fumarate hydratase gene.

Leiomyosarcomas (p. 1254)

Leimyosarcomas account for 10% to 20% of soft tissue sarcomas; they are more common in women than men, and they typically occur in the skin and deep soft tissues of the extremities and retroperitoneum. Superficial leiomyosarcomas are usually small and have a good prognosis; tumors of the retroperitoneum are usually large and non-resectable, and they cause death through local extension and metastasis.

Morphology (p. 1254)

- *Grossly:* Tumors are usually painless, firm masses.
- *Microscopically:* Lesions consist of malignant spindle cells in interweaving fascicles; bundles of muscle filaments can be demonstrated ultrastructurally and by immunohistochemistry.

Synovial Sarcoma (p. 1254)

Despite the name, the cell of origin is not clear; moreover, less than 10% are intra-articular. These account for 10% of soft tissue tumors; most occur between ages 20 and 50 years, and most arise in the deep soft tissues of the lower extremity (knee and thigh). Tumors often exhibit a characteristic t(x;18) translocation that produces a chimeric transcription factor (see Table 26-3). Lesions are treated surgically and with chemotherapy; 5-year survivals are between 25% and 62%, while 10-year survivals are between 11% and 30%.

Morphology (p. 1254)

Histologically, lesions can be biphasic (with both cuboidal epithelial and spindled mesenchymal differentiation) or monophasic (mostly mesenchymal). Occasionally, there are calcified concretions that can be detected radiologically.

27

Peripheral Nerve and Skeletal Muscle

Neuromuscular diseases are typically characterized by weakness; most are due to disorders of some aspect of the *motor unit*. Motor units comprise (Fig. 27-1):

- A single *lower motor neuron* (spinal anterior horn cell or brain stem cranial nerve motor neuron)
- *Axon* of the neuron
- *Muscle fibers* innervated by the neuron

Nerve fibers, which are composed of axons and their associated Schwann cells and myelin sheath; *peripheral nerves* consist of multiple fibers grouped into fascicles by connective tissue sheaths. *Myelinated* and *unmyelinated* nerves intermingle within each fascicle.

- Unmyelinated fibers far outnumber myelinated fibers.
- In myelinated fibers, single Schwann cells myelinate each axonal segment (internode) separated by *nodes of Ranvier.*
- In unmyelinated fibers, each Schwann cell can envelop 5 to 20 fibers.

Connective tissue of peripheral nerve is composed of:

- *Epineurium* encasing all the fascicles of the entire nerve
- *Perineurium* encircling each fascicle
- *Endoneurium* surrounding individual nerve fibers

Motor and sensory fibers—separated in the spinal cord anterior and posterior roots, respectively—intermingle within the nerves that exit the spinal canal.

Skeletal muscles (muscle fibers) are multinucleated syncytial cells delimited by a plasma membrane *(sarcolemma);* they contain identical repeating units *(sarcomeres)* of actin and myosin contractile elements (and associated proteins). Normal human skeletal muscle contains two major fiber types with different functional characteristics and staining patterns (Table 27-1); the mneumonic— *one* (type 1), *slow* (twitch), *fat* (lipid-rich), *red* (gross appearance), *ox* (oxidative)—can help with remembering the physiologic and histochemical distinctions. All fibers of a given motor unit are of the same type, with the characteristics imparted by the nature of the innervation. However, different motor units (and thus different fiber types) are intermingled within any given muscle; when visualized by special stains, this intermingling yields a checkerboard pattern.

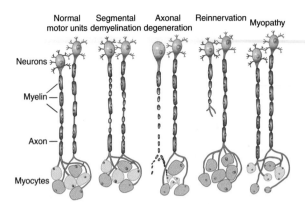

FIGURE 27-1 Normal and abnormal motor units. *Normal motor units*: two adjacent motor units are shown (light and dark). *Segmental demyelination*: random myelin internodes are injured and remyelinated by multiple Schwann cells; axons and myocytes are intact. *Axonal degeneration*: axon and myelin sheath both undergo anterograde degeneration, causing denervation atrophy of the associated myocytes in the motor unit. *Reinnervation*: sprouting of adjacent uninjured motor axons leads to myocyte fiber *type grouping*; meanwhile, the injured axon attempts sprouting. Note that new injury of the previously undamaged nerve will lead to *grouped atrophy*. *Myopathy*: scattered myocytes of different motor units are small (degenerating or regenerating), while the neurons and nerve fibers are normal.

TABLE 27-1 Muscle Fiber Types

Feature	Type 1	Type 2
Action	Sustained force	Sudden movements
Strength	Weight bearing	Purposeful motion
Enzyme content	NADH dark staining ATPase at pH 4.2, dark staining ATPase at pH 9.4, light staining	NADH light staining ATPase at pH 4.2, light staining ATPase at pH 9.4, dark staining
Lipids	Abundant	Scant
Glycogen	Scant	Abundant
Ultrastructure	Many mitochondria Wide Z-band	Few mitochondria Narrow Z-band
Physiology	Slow-twitch	Fast-twitch
Color	Red	White
Prototype	Soleus (pigeon)	Pectoral (pigeon)

ATPase, Adenosine triphosphatase; *NADH*, nicotinamide adenine dinucleotide, reduced form.

General Reactions of the Motor Unit (p. 1258)

Segmental Demyelination (p. 1259)

Myelin loss is caused by Schwann cell dysfunction or by primary myelin sheath damage (see Fig. 27-1); the underlying axon is normal. Denuded axons stimulate remyelination, and precursor cells within the endoneurium can replace injured Schwann cells; the repair is not perfect—the internode distances are shorter and the myelin sheath is thinner. If a nerve suffers recurrent demyelination and remyelination, layers of Schwann cell processes accumulate around the axon *(onion bulbs);* chronic demyelinating disorders can also eventually result in axonal injury.

Axonal Degeneration and Muscle Fiber Atrophy (p. 1259)

Primary axonal injury can be focal (e.g., trauma or ischemia) or more generalized *(neuronopathy* or *axonopathy);* axonal damage precipitates secondary myelin sheath dissolution (see Fig. 27-1). *Wallerian degeneration* is the reaction distal to a transected axon; it reflects axonal and myelin breakdown with macrophage recruitment and phagocytosis. The proximal uninjured nerve may show focal degeneration of the most distal two to three internodes before undergoing regenerative activity. Muscle fibers of the affected motor unit undergo *denervation atrophy;* myocytes become smaller and more angular, but they are still viable.

Nerve Regeneration and Reinnervation of Muscle (p. 1260)

Proximal stumps of injured axons can regrow, guided by Schwann cells; regeneration proceeds at roughly 1 mm/day, largely limited by the slow component of axonal transport.

Reinnervation of atrophic muscle fibers occurs when axons of neighboring undamaged motor units extend sprouts and incorporate the muscle fibers into the healthy motor unit. The numbers of muscle fibers in the motor unit thus increase; moreover, the newly adopted fibers assume the fiber type imparted by the nature of the innervating neuron. This leads to a confluent patch of myocytes all of the same histologic and physiologic type *(type grouping;* see Fig. 27-1); subsequent injury of the nerve innervating that patch will lead to *group atrophy.*

Type-specific atrophy is a feature of some disease states; thus type 2 fiber atrophy occurs in *disuse atrophy* and is characteristic of *corticosteroid myopathy.*

Reactions of the Muscle Fiber (p. 1260)

Besides the various patterns of atrophy (see preceding discussion), the pathologic changes of skeletal myocytes include:

- *Segmental necrosis:* Myofiber damage is followed by *myophagocytosis* as macrophages infiltrate the region; fibers may be replaced with collagen and fat.
- *Vacuolation, alterations in structural proteins or organelles, and intracytoplasmic deposits.*
- *Regeneration:* Satellite cells proliferate to reconstitute destroyed fibers. Regenerating fibers exhibit large internalized nuclei, prominent nucleoli, and basophilic cytoplasm laden with RNA.
- *Hypertrophy:* Increased loads lead to enlarged fibers; these can divide longitudinally *(muscle fiber splitting),* yielding a single large fiber with a central membrane, often with adjacent nuclei.

Diseases of Peripheral Nerve (p. 1261)

Inflammatory Neuropathies (p. 1261)

Immune-Mediated Neuropathies (p. 1261)

Guillain-Barré syndrome (acute inflammatory demyelinating polyradiculoneuropathy) (p. 1261) is an acute life-threatening ascending paralysis; the annual incidence is one to three cases per 100,000 population.

Pathogenesis (p. 1261)

Guillain-Barré syndrome is likely an immune-mediated disorder; 60% to 70% of cases are preceded by vaccination or by a viral (cytomegalovirus, Epstein-Barr virus [EBV]) or bacterial *(Campylobacter, Mycoplasma)* infection; T cells and/or circulating antibodies can be responsible for the demyelination.

Morphology (p. 1262)

Lesions show segmental demyelination with chronic inflammation involving the nerve roots and peripheral nerves; axonal damage can also be present in severe disease.

Clinical Course (p. 1262)

The clinical picture is dominated by muscle weakness; deep tendon reflexes disappear early in the process. Sensory involvement is usually less dramatic. Weakness begins in the distal limbs but rapidly includes proximal muscles. Nerve conduction velocity is slowed; although cerebrospinal fluid protein is elevated, there is no pleocytosis. Death occurs in 2% to 5% of patients due to respiratory paralysis, autonomic instability, or cardiac arrest; 20% of patients can have permanent disability.

Chronic inflammatory demyelinating polyradiculoneuropathy (p. 1262) is a mixed sensorimotor polyneuropathy similar to Guillain-Barré syndrome, but it follows a subacute or chronic course with relapses and remissions. Peripheral nerves show evidence of recurrent demyelination and remyelination ("onion bulb" changes).

Infectious Polyneuropathies (p. 1262)

Leprosy (Hansen's Disease) (p. 1262)

Mycobacterium leprae directly invade Schwann cells where they proliferate and eventually infect other cells (Chapter 8); lesions include segmental demyelination and remyelination, with axonal loss and endoneurial and epineurial fibrosis.

- *Lepromatous leprosy:* Disease tends to be more severe and diffuse; patients develop a symmetric polyneuropathy, mostly in the extremities (lower temperatures favor mycobacterial growth). A predilection for pain fibers renders patients relatively insensitive to injurious stimuli, and large traumatic ulcers are common.
- *Tuberculous leprosy:* Better host responsiveness, reflected by nodules of granulomatous inflammation, leads to more localized nerve injury.

Diphtheria (p. 1262)

Diphtheritic neuropathy results from the effects of the diphtheria exotoxin (Chapter 8). Clinical manifestations are paresthesias and weakness; pathologically, there is segmental demyelination.

Varicella-Zoster Virus (p. 1262)

Following varicella (chickenpox) infection, virus persists as a latent infection of spinal cord and brain stem sensory ganglia. Subsequent reactivation leads to a painful vesicular skin eruption in the distribution of sensory dermatomes *(shingles)*, most frequently thoracic or trigeminal. Affected ganglia exhibit neuronal destruction with associated mononuclear cell infiltrates, and peripheral nerves show axonal degeneration.

Hereditary Neuropathies (p. 1263)

These are a heterogeneous group of progressive and disabling syndromes of peripheral nerves. The most common—hereditary motor and sensory neuropathy type I (see later discussion)—is a demyelinating disorder; the others are primary axonopathies characterized by fiber loss:

- *Hereditary and sensory autonomic neuropathies (HSANs)* are summarized in Table 27-2; these typically present with numbness, pain, and autonomic dysfunction, but not weakness.
- *Familial amyloid polyneuropathies* are characterized by the deposition of amyloid in the peripheral nervous system; the clinical presentation is similar to HSAN. Most kindreds have mutations of *transthyretin* (a serum protein that *trans*ports *thy*roxine and *retin*ol), and the amyloid fibrils (Chapter 6) are composed of transthyretin (Table 27-3).
- Peripheral neuropathies accompanying inherited metabolic disorders are summarized in Table 27-3.
- *Hereditary motor and sensory neuropathies (HMSNs)* impact both strength and sensation and are caused by mutations affecting peripheral nerve function.

Hereditary Motor and Sensory Neuropathy Type I (p. 1263)

Hereditary motor and sensor neuropathy type I (HMSN I) is also known as *Charcot-Marie-Tooth disease*; it is most often an autosomal dominant disease, typically presenting in young adults with distal muscle weakness and calf atrophy.

TABLE 27-2 Hereditary Sensory and Autonomic Neuropathies (HSANs)		
Disease and Inheritance	**Gene and Locus**	**Clinical and Pathologic Findings**
HSAN I; autosomal dominant	Serine palmitoyl transferase, long-chain base, subunit 1 (*SPTLC1*) gene; 9q22.1–q22.3	Predominantly sensory neuropathy, presenting in young adults; axonal degeneration (mostly myelinated fibers)
HSAN II; autosomal recessive (some cases are sporadic)	*HSN2* gene; 12q13.3	Predominantly sensory neuropathy, presenting in childhood; axonal degeneration (mostly myelinated fibers)
HSAN III; (Riley-Day syndrome; familial dysautonomia; most often in Jewish children); autosomal recessive	IKAP histone acetyltransferase (*IKAP*) gene; 9q31	Predominantly autonomic neuropathy, presenting in infancy; axonal degeneration (mostly unmyelinated fibers); atrophy and loss of sensory and autonomic ganglion cells
HSAN IV; autosomal recessive dysautonomia, type II	Neurotrophic tyrosine kinase receptor, type 1, (*NTRK1* gene); 1q21–q22	Congenital insensitivity to pain and anhidrosis; presentation in infancy; nearly complete loss of small myelinated and unmyelinated fibers
HSAN V; autosomal recessive	Nerve growth factor β subunit (*NGFB*) gene; 1p13.1	Congenital insensitivity to pain and temperature; presentation in infancy; nearly complete loss of small myelinated fibers

TABLE 27-3   Hereditary Neuropathies Accompanying Inherited Metabolic Disease

Disease	Metabolic Defect	Inheritance	Clinical Findings	Pathologic Findings
Adrenoleukodystrophy	ATP-binding cassette (ABC) transporter protein, subfamily D, member 1 (ABCD1); Xq28	X-linked; 4% of female carriers are symptomatic	Mixed motor and sensory neuropathy, adrenal insufficiency, spastic paraplegia; onset between 10 and 20 years for males with leucodystrophy, between 20 and 40 years for females with myeloneuropathy	Segmental demyelination, with onion bulbs; axonal degeneration (myelinated and unmyelinated); electron microscopy shows linear inclusions in Schwann cells
Familial amyloid polyneuropathies	Transthyretin (TTR) gene (rarely other genes); 18q11.2–q12.1	Autosomal dominant	Sensory and autonomic dysfunction; age at onset varies with site of mutation	Amyloid deposits in vessel walls and connective tissue with axonal degeneration
Porphyria, acute intermittent (AIP) or variegate coproporphyria	Enzymes involved in heme synthesis (acute intermittent porphyria—porphobilinogen deaminase deficiency; 11q24.1–q24.2)	Autosomal dominant	Acute episodes of neurologic dysfunction, psychiatric disturbances, abdominal pain, seizures, proximal weakness, autonomic dysfunction; attacks may be precipitated by drugs	Acute and chronic axonal degeneration; regenerating clusters
Refsum disease	Peroxisomal enzyme phytanoyl CoA α-hydroxylase (PAHX) gene; 10pter–p11.2	Autosomal recessive	Mixed motor and sensory neuropathy with palpable nerves; ataxia, night blindness, retinitis pigmentosa, ichthyosis; age at onset before 20 years (a genetically distinct infantile form also exists)	Severe onion bulb formation

ATP, Adenosine triphosphate; CoA, coenzyme A.

Pathogenesis (p. 1263)

HMSN I is a group of demyelinating disorders caused by a host of different mutations. The most common variant (HMSN IA) has a duplicated segment of chromosome 17, leading to increased expression of the myelin-specific protein gene (*PMP-22*) involved in the normal compaction of myelin as Schwann cells wrap around axons. Less commonly (HMSN IB), mutations of myelin protein zero (MPZ) have the same outcome. Additional pedigrees with hereditary demyelinating neuropathy have mutations in connexin 32, protein degradation pathways, and myelination induction genes.

Morphology (p. 1264)

Histology reveals segmental demyelination and "onion bulb" changes due to repetitive cycles of remyelination.

Other Hereditary Motor and Sensory Neuropathies (p. 1264)

* *HMSN II* (p. 1264) is an autosomal dominant disorder clinically similar to HMSN I, but it exhibits axonal loss without demyelination, and presents at a slightly later age. Mutations in kinesin family members (important in axonal transport) are implicated in some cases.
* *Déjérine-Sottas neuropathy (HMSN III)* (p. 1264) is an infantile, autosomal recessive neuropathy with progressive upper and lower extremity weakness and muscle atrophy and greatly enlarged palpable nerves. Mutations in *PMP-22* or *MPZ* are seen in many cases. Segmental demyelination is severe, with prominent onion bulbs and axonal loss.

Acquired Metabolic and Toxic Neuropathies (p. 1265)

Peripheral Neuropathy in Adult-Onset Diabetes Mellitus (p. 1265)

The prevalence of peripheral neuropathy in diabetes depends on disease duration; half of all diabetics have some manifestation. Nonenzymatic protein glycation and polyol-mediated damage are both causally implicated, as is diabetic microvascular disease with secondary ischemic injury.

* *Distal symmetric sensory or sensorimotor neuropathy* (typically an axonal neuropathy with loss of small fibers). Sensory loss is greater than motor dysfunction; loss of pain sensation can result in development of cutaneous ulcers that heal poorly due to diabetic microvascular disease.
* *Autonomic neuropathy* affects about 20% to 40% of diabetics; clinical sequelae include postural hypotension, incomplete bladder emptying, and sexual dysfunction.
* *Focal or multifocal asymmetric neuropathy* (e.g., unilateral ocular nerve palsy) are presumed secondary to vascular insufficiency of peripheral nerves.

Metabolic and Nutritional Peripheral Neuropathies (p. 1266)

Axonal degeneration can occur secondary to renal failure; it typically presents with distal symmetric sensory and motor neuropathy. Chronic liver disease, respiratory insufficiency, and thyroid dysfunction can also cause peripheral neuropathies; axonal neuropathies occur with deficiencies of thiamine and vitamins B_{12}, B_6, or E. The neuropathy caused by excessive alcohol consumption is due to a combination of ethanol toxicity and thiamine deficiency.

Neuropathies Associated with Malignancy (p. 1266)

- *Direct infiltration or nerve compression* by tumor can cause mononeuropathy, brachial plexopathy, cranial nerve palsy, or polyradiculopathy of lower extremities (meningeal carcinomatosis of cauda equina).
- *Paraneoplastic syndromes:*

  A progressive sensorimotor neuropathy (mostly of lower extremities) is present in 2% to 5% of patients with lung cancer (especially small cell carcinoma). Less commonly, a pure sensory neuropathy results from loss of dorsal root ganglia; it is associated with circulating antibodies directed against an RNA-binding protein shared by neurons and tumor cells.

  Peripheral neuropathy can be caused by deposition of light-chain amyloid in patients with plasma cell dyscrasias; neuropathy can also develop secondary to autoantibodies that develop against myelin-associated glycoprotein.

Toxic Neuropathies (p. 1266)

Toxic neuropathies can occur after exposure to industrial or environmental chemicals, biologic toxins, heavy metals (e.g., lead, arsenic), or therapeutic drugs.

Traumatic Neuropathies (p. 1266)

- *Lacerations* occur with slicing injuries or bone fractures where sharp fragments cut a nerve.
- *Avulsions* occur when a nerve is put under tension (e.g., with force applied to a limb).
- *Traumatic neuromas* can occur after nerve transection or damage; these are painful nodules of tangled axons and connective tissue from regenerating axonal sprouts.
- *Compression neuropathy (entrapment neuropathy)* occurs when a nerve is compressed, often within an anatomic compartment. *Carpal tunnel syndrome*—involving the median nerve at the level of the wrist—is the most common entrapment neuropathy. It occurs with conditions that reduce the space beneath the transverse carpal ligament (e.g., edema, pregnancy, degenerative joint disease, hypothyroidism, amyloidosis, and excessive wrist use). Other nerves prone to compression neuropathies are the ulnar nerve at the level of the elbow, the peroneal nerve at the level of the knee, and the radial nerve in the upper arm. Compression neuropathy of the foot is most common in women; involvement of the interdigital nerve at intermetatarsal sites leads to pain from a traumatic (*Morton*) *neuroma.*

Diseases of Skeletal Muscle (p. 1267)

Denervation Atrophy (p. 1267)

Denervation atrophy of skeletal muscle occurs with any disorder that affects motor neurons (see Fig. 27-1).

Spinal Muscular Atrophy (Infantile Motor Neuron Disease) (p. 1267)

Spinal muscular atrophy (SMA) refers to a group of autosomal recessive motor neuron diseases with onset in childhood or adolescence. All forms of SMA are associated with mutations of the

SMN1 gene on chromosome 5; the numbers of copies of the adjacent homologous *SMN2* gene modifies disease severity (more copies means a milder phenotype). The SMN protein is important in axonal transport and neuromuscular junction integrity, so that loss leads to neuronal cell death.

Morphology (p. 1267)

Histology typically exhibits large numbers of extremely atrophic muscle fibers, often involving an entire fascicle of a muscle.

Clinical Course (p. 1267)

The most common form *(Werdnig-Hoffmann disease, SMA type 1)* presents within the first 4 months of life with hypotonia and death within the first 3 years. SMA 2 and SMA 3 present at later ages; SMA 2 patients usually die in childhood (after age 4 years), whereas SMA 3 patients survive into adulthood.

Muscular Dystrophies (p. 1268)

These are a heterogeneous group of inherited disorders, often beginning in childhood and characterized clinically by progressive muscular weakness and wasting.

X-Linked Muscular Dystrophy (Duchenne Muscular Dystrophy and Becker Muscular Dystrophy) *(p. 1268)*

Duchenne muscular dystrophy (DMD) is the most severe and most common form of muscular dystrophy; the incidence is 1 in 3500 live-born males. It is clinically manifest by age 5 years; and patients are wheelchair bound by age 10 to 12 years; the disease progresses relentlessly until death in the early 20s. *Becker muscular dystrophy (BMD)* involves the same genetic locus but is less common and less severe, with later onset and a slower rate of progression.

Pathogenesis (p. 1268)

The responsible *DMD* gene at Xp21 encodes the 427-kD *dystrophin* protein responsible for transducing contractile forces from the intracellular sarcomeres to the extracellular matrix. Most mutations are deletions, with frameshift and point mutations accounting for the rest; two-thirds are familial and the remainder are new mutations. Muscle from DMD patients has almost no detectable dystrophin; muscle from BMD patients has diminished amounts of dystrophin, usually of an abnormal molecular weight, reflecting mutations that allow synthesis of some protein.

Morphology (p. 1268)

DMD cases can exhibit enlarged, rounded, hyaline fibers lacking normal cross striations. Both DMD and BMD muscles show:

- *Variation in myofiber diameter*, with both small and giant fibers, sometimes with fiber splitting
- Increased numbers of internalized nuclei
- Degeneration, necrosis, and phagocytosis of muscle fibers
- Regeneration of muscle fibers
- Proliferation of endomysial connective tissue
- In late stages, muscles are entirely replaced by fat and connective tissue
- Both type 1 and type 2 fibers are involved, without change in relative distribution.

Clinical Course (p. 1268)

Weakness begins in the pelvic girdle muscles, extending to the shoulder girdle; the lower leg is hypertrophied associated with weakness *(pseudohypertrophy)*. Pathologic changes are also found in the heart (failure and arrhythmia), and cognitive impairment is a component of the disease. Female carriers and affected males are at risk for developing dilated cardiomyopathy. Death results from respiratory insufficiency, pulmonary infection, and cardiac decompensation.

Other Muscular Dystrophies (p. 1269)

Other muscular dystrophies are caused by mutations affecting genes besides dystrophin; specific diagnosis is based largely on the patterns of inheritance and muscle weakness (Table 27-4). *Limb girdle muscular dystrophies* are a group of autosomal muscular dystrophies that affect the proximal trunk and limb musculature; they are frequently caused by mutations of the transmembrane *sarcoglycan complex of proteins* that link dystrophin with the extracellular matrix.

Myotonic Dystrophy (p. 1269)

Myotonic dystrophy is an autosomal dominant disease that tends to increase in severity and appear at a younger age in succeeding generations (the phenomenon is called *anticipation*). *Myotonia*— a sustained involuntary muscular contraction—is the cardinal neuromuscular symptom.

Pathogenesis (p. 1269)

Myotonic dystrophy is associated with a CTG trinucleotide repeat expansion on chromosome 19q13; it affects the mRNA for the dystrophia myotonia protein kinase (DMPK). The disease state is caused by expansion of the repeat sequence, which is inversely correlated to the concentration of the protein product; normal persons have less than 30 repeats, whereas several thousand repeats may be present in severely affected individuals. The repeat number increases with each succeeding generation, explaining successively earlier onset and more severe disease.

Morphology (p. 1269)

Histology reveals striking fiber size heterogeneity, with increased numbers of internal nuclei and *ring fibers* (i.e., a subsarcolemmal band of cytoplasm exhibiting a rim of myofibrils that appear to wrap around the normal longitudinally oriented fibrils). Myotonic dystrophy is also unique in exhibiting pathologic changes in muscle spindles (fiber splitting, necrosis, and regeneration).

Clinical Course (p. 1270)

Myotonic dystrophy presents with abnormalities in gait secondary to foot dorsiflexor weakness; weakness of intrinsic hand muscles and wrist extensors also occurs, with facial muscle atrophy and ptosis. Other findings include cataracts, frontal balding, gonadal atrophy, cardiomyopathy, smooth muscle involvement, decreased plasma immunoglobulin G (IgG), and an abnormal glucose tolerance test.

Ion Channel Myopathies (Channelopathies) (p. 1270)

These are a group of familial diseases associated featuring myotonia and/or hypotonic paralysis; hypotonia variants are associated with hyperkalemia, hypokalemia, or normokalemia.

Pathogenesis (p. 1270)

These disorders are caused by mutation in genes encoding ion channels:

- *Hyperkalemic periodic paralysis* involves mutations in the SCN4A sodium channel protein that regulates sodium entry during muscle contraction.

TABLE 27-4 Other Selected Muscular Dystrophies

Disease and Inheritance	Gene and Locus	Clinical Findings	Pathologic Findings
Facioscapulohumeral muscular dystrophy; autosomal dominant	Type 1A—deletion of variable number of 3.3-kilobase subunits of a tandemly arranged repeat (DZ4) on 4q35 Type 1B (FSHMD1B)—locus unknown	Variable age at onset (most commonly 10-30 years); weakness of muscles of face, neck, and shoulder girdle	Dystrophic myopathy, often associated with inflammatory infiltrates in muscle
Oculopharyngeal muscular dystrophy; autosomal dominant	Poly(A)-binding protein-2 (PABP2) gene; 14q11.2-q13	Onset in mid-adult life; ptosis and weakness of extraocular muscles; difficulty in swallowing	Dystrophic myopathy, but often including rimmed vacuoles in type 1 fibers
Emery-Dreifuss muscular dystrophy; X-linked	Emerin (EMD1) gene; Xq28	Variable onset (most commonly 10-20 years); prominent contractures, especially of elbows and ankles	Mild myopathic changes; absent emerin by immunohistochemistry
Congenital muscular dystrophies; autosomal recessive (also called congenital, muscular dystrophy, subtypes MDC1A, MDC1B, MDC1C)	Type 1A (merosin-deficient type)—laminin α2 (merosin) gene; 6q22-q23 Type 1B—locus at 1q42; gene unknown Type 1C; fukutin-related protein gene; 19q13.3	Neonatal hypotonia, respiratory insufficiency, delayed motor milestones	Variable fiber size and extensive endomysial fibrosis
Congenital muscular dystrophy with CNS malformations (Fukuyama type); autosomal recessive	Fukutin; 9q31	Neonatal hypotonia and mental retardation	Variable muscle fiber size and endomysial fibrosis; CNS malformations such as polymicrogyria
Congenital muscular dystrophy with CNS and ocular malformations (Walker-Warburg type)	Protein O-mannosyl transferases (POMT1, 9q34.1; POMT2, 14q24.3)	Neonatal hypotonia and mental retardation with cerebral and ocular malformations	Variable muscle fiber size and endomysial fibrosis; CNS and ocular malformations

CNS, Central nervous system.

- *Hypokalemic periodic paralysis* involves the gene encoding a voltage-gated, L-type calcium channel.
- *Malignant hyperpyrexia (malignant hyperthermia)* presents as a dramatic hypermetabolic state (e.g., tachycardia, tachypnea, muscle spasms, and later hyperpyrexia) triggered by anesthesia (usually succinylcholine or halogenated inhalational agents). Although it can occur in a number of settings (e.g., congenital myopathies, metabolic myopathies, and dystrophinopathies), it is also associated with mutations of genes encoding L-type voltage-dependent calcium channels (notably the ryanodine receptor, RyR1). Upon exposure to anesthetic, the mutant receptor allows uncontrolled sarcoplamic calcium efflux. This in turn causes tetany, increased muscle metabolism, and excess heat production.

Congenital Myopathies (p. 1271)

These muscle diseases are characterized by early onset of nonprogressive or slowly progressive, proximal or generalized muscle weakness, and hypotonia *(floppy babies)*, or severe joint contractures *(arthrogryposis)* (Table 27-5).

Myopathies Associated with Inborn Errors of Metabolism (p. 1271)

Myopathies associated with disorders of glycogen synthesis and degradation are discussed in Chapter 5.

Lipid Myopathies (p. 1271)

Abnormalities of the carnitine transport system or deficiencies of the mitochondrial dehydrogenase enzyme systems lead to blocks in fatty acid catabolism and muscle lipid accumulation. Reduced fatty acid oxidation limits adenosine triphosphate (ATP) generation in exercising muscle, leading to pain, tightness, and myoglobinuria; cardiomyopathies and fatty liver can also occur.

Mitochondrial Myopathies (Oxidative Phosphorylation Diseases) (p. 1271)

The mitochondrial genome (mtDNA) encodes one fifth of the proteins involved in mitochondrial oxidative phosphorylation as well as mitochondrial tRNA and rRNA; the remainder of the mitochondrial proteins are encoded in the nuclear genome, so that mutations in both nuclear and mitochondrial genes can cause *mitochondrial myopathies.*

Morphology (p. 1271)

Findings include aggregates of abnormal mitochondria, causing irregular muscle fiber contour *(ragged red fibers* on trichrome stains). There are increased numbers of and abnormalities in the shape and size of mitochondria, some of which contain paracrystalline arrays (called *parking lot inclusions*) or alterations in the structure of cristae.

Clinical Course (p. 1272)

Mitochondrial myopathies typically present in young adulthood, manifesting with proximal muscle weakness, and occasionally severe eye muscle dysfunction *(external ophthalmoplegia).* Other neurologic symptoms, lactic acidosis, and cardiomyopathy can also occur.

- Disorders due to mtDNA mutations exhibit maternal inheritance since the oocyte contributes the mitochondria to the embryo. Disease expression can be variable due to unequal distribution of mtDNA in various cells.

TABLE 27-5 Congenital Myopathies

Disease and Inheritance	Gene and Locus	Clinical Findings	Pathologic Findings
Central core disease: autosomal dominant	Ryanodine receptor-1 (RYR1) gene; 19q13.1	Early-onset hypotonia and nonprogressive weakness; associated skeletal deformities; may develop malignant hyperthermia	Cytoplasmic cores are lightly eosinophilic and distinct from surrounding sarcoplasm; found only in type 1 fibers, which usually predominate, best seen on NADH stain
Nemaline myopathy; autosomal dominant or autosomal recessive	Autosomal dominant (NEM1)—Tropomyosin 3 (TPM3) gene; Autosomal recessive (NEM2)—nebulin (NEB) gene; 2q22 Autosomal dominant or recessive—skeletal muscle actin, α chain-1 (ACTA1) gene; 1q42.1	Weakness, hypotonia, and delayed motor development in childhood; may also be seen in adults; usually nonprogressive; involves proximal limb muscles most severely; skeletal abnormalities may be present	Aggregates of subsarcolemmal spindle-shaped particles (nemaline rods); occur predominantly in type 1 fibers; derived from Z-band material (α-actinin) and best seen on modified Gomori stain
Myotubular (centronuclear) myopathy; X-linked (MTM1), autosomal recessive, or autosomal dominant	X-linked—myotubularin (MTM1) gene; Xq28 Autosomal dominant—myogenic factor 6 (MYF6) gene; 12q21 Autosomal recessive—locus and gene unknown	X-linked form presents in infancy with prominent hypotonia and poor prognosis; autosomal forms have limb weakness and are slowly progressive; autosomal recessive form is intermediate in severity and prognosis	Abundance of centrally located nuclei involving the majority of muscle fibers; central nuclei are usually confined to type 1 fibers, which are small in diameter but can occur in both fiber types

NADH, Nicotinamide adenine dinucleotide, reduced form.

Disorders due to *point mutations* in the mtDNA include myoclonic epilepsy with ragged red fibers, Leber hereditary optic neuropathy, and mitochondrial encephalomyopathy with lactic acidosis and stroke-like episodes (MELAS).

Disorders due to *deletions* or *duplications* of mtDNA include chronic progressive external ophtlamoplegia and Kearns-Sayre syndrome.

• Mutations encoded in nuclear DNA show X-linked or autosomal dominant or recessive inheritance. Examples include subacute necrotizing encephalopathy, exertional myoglobinuria, and X-linked cardioskeletal myopathy.

Inflammatory Myopathies (p. 1273)

Covered elsewhere are infectious myositis (Chapter 8) and systemic inflammatory diseases that involve muscle (Chapter 6).

Noninfectious Inflammatory Myopathies (p. 1273)

Noninfectious inflammatory myopathies are a heterogeneous group of immune-mediated disorders characterized by skeletal muscle inflammation and injury.

• *Dermatomyositis* (p. 1273) involves skin and muscle. Classically, a lilac discoloration of upper eyelids and periorbital edema accompanies or precedes weakness; scaling, erythematous patches are also present over knuckles, elbows, and knees *(Grotton lesions)*. Muscle weakness is slow in onset and bilaterally symmetric, affecting proximal muscles first; dysphagia occurs in a third of patients. Interstitial lung disease, vasculitis, and myocarditis can also be present. Nearly 25% of adult patients have cancer; juvenile patients more characteristically exhibit gastrointestinal symptoms, and a third have calcinosis. Capillaries appear to be the primary target of immunologic attack. Immune suppressive therapy is beneficial.

• *Polymyositis* (p. 1273) is similar to dermatomyositis but lacks cutaneous involvement; it occurs primarily in adults. The pathogenesis involves cytotoxic T-cell–driven myocyte damage; various autoantibodies against tRNA synthetases are also present. Immune suppressive therapy is beneficial.

• *Inclusion body myositis* (p. 1273) begins with *distal muscle* involvement, especially extensors of the knee and flexors of the wrists, and can be asymmetric. It has an insidious onset, typically affecting individuals older than 50 years. Although cytotoxic CD8+ T cells are present, immunosuppressive therapy is generally not beneficial. Intracellular depositions of β-amyloid protein and hyperphosphorylated tau proteins suggest abnormal protein folding as an etiology.

Morphology (p. 1274)

• *Dermatomyositis:* Perivascular inflammatory infiltrates are associated with scattered necrotic muscle fibers and muscle fiber atrophy, especially at the periphery of fascicles ("perifascicular atrophy")—likely related to hypoperfusion.

• *Polymyositis:* There is endomysial inflammation and scattered necrotic muscle fibers, but no apparent vascular injury (perifascicular atrophy).

• *Inclusion body myositis:* Endomysial inflammatory infiltrates are associated with diagnostic "rimmed vacuoles"—clear cytoplasmic vacuoles in myocytes surrounded by a thin rim of basophilic material; myocytes can also contain amyloid deposits highlighted by Congo red staining.

Toxic Myopathies (p. 1275)

Thyrotoxic Myopathy (p. 1275)

Thyrotoxic myopathy presents as proximal muscle weakness that can precede clinical thyroid dysfunction; myofiber necrosis, regeneration, and interstitial lymphocytosis can be present. In *hypothyroidism,* muscle cramping and slowed movements are associated with fiber atrophy, increased numbers of internal nuclei, and glycogen aggregates.

Ethanol Myopathy (p. 1275)

Binge drinking can produce an acute toxic syndrome of painful rhabdomyolysis with accompanying myoglobinuria; it can lead to renal failure.

Drug-Induced Myopathies (p. 1275)

- Proximal muscle weakness and atrophy predominantly of type 2 fibers can occur in *Cushing syndrome* or during *corticosteroid administration.*
- *Chloroquine* can produce a proximal myopathy, histologically marked by autophagic membrane-bound vacuoles and intracellular curvilinear lamellar bodies.
- *Statin-induced myopathy* occurs in 1% to 2% of recipients.

Diseases of the Neuromuscular Junction (p. 1275)

Myasthenia Gravis (p. 1275)

Myasthenia gravis is due to autoantibodies directed against skeletal muscle acetylcholine receptors (AChR); it is more common in women younger than 40 years, but it has equal gender predilection in older age groups.

Pathogenesis (p. 1275)

AChR autoantibodies can mediate complement fixation and direct postsynaptic membrane damage, accelerate internalization and down-regulation of the AChR, or block ACh binding.

Morphology (p. 1276)

Light microscopic examination of muscle is ordinarily unremarkable; ultrastructurally, junctional folds are greatly reduced or abolished at the neuromuscular junction, and there is diminished AChR expression.

Clinical Course (p. 1276)

Patients classically present with easy fatigability, ptosis, and diplopia; symptoms worsen with repeated stimulation. Treatments include anticholinesterase agents, prednisone, and plasmapheresis. Thymic hyperplasia occurs in 65% of patients and thymomas in 15%; thymic resection can improve symptoms.

Lambert-Eaton Myasthenic Syndrome (p. 1276)

Lambert-Eaton myasthenic syndrome presents with weakness and autonomic dysfunction. Most cases (i.e., 60%) are paraneoplastic and are classically associated with small cell lung carcinoma; the syndrome can also occur in the absence of malignancy. The causal autoantibody is directed against a pre-synaptic voltage-gated calcium channel; each presynaptic action potential releases fewer synaptic vesicles than normal; as compared to myasthenia gravis, neurotransmission improves with repeated stimulation.

28

The Central Nervous System

Features that influence the manifestations of central nervous system (CNS) disorders include the following:

- Specific neurologic functions are typically localized to distinct (often spatially clustered) neurons; the clinical effects of injury therefore frequently are site-specific and may not be corrected by other neurons.
- CNS stem cell populations exist but have limited restorative capacity; destructive lesions thus typically cause permanent deficits.
- Certain neurons have selective vulnerability to injury.
- Physical restrictions of the skull and spine render the brain and spinal cord vulnerable to expansile pressure.
- The CNS has a distinct cerebrospinal fluid (CSF) circulation, lacks lymphatics, and has a selective blood-brain barrier.
- Some responses to injury are unique to the CNS (see later discussion).

Cellular Pathology of the Central Nervous System (p. 1281)

Reactions of Neurons to Injury (p. 1281)

- *Acute neuronal injury* encompasses a spectrum of changes secondary to hypoxia/ischemia (or other insults), leading to cell necrosis or apoptosis; there is intense cytoplasmic eosinophilia and nuclear pyknosis (as reflected by "*red neurons*").
- *Subacute and chronic neuronal injury ("degeneration")* refers to neuronal death (mostly apoptosis) and accompanying reactive gliosis, occurring as a consequence of progressive degenerative disorders. *Trans-synaptic degeneration* occurs when the afferent inputs to a neuron are lost.
- *Axonal reaction* reflects the response of a neuronal cell body to the challenge of regenerating damaged axons. The cell body rounds up and nucleoli enlarge; Nissl substance dispersal and perinuclear cytoplasmic pallor *(central chromatolysis)* are associated with increased protein synthesis and axonal sprouting.
- *Neuronal inclusions* can be manifestations of aging (lipofuscin), disorders of metabolism (storage material), viral diseases (inclusion bodies), or neurodegenerative diseases associated with aggregated proteins.

Reactions of Astrocytes to Injury (p. 1281)

Astrocytes are the principal cells responsible for repair and scar formation in the brain; they are also important cellular elements of the blood-brain barrier.

- In areas of CNS damage, astrocytes develop enlarged vesicular nuclei and conspicuous eosinophilic cytoplasm *(gemistocytic astrocytes)*; such astrocyte hypertrophy and hyperplasia culminates in tissue *gliosis.*
- When directly injured, astrocytes can also exhibit characteristic changes:

    Rosenthal fibers are elongated, eosinophilic structures within astrocytic processes; these contain αB-crystallin and hsp27 (heat shock proteins) and are seen in long-standing gliosis or pilocytic astrocytomas.

    Corpora amylacea are lamellated polyglucosan bodies (also containing heat shock proteins); these increase in number with advancing age and represent a degenerative change.

    Alzheimer type II astrocytes exhibit an enlarged nucleus with intranuclear glycogen and pale chromatin; these occur in the setting of hyperammonemia.

Reactions of Other Glial Cells to Injury (p. 1282)

- *Oligodendroglial cell* apoptosis is a feature of demyelinating disorders and leukodystrophies; viral inclusions can be seen in progressive multifocal leukoencephalopathy, and α-synuclein inclusions can be seen in multiple system atrophy (MSA).
- *Ependymal cells* do not regenerate; any damage results in proliferation of subependymal astrocytes, forming *ependymal granulations.*

Reactions of Microglia to Injury (p. 1282)

Following injury, microglia proliferate, develop elongated nuclei *(rod cells)*, form aggregates around necrotic foci *(microglial nodules)*, and/or aggregate around dying neurons *(neuronophagia)*.

Cerebral Edema, Hydrocephalus, and Raised Intracranial Pressure and Herniation (p. 1282)

The volume of the intracranial contents is fixed by the skull. Generalized CNS edema, increased CSF volume *(hydrocephalus)*, and hemorrhage or expanding mass lesions can thus increase intracranial pressure; consequences range from subtle neurologic deficits to death.

Cerebral Edema (p. 1282)

Brain parenchymal edema can be:

- *Vasogenic:* Increased vascular permeability leads to the accumulation of *intercellular fluid*; it can be focal or generalized. The absence of lymphatics impairs resorption.
- *Cytotoxic:* Increased *intracellular fluid* is secondary to endothelial, neuronal, or glial injury (e.g., after anoxia or toxic/metabolic disturbances).
- *Interstitial:* Fluid from the ventricular system transudates across the ependymal lining secondary to increased intraventricular pressure.

Hydrocephalus (p. 1283)

Obstruction of CSF flow leads to ventricular enlargement and increased CSF volume. Most cases are due to impaired flow or resorption; overproduction is an uncommon cause.

- When hydrocephalus occurs prior to cranial suture closure, the head is enlarged; hydrocephalus after bone fusion leads to ventricular expansion and increased intracranial pressure.

- *Non-communicating hydrocephalus* refers due enlargement of only a portion of the ventricle system (e.g., due to blockage of the third ventricle); in *communicating hydrocephalus*, the entire system is expanded.
- In diseases associated with extensive tissue loss, compensatory expansion of the entire CSF compartment results in *hydrocephalus ex vacuo.*

Raised Intracranial Pressure and Herniation (p. 1283)

Increased intracranial pressure leads to compression of brain parenchyma; vascular perfusion can also be compromised, further exacerbating cerebral edema. Because the cranial vault is divided by rigid dural folds *(falx* and *tentorium)*, localized expansion can cause displacement relative to the partitions with associated *herniation syndromes* (Fig. 28-1):

- *Subfalcine (cingulate) herniation* can compromise branches of the anterior cerebral artery.
- *Transtentorial (uncinate, mesial temporal) herniation* can distort the adjacent midbrain and pons; third cranial nerve compromise causes pupillary dilation, and compression of the posterior cerebral artery can cause visual cortex ischemia. Substantial herniation causes ipsilateral hemiparesis and is often accompanied by tearing of feeding vessels *[Duret hemorrhages].*
- *Tonsillar herniation* through the foramen magnum can compress the medulla and compromise cardiac and respiratory centers.

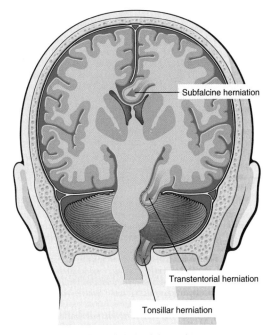

Subfalcine herniation

Transtentorial herniation

Tonsillar herniation

FIGURE 28-1 Major herniation syndromes.

Malformations and Developmental Diseases (p. 1284)

The nature of developmental malformation depends on when injury occurs during gestation; maternal and fetal infections, drugs, anoxia, ischemia, and genetic disorders can all be involved.

Neural Tube Defects (p. 1284)

These malformations reflect primary failure to close, or secondary reopening of the neural tube after successful closure. All are associated with abnormalities in some combination of neural tissue, meninges, and overlying bone and soft tissue. The frequency varies among ethnic groups and has both genetic and environmental influences; folate deficiency is a major risk factor; some population differences are secondary to polymorphisms in folate metabolism. Antenatal diagnosis can be made by imaging and maternal screening for α-fetoprotein.

- *Encephalocele* is a malformed CNS diverticulum extending through a defect in the cranium, typically in the occiput or posterior fossa.
- *Anencephaly* is a malformation of the anterior neural tube, resulting in failure of development of the cerebrum.
- *Spina bifida* can be an asymptomatic bony defect *(spina bifida occulta)* or a severe malformation with a flattened, disorganized cord segment with overlying meningeal outpouching.
- *Myelomeningocele* represents CNS outpouching through a vertebral column defect; most occur in the lumbosacral region associated with lower extremity motor and sensory deficits and disturbed bowel and bladder control.

Forebrain Anomalies (p. 1284)

- *Brain size* is influenced by the duration of periventricular cell proliferation relative to the onset of their migration into the cortex. If too many cells exit the proliferating population too soon, the result is *microencephaly* (small brain) and simplification of gyral folding—including complete absence of gyri *(lissencephaly* or *agyria)*. Chromosomal abnormalities, fetal alcohol syndrome, and *in utero* HIV infection can be causal. Conversely, if too few cells exit the proliferating pool at early stages (much less common), there is an eventual overproduction of neurons; *megalencephaly* (large brain) ensues.
- *Gyral formation* and overall *organization* are influenced by the patterns of neuronal movement following cell division.

  Polymicrogyria are small, overabundant cerebral convolutions due to focal injury near the end of neuronal migration; there are also genetic causes.

  Neuronal heterotopias are abnormal clusters of neurons in inappropriate locations along normal migratory routes; they are commonly associated with epilepsy. Mutations in cytoskeletal (e.g., filamin A) or microtubule-associated proteins can be causal.

  Holoprosencephaly is characterized by incomplete separation of the cerebral hemispheres; it is also associated with midline facial abnormalities (including cyclopia). Holoprosencephaly can result from mutations of *sonic hedgehog* or other genes involved in neural development.

  In *agenesis of the corpus callosum*, normal white matter interhemispheric bundles are not formed; although mental retardation can occur, individuals are often clinically normal.

Posterior Fossa Anomalies (p. 1285)

- *Dandy-Walker malformation* is characterized by an enlarged posterior fossa, absent cerebellar vermis, and large midline cyst, with brainstem nuclei dysplasias.
- *Arnold-Chiari malformation (Chiari II malformation)* consists of a small posterior fossa, a malformed midline cerebellum with extension of the vermis through the foramen magnum, hydrocephalus, and a lumbar myelomeningocele.
- *Chiari I malformation* is associated with low-lying cerebellar tonsils extending into the vertebral canal; it is often clinically silent, but it can present with CSF flow obstruction.

Syringomyelia and Hydromyelia (p. 1286)

These are expansions of the central canal *(hydromyelia)* or formation of a cleftlike cavity *(syringomyelia)* in the spinal cord. Histologically, there is associated gray and white matter destruction surrounded by reactive gliosis. Patients present with loss of pain and temperature sensation in the upper extremities.

Perinatal Brain Injury (p. 1286)

Cerebral palsy is the broad term for nonprogressive motor deficits related to pre- and perinatal neurologic insults; prematurity is a major risk factor. Depending on the location of the injury, lesions are clinically manifested by dystonia, spasticity, ataxia/athetosis, and/or paresis:

- *Intraparenchymal hemorrhage* within the germinal matrix often occurs between the thalamus and caudate nucleus and can extend into the ventricular system.
- *Ischemic infarcts* can occur in the periventricular white matter *(periventricular leukomalacia)* or within the hemispheres *(multicystic encephalopathy)*.
- *Ulegyria* is the term for thin, gliotic gyri due to perinatal cortical ischemia; *status marmoratus* reflects ischemic neuronal loss and gliosis in the basal ganglia and thalamus associated with aberrant and irregular myelin formation.

Injury during gestation can destroy brain tissue without evoking any reactive gliosis.

Trauma (p. 1287)

Skull Fractures (p. 1287)

Fracture resistance varies with skull bone thickness; *displaced fracture* is the term used when bone shifts into the cranial vault by more than its thickness. Accidental falls tend to involve the occiput; they can have secondary basal skull involvement with lower cranial nerve or cervicomedullary symptoms, CSF discharge, and/or meningitis. Trauma occurring as a consequence of syncope tends to involve the frontal skull. Although the kinetic energy that causes fractures tends to be dissipated at sutures, fractures can nevertheless traverse sutures *(diastatic fractures)*.

Parenchymal Injuries (p. 1287)

Concussion (p. 1287)

Concussion is a transient trauma-related clinical syndrome associated with loss of consciousness, temporary respiratory arrest, and loss of reflexes; there is amnesia for the event. Postconcussive neuropsychiatric syndromes, commonly associated with repetitive injuries, are well recognized.

Direct Parenchymal Injury (p. 1287)

Direct parenchymal injury takes the form of *lacerations* (penetrating injury causing tissue tearing) and *contusions* (essentially CNS bruises). Gyral crests are most susceptible to contusion, for example, at the site of impact *(coup contusion)* or the point in the cranium opposite the impact *(contrecoup)*. Microscopically, there is brain hemorrhage and edema that eventually resolves as a depressed, yellow-brown glial scar extending to the pial surface *(plaque jaune)*.

Diffuse Axonal Injury (p. 1288)

Diffuse axonal injury occurs when mechanical forces, including angular acceleration even in the absence of impact, disrupt axonal integrity and subsequent axoplasmic flow. Microscopically, there is widespread axonal swelling and focal hemorrhage, subsequently replaced by degenerated fibers and gliosis. Up to half of patients who become comatose after trauma have diffuse axonal injury, even in the absence of cerebral contusions.

Traumatic Vascular Injury (p. 1288)

Depending on the anatomy of ruptured vessels, trauma-related hemorrhages are *epidural, subdural, subarachnoid,* and *intraparenchymal* (Fig. 28-2).

Subarachnoid and intraparenchymal hemorrhages are most often associated with superficial contusions and lacerations.

Epidural Hematoma (p. 1289)

Epidural hematomas result from rupture of dural arteries, most commonly the middle meningeal artery; blood collects between the dura and skull, compressing the brain. Depending on the tempo of accumulation, patients can be lucid for several hours after trauma. Lesions can also expand rapidly, mandating prompt drainage.

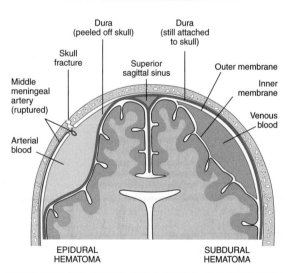

FIGURE 28-2 Epidural hematoma *(left):* A meningeal artery rupture (usually associated with a skull fracture) leads to accumulation of arterial blood between the dura and skull. Subdural hematoma *(right):* Damage to bridging veins between the brain and superior sagittal sinus leads to blood accumulation between the dura and the arachnoid.

Subdural Hematoma (p. 1289)

Subdural hematomas result from tearing of veins that stretch from the cortical surface through the subarachnoid and subdural spaces and into draining veins (e.g., superior sagittal sinus). While the brain "floats" freely in the CSF, the veins are tethered and thus prone to rupture with traumatic shifting of the brain within the skull. Geriatric patients with cerebral atrophy are particularly susceptible, even after minor trauma. Slowly progressive symptoms (often, non-localizing headache and confusion) usually occur within 48 hours of injury, although acute decompensation can occur. Frequently, subdural hematomas exhibit recurrent episodes of bleeding, attributed to hemorrhage from thin-walled vessels of granulation tissue *(chronic subdural hematoma)*. Treatment involves surgical drainage and removal of the associated granulation tissue.

Sequelae of Brain Trauma (p. 1290)

Sequelae include epilepsy, meningiomas, infectious diseases, and psychiatric disorders:

- *Post-traumatic hydrocephalus* occurs when hemorrhage into the subarachnoid space obstructs CSF resorption.
- *Post-traumatic dementia (dementia pugilistica)* is the consequence of repeated head trauma; findings include hydrocephalus, corpus callosum thinning, diffuse axonal injury, amyloid plaques, and neurofibrillary tangles.

Spinal Cord Trauma (p. 1290)

Cord injuries are associated with displacement of the spinal column; the level of injury determines the neurologic outcome:

- Thoracic vertebrae or below: paraplegia
- Cervical vertebrae: quadriplegia; with lesions at C4 and above, respiratory compromise due to diaphragm paralysis

Hemorrhage, necrosis, and white matter axonal swellings are acute findings. With time, necrotic lesions become cystic and gliotic; affected ascending and descending white matter tracts undergo secondary degeneration.

Cerebrovascular Diseases (p. 1290)

Cerebrovascular disease is the third leading cause of death in the United States (i.e., after heart disease and cancer); it is the most common cause of neurologic morbidity and mortality. Disease is a consequence of *hemorrhage* due to vessel rupture or of *ischemia* and *infarction* due to impaired perfusion or oxygenation.

Hypoxia, Ischemia, and Infarction (p. 1291)

Brain oxygen deprivation causes either global *(ischemic* or *hypoxic encephalopathy)* or focal ischemic necrosis *(cerebral infarction)*. At sites of diminished perfusion, outcomes depend on collateral circulation, duration of ischemia, and the magnitude and rapidity of flow reduction. *Stroke* is the clinical designation for these events, particularly with acute symptom onset.

Hypotension, Hypoperfusion, and Low-Flow States (Global Cerebral Ischemia) (p. 1291)

Hypoxia can occur secondary to reduced blood oxygen content or to hypotension; neurons are more sensitive than astrocytes and oligodendrocytes, and some neurons are more susceptible than others due to differences in regional blood flow and/or metabolic demand.

Severe global ischemia leads to widespread neuronal cell death; patients who survive can remain in a persistent vegetative state or meet "brain death" criteria: "flat" electroencephalogram and absent reflexes, respiratory drive, and cerebral perfusion. When maintained on mechanical ventilation, the brain of such patients eventually autolyzes ("respirator brain").

If oxygenation is only incompletely compromised, *watershed (border zone) infarcts* can occur at the interface between major vascular supplies; the territory between the anterior and middle cerebral artery is most vulnerable.

Morphology (p. 1291)

- *Grossly:* Ischemic areas are edematous with widened gyri and narrowed sulci; there is poor gray/white matter demarcation.
- *Microscopically:* Between 12 and 24 hours after injury, cellular ischemia is highlighted by the presence of *red neurons*; pyramidal neurons in the hippocampus CA1 (Sommer sector), cerebellar Purkinje cells, and cortical pyramidal neurons are most susceptible. Subsequent neutrophil infiltration is followed by macrophage influx, neovascularization, and reactive gliosis. Uneven cortical neuronal loss and gliosis alternating with preserved zones generates a pattern termed *pseudolaminar necrosis.*

Infarction from Obstruction of Local Blood Supply (Focal Cerebral Ischemia) (p. 1292)

Infarction from obstruction of local blood supply can result from thrombotic or embolic arterial occlusion. The clinical manifestations depend on the anatomic location of the lesion; deficits evolve with time and can be permanent or can slowly improve.

- *Thrombosis* (usually due to underlying atherosclerosis) most frequently affects the extracerebral carotid system and the basilar artery.
- *Embolism* most commonly involves the intracerebral arteries and particularly the middle cerebral artery distribution. Emboli originate from atheromatous cerebrovascular plaques, cardiac mural thrombi (especially in the setting of atrial fibrillation), valvular lesions, or paradoxically through atrial or ventricular septal defects.
- *Inflammatory* lesions, including infectious vasculitis (e.g., syphilis or tuberculosis) and other vasculitides (e.g., polyarteritis nodosa) can also cause luminal narrowing and cerebral infarction.
- *Venous infarcts* occur after occlusion of the superior sagittal sinus, other sinuses, or deep cerebral veins and are characteristically hemorrhagic.

Morphology (p. 1293)

- *Nonhemorrhagic infarcts (bland or anemic infarcts)* are evident at 48 hours as pale, soft regions of edematous brain, with neutrophilic infiltration. The tissue then liquefies, and a fluid-filled cavity containing macrophages is lined by reactive glia.
- *Hemorrhagic infarcts*—characteristic of embolic occlusion with reperfusion injury—exhibit blood extravasation, but otherwise they evolve in a fashion comparable to bland infarcts.

Hypertensive Cerebrovascular Disease (p. 1295)

Lacunar Infarcts (p. 1295)

Lacunar infarcts are small (less than 15 mm) cystic infarcts resulting from cerebral arteriolar sclerosis and occlusion; tissue loss is accompanied by lipid-laden macrophages and surrounding gliosis. The lenticular nucleus, thalamus, internal capsule, deep white matter, caudate nucleus, and pons are most commonly affected. Clinically, they can be silent or cause serious impairment.

Slit Hemorrhages *(p. 1295)*

Slit hemorrhages occur when hypertension causes small vessel rupture; these eventually resorb, leaving residual hemosiderin-laden macrophages and associated gliosis.

Hypertensive Encephalopathy *(p. 1295)*

- *Acute hypertensive encephalopathy:* This is a clinicopathologic syndrome caused by increased intracranial pressure and manifesting as diffuse cerebral dysfunction (e.g., headaches, confusion, vomiting, convulsions, and occasionally coma). Rapid therapeutic intervention is required; postmortem examination reveals an edematous brain (occasionally with herniation) with petechiae and arteriolar fibrinoid necrosis.
- *Chronic hypertensive injury:* Recurrent small infarcts (hypertensive, atherosclerotic, and/or embolic) can lead to *vascular (multi-infarct) dementia,* a syndrome characterized by dementia, gait abnormalities, pseudobulbar signs, and other focal neurologic deficits. *Binswanger disease* is the designation when the pattern of recurrent ischemic injury preferentially involves subcortical white matter with myelin and axonal loss.

Intracranial Hemorrhage *(p. 1295)*

Intracerebral (Intraparenchymal) Hemorrhage *(p. 1295)*

Intracerebral (intraparenchymal) hemorrhage typically involves spontaneous rupture of a small intraparenchymal vessel; peak incidence is age 60 years.

- *Hypertension* is the predisposing factor in half, accounting for 15% of deaths among patients with chronic hypertension. Hypertension leads to vessel weakening through hyaline arteriosclerosis, focal vessel necrosis, and the formation of microaneurysms *(Charcot-Bouchard aneurysms).* Lesions occur in the putamen (50% to 60% of cases), thalamus, pons, and rarely the cerebellar hemispheres.
- *Cerebral amyloid angiopathy (CAA):* CAA is the second most common etiology; amyloidogenic peptides identical to those seen in Alzheimer disease (see later) deposit in vessel walls, leading to weakening. Lesions characteristically comprise "stiff" amyloid deposition involving the leptomeningeal and cerebral cortical vessels.
- *Cerebral autosomal dominant arteriopathy with subcortical infarcts and leukoencephalopathy (CADASIL)* is a rare form of stroke caused by mutations in the Notch3 receptor. Affected vessels exhibit concentric medial and adventitial thickening with basophilic granular deposits and smooth muscle drop-out.

Subarachnoid Hemorrhage and Ruptured Saccular Aneurysms *(p. 1297)*

The most common cause of clinically significant subarachnoid hemorrhage is *berry (saccular) aneurysm* rupture; subarachnoid hemorrhages can also result from traumatic hematomas, vascular malformations, hypertensive intracerebral hemorrhage, tumors, and hematologic disturbances.

Pathogenesis *(p. 1297)*

Berry aneurysms occur in 2% of the population, with 20% to 30% of patients having multiple aneurysms; 90% of berry aneurysms occur in the anterior circulation near arterial branch points. Although most are sporadic, aneurysms can also be associated with autosomal dominant polycystic kidney disease (Chapter 20), hypertension, aortic coarctation, collagen disorders (e.g., Ehlers-Danlos syndrome type IV, Marfan syndrome), neurofibromatosis type 1, and fibromuscular dysplasia.

Morphology (p. 1297)

Lesions are a few mm to 2 to 3 cm in diameter with a red shiny translucent wall. At the aneurysm neck, the muscular wall and intimal elastic lamina are absent or fragmentary; the sac wall is composed of only thickened hyalinized intima.

Clinical Features (p. 1297)

Rupture risk increases with lesion size; aneurysms more than 10 mm have a 50% annual risk of bleeding. Rupture often occurs with elevated intracranial pressure (e.g., straining at stool or sexual orgasm). Symptoms include excruciating headache and rapid loss of consciousness. Between 25% and 50% die with the first rupture; in survivors, re-bleeding is common with progressively worsening prognosis with each episode. Blood in the subarachnoid space can lead to arterial vasospasm, and blood resorption can cause meningeal fibrosis and hydrocephalus.

Vascular Malformations (p. 1298)

- *Arteriovenous malformations (AVM)* are tangles of abnormally tortuous and misshapen vessels, shunting arterial blood directly into the venous circulation; middle cerebral artery territory is most commonly involved. The male to female ratio is 2:1; most cases manifest between ages 10 and 30 years as a seizure disorder, intracerebral hemorrhage, or subarachnoid hemorrhage.
- *Cavernous hemangiomas* are distended, loosely organized vascular channels with thin, collagenized walls; they occur most often in the cerebellum, pons, and subcortical regions and have low flow without arteriovenous shunting.
- *Capillary telangiectasias* are microscopic foci of dilated, thin-walled vascular channels separated by relatively normal brain parenchyma; they occur most frequently in the pons.
- *Venous angiomas (varices)* consist of aggregates of ecstatic veins. *Foix-Alajouanine disease* is a venous angiomatous malformation typically seen in the lumbosacral region, associated with slowly progressive ischemia and neurologic symptoms.

Infections (p. 1299)

Infectious injury to the CNS can occur by direct microbial damage, through elaboration of microbial toxins, or by the effects of the host immune response. Microbes can access the CNS by:

- *Hematogenous spread:* Most common, usually arterial
- *Direct implantation:* Usually traumatic
- *Local extension:* From an established infection in an air sinus
- *Axonal transport:* Along peripheral nerves (e.g., rabies and herpes zoster)

Acute Meningitis (p. 1299)

Acute Pyogenic (Bacterial) Meningitis (p. 1299)

Pathogens differ across age groups:

- Neonates: *E. coli* and the group B streptococci
- Infants and children: *S. pneumoniae* (The incidence of *Haemophilus influenzae* as an agent has been reduced by immunization.)

- Adolescents and young adults: *Neisseria meningitidis*
- Elderly: *S. pneumoniae* and *Listeria monocytogenes*

Affected individuals present with fever, headache, photophobia, irritability, clouded sensorium, and neck stiffness. The CSF is purulent with neutrophils and organisms, increased protein, and decreased glucose.

Morphology (p. 1299)

- *Grossly:* Meningeal vessels are engorged, and there is a purulent exudate.
- *Microscopically:* Neutrophils fill the subarachnoid space; in fulminant cases, inflammation may focally extend into the underlying CNS (cerebritis). Phlebitis can cause venous thrombosis and hemorrhagic infarction. Resolution can lead to leptomeningeal fibrosis and hydrocephalus.

Acute Aseptic (Viral) Meningitis (p. 1300)

Acute aseptic (viral) meningitis is characterized by meningeal irritation, a CSF lymphocytic pleocytosis, with moderate protein elevation, and normal glucose; the course is usually less fulminant than for pyogenic meningitis and is self-limited. Causal pathogens are infrequently identified.

Acute Focal Suppurative Infections (p. 1300)

Brain Abscess (p. 1300)

Brain abscess is a destructive lesion arising in the setting of bacterial endocarditis, congenital heart disease (with right-to-left shunting), chronic pulmonary sepsis, or immunosuppression. Streptococci and staphylococci are the principal organisms. Patients present with progressive focal neurologic deficits and signs of increased intracranial pressure. If the subdural space becomes infected, thrombophlebitis can develop, resulting in venous occlusion and brain infarction.

Morphology (p. 1300)

There is a central region of liquefactive necrosis; older lesions have a fibrous capsule surrounded by reactive gliosis and marked vasogenic edema.

Chronic Bacterial Meningoencephalitis (p. 1301)

Tuberculosis (p. 1301)

Tuberculous meningitis causes headache, malaise, mental confusion, and vomiting. There is moderate CSF mononuclear cell pleocytosis (occasionally with neutrophils), elevated protein, and moderately reduced or normal glucose. Tuberculous meningitis can cause arachnoid fibrosis, hydrocephalus, and obliterative endarteritis. Tuberculomas present as typical space-occupying lesions. *Mycobacterium avium-intracellulare* infections can also occur in patients with acquired immunodeficiency syndrome (AIDS) but typically provoke little granulomatous response.

Morphology (p. 1301)

Diffuse meningoencephalitis is the most common pattern of disease. The subarachnoid space contains a gelatinous or fibrinous exudate of chronic inflammatory cells and, rarely, well-formed granulomas, most often at the base of the brain, obliterating the cisternae and encasing the cranial nerves. Arteries running through the subarachnoid space may show *obliterative endarteritis*.

Neurosyphilis (p. 1301)

Neurosyphilis is a manifestation of the tertiary stage of disease; it occurs in 10% of patients with untreated infections. Human immunodeficiency virus (HIV)-infected patients are at increased risk for neurosyphilis related to impaired cell-mediated immunity; the severity and tempo of disease is also accelerated.

- *Meningovascular neurosyphilis* is a chronic meningitis sometimes associated with obliterative endarteritis.
- *Paretic neurosyphilis* results from brain invasion by spirochetes, with neuronal loss and microglial proliferation. Patients exhibit insidious loss of mental and physical capacity with mood alterations (including delusions of grandeur), terminating in severe dementia.
- *Tabes dorsalis* results from spirochete damage to dorsal root sensory neurons, leading to impaired joint position sense, locomotor ataxia, loss of pain sensation with secondary skin and joint damage (Charcot joints), and absent deep tendon reflexes.

Patients with HIV (human immunodeficiency virus) infection are at increased risk for neurosyphilis due to impaired cell-mediated immunity; disease progression and severity is also worse relative to immunocompetent hosts.

Neuroborreliosis (Lyme Disease) (p. 1302)

The neurologic manifestations of Lyme disease are highly variable but can include aseptic meningitis, facial nerve palsies (and other polyneuropathies), and encephalopathy. Microscopically, there is microglial proliferation and scattered organisms.

Viral Meningoencephalitis (p. 1302)

Viral parenchymal infections of the CNS *(encephalitis)* are almost invariably associated with inflammation of the meninges *(meningoencephalitis)* and occasionally with the spinal cord *(encephalomyelitis)*. Viruses can exhibit specific cellular tropisms or can have a predilection for particular brain regions. Latency is a common feature of several CNS viral infections; non-CNS systemic infections can also precipitate immune-mediated neurologic injury.

Arthropod-Borne Viral Encephalitis (p. 1302)

Arthropod-borne viral encephalitis is the etiology of most epidemic encephalitides (e.g., Eastern and Western equine, Venezuelan, St. Louis, La Crosse, and West Nile viruses). All have animal hosts and mosquito or tick vectors. Typical clinical manifestations are seizures, confusion, delirium, and stupor or coma.

Herpes Simplex Virus Type 1 (p. 1302)

Herpes simplex virus-1 (HSV-1) is most common in children and young adults; only 10% of patients have prior herpes infection. Patients classically present with alterations in affect, mood, memory, and behavior; some cases follow a more protracted course with weakness, lethargy, ataxia, and seizures.

Morphology (p. 1302)

Severe cases exhibit hemorrhagic, necrotizing encephalitis of the inferomedial temporal lobes and the orbital gyri of the frontal lobes. There are perivascular infiltrates, with Cowdry A intranuclear viral inclusion bodies in neurons and glia.

Herpes Simplex Virus Type 2 (p. 1303)

Herpes simplex virus-2 (HSV-2) causes a severe, generalized, encephalitis in 50% of neonates born vaginally to women with primary HSV-2 infection. It can cause meningitis in adults and a severe henorrhagic, necrotizing encephalitis in HIV-infected individuals.

Varicella-Zoster Virus (Herpes Zoster) *(p. 1303)*

Latent chickenpox infections in dorsal root ganglia can be reactivated, leading to painful vesicular skin eruptions in a dermatomal distribution *(shingles)*. These are usually self-limited, but patients can develop a persistent painful post-herpetic neuralgia syndrome. Herpes zoster can also cause a granulomatous arteritis or a necrotizing encephalitis in immunosuppressed patients.

Cytomegalovirus *(p. 1304)*

In utero infection leads to periventricular necrosis, microcephaly, and periventricular calcification. In patients with AIDS, cytomegalovirus (CMV) is a common opportunistic viral pathogen; it causes a subacute encephalitis with microglial nodules or a periventricular hemorrhagic necrotizing encephalitis and choroid plexitis. Classic CMV inclusions are readily identified.

Poliomyelitis *(p. 1304)*

Poliomyelitis presents with meningeal irritation and a CSF picture of aseptic meningitis; involvement of lower motor neurons can cause flaccid paralysis with hyporeflexia and secondary muscle wasting. Patients can also develop myocarditis, and death can result from paralysis of the respiratory muscles. Inflammation is usually confined to the anterior horns but can extend into the posterior horns. The *post-polio syndrome* typically develops 25 to 35 years after the initial illness; it is characterized by progressive weakness associated with pain and decreased muscle mass.

Rabies *(p. 1304)*

Rabies is a severe encephalitis transmitted by the bite of a rabid animal or exposure to certain bat species even without a bite. Over the course of 1 to 3 months, the virus ascends from the wound site to the CNS along the peripheral nerves. It causes extraordinary CNS excitability, hydrophobia, and flaccid paralysis; death ensues from respiratory center failure. Widespread neuronal necrosis and inflammation are present, most severe in the basal ganglia, midbrain, and medulla. Pathognomonic *Negri bodies* (intracytoplasmic eosinophilic inclusions) are found in hippocampal pyramidal cells and Purkinje cells, usually without associated inflammation.

Human Immunodeficiency Virus *(p. 1305)*

An *aseptic meningitis* occurs in 10% of patients within 1 to 2 weeks of a primary HIV infection; during the chronic phase of infection, *HIV encephalitis* is commonly found in symptomatic individuals. Notably, only microglia express the appropriate CD4 and chemokine receptors necessary for efficient HIV infection. In the absence of antiretroviral therapy, 80% to 90% of AIDS patients eventually develop direct CNS lesions, including direct viral pathogenic effects, opportunistic infections, and/or CNS lymphomas; intensive multidrug therapy has substantially reduced this incidence. *HIV-associated dementia* is related to the extent of activated CNS microglia; cytokines and other inflammatory mediators are causally implicated.

Morphology *(p. 1305)*

HIV encephalitis exhibits a chronic inflammatory reaction with widely distributed microglial nodules (and multinucleated giant cells) sometimes with associated necrosis and gliosis. The subcortical white matter, diencephalon, and brain stem are typically most affected.

Progressive Multifocal Leukoencephalopathy (p. 1305)

Progressive multifocal leukoencephalopathy (PML) is due to oligodendrocyte infection by the JC polyomavirus, typically in immunosuppressed patients. Most adults have serologic evidence of prior JC exposure; thus, PML likely represents viral reactivation. Patients develop progressive neurologic manifestations caused by focal myelin destruction.

Morphology (p. 1305)

Lesions consist of demyelinated patches, greatly enlarged oligodendrocyte nuclei with viral inclusions, and astrocytes with greatly enlarged atypical nuclei.

Subacute Sclerosing Panencephalitis (p. 1306)

Subacute sclerosing panencephalitis (SSPE) is a progressive syndrome of cognitive decline, limb spasticity, and seizures. It occurs months to years after an early-age measles infection and represents a persistent but nonproductive CNS infection by an altered measles virus. Widespread gliosis and myelin degeneration is associated with viral nuclear inclusions in oligodendrocytes and neurons; there is also variable inflammation with neurofibrillary tangles.

Fungal Meningoencephalitis (p. 1306)

Fungal CNS infections are typically encountered in immunocompromised patients, usually in the setting of widespread hematogenous dissemination (e.g., with *Candida albicans, Mucor, Aspergillus fumigatus,* and *Cryptococcus neoformans*). In endemic areas, *Histoplasma, Coccidioides,* and *Blastomyces* can involve the CNS after primary pulmonary or cutaneous infections.

* *Meningitis* is caused most frequently by *Cryptococcus;* it can be fulminant and fatal within 2 weeks, or it can be chronic and indolent, evolving over months or years.
* *Vasculitis* occurs most frequently with *Mucor* and *Aspergillus;* there is vessel invasion with associated thrombosis and hemorrhagic infarction.
* *Parenchymal involvement* can manifest with granulomas or abscesses and is most commonly encountered with *Candida* and *Cryptococcus.*

Other Infectious Diseases of the Nervous System (p. 1306)

Protozoal (i.e., malaria, toxoplasmosis, amebiasis, and trypanosomiasis), rickettsial (i.e., typhus, Rocky Mountain spotted fever), and metazoal (i.e., cysticercosis and echinococcosis) organisms can all infect the CNS (Chapter 8); some are opportunistic while others occur in immunocompetent hosts.

* *Toxoplasma gondii* is one of the most common CNS organisms seen in HIV-infected patients. Clinical symptoms occur over 1 to 2 weeks and are typically focal; imaging studies show multiple ring-enhancing lesions. Abscesses contain free tachyzoites and encysted bradyzoites. Primary maternal infection can be followed by a fetal cerebritis with multifocal necrotizing lesions that calcify.
* *Naegleria* is an amoeba that causes a rapidly fatal necrotizing encephalitis; *acanthamoeba* is associated with a chronic granulomatous meningoencephalitis.

Transmissible Spongiform Encephalopathies (Prion Diseases) (p. 1308)

These progressively dementing disorders are characterized by *spongiform changes* (neuronal and glial intracellular vacuoles) caused by abnormal forms of the *prion protein (PrP)*. Prion diseases are transmissible and can be infectious, sporadic, or familial; disorders include Creutzfeldt-Jakob disease (CJD), Gerstmann-Straussler-Scheinker syndrome (GSS), fatal familial insomnia, and kuru in humans, scrapie in sheep and goats, mink-transmissible encephalopathy, chronic wasting disease in elk and deer, and bovine spongiform encephalopathy *(mad cow disease)*.

Pathogenesis (p. 1308)

PrP is a normal 30-kD neuronal protein; disease occurs when PrP undergoes a conformational change from its native α-helical isoform (PrP^c) to an abnormally folded (and protease-resistant) β-pleated sheet configuration, called PrP^{sc} (for scrapie). The PrP^{sc} conformational change occurs spontaneously at a very low rate (sporadic disease); it occurs more readily if certain mutations are present (familial disease). The transmissible/infectious nature of PrP^{sc} derives from its ability to induce the conformational change of PrP^c, thereby corrupting the integrity of normal cellular PrP. The *PRNP* gene encoding PrP is highly conserved across species, underlying some of the ability of PrP from other sources to cause human disease. Polymorphisms at codon 129 (encoding methionine or valine) also influence disease susceptibility or incubation period; heterozygosity at codon 129 is protective.

CREUTZFELDT-JAKOB DISEASE (p. 1309)

CJD is sporadic in 85% of cases with a worldwide incidence of one in a million, and peak occurrence in the seventh decade; cases can also be familial or iatrogenic (e.g., through corneal transplantation or electrode implantation). Patients present with subtle memory and behavior changes, followed by a rapidly progressive dementia, often with involuntary jerking muscle contractions. The disease is uniformly fatal, with an average duration of only 7 months after symptom onset.

VARIANT CREUTZFELDT-JAKOB DISEASE (p. 1309)

Variant Creutzfeldt-Jakob Disease (vCJD) came to medical attention in the United Kingdom in 1995; it occurs in young adults, with early behavioral manifestations and slower neurologic progression than for classic CJD. No *PRNP* mutations are present, and vCJD has been linked to bovine spongiform encephalopathy. Extensive cortical plaques are present, with a surrounding halo of spongiform change.

GERSTMANN-STRAUSSLER-SCHEINKER SYNDROME

GSS is an inherited disease due to *PRNP* mutations; it typically begins with a chronic cerebellar ataxia, followed by a progressive dementia. The clinical course is usually slower than that of CJD, with progression to death several years after the onset of symptoms.

Morphology (p. 1309)

The pathologic finding is a spongiform transformation of the cerebral cortex and, often, deep gray matter structures (e.g., caudate and putamen). In advanced cases, there is severe neuronal loss, reactive gliosis, and sometimes expansion of the vacuolated areas into cystlike spaces *(status spongiosus)*. No inflammatory infiltrate is present. *Kuru plaques* are extracellular aggregates of aggregated abnormal PrP^{sc} proteins; they are Congo red- and PAS-positive.

FATAL FAMILIAL INSOMNIA (p. 1309)

Fatal familial insomnia (FFI) is named, in part, for the sleep disturbances that characterize its initial stages; it is caused by *PRNP* mutations substituting aspartate for asparagine at residue 178 of PrP^{c}. When the mutations are present in alleles with methionine at position 129, FFI results; when a valine is present at position 129, CJD occurs.

Morphology (p. 1309)

Unlike other prion diseases, FFI does not exhibit spongiform changes; instead, there is neuronal loss and reactive gliosis in the inferior olivary nuclei and anterior ventral and dorsomedial nuclei of the thalamus.

Demyelinating Diseases (p. 1309)

These inherited or acquired disorders are characterized by myelin damage with relative preservation of axons; neurologic deficits are secondary to loss of electric impulse transmission.

Multiple Sclerosis (p. 1309)

Multiple sclerosis (MS) is an autoimmune demyelinating disorder characterized by *distinct episodes of neurologic deficit separated in time and attributable to white matter lesions that are separated in space.* Women are affected twice as frequently as men; peak onset is between childhood and age 50 years. The natural course is variable but is characteristically relapsing and remitting with acute (i.e., days to weeks) deficit onset and slow, gradual partial remission. Relapse frequency tends to decrease over time, but most patients exhibit steady neurologic deterioration.

Pathogenesis (p. 1310)

MS is attributed to cellular immune responses directed against myelin. Genetic and environmental factors are both implicated, although the inciting stimulus (e.g., Epstein-Barr virus [EBV] infection) is uncertain in most cases; MS susceptibility is linked to the DR2 locus of the major histocompatibility complex and to polymorphisms in the IL-2 and IL-7 receptor genes. Disease is initiated by CD4+ T$_H$1 and T$_H$17 cells responding to myelin components. T$_H$1 cell interferon-γ secretion activates macrophages, and T$_H$17 cells help recruit additional leukocytes; the resulting inflammatory infiltrate causes myelin destruction. The CSF in affected patients exhibits an oligoclonal immunoglobulin response, suggesting a contribution from B-cell immunity.

Morphology (p. 1311)

- *Grossly:* Lesions *(plaques)* are sharply defined areas of gray discoloration of white matter occurring especially around the ventricles but potentially located anywhere in the CNS.
- *Microscopically:* Active plaques show myelin breakdown, lipid-laden macrophages, and relative axonal preservation. Lymphocytes and mononuclear cells are prominent at plaque edges and around venules. *Inactive plaques* lack the inflammatory cell infiltrate and show gliosis; most axons within the lesion persist but remain unmyelinated.

Clinical Features (p. 1312)

Although neurologic manifestations can be diverse (depending on the site of demyelination), certain features are more common:

- Unilateral vision impairment due to optic neuritis is a frequent initial manifestation, although only 10% to 50% of patients with optic nerve involvement progress to full-blown MS.
- Brainstem involvement produces cranial nerve signs, ataxia, nystagmus, and internuclear ophthalmoplegia.
- Spinal cord lesions cause limb and trunk motor and sensory impairment, spasticity, and bladder dysfunction.

Neuromyelitis Optica (Devic Disease) (p. 1312)

This disorder is characterized by bilateral optic neuritis and spinal cord demyelinating lesions. White matter lesions exhibit necrosis with acute inflammation, as well as vascular immunoglobulin and complement deposition; many patients have antibodies directed against aquaporins, which are important in maintaining astrocyte foot processes and thus blood-brain barrier integrity.

Acute Disseminated Encephalomyelitis and Acute Necrotizing Hemorrhagic Encephalomyelitis (p. 1312)

- Acute disseminated encephalomyelitis (ADEM) is a diffuse demyelinating disease occurring after viral infection (or rarely, a viral immunization); patients present with headache, lethargy, and coma, but no focal deficits. The clinical course is rapid; up to 20% die. All lesions appear similar, consistent with a single initiating insult, and exhibit perivenular demyelination with axonal preservation; early neutrophil infiltrates are followed by mononuclear cell inflammation and lipid-laden macrophages.
- Acute necrotizing hemorrhagic encephalomyelitis (ANHE) is a more fulminant, frequently fatal, demyelinating syndrome typically affecting children and young adults after an upper respiratory tract infection. Lesions are similar to ADEM, but they are more severe and often confluent, with small vessel destruction and disseminated CNS necrosis.

Other Diseases with Demyelination (p. 1313)

Central pontine myelinolysis is characterized by myelin damage (with axonal preservation) without inflammation in the basis pontis and portions of the pontine tegmentum, often leading to spastic paresis. It is most commonly associated with a rapid correction of a hyponatremic state, although it can occur with other electrolyte abnormalities or following liver transplantation.

Degenerative Diseases (p. 1313)

These are gray matter diseases, characterized by progressive loss of specific neurons with secondary white matter tract changes. *A common theme is the presence of protein aggregates resistant to proteasome degradation.* Degenerative CNS disorders are grouped according to the anatomic site of neuronal loss (and/or related clinical manifestations), as well as the nature of the associated inclusions or abnormal structures.

Degenerative Diseases Affecting the Cerebral Cortex (p. 1313)

The principal clinical manifestation of these disorders is dementia.

Alzheimer Disease *(p. 1313)*

Alzheimer disease (AD) is the most common dementing illness of the elderly, reaching a prevalence of more than 40% in the 85- to 89-year-old cohort. It usually begins after age 50 years, with progressive, insidious impairment of higher intellectual function over 5 to 10 years. Most cases are sporadic, although at least 5% to 10% of cases are familial. Intercurrent disease (often pneumonia) is the cause of death in most AD patients.

Morphology (p. 1314)

- *Grossly:* There is cortical atrophy with narrowed gyri and widened sulci especially in the frontal, temporal, and parietal lobes; hydrocephalus *ex vacuo* also occurs. Medial temporal lobe structures (i.e., hippocampus, entorhinal cortex, and amygdala) are involved early and are severely atrophied in later stages.
- *Microscopically:* There are no unique pathognomonic findings in AD; *neuritic plaques* and *neurofibrillary tangles* are characteristic, but since these (and other histologic findings) can occur in nondemented individuals, the formal diagnosis of AD is based on both clinical and pathologic features.

  Neuritic plaques are spherical collections of dilated, tortuous, neuritic processes (dystrophic neurites) around a central amyloid core; microglia and reactive astrocytes are at the periphery. The amyloid core predominantly contains Aβ, a 40- or 42-amino acid peptide processed from a larger amyloid precursor protein (APP). Aβ can also be deposited in the absence of the neuritic reaction *(diffuse plaques)*, likely representing an early stage of plaque development.

  Neurofibrillary tangles are bundles of paired helical filaments in neuronal cytoplasm, largely containing hyperphosphorylated tau (a microtubule-associated protein that enhances microtubule assembly), as well as ubiquitin and other microtubule-associated molecules.

  Cerebral amyloid angiopathy (CAA) almost invariably accompanies AD; there is vascular wall deposition of Aβ (predominantly $A\beta_{40}$). *Granulovacuolar degeneration* is the formation of small, clear intraneuronal cytoplasmic vacuoles, and *Hirano bodies* are elongated, glassy eosinophilic paracrystalline arrays of beaded filaments, primarily composed of actin.

Pathogenesis (p. 1316)

Aβ deposition constitutes the fundamental AD abnormality; Aβ peptides readily aggregate and can be directly neurotoxic, resulting in synaptic dysfunction. Aggregates also elicit inflammatory responses that can cause damage through mediator release. Although neurofibrillary tangles are associated with AD, they do not appear to be causal.

Aβ derives from the processing of APP, a normal transmembrane protein (Fig. 28-3). Cleavage by β- and γ-secretase generates peptide fragments that form amyloidogenic aggregates; the variation in peptide length (i.e., 40 or 42 amino acids) depends on the exact location of the intramembranous γ-secretase cleavage. If the initial cleavage is by α-secretase, no Aβ will be formed. The various familial forms of AD are related to mutations in APP or alterations in its processing:

- The gene for APP resides on chromosome 21; Down syndrome patients (i.e., trisomy 21) experience early-onset AD secondary to a gene dosage effect.

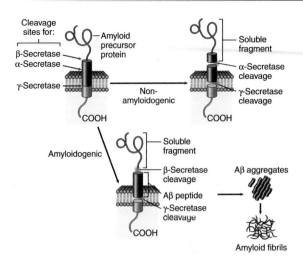

FIGURE 28-3 Mechanisms of amyloid precursor protein (APP) processing. Sequential cleavage by β-secretase and γ-secretase results in Aβ generation and ultimately formation of amyloid fibrils. Cleavage by α-secretase leads to non-amyloidogenic peptide fragments.

- APP point mutations can affect secretase sensitivity or influence the propensity to aggregate.
- Early-onset familial AD is often due to gain-of-function mutations in the presenilin genes *(PS1* or *PS2)*, causing enhanced γ-secretase activity.
- The apolipoprotein ε4 allele is associated with increased AD risk; the mechanism is unknown.

Frontotemporal Dementias (p. 1317)

Frontotemporal dementias constitute a group of disorders that share clinical features—progressive deterioration of language and changes in personality—corresponding to temporal and frontal lobe degeneration; many are characterized by tau inclusions *(tauopathy).*

FRONTOTEMPORAL DEMENTIA WITH PARKINSONISM LINKED TO TAU MUTATIONS (p. 1317)

- This is typically associated with parkinsonian symptoms; it is linked to mutations in the *MAPT* (tau) gene, affecting tau association with microtubules.

Morphology (p. 1318)

- *Grossly:* Frontal and temporal lobe atrophy is seen in various combinations and to various degrees.
- *Microscopically:* Atrophic regions exhibit neuronal loss and gliosis as well as tau-containing neurofibrillary tangles. Nigral degeneration may also occur. Glial cell inclusions occur in some forms.

PICK DISEASE (p. 1318)

Pick disease is much rarer than AD; it causes dementia, often with prominent frontal signs.

Morphology (p. 1318)

- *Grossly:* Brains exhibit frontal and temporal lobe atrophy, with sparing of the posterior two thirds of the superior temporal gyrus; caudate and putamen atrophy can also occur.
- *Microscopically:* Lesions show large ballooned neurons (Pick cells) and smooth argyrophilic inclusions composed of straight and paired helical filaments (Pick bodies).

PROGRESSIVE SUPRANUCLEAR PALSY (p. 1318)

Progressive supranuclear palsy is characterized by loss of vertical gaze, truncal rigidity, dysequilibrium, loss of facial expression, and mild progressive dementia. It typically affects men older than 50 years; death usually occurs within 5 to 7 years. Although no *MAPT* mutations are associated with the disease, certain gene polymorphisms are highly over-represented.

Morphology (p. 1318)

There is widespread neuronal loss and neurofibrillary tangles in the globus pallidus, subthalamic nucleus, substantia nigra, colliculi, periaqueductal gray matter, and dentate nucleus of the cerebellum. Tau pathology can be found in glial cells as well.

CORTICOBASAL DEGENERATION (p. 1318)

Corticobasal degeneration is a disease of the elderly characterized by extrapyramidal rigidity, asymmetric motor disturbances, and sensory cortical dysfunction; this disorder is highly associated with the same *MAPT* haplotype as progressive supranuclear palsy.

Morphology (p. 1319)

Motor, premotor, and anterior parietal cortex exhibit neuronal loss, gliosis, and ballooned neurons. The substantia nigra and locus ceruleus show loss of pigmented neurons and argyrophilic inclusions. Tau immunoreactivity is present in astrocytes ("tufted astrocytes") and oligodendrocytes ("coiled bodies").

FRONTOTEMPORAL DEMENTIAS WITHOUT TAU PATHOLOGY (p. 1319)

In frontotemporal dementias without tau pathology, neurons exhibit tau-negative, ubiquitin-positive inclusions in the dentate gyrus and superficial temporal and frontal lobes.

Vascular Dementia (p. 1319)

CNS vascular injury can also cause dementia; moreover, vascular injury lowers the threshold for the dementing effects of other disorders (e.g., AD). Etiologies include: multiple lacunar infarcts, hypertensive injury (e.g., *Binswanger disease*), strategically located large infarcts (involving hippocampus, dorsomedial thalamus, or frontal cortex, including cingulate gyrus), and vasculitis.

Degenerative Diseases of Basal Ganglia and Brainstem (p. 1319)

These diseases are associated with movement disorders, tremor, and rigidity; typically there is either a paucity of voluntary movement or increased involuntary movement.

Parkinsonism (p. 1319)

Parkinsonism is a clinical syndrome characterized by diminished facial expression, stooped posture, slowed voluntary movement, festinating gait (progressively shortened, accelerated steps), rigidity, and a pill-rolling tremor, associated with decreased function of the nigrostriatal dopaminergic system. Causes include:

- Parkinson disease
- Multiple system atrophy
- Postemcephalitic parkinsonism (e.g., associated with the 1918 influenza pandemic)
- Frontotemporal dementias associated with movement disorders (discussed previously)
- Dopamine antagonists or toxins (e.g., pesticides, or 1-methyl-4-prenyl-1,2,3,6 tetrahydroperidine [MPTP], a contaminant in the illicit synthesis of meperidine analogues)

Parkinson Disease (p. 1319)

Parkinson disease (PD) is diagnosed in individuals with progressive l-dihydroxyphenylalanine (L-DOPA)-responsive parkinsonism in the absence of toxic or other known etiology.

Morphology (p. 1319)

There is pallor of the substantia nigra and locus ceruleus with loss of pigmented, catecholaminergic neurons and gliosis; *Lewy bodies* (intracytoplasmic, eosinophilic inclusions, containing α-synuclein) occur in the remaining neurons.

Pathogenesis (p. 1320)

More than a dozen genetic loci are associated with PD. Autosomal dominant forms of the disease include mutations causing over-expression of α-synuclein (a lipid-binding protein associated with synapses) or gain-of-function in the *LRRK2* gene (encoding a kinase). A juvenile recessive form of PD is caused by loss-of-function mutations in the *parkin* gene (encoding an E3 ubiquitin ligase). Other recessive forms involve mutations in DJ-1 (a protein that regulates redox responses to stress) and the PINK1 kinase (regulating mitochondrial function).

Dopaminergic neurons in the substantia nigra are lost secondary to several mechanisms: misfolded protein stress responses triggered by α-synuclein aggregation, proteasome dysfunction, or altered mitochondrial activity. Nigral dopaminergic neuronal depletion leads to striatal dopamine deficiency that correlates with the severity of the motor syndrome.

Clinical Features (p. 1321)

In addition to parkinsonism, autonomic and cognitive dysfunction can occur. L-DOPA replacement therapy can provide transient symptomatic relief but does not reverse the neuronal destruction or arrest disease progression; with time, patients become increasingly refractory to treatment. Neural transplantation, gene therapy, neurosurgical lesions in the extrapyramidal system, and deep brain stimulation are additional therapeutic approaches.

Dementia with Lewy Bodies (p. 1321)

Dementia develops in 10% to 15% of PD patients, often with a fluctuating course and associated hallucinations and frontal signs. Some patients have concurrent AD, but most have α-synuclein-containing Lewy bodies as the major histologic correlate.

Multiple System Atrophy (p. 1321)

MSA reflects a group of disorders characterized by atrophy in specific CNS regions associated with glial (predominantly oligodendrocyte) tubular cytoplasmic inclusions composed of α-synuclein, ubiquitin, and αB-crystallin.

- *Striatonigral degeneration* is dominated by parkinsonism; there is prominent atrophy of the substantia nigra and striatum.
- *Olivopontocerebellar atrophy* presents with cerebellar ataxia, eye and somatic movement abnormalities, dysarthria, and rigidity; atrophy involves the cerebellar peduncles, basis pontis, and inferior olives.
- *Shy-Drager syndrome* is marked by autonomic dysfunction, with loss of the sympathetic neurons of the intermediolateral column of the spinal cord.

Pathogenesis (p. 1321)

The glial inclusions are likely pathogenic, but no α-synuclein mutations have been identified in MSA, and the mechanism of injury is obscure.

Huntington Disease (p. 1322)

Huntington disease (HD) is an autosomal dominant movement disorder clinically manifesting between ages 20 and 50 years. Patients develop *chorea* (jerky, hyperkinetic, dystonic movements) that can evolve into parkinsonism; motor symptoms precede cognitive impairment, and disease is progressive, leading to death within 15 years.

Morphology (p. 1322)

There is striking atrophy of the caudate nucleus and putamen, with loss of medium-sized, spiny striatal neurons that use γ-aminobutyric acid as their neurotransmitter; gliosis is prominent, and intraneuronal *huntingtin* aggregates are seen in the striatum and cerebral cortex. Neurons containing nitric oxide synthase and cholinesterase are spared.

Pathogenesis (p. 1322)

HD is associated with expansion of a CAG trinucleotide repeat encoding a polyglutamine tract in *huntingtin*. The normal *HD* gene has 6 to 35 copies of the repeat; increases beyond this are associated with disease. Since longer stretches generally lead to earlier disease onset, and repeats expand during spermatogenesis, paternal transmission is associated with earlier expression in the next generation *(anticipation)*. Polyglutamine expansion appears to bestow a toxic gain-of-function on huntingtin, with protein aggregation, sequestration of various transcriptional regulators, and potential dysregulation of transcription pathways involved in mitochondrial biogenesis or protection against oxidative injury.

Spinocerebellar Degenerations (p. 1323)

These are genetically distinct disorders characterized by neuronal loss in specific regions, with secondary white matter tract degeneration.

Spinocerebellar Ataxias (p. 1323)

Spinocerebellar ataxias (SCAs) are a group of at least 29 different diseases involving the cerebellum, brain stem, spinal cord, and peripheral nerves. Some forms are caused by unstable expansions of CAG repeats, encoding polyglutamine tracts in different proteins (analogous to HD); others are caused by repeat expansions in non-coding regions or by point mutations in cytoskeletal proteins, ion channels, kinases, or growth factors.

FRIEDREICH ATAXIA (p. 1323)

Friedreich ataxia is autosomal recessive; patients present with gait ataxia, hand clumsiness, dysarthria, depressed tendon reflexes, and sensory loss, rendering most individuals wheelchair-bound within 5 years. Death occurs secondary to associated cardiac arrhythmias or pulmonary infections. Disease is caused by expansion of an intronic GAA repeat in the gene encoding *frataxin*, an inner mitochondrial membrane protein involved in iron regulation; depressed frataxin is associated with generalized mitochondrial dysfunction.

Morphology (p. 1323)

There is axonal loss and gliosis in the posterior columns of the spinal cord and the distal corticospinal and spinocerebellar tracts. Neuronal degeneration is also seen in the VIII, X, and XII cranial nerve nuclei, dentate nucleus, Purkinje cells of the superior vermis, and dorsal root ganglia.

ATAXIA-TELANGIECTASIA (p. 1323)

Ataxia-telangiectasia is autosomal recessive; patients present in childhood with cerebellar dysfunction, telangiectatic lesions in the skin and conjunctiva (and CNS), and immunodeficiency (lymph nodes and thymus are hypoplastic). The relevant *ATM* gene encodes a kinase involved in repairing double-stranded DNA breaks (Chapter 7); in addition to increasing the risk of malignancy, ineffective DNA repair may make neurons more degeneration-prone. The disease is relentlessly progressive, with death in the second decade.

Morphology (p. 1324)

Cerebellar Purkinje and granule cells are lost, with degeneration of the dorsal columns, spinocerebellar tracts, and anterior horn cells; Schwann cell nuclei in dorsal root ganglia and peripheral nerves can be enlarged two- to five-fold.

Degenerative Diseases Affecting Motor Neurons (p. 1324)

These are inherited or sporadic disorders. Involvement of lower motor neurons of the anterior horn and brainstem leads to muscular atrophy, weakness, and fasciculations; involvement of the cortical upper motor neurons manifests as paresis, hyperreflexia, and spasticity.

Amyotrophic Lateral Sclerosis (Motor Neuron Disease) (p. 1324)

Amyotrophic lateral sclerosis (ALS) is characterized by loss of both lower motor neurons and upper motor neurons.

Pathogenesis (p. 1324)

The minority of cases (5% to 10%) are familial, mostly with autosomal dominant inheritance; 25% of these are due to adverse gain-of-function mutations in the copper-zinc superoxide dismutase *(SOD1)* gene, believed to yield misfolded proteins that engender an injurious unfolded protein response. Abnormal axonal transport, protein aggregation, and glutamate neurotransmitter toxicity have also been implicated.

Morphology (p. 1324)

Degeneration of the upper motor neurons results in loss of myelinated fibers in the corticospinal tracts and reactive gliosis; occasionally, there is atrophy of the precentral gyrus. Remaining neurons can contain PAS-positive cytoplasmic inclusions *(Bunina bodies)*. The affected skeletal muscle shows neurogenic atrophy.

Clinical Features (p. 1325)

ALS is slightly more common in men, usually with onset after age 40 years. Early clumsiness gives way to muscle weakness and fasciculations, eventually involving the respiratory muscles with recurrent bouts of pneumonia. Some patients have predominantly bulbar manifestations (involvement of motor cranial nerves) with complications related to deglutition and phonation. ALS is typically relentlessly progressive, with death from respiratory complications.

Bulbospinal Atrophy (Kennedy Syndrome) (p. 1325)

Bulbospinal atrophy is an X-linked disorder; lower motor neuron loss is also associated with androgen insensitivity (gynecomastia, testicular atrophy, and oligospermia). The gene defect is expansion of a CAG/polyglutamine trinucleotide repeat in the androgen receptor gene, associated with intranuclear receptor aggregation.

Genetic Metabolic Diseases (p. 1325)

* *Neuronal storage diseases* are primarily due to mutations affecting the synthesis or degradation of sphingolipids, mucolipids, or mucopolysaccharides. These result in intraneuronal accumulation of the enzyme substrates, with eventual neuronal death.
* *Leukodystrophies* are caused by defects in myelin synthesis or turnover, with resulting hypomyelination.
* *Mitochondrial encephalomyelopathies* are disorders of oxidative phosphorylation; most are due to mutations in the mitochondrial genome.

Neuronal Storage Diseases (p. 1326)

Neuronal Ceroid Lipofuscinoses (p. 1326)

Neuronal ceroid lipofuscinoses are a group of inherited lysosomal storage disorders characterized by the neuronal accumulation of lipofuscin. More than eight genetic loci are known and associated with defective protein degradation and neuronal dysfunction, including blindness, mental and motor deterioration, and seizures.

Leukodystrophies (p. 1326)

Krabbe Disease (p. 1326)

Krabbe disease is an autosomal recessive deficiency of galactocerebroside β-galactosidase (catalyzing the breakdown of galactocerebroside to ceramide and galactose). An alternate catabolic pathway acts on the excess accumulated substrate to generate galactosylsphingosine, which is toxic to oligodendrocytes. Patients present with weakness and stiffness by 3 to 6 months of age; survival beyond age 2 years is uncommon. There is diffuse loss of myelin and oligodendrocytes; aggregates of glycolipid-engorged macrophages around blood vessels *(globoid cells)* are characteristic.

Metachromatic Leukodystrophy (p. 1326)

Metachromatic leukodystrophy is an autosomal recessive disease caused by deficiency of arylsulfatase. Sulfatides (especially cerebroside sulfate) accumulate and may block oligodendrocyte differentiation. Findings include myelin loss and gliosis with macrophages containing metachromatic material.

Adrenoleukodystrophy (p. 1327)

Adrenoleukodystrophy has several clinically and genetically distinct forms; it is a progressive disorder caused by myelin loss and adrenal insufficiency, attributable to the inability to catabolize very long chain fatty acids.

Pelizaeus-Merzbacher Disease (p. 1327)

Pelizaeus-Merzbacher disease is an X-linked leukodystrophy typically caused by mutations in a gene encoding two alternatively spliced myelin proteins (i.e., PLP and DM20).

Mitochondrial Encephalomyopathies (p. 1327)

Inherited disorders of mitochondrial oxidative phosphorylation present as muscle diseases (Chapter 27), and secondarily as CNS disorders.

Mitochondrial Encephalomyopathy, Lactic Acidosis, and Strokelike Episodes (p. 1327)

Mitochondrial encephalomyopathy with lactic acidosis and stroke-like episodes (MELAS) is the most common neurologic syndrome associated with mitochondrial abnormalities. Besides the muscle and metabolic findings, patients present with recurrent neurologic dysfunction and cognitive changes; although areas of infarction do occur, the stroke-like episodes are typically associated with reversible deficits that do not correspond to specific vascular territories. Most of the MELAS mutations involve mitochondrial tRNA.

Leigh Syndrome (Subacute Necrotizing Encephalopathy) (p. 1328)

Leigh syndrome typically presents between 1 and 2 years of age with developmental arrest, feeding problems, seizures, extraocular palsies, hypotonia, and lactic academia; mutations in diverse elements of the oxidative phosphorylation pathways have been demonstrated. The brain reveals bilateral damage with vascular proliferation and spongiform changes, usually symmetrically involving the midbrain periventricular gray matter, pontine tegmentum, and thalamus and hypothalamus.

Toxic and Acquired Metabolic Diseases (p. 1328)

Vitamin Deficiencies (p. 1328)

Thiamine (Vitamin B_1) Deficiency (p. 1328)

Beriberi was discussed in Chapter 9; thiamine deficiency can also manifest as sudden onset of psychosis and/or ophthalmoplegia *(Wernicke encephalopathy)*, potentially followed by a largely irreversible memory disorder associated with confabulation *(Korsakoff syndrome)*. Chronic alcoholism is a common substrate, but thiamine deficiency can also result from gastric disease (carcinoma, chronic gastritis, or persistent vomiting). Mamillary body (and third and fourth ventricle) hemorrhage and necrosis are common; thalamic dorsomedial nucleus lesions correlate best with the memory disturbances.

Vitamin B_{12} Deficiency (p. 1328)

Vitamin B_{12} deficiency causes anemia and nervous system injury; the latter begins with slight ataxia and lower extremity paresthesias but can rapidly progress to lower extremity spastic weakness and paraplegia, which can be permanent. Vacuolar swelling of myelin *affects both ascending and descending tracts* starting at the midthoracic cord, with the eventual degeneration of both.

Neurologic Sequelae of Metabolic Disturbances (p. 1329)

Hypoglycemia (p. 1329)

Neurons that are relatively sensitive to hypoglycemia include large cerebral pyramidal cells, hippocampal pyramidal cells in area CA1, and Purkinje cells. With prolonged, severe hypoglycemia, there can be global neuronal injury.

Hyperglycemia (p. 1329)

Hyperglycemia occurs most commonly with inadequately controlled diabetes mellitus; ketoacidosis can also occur. In the hyperosmolar state, dehydration results in confusion, stupor, and eventually coma; fluid depletion must be corrected gradually to minimize the risk of cerebral edema.

Toxic Disorders (p. 1329)

Carbon Monoxide (p. 1329)

Injury is largely related to the hypoxia that occurs secondary to reduced hemoglobin oxygen-carrying capacity. There is selective injury of the layer III and V neurons of the cerebral cortex, hippocampal Sommer sector, and Purkinje cells. Bilateral necrosis of the globus pallidus is more common in carbon monoxide–induced hypoxia than for other hypoxia causes.

Methanol (p. 1329)

Methanol toxicity preferentially affects the retina; degeneration of ganglion cells will cause blindness. The methanol metabolite formic acid is causally implicated.

Ethanol (p. 1329)

In addition to the nutritional effects of chronic alcoholism (discussed previously), cerebellar dysfunction (manifesting as truncal ataxia, unsteady gait, and nystagmus) occurs in up to 1%. Atrophy and granule cell loss in the anterior cerebellar vermis are followed by Purkinje cell drop-out and astrocyte proliferation *(Bergmann gliosis)*.

Radiation (p. 1329)

Radiation can cause acute CNS decompensation (Chapter 9) as well as damage that can precipitously develop months to years later. Late radionecrosis is associated with large zones of coagulative necrosis and edema in white matter; blood vessels show thickened walls with intramural fibrin-like material, and proteinaceous spheroids may be present in adjacent tissue. Radiation and methotrexate administration may act synergistically to cause damage.

Tumors (p. 1330)

The annual incidence of intracranial CNS tumors is 10 to 17 per 100,000 population; the intraspinal tumor incidence is 1 to 2 per 100,000. Primary CNS tumors account for 20% of all childhood cancers; 70% of these arise in the posterior fossa. In adults, 70% of CNS tumors occur above the tentorium.

- *Consequences of location:* The ability to resect CNS tumor resection can be constrained by functional anatomic considerations; thus, even benign lesions can have fatal consequences due to location.
- *Patterns of growth:* Most glial tumors, including many with histologic features of a benign neoplasm, infiltrate entire regions of the brain, leading to clinically malignant behavior.
- *Patterns of spread:* Some tumors spread through the CSF; however, even the most malignant gliomas rarely metastasize outside the CNS.

Gliomas (p. 1330)

Astrocytoma (p. 1330)

PILOCYTIC ASTROCYTOMA (p. 1332)

Pilocytic astrocytoma occurs in children and young adults, usually in the cerebellum but also in the floor and walls of the third ventricle, the optic nerves, and, occasionally, the cerebral hemispheres. These tumors have a relatively benign behavior; they grow slowly and are rarely infiltrative. They uncommonly exhibit *p53* mutations or other genetic changes associated with more aggressive astrocytomas.

Morphology (p. 1333)

These are World Health Organization (WHO) grade I/IV tumors.

* *Grossly:* Lesions are often cystic with a mural nodule in the wall of the cyst.
* *Microscopically:* Tumors are composed of bipolar cells with long, thin, hairlike processes; *Rosenthal fibers* and microcysts are often present. There is a narrow infiltrative border with the surrounding brain.

INFILTRATING ASTROCYTOMAS (p. 1330)

Infiltrating astrocytomas account for 80% of adult primary brain tumors; most occur between ages 30 and 60 years. Certain genetic alterations correlate with progression from low- to high-grade lesions; low-grade tumors typically over-express platelet-derived growth factor-α and its receptor and carry mutations that affect *p53* function. Higher-grade lesions are associated with abnormalities of the tumor suppressor genes *RB* and *p16/CDKNaA*. Most mutations influence cellular proliferation; combinations that activate RAS and PI-3 kinase pathways and inactivate *p53* and *RB* occur in 80% to 90% of high-grade tumors.

Morphology (p. 1330)

Histologic differentiation (WHO grades II–IV) correlates well with the clinical course:

* *Diffuse astrocytomas (grade II/IV)* are poorly defined, gray-white, infiltrative tumors that expand and distort a region of the brain; they show hypercellularity and some nuclear pleomorphism, and the transition from normal to neoplastic cells is indistinct.
* *Anaplastic astrocytomas (grade III/IV)* exhibit increased nuclear anaplasia with numerous mitoses.
* *Glioblastomas (grade IV/IV; previously called glioblastoma multiforme or GBM)* are composed of a mixture of firm white areas, softer yellow foci of necrosis, cystic change, and hemorrhage; there is also increased vascularity. Increased tumor cell density along the necrotic edges is termed *pseudopalisading.*

Clinical Consequences (p. 1332)

Patients typically present with focal neurologic deficits, headaches, or seizures, attributable to mass effects and/or cerebral edema; high-grade lesions have leaky vessels that exhibit contrast enhancement on imaging. The prognosis for glioblastoma is poor; despite resection and chemotherapy, mean survival is only 15 months and only 25% are alive at 2 years.

PLEOMORPHIC XANTHOASTROCYTOMAS (p. 1333)

Pleomorphic xanthoastrocytomas typically occur in the temporal lobes of young patients, often with a history of seizures. The tumor (usually WHO grade II/IV) exhibits neoplastic, occasionally bizarre astrocytes, abundant reticulin and lipid deposits, and chronic inflammatory cell infiltrates; 5-year survival nears 80%.

BRAINSTEM GLIOMAS (p. 1333)

Brainstem gliomas occur mostly in the first two decades of life. Their course depends on location, with pontine gliomas (most common) having an aggressive course, tectal gliomas with a relatively benign course, and corticomedullary junction tumors somewhere intermediate.

Oligodendroglioma (p. 1333)

Oligodendrogliomas constitute 5% to 15% of gliomas and are most common in middle life. Loss of heterozygosity (LOH) in chromosomes 1p and 19q occurs in 80% of cases; additional mutations accrue in more anaplastic lesions.

Morphology (p. 1333)

- *Grossly:* Tumors have a white matter predilection; they are well-circumscribed, gelatinous gray masses, often with cysts, focal hemorrhage, and calcification.
- *Microscopically:* Tumors consist of sheets of regular cells with round nuclei containing finely granular chromatin, often surrounded by a clear halo of cytoplasm and sitting in a delicate capillary network. Calcification is present in 90% and ranges from microscopic to massive.

Clinical Features (p. 1334)

Prognosis is typically better than for astrocytomas, and current therapies yield an average survival of 5 to 10 years; lesions with only 1p and 19q LOH usually have durable responses to chemo- and radiotherapy. Progression from low- to high-grade lesions can occur; anaplastic oligodendrogliomas (WHO grade III/IV) have a worse prognosis.

Ependymoma (p. 1334)

Ependymomas are tumors arising from the ependymal lining. In the first two decades of life, the fourth ventricle is the most common site; the spinal cord central canal is a common location in middle age and in neurofibromatosis type 2.

Morphology (p. 1334)

- *Grossly:* Tumors are moderately well-demarcated solid or papillary lesions.
- *Microscopically:* Lesions have regular, round-oval nuclei with abundant granular chromatin; they can form elongated ependymal canals or perivascular pseudorosettes. Most are WHO grade II/IV; anaplastic lesions (grade III/IV) exhibit greater cell density, mitoses, and necrosis with less evident ependymal differentiation.

    Myxopapillary ependymomas are distinct but related lesions arising in the filum terminale of the spinal cord. Cuboidal cells, sometimes with clear cytoplasm, are arranged around papillary cores; myxoid areas contain neutral and acidic mucopolysaccharides.

Clinical Features (p. 1335)

Posterior fossa ependymomas often present with hydrocephalus; CSF dissemination is common, and 5-year survival is only 50%. Spinal cord lesions usually do better.

Related Paraventricular Mass Lesions (p. 1334)

- *Subependymomas* (p. 1335) are solid, sometimes calcified, slow-growing nodules attached to the ventricular lining and protruding into the ventricle; they are usually asymptomatic but can cause hydrocephalus. Lesions exhibit clumps of ependymal-appearing nuclei scattered in a dense, finely fibrillar background.
- *Choroid plexus papillomas* (p. 1335) recapitulate the normal choroid plexus; they exhibit connective tissue papillae covered with

a cuboidal-columnar ciliated epithelium. Hydrocephalus is common, either due to obstruction or CSF overproduction. *Choroid plexus carcinomas* are typically adenocarcinomas and are much rarer; they mainly arise in children.

- *Colloid cysts of the third ventricle* (p. 1335) are non-neoplastic lesions of young adults; they are located at the foramina of Monro and can result in noncommunicating hydrocephalus, sometimes rapidly fatal. The cyst contains gelatinous proteinaceous material within a thin, fibrous capsule lined by cuboidal epithelium.

Neuronal Tumors (p. 1335)

Ganglioglioma is the most common CNS tumor of mature-appearing neurons (ganglion cells); it is slow-growing, although the glial component can become frankly anaplastic and the tumor more aggressive. Lesions often present with seizures that remit after resection.

Morphology (p. 1335)

- *Grossly:* Most occur in the temporal lobe and have a cystic component.
- *Microscopically:* Neoplastic ganglion cells are irregularly clustered with randomly oriented neurites; the glial component resembles a low-grade astrocytoma but lacks mitotic activity and necrosis.

Dysembryoplastic neuroepithelial tumor (p. 1335) is a rare, low-grade childhood neoplasm often presenting as a seizure disorder; prognosis after resection is good.

Morphology (p. 1336)

Features include intracortical location, cystic changes, nodular growth, "floating neurons" in a pool of mucopolysaccharide-rich fluid, and surrounding neoplastic glia without anaplastic features.

Central neurocytoma (p. 1336) is a low-grade neuronal neoplasm within the ventricles consisting of evenly spaced, round, uniform nuclei and islands of neuropil.

Poorly Differentiated Neoplasms (p. 1336)

Some neuroectodermal tumors express few mature phenotypic markers and are described as poorly differentiated or embryonal.

Medulloblastoma (p. 1336)

Medulloblastomas account for 20% of childhood brain tumors; they occur exclusively in the cerebellum. The most common genetic alteration is loss of material from 17p with an isochromosome of 17q; *MYC* amplifications are associated with a more aggressive clinical course. Conversely, tumors with increased neurotropin receptor TRKC or elevated intranuclear β-catenin have better outcomes.

Morphology (p. 1336)

- *Grossly:* Tumors are well-circumscribed, gray, and friable.
- *Microscopically:* Lesions are usually extremely cellular, with sheets of anaplastic cells exhibiting hyperchromatic nuclei and abundant mitoses; cells have little cytoplasm and are often devoid of specific markers of differentiation, although glial and neuronal features (e.g., Homer-Wright rosettes) can occur. Extension into the subarachnoid space can elicit prominent desmoplasia.

Clinical Features (p. 1337)

Tumors tend to be midline in children and in lateral locations in adults. Rapid growth can occlude CSF flow, leading to hydrocephalus; CSF dissemination is common. The tumor is highly malignant, and if untreated, the prognosis is dismal. However, it is exquisitely radiosensitive, and with excision and radiation, the 5-year survival rate is 75%.

Atypical Teratoid/Rhabdoid Tumor (p. 1337)

Atypical teratoid/rhabdoid tumor is a highly malignant tumor of the posterior fossa and supratentorium of young children; survival is usually less than 1 year. Chromosome 22 deletions occur in more than 90%; the relevant gene is *hSNF5/INI1*, encoding a protein involved in chromatin remodeling. These are large, soft tumors that spread over the brain surface; they are highly mitotic lesions histologically characterized by rhabdoid cells resembling those seen in rhabdomyosarcoma.

Other Parenchymal Tumors (p. 1337)

Primary Central Nervous System Lymphoma (p. 1337)

Primary CNS lymphoma accounts for 2% of extranodal lymphomas and 1% of intracranial tumors; it is the most common CNS neoplasm in immunocompromised hosts. Primary brain lymphoma is often multifocal within the CNS; involvement outside the CNS is a rare and late complication. Most primary brain lymphomas are of B-cell origin and nearly all are latently infected by EBV; these are aggressive tumors and respond poorly to chemotherapy compared with their peripheral counterparts.

Morphology (p. 1337)

Diffuse large-cell B-cell lymphomas are the most common histologic group; malignant cells diffusely involve the parenchyma of the brain and typically accumulate around blood vessels.

Germ Cell Tumors (p. 1338)

Germ cell tumors occur along the midline in adolescents and young adults; they constitute 0.2% to 1% of CNS tumors in European populations but up to 10% of Japanese CNS tumors. Tumors most commonly occur in the pineal (male predominance) and suprasellar regions. The histologic classification and therapeutic responsiveness of CNS germ cell tumors mirror those of their non-CNS counterparts (Chapter 21).

Meningiomas (p. 1338)

Meningiomas are predominantly benign tumors of adults that arise from arachnoid meningothelial cells and are attached to the dura. LOH of the long arm of chromosome 22 is a common finding. Deletions include the *NF2* gene (encoding *merlin* protein); more than half of sporadic tumors have mutations that lead to loss of functional merlin.

Morphology (p. 1338)

- *Grossly:* Tumors are usually rounded masses with well-defined dural bases that compress underlying brain but easily separate from it; lesions are usually firm, lack necrosis or extensive hemorrhage, and may be gritty due to calcified psamomma bodies.
- *Microscopically:* Several histologic patterns exist (e.g., synctytial, fibroblastic, transitional, psammomatous, secretory, and microcystic) all with roughly comparable favorable prognoses (WHO grade I/IV); among these, the proliferation index is the best predictor of biologic behavior.
- *Anaplastic (malignant) meningiomas* (WHO grade III/IV): These are aggressive tumors that resemble sarcomas; mitotic rates are high (i.e., more than 20 per 10 high powered fields). *Papillary*

meningiomas (pleomorphic cells arranged around fibrovascular cores) and *rhabdoid meningiomas* (sheets of cells with hyaline eosinophilic cytoplasms composed of intermediate filaments) also have a high recurrence rate (WHO grade III/IV tumors).

Clinical Features (p. 1339)

These are typically solitary, slow-growing lesions that manifest due to CNS compression, or with vague non-localizing symptoms; multiple lesions suggest *NF2* mutations. They are uncommon in children and have a slight (3:2) female predominance; they often express progesterone receptors and can grow more rapidly during pregnancy.

Metastatic Tumors (p. 1339)

Metastatic lesions (mostly carcinomas) account for approximately half of intracranial tumors. Common primary sites are lung, breast, skin (melanoma), kidney, and gastrointestinal tract; meninges are also a frequent site.

Morphology (p. 1339)

Metastases are usually sharply demarcated, often at the gray-white junction, and surrounded by edema. *Meningeal carcinomatosis* (tumor nodules studding brain surface, spinal cord, and nerve roots) is particularly associated with lung and breast carcinoma.

Paraneoplastic Syndromes (p. 1339)

Paraneoplastic syndromes result from malignancy elsewhere in the body; most are due to anti-tumor immune responses that cross-react with central or peripheral nervous system antigens.

- *Subacute cerebellar degeneration* is most common, associated with Purkinje cell loss, gliosis, and inflammatory infiltrates.
- *Limbic encephalitis* is a subacute dementia associated with perivascular inflammation, microglial nodules, neuronal loss, and gliosis, most evident in the anterior and medial temporal lobe.
- *Eye movement disorders* (e.g., opsoclonus) are often associated with childhood neuroblastomas.
- *Subacute sensory neuropathy* plus/minus limbic encephalitis is marked by dorsal root ganglia inflammation and neuronal loss.
- *Lambert-Eaton myasthenic syndrome* (Chapter 27).

Peripheral Nerve Sheath Tumors (p. 1340)

These can arise within the dura, as well as along the peripheral course of nerves.

Schwannomas (p. 1340)

Schwannomas are benign tumors of Schwann cells; these are commonly associated with the vestibular branch of the eighth nerve at the cerebellopontine angle (vestibular schwannoma or acoustic neuroma), with patients experiencing tinnitus and hearing loss. When extradural, schwannomas are commonly associated with large nerve trunks. Most are associated with inactivating mutations of *NF2* with loss of *merlin* expression, leading to hyperproliferation. Malignant change is rare.

Morphology (p. 1340)

- *Grossly:* Tumors are well-circumscribed, encapsulated firm gray masses with cystic and xanthomatous changes; they are typically attached to the nerve but separable from it. Spinal tumors mostly arise from dorsal roots and can extend through the vertebral foramen, acquiring a dumbbell configuration.

- *Microscopically:* Lesions exhibit two patterns:

  Antoni A: Elongated cells with cytoplasmic processes arranged in fascicles in areas of moderate-to-high cellularity with little stromal matrix

  Antoni B: Less densely cellular tissue with microcysts and myxoid changes

  Electron microscopy shows basement membrane deposition encasing single cells and collagen fibers.

Neurofibroma *(p. 1341)*

Neurofibromas can present as discrete localized masses (e.g., *cutaneous neurofibroma* or *solitary neurofibroma*). Skin lesions grow as (occasionally hyperpigmented) nodules and can be large and pedunculated; malignant transformation is rare. Infiltrating lesions that expand peripheral nerve constitute *plexiform neurofibromas;* in contrast to schwannomas, separation from the nerve is difficult. Lesions have loose myxoid background with a low cellularity. Multiple or plexiform lesions suggest a diagnosis of neurofibromatosis type 1 (NF1). NF1 lesions are difficult to remove from nerve trunks, and also have increased risk for malignant transformation. In plexiform neurofibromas, loss of both copies of the *NF1* gene (encoding neurofibromin) leads to decreased RAS GTPase activity, and thus increased RAS function.

Malignant Peripheral Nerve Sheath Tumors *(p. 1341)*

Malignant peripheral nerve sheath tumors are highly malignant, locally invasive sarcomas; they do not arise from malignant degeneration of schwannomas but rather arise de novo or from plexiform neurofibroma transformation, often in the setting of NF1. Lesions are ill-defined masses infiltrating the parent nerve and adjacent soft tissues. Tumor cells resemble Schwann cells; fascicle formation can be present, and mitosis, necrosis, and anaplasia are common.

Familial Tumor Syndromes *(p. 1342)*

These are primarily autosomal dominant disorders caused by loss of tumor suppressor genes; the bulk of disease manifestations are outside the CNS:

- *Cowden syndrome:* dysplastic cerebellar gangliocytomas due to *PTEN* mutation
- *Li-Fraumeni syndrome:* medulloblastomas due to *p53* mutation (Chapter 7)
- *Turcot syndrome:* medulloblastomas or glioblastomas due to *APC* or mismatch repair gene mutation (Chapter 17)
- *Gorlin syndrome:* medulloblastomas due to *PTCH* mutation (Chapter 25)

Neurofibromatosis Type 1 *(p. 1342)*

Neurofibromatosis type 1 (NF1) is an autosomal dominant disorder characterized by neurofibromas (plexiform and cutaneous), optic nerve gliomas, meningiomas, pigmented nodules of the iris *(Lisch nodules),* and cutaneous hyperpigmented macules *(café au lait spots).* Even without malignant transformation, lesions can be disfiguring and can create spinal deformities. Tumor cells in NF1-related lesions lack neurofibromin due to biallelic gene inactivation.

Neurofibromatosis Type 2 *(p. 1342)*

Neurofibromatosis type 2 (NF2) is an autosomal dominant disorder (due to inactivating mutations of *NF2*) with a propensity for forming bilateral eighth nerve schwannomas or multiple meningiomas.

Tuberous Sclerosis Complex (p. 1342)

This is an autosomal dominant disorder characterized by angio-fibromas, seizures, and mental retardation. CNS hamartomas include *cortical tubers* (haphazardly arranged neurons and cells expressing phenotypes intermediate between glia and neurons) and subependymal hamartomas (large astrocytic and neuronal clusters forming subependymal giant cell astrocytomas). In addition, renal angiomyolipomas, retinal glial hamartomas, cardiac rhabdomyomas, and pulmonary lymphangioleiomyomatosis can occur; cutaneous lesions include angiofibromas, leathery thickenings *(shagreen patches)*, sun-ungual fibromas, and hypopigmented areas *(ash-leaf patches)*. One tuberous sclerosis locus *(TSC1)* encodes *hamartin;* the more commonly mutated *TSC2* locus encodes *tuberin.* Both proteins form a complex that inhibits the mTOR kinase; mutations lead to increased mTOR activity, leading to increased protein synthesis and impressive increases in cell size.

Von Hippel–Lindau Disease (p. 1343)

This is an autosomal dominant disorder; affected individuals develop hemangioblastomas in the cerebellum, retina, or brain stem and spinal cord, as well as cysts involving the pancreas, liver, and kidney. There is also a propensity for renal cell carcinoma and pheochromocytomas. The causal gene is *VHL,* a tumor suppressor gene that encodes a component of a ubiquitin-ligase complex that down-regulates hypoxia-induced factor-1 expression (HIF-1); dysregulated HIF-1 in turn, leads to increased expression of vascular endothelial growth factor, erythropoietin, and other growth factors.

29

The Eye

Orbit (p. 1346)

Functional Anatomy and Proptosis (p. 1346)

Because the orbit (Fig. 29-1) is bounded by bone medially, laterally, and posteriorly, any process that increases orbital contents causes forward eye displacement, or *proptosis*.

Thyroid Ophthalmopathy (Graves Disease) (p. 1347)

Proptosis in *Graves disease* is caused by extracellular matrix (ECM) accumulation and rectus muscle fibrosis; the severity is independent of thyroid status.

Other Orbital Inflammatory Conditions (p. 1347)

The floor and medial aspects of the orbit are bounded by the maxillary and ethmoid sinuses, respectively; thus orbits can be involved by sinus infections evolving into *cellulitis* or as part of a fungal infection (e.g., *mucormycosis*). Orbital involvement by *Wegener granulomatosis* can be primary or can be a secondary extension from the sinuses. Idiopathic orbital inflammation *(orbital inflammatory pseudotumor)* is characterized by chronic inflammation and variable fibrosis.

Neoplasms (p. 1348)

The most common primary orbital tumors are vascular in origin (e.g., lymphangiomas, capillary and cavernous hemangiomas); most orbital tumors are benign. Malignant tumors of the orbit can derive from any of the orbital tissues (e.g., lacrimal gland); lymphomas and metastases also affect this site.

Eyelid (p. 1348)

Eyelids are composed of skin externally and mucosa *(conjunctiva)* adjacent to the eye (Fig. 29-2). Besides covering and protecting the eye, eyelids generate lipids that retard tear evaporation. If sebaceous drainage is blocked by inflammation *(blepharitis)* or neoplasm, extravasated lipid provokes a lipogranulomatous response *(chalazion)*.

Neoplasms (p. 1348)

Eyelid neoplasms can distort the eyelid and impede closure; subsequent corneal exposure is painful and predisposes to corneal ulceration. Prompt treatment is imperative to preserve vision.

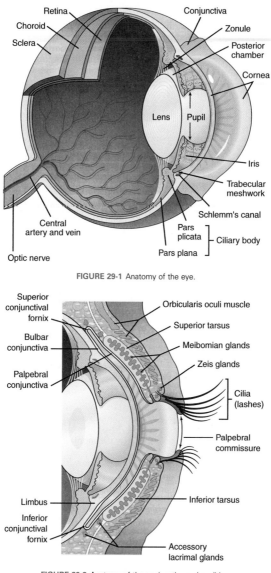

FIGURE 29-1 Anatomy of the eye.

FIGURE 29-2 Anatomy of the conjunctiva and eyelids.

- *Basal cell carcinoma* is the most common eyelid malignancy; it has a predilection for lower eyelids and medial canthi.
- *Sebaceous carcinoma* is the second most common eyelid malignancy; it metastasizes first to parotid and submandibular lymph nodes, and it can exhibit intraepithelial pagetoid spread into the nasopharynx and lacrimal glands; overall mortality rate can be more than 20%.
- *Squamous cell carcinoma* is the third most common lesion; melanomas are rare.

Conjunctiva (p. 1349)

The conjunctiva has topologic zones (see Fig. 29-2) with distinctive histology and disease responses:

- *Palpebral conjunctiva* is nonkeratinizing stratified squamous epithelium; it responds to inflammation by forming minute papillary folds.
- *Fornix conjunctiva* is a pseudostratified columnar epithelium rich in goblet cells; its associated lacrimal and lymphoid tissues can be expanded in *viral conjunctivitis* or lymphoid malignancy.
- *Bulbar conjunctiva* is a nonkeratinizing stratified squamous epithelium that covers the surface of the eye.

The aqueous component of tears is generated by accessory lacrimal glands embedded in the eyelid and fornix; conjunctival goblet cell mucin production is essential for adhering tears to corneal epithelium. *Dry eyes* occur when either the lacrimal gland (most commonly) or goblet cell production is insufficient; the condition is painful and predisposes to corneal ulceration and opacification.

Conjunctival Scarring (p. 1349)

Conjunctival scarring causes goblet cell loss; dry eyes result even with adequate aqueous tear film production. Bacterial or viral *conjunctivitis* typically causes only redness and itching, and it heals without sequelae. However, conjunctival scarring can occur with:

- *Chlamydia trachomatis* infections
- Immune-mediated conditions, such as ocular cicatricial pemphigoid
- Chemical agents, especially alkalis
- Excessive surgical resection of conjunctival tissue

Pinguecula and Pterygium (p. 1349)

Pinguecula and pterygium are submucosal conjunctival elevations; they are a consequence of actinic damage and thus occur in sun-exposed regions (e.g., the interpalpebral fissure).

- *Pterygium:* Growth of conjunctival mucosa and fibrovascular connective tissue originating in the limbus and invading the cornea; vision is usually unaffected. Resections are performed for irritation or cosmetic reasons; rarely melanoma or squamous cell carcinoma may be present.
- *Pinguecula:* This does not invade the cornea, but it can affect tear film distribution and result in focal dehydration with corneal depression *(dellen)*.

Neoplasms (p. 1349)

Neoplasms tend to develop at the limbus, likely related to sun exposure; they exhibit a spectrum of changes from mild dysplasia to carcinoma *in situ (conjunctival intraepithelial neoplasia)* to frank malignancy.

- *Squamous cell carcinomas* tend to follow an indolent course; they can be associated with human papillomavirus (HPV) types 16 and 18. *Mucoepidermoid carcinoma* is much more aggressive.
- *Conjunctival nevi* are common and typically benign, rarely involving the cornea, fornix, or palpebral conjunctiva (pigmented lesions in those locations are more likely melanomas). Chronic inflammation can occur during adolescence *(inflamed juvenile nevus)*.
- *Conjunctival melanomas* are unilateral, typically affecting middle-aged, fair-complexioned individuals; there is a 25% mortality rate. Most have an intraepithelial phase called *primary acquired*

melanosis with atypia (analogous to *melanoma in situ*); melanomas develop in 50% to 90% of these lesions. Parotid or submandibular lymph nodes are favored initial metastatic sites.

Sclera (p. 1350)

Because the sclera has relatively scant numbers of blood vessels and
fibroblasts, wounds and surgical incisions heal poorly. Scleral "blue-
ness" can be due to thinning caused by inflammation *(scleritis)*,
increased intraocular pressure, or defective collagen synthesis (e.g.,
in *osteogenesis imperfecta*), or it can result from a pigmented nevus
in the underlying uvea *(congenital melanosis oculi)*.

Cornea (p. 1351)

The cornea and its overlying tear film (and *not* the lens) compose
the major refractive eye surface (see Fig. 29-1). *Myopia* occurs when
the eye is too long for the corneal refractive power, and *hyperopia*
occurs when the globe is too short; laser sculpting of the cornea
(e.g., LASIK) can accommodate for these disproportions.

The cornea is transparent because its stroma lacks blood vessels
and lymphatics; this also markedly attenuates rejection in corneal
transplants. Precise collagen alignment is also necessary to maintain corneal transparency; the stroma is normally maintained in a
relatively dehydrated state by the action of corneal endothelium
pumping fluid into the anterior chamber. Thus, corneal scarring
or edema markedly affects vision.

Anteriorly, the cornea is covered by epithelium overlying basement membrane and an acellular *Bowman's layer*. Posteriorly, the
cornea is bounded by *corneal endothelium* derived from neural
crest (and unrelated to vascular endothelium); it sits on a basal
lamina *Descemet membrane.*

Keratitis and Ulcers (p. 1351)

Bacteria, fungi, viruses (especially herpes simplex and zoster), and
protozoa *(Acanthamoeba)* can cause corneal ulceration; stroma dissolution is accelerated by collagenase activation. Some forms of
keratitis have distinctive features (herpes simplex is associated with
granulomatous responses involving the Descemet membrane).

Corneal Degenerations and Dystrophies (p. 1351)

Degenerations may be uni- or bilateral and are typically nonfamilial; *dystrophies* are typically bilateral and hereditary.

Band Keratopathies (p. 1351)

Calcific band keratopathy, a common complication of chronic uveitis, is characterized by calcium deposition in Bowman's layer.
Actinic band keratopathy involves ultraviolet-induced corneal collagen degeneration.

Keratoconus (p. 1352)

Corneal thinning and ectasia cause the cornea to become conical
(rather than spherical), and they distort vision. Bowman's layer
fractures are histologic hallmarks; metalloproteinase activation
may be causal, but inflammation is usually absent.

Fuchs Endothelial Dystrophy (p. 1352)

A primary loss of corneal endothelial cells causes *stromal edema*
and *bullous keratopathy* (epithelial detachment from Bowman's
layer, forming bullae). There is blurring and loss of vision.

Stromal Dystrophies (p. 1353)

Deposits of various stromal proteins (resulting from mutations that affect folding) form discrete opacities in the cornea, compromising vision; deposits adjacent to epithelium or Bowman's layer can also cause painful erosions and scarring.

Anterior Segment (p. 1353)

The eye is divided into two compartments (Fig. 29-3):

- *Anterior segment* comprising cornea, anterior chamber, posterior chamber, iris, and lens.

  The basement membrane of the lens epithelium *(lens capsule)* totally envelops the lens. Thus, lens epithelium and associated proteins progressively accumulate within the confines of the lens capsule ("infoliation"), and the lens size increases with age.

  The ciliary body forms the aqueous humor that enters the posterior chamber, bathes the lens, and circulates through the pupil into the anterior chamber.

- *Posterior pole* (remainder of the eye; see Fig. 29-1).

Cataract (p. 1353)

Cataracts are congenital or acquired lens opacities. Systemic diseases (e.g., diabetes mellitus, atopic dermatitis), drugs (especially corticosteroids), radiation, trauma, and many intraocular disorders (e.g., uveitis) cause cataracts. Age-related cataracts typically result from lens nucleus opacification; accumulation of urochrome pigments causes the nucleus to become brown and distorts the perception of blue colors. Lens epithelium migration and hyperplasia posterior to the lens can cause *posterior subcapsular cataracts.* Opacification can also occur through lens cortex liquefaction; leakage of the liquid through the lens capsule *(phacolysis)* can clog the trabecular meshwork and be a cause of open-angle glaucoma (see below).

The Anterior Segment and Glaucoma (p. 1353)

Glaucoma has distinctive visual field changes and optic nerve cup alterations. Most glaucoma is associated with elevated intraocular pressure (see Fig. 29-3 for normal flow patterns), although some patients have normal intraocular pressure *(normal- or low-tension glaucoma).* There are two major categories of glaucoma:

- *Open-angle glaucoma* is most common; intraocular pressures are elevated despite an open angle and normal-appearing structures; presumably there is some *functional* increase in resistance to aqueous humor outflow. Some hereditary *(primary)* forms of glaucoma are associated with *MYOC* mutations encoding the protein myocilin; however, the pathogenesis is obscure. By physically clogging the trabecular meshwork, particulate matter (e.g., senescent erythrocytes after trauma, or iris pigment epithelial granules) can be a cause of *secondary open-angle glaucoma.*

- *Angle-closure glaucoma* occurs when the peripheral zone of the iris (or associated tissue) adheres to the trabecular meshwork and physically impedes the aqueous outflow from the eye. It may occur as *primary angle-closure glaucoma* in eyes with shallow anterior chambers (patients are often hyperopic) or can occur subsequent to neovascular membrane formation (e.g., after trauma) or ciliary body tumors (see Fig. 29-3).

Endophthalmitis and Panophthalmitis (p. 1355)

Anterior chamber inflammation results in increased permeability of the vessels in the ciliary body and iris, with accumulation of cells and exudate. Such exudates can induce adhesions between the iris and corneal meshwork (causing glaucoma) or lens (causing fibrous cataracts).

- *Endophthalmitis* is inflammation involving the vitreous humor. The retina does not tolerate endophthalmitis; only a few hours of acute inflammation can cause irreversible damage. Endophthalmitis can be *exogenous* (e.g., following a wound) or *endogenous* (delivered hematogenously).
- *Panophthalmitis* is eye inflammation involving the retina, choroid, and sclera and extending into the orbit.

ANTERIOR AND POSTERIOR CHAMBERS

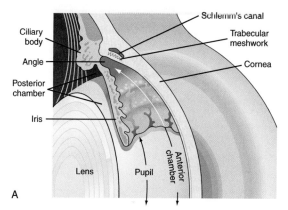

A

MAJOR AQUEOUS OUTFLOW PATHWAY

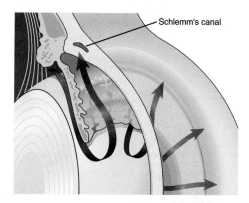

B

FIGURE 29-3 **A,** Normal eye; note the iris surface is highly textured with crypts and folds. **B,** The normal flow of an aqueous humor. Aqueous humor flows from the posterior chamber (site of production) through the pupil into the anterior chamber, and through the trabecular meshwork into Schlemm's canal; minor outflow pathways through the uveosclera and iris are not depicted.

Continued

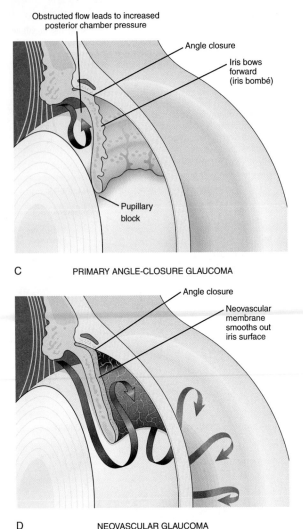

C   PRIMARY ANGLE-CLOSURE GLAUCOMA

D   NEOVASCULAR GLAUCOMA

FIGURE 29-3, cont'd C, *Primary angle-closure glaucoma* occurs in anatomically predisposed eyes by transient iris apposition to the lens, blocking aqueous humor passage from the posterior to anterior chambers. Pressure builds in the posterior chamber, bowing the iris forward (*iris* bombé) and occluding the trabecular meshwork. D, *Neovascular glaucoma* occurs when an angiogenic membrane grows over the iris, smoothing the folds and crypts; contracture of this membrane causes tissue apposition over the trabecular meshwork, blocking aqueous humor outflow and increasing intraocular pressure.

Uvea (p. 1355)

The iris, the choroid, and the ciliary body constitute the *uvea* (see Fig. 29-1). Although highly vascularized, the uvea has no lymphatics.

Uveitis (p. 1355)

Uveitis can be infectious, idiopathic (e.g., *sarcoidosis*), or autoimmune (e.g., *sympathetic ophthalmia*); it can be part of a systemic process or involve only the eye. Although inflammation in one compartment typically extends into others, uveitis can involve only the anterior segment (e.g., in *juvenile rheumatoid arthritis*).

Sympathetic ophthalmia is a noninfectious uveitis limited to the eye. It is a consequence of penetrating eye injury, developing within 2 weeks (to many years) after the insult. Presumably, previously sequestered retinal antigens released from the injured eye establish a delayed hypersensitivity response that affects not only the injured eye but also the contralateral, uninjured eye. Histologically, there is bilateral granulomatous inflammation affecting all uveal components.

Neoplasms (p. 1356)

The most common intraocular malignancy in adults is metastasis of some other primary tumor (the uvea is the favored site, typically in the choroid).

Uveal Nevi and Melanomas (p. 1356)

Uveal melanoma is the most common *primary* intraocular adult malignancy. Uveal nevi are common (seen in 10% of the Caucasian population), but progression to melanoma is exceptionally uncommon. The eye lacks lymphatics; thus, uveal melanomas typically spread hematogenously and favor the liver. Five-year survival rates approach 80%, but mortality is 40% at 10 years, increasing 1% per year thereafter. Prognostic variables include extraocular extension, large basal diameter, location within the eye, cell type, extent of tumor-infiltrating lymphocytes, monosomy 3 and trisomy 8, and the patterns of extracellular matrix protein deposition.

Retina and Vitreous (p. 1357)

The neurosensory retina is embryologically derived from the diencephalon, and injury causes gliosis. The retinal architecture explains the ophthalmoscopic appearance of ocular disorders (Fig. 29-4). There are no retinal lymphatics. The adult vitreous is avascular, but it can be opacified by hemorrhage from trauma or retinal neovascularization. Age-related liquefaction and collapse of the vitreous gives rise to "floaters" in the visual field.

Retinal Detachment (p. 1357)

Separation *(retinal detachment)* of the neurosensory retina from the retinal pigmented epithelium (RPE) is classified based on the presence or absence of a break in the retina.

- *Rhegmatogenous retinal detachment* is associated with a full-thickness retinal defect developing when structural collapse of the vitreous exerts traction on the retinal internal limiting membrane; liquefied viteous humor then seeps through the tear and separates the neurosensory retina and RPE.
- *Non-rhegmatogenous retinal detachment* (without a retinal break) occurs when exudates accumulate or fluid leaks from the choroidal circulation beneath the retina (e.g., with choroidal tumors or malignant hypertension).

Retinal Vascular Disease (p. 1359)

Retinal vasculopathy *(neovascularization)* is a common end-point of numerous insults (see following topics); it can occur secondary to vessel occlusion, hypoxia, or primary angiogenic factor production.

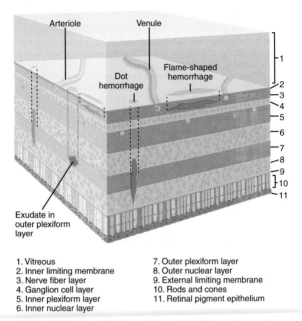

FIGURE 29-4 Clinicopathologic correlations of retinal hemorrhages and exudates; location within the retina determines the ophthalmoscopic appearance. Hemorrhages of the retinal nerve fiber layer (oriented parallel to the internal limiting membrane) appear flame shaped. Hemorrhages of the deeper retinal layers (oriented perpendicular to the internal limiting membrane) appear as "dots." Exudates from leaky retinal vessels accumulate in the outer plexiform layer.

Retinal hypoxia causes growth factor production (e.g., vascular endothelial growth factor [VEGF]), leading to angiogenesis; bleeding, increased vascular permeability, or subsequent contraction of the neovascular membrane can cause retinal detachment.

Hypertension (p. 1359)

Hypertension results in retinal arteriosclerosis with wall thickening. In malignant hypertension, damaged choroidal vessels can cause choroidal infarcts *(Elschnig pearls)* or exudate accumulation between the neurosensory retina and RPE (causing detachment). Occlusion of retinal arteries causes infarcts of the retinal nerve fiber layer, and exudates from damaged retinal vessels accumulate in the outer plexiform layer (see Fig. 29-4).

Diabetes Mellitus (p. 1359)

Diabetes mellitus causes microvascular injury with thickened basement membrane (and physiologic breakdown of the blood-retina barrier with edema and hemorrhage), as well as pericyte, loss leading to characteristic microaneurysms.

- *Background (pre-proliferative) diabetic retinopathy* constitutes a spectrum of structural and functional abnormalities of angiogenesis restricted to the retina (i.e., beneath the internal limiting membrane).
- *Proliferative diabetic retinopathy* reflects new vessels *(retinal neovascularization)* that breach the retinal internal limiting membrane. Retinal neovascularization can be accompanied a neovascular

membrane on the iris secondary to elevated aqueous humor VEGF levels; contraction of this membrane leads to adhesions that occlude aqueous outflow and precipitate glaucoma.

Retinopathy of Prematurity (Retrolental Fibroplasia) *(p. 1361)*

Immature retinal vessels respond to increased oxygen tension (administered to premature infants) by constricting, resulting in local ischemia.

Sickle Retinopathy, Retinal Vasculitis, Radiation Retinopathy *(p. 1361)*

Reduced oxygen tension leads to erythrocyte sickling and microvascular occlusions. Vasculitis and ocular radiation both damage vessels, producing zones of retinal ischemia.

Retinal Artery and Vein Occlusions *(p. 1362)*

Arterial occlusions due to atherosclerosis or to atheroembolism cause retinal infarction; since onset is typically sudden, there is no prolonged ischemia and hence no significant neovascularization. Retinal vein occlusion (e.g., due to arteriolar thickening in hypertension that compromises the venous lumen where the vessels cross) typically leads to ischemia and subsequent neovascularization.

Age-Related Macular Degeneration *(p. 1363)*

Age-related macular degeneration (ARMD) is the most common cause of irreversible visual loss in the United States; more than 70% of cases are hereditary; onset is also influenced by environmental exposures (e.g., smoking). Any disruption of RPE, its basement membrane *(Bruch membrane)*, or the associated choroidal vasculature affects the overlying photoreceptors and causes visual loss.

- *Atrophic (dry) ARMD* is most common (80% to 90% of cases); it is associated with geographic atrophy of the retinal pigment epithelium and deposits *(drusen)* in the Bruch membrane.
- *Exudative (wet) ARMD* (10% to 20% of cases) is associated with overall greater vision loss; it is caused by leaky choroidal neovascular membranes. Therapy involves VEGF antagonists to block the vessel formation.

Other Retinal Degenerations *(p. 1364)*

Retinitis Pigmentosa *(p. 1364)*

Retinitis pigmentosa is a collection of fairly common (1 in 3600 individuals) inherited disorders that affect various aspects of vision including visual cascade and cycle, structural genes, transcription factors, catabolic pathways, and mitochondrial metabolism. Despite the name, these disorders are *not* primarily inflammatory; both rods and cones are lost to apoptosis and there is retinal atrophy, with perivascular retinal pigment accumulation.

Retinal Neoplasms *(p. 1365)*

Retinoblastoma *(p. 1365)*

Retinoblastoma is the most common primary intraocular malignancy of children. Prognosis is worsened with extraocular extension or optic nerve or choroidal invasion. In 40% of cases, retinoblastoma is associated with a germ-line *RB* mutation (Chapter 7); such cases are often bilateral and are associated with pinealoblastoma ("trilateral" retinoblastoma) with a dismal outcome. Retinoblastoma tends to spread to brain and marrow, with rare dissemination to the lung.

Morphology (p. 1365)

Tumors contain undifferentiated (i.e., small, round cells) and differentiated elements encircling blood vessels with zones of necrosis and dystrophic calcification. Well-differentiated tumors exhibit *Flexner-Wintersteiner* rosettes, reflecting abortive photoreceptor development. The degree of differentiation does not influence prognosis.

Optic Nerve (p. 1365)

Optic nerve pathology is similar to brain pathology; cerebrospinal fluid circulates around the nerve and it is surrounded by meninges. The most common primary neoplasms are gliomas (typically *pilocytic astrocytomas*) and meningiomas.

Anterior Ischemic Optic Neuropathy (p. 1366)

The optic nerve blood supply can be interrupted by vascular inflammation (e.g., temporal arteritis; Chapter 11) or by embolism or thrombosis.

Papilledema (p. 1366)

Optic nerve edema can be caused by compression (e.g., by neoplasm) or by elevated cerebrospinal fluid pressure; the latter is typically bilateral *(papilledema)*. Papilledema associated with increased intra-cranial pressure is not typically associated with visual loss.

Glaucomatous Optic Nerve Damage (p. 1366)

Glaucomatous optic nerve damage is characterized by atrophy (due to increased intraocular pressures; see earlier discussion) accompanied by optic nerve head cupping. In *normal-tension glaucoma*, the same changes are seen without increased intra-ocular pressures; mutations in the *optineurin* gene are implicated.

Other Optic Neuropathies (p. 1367)

Other optic neuropathies can be inherited (e.g., *Leber hereditary optic neuropathy* due to mitochondrial gene mutations) or result from toxins (e.g., methanol) or nutritional deficiency.

Optic Neuritis (p. 1367)

This represents several unrelated entities, not all of which are inflammatory; the common feature is instead visual loss secondary to optic nerve demyelinization. Multiple sclerosis (Chapter 28) is the most important cause of optic neuritis.

The End-Stage Eye: Phthisis Bulbi (p. 1368)

Trauma, intraocular inflammation, chronic retinal detachment, and many other conditions give rise to a small (atrophic) and internally disorganized eye: *phthisis bulbi*.

Index

Note: Page numbers followed by *f* indicate figures; *t* indicate tables.